Introduction to Clinical Ethics

Second Edition

General Editors:
John C. Fletcher, Ph.D.
Paul A. Lombardo, Ph.D., J.D.
Mary Faith Marshall, Ph.D.
Franklin G. Miller, Ph.D.

Contributing Authors:
Robert Boyle, M.D.
Joseph J. Fins, M.D.
Joanne D. Pinkerton, M.D.
Mary V. Rorty, Ph.D.
Edward M. Spencer, M.D.

This textbook is dedicated to those whose vision and labors
helped to lay the foundations for the field of biomedical ethics
in the United States and at the University of Virginia.

James F. Childress, Ph.D.
Kenneth R. Crispell, M.D.
Joseph F. Fletcher, S.T.D.
Edward W. Hook, M.D.
Thomas H. Hunter, M.D.
Lockhart McGuire, M.D.
E. Haavi Morreim, Ph.D.
Oscar A. Thorup, Jr., M.D.
Clyde M. Watson, Jr., Ph.D.

University Publishing Group, Inc.
Frederick, Maryland 21701

ISBN 1-55572-050-1

CONTENTS

III. RESOURCES FOR ETHICS COMMITTEES

IV. APPENDICES

FOREWORD
TO THE SECOND EDITION

The field of bioethics continues to be in creative ferment. Especially noteworthy are developments in clinical ethics, that is, ethics at the bedside. To keep pace in this rapidly changing arena, the second edition of *Introduction to Clinical Ethics* carries forward an approach carefully tested over time with clinicians, students in the health professions, and members of ethics committees.

The authors understand clinical ethics as a "bridge" between theoretical bioethics and the bedside. Ideas move both ways on the bridge--not merely from theorists to practitioners, but also from practitioners to theorists. In the process, both activities are enriched. While making a contribution to bioethics in general, this volume is primarily intended to provide a thoughtful, imaginative, and helpful introduction to ethics at the bedside.

Compared with the first edition, the first and second chapters have been strengthened theoretically by the development of a perspective of "clinical pragmatism." This perspective and a case method derived from it build especially upon the work of John Dewey, an American philosopher whose importance for bioethics is only now being appreciated more fully.

Consistent with Dewey's approach to ethics, the text stresses a case method of planning for the care of patients, but does not ignore general moral norms. Without resolving the debate about the respective roles of casuistry and principles or rules, this text attends to both cases and general moral considerations, for example, in the form of enduring duties to respect privacy and confidentiality and to support and respect the informed consents and refusals of patients who have the capacity to make their own decisions. In addition, the authors show how virtues are central in clinical ethics. This work is further enriched by such critical perspectives as feminism, by close attention to the legal context of moral problems, and by a recognition of the history of these problems. The second edition is also stronger at the interface between clinical ethics and business ethics, particularly as it addresses issues posed by managed care and other techniques to limit the costs of healthcare.

The main body of the text addresses the major problem areas that any clinician and ethics committee can be expected to encounter. The second edition is admirably current with, and informed by, the extensive literature in clinical, ethical, and legal topics relevant to these problems.

In many ways this text serves as an important model for creative work in bioethics. First, it is interdisciplinary and interprofessional, not merely multidisciplinary and multiprofessional. Members of different disciplines and professions talked, taught, and wrote with each other to develop clear and compelling ideas about clinical ethics. This text provides the fruits of their conversations.

Second, as their conversation extended over time, so their book has now evolved to a second edition, and the conversation has matured. This text displays major changes and improvements that have occurred over the ten years or so of its development.

Third, this product is the result of careful testing and assessment. Its approached and its substantive ideas were tested in the classroom as well as in practice. Some prior approaches failed, while others succeeded; some ideas flourished, while others floundered.

In short, this book reflects an ideal approach to both teaching and scholarship in bioethics. It involved a community--a small community of teachers and practitioners interested in ethics in healthcare; the members of this community worked together over time on the first and second editions; and finally, their ideas grew out of and were tested in both the classroom and the clinical setting.

I have greatly benefited from my own conversations with my colleagues as they revised and prepared this second edition, and I congratulate them on this version, knowing they will continue to develop and test their approaches and ideas for years to come.

James F. Childress, Ph.D.
Kyle Professor of Religious Studies
Professor of Medical Education
University of Virginia
July 1997

PREFACE

John C. Fletcher, Ph.D.

The second edition of this book is an updated introduction to clinical ethics. Clinical ethics is concerned with the ethics of clinical practice and with ethical problems that arise in the care of patients. We developed this book for clinicians,[1] students preparing for health professions, and members of ethics committees in healthcare organizations (HCOs) who work on ethical issues in patient care. We intend to reach a wide variety of HCOs--hospitals, ambulatory and home-healthcare organizations, long-term-care and hospice-care organizations, and various types of managed-care organizations.

We emphasize the word *introduction* in the title of this book. Readers may have had little exposure to the literature and language of ethics or bioethics. Or, after some exposure, they may feel a need for more specific discussion of their concerns about ethical issues in caring for patients, preparing to be a clinician, or serving on an ethics committee.

I. "Doing Ethics" in a Healthcare Organization

Our overall purpose is to provide a clear framework and some resources for "doing ethics" in a HCO. These resources include ethically informed healthcare professionals, ethical concepts, and specific services in clinical ethics. Clinical ethics builds upon the ethical obligations of clinicians and requires practical deliberation and action when ethical problems arise in the care of patients. Decisions must be made. Because clinicians--physicians, nurses, and their colleagues in the allied health professions--are those who actually care for patients, they are our primary audience. Informed clinicians are society's main human resources for clinical ethics. Ethics services exist primarily to serve decision makers--clinicians, patients, and surrogates.

In this vein, the book's main educational aim is to engage readers in a case-based examination of three aspects of clinical ethics:

1. the four ethical obligations of clinicians that apply in all cases (to respect the patient's privacy and maintain confidentiality; to communicate honestly about patient's diagnosis, treatment, and prognosis; to determine whether the patient is capable of sharing in decision making; to participate in the process of informed consent [Chapters 3 through 6]);
2. the most frequent ethical problems about which all clinicians must be informed to be competent in practice (Chapters 7 through 13); and
3. the conceptual (Chapters 1 and 2), institutional (Chapter 14), and professional (Chapter 15) resources needed to address these ethical problems.

The book also provides a case method of moral problem solving in the context of planning for the care of patients, which is discussed in Chapter 2. We call this method *clinical pragmatism*.

Clinicians need knowledge and skills in clinical ethics to care competently for patients. Reflection on the four ethical obligations of clinicians that apply in all cases is as much a part of the "workup" of the patient as clinical tests and steps in diagnosis. Attention to these obligations aims at a goal of ethically sound dialogue between clinicians and patients. In educational programs that prepare individuals to practice medicine, nursing, or one of the allied health professions, clinical ethics belongs in the curriculum as much as anatomy, physiology, pathology, epidemiology, and so forth. Most medical and nursing schools have adopted this position and offer or require courses in this area.

HCOs are also crucial resources for clinical ethics. Concern for the well-being of HCOs is important in this time of conflict about access for everyone to basic healthcare, containment of spiraling costs, and concern for quality. Patterns of organization and reimbursement for physicians' services have rapidly changed due to managed care and alternatives to traditional fee-for-service medicine. If our society neglects examination of the ethical issues raised by managed care, we do so at our moral peril, because managed care confronts clinicians with difficult ethical problems and conflicts of interest. We trust that managed care is not a finished product and will evolve morally in our open society in response to legitimate criticism.

The culture of particular HCOs can be supportive, dismissive, or even hostile to clinical ethics. In our experience, working closely with leaders in HCOs to strengthen their support of clinical ethics services is as important as providing ethics education for clinicians and ethics committee members. It is self-defeating to pursue the latter task with great energy and ignore the need to develop a real plan to support a program of ethics services. Education is useful, but if newly motivated clinicians go back into an unreceptive or "cold" HCO, they will accomplish little. A better strategy is to help administrative leaders gain a vision of ethics services and to help them select resource persons for the HCO's ethics program. This textbook discusses the service dimension of clinical ethics: education for clinicians, patients, and the community; policy studies; ethics consultation at the bedside; targeted research on the causes of ethical problems; and outreach to HCOs that do not have ethics programs.

Further, we hope to overcome any perception that "ethics" is one more alien force, outside of clinical practice, to be resisted and feared along with other bureaucratic forces that impede the care of patients. The origin of this perception was probably in an earlier "backlash to bioethics" in the 1970s--a justified criticism of abstract, overly academic approaches used in education among clinicians and students.[2] We hope that this book supports clinicians who want to address and prevent ethical problems in the context of practical planning for the care of patients.

II. Bioethics, Medical Humanities, and Clinical Ethics

Other texts or anthologies will be more useful to readers who are broadly interested in bioethics and medical humanities.[3] *Bioethics*, a new branch of ethics, began to emerge in the late 1960s. It involves systematic reflection on ethical issues and problems in healthcare, biomedical research, public health, and environmental issues that affect health. *Medical humanities* involves interdisciplinary studies of medicine and the arts, literature, history, and law. *Clinical ethics* can be seen as a bridge between the world of bioethics and medical humanities and the world of clinicians and patients. Chapter 1 has a section on the evolution of clinical ethics and its bridging role.

Readers who want to examine the claims of ethical theories, which are mainly shaped by moral or political philosophers or theologians, will also need to go to other sources. These sources discuss some of the major ethical theories that compete for attention today.[4] In addition, some physicians and nurses are creative contributors to theoretical resources for bioethics.[5]

Chapter 13, supplemented by other sources, addresses some of the ethical aspects of health policy. There is a need to link clinical ethics with health policy, as Annette Baier indicates: "The ethics of health care goes beyond the ethics of all relationships within hospitals to all physician-patient relationships, and to all the community-health measures, preventive and remedial, that we as a society arrange to have taken."[6] Baier urges that the boundaries of bioethics be pushed far beyond the clinical setting to the choices about healthcare policy that are facing society. This is necessary to supplement a course on clinical ethics with studies of the social, economic, and political realities of health policy and delivery. This is a task that deserves attention by all teachers of clinical ethics.

III. A Note on Ethics and Law

Clinical ethics and health law evolve together in a dynamic and interactive relationship. Because of the diversity of moral traditions in this society, among other reasons, citizens look to the law to articulate both settled and developing norms of conduct in healthcare. Accordingly, some famous legal cases have helped to clarify norms in clinical practice. These cases, along with other forces at work since the early 1960s, have helped to create a new field of biomedical ethics. One thinks especially of court disputes about withdrawing life support--for example, the cases of Karen Ann Quinlan and Nancy Beth Cruzan (Chapter 9). Disputes about reproductive rights have often been taken to court in cases such as *Buck v. Bell*, *Griswold v. Connecticut*, *Roe v. Wade*, and *Planned Parenthood of Pennsylvania v. Casey* (Chapter 11). Another heavily contested area in law involves how to resolve disagreement between parents and physicians regarding choices about treatment of newborns and children (Chapter 10). Chapter 1 discusses in more detail the rich interaction between law and ethics in this morally pluralistic society. Clinicians need to know about this society's legal institutions and their own institution's legal process in order to practice wisely.

Notwithstanding the importance of the relationship between law and clinical ethics, a very poor, even antagonistic, understanding of this relationship exists in many clinical settings. The threat of lawsuits and the costs of defending against them have sadly bent this relationship out of shape. The anger that many good clinicians feel about being sued and their defensive posture can pose many roadblocks to a simpler and less costly process of resolving ethical problems in the clinical setting. Ironically, if such ethical problems remain unresolved, they can flare into legal problems. Fear of the law and lawyers makes some clinicians ask about legal liability before asking about what is ethically sound. Furthermore, ignorance about what the law requires or permits may lead clinicians to make ethically inappropriate decisions. This distorted situation does not exist everywhere, to be sure, but it can be found in many hospitals and nursing homes. Where it does exist, it poses the single greatest obstacle, in our experience, for ethics committees to carry out their mandated tasks in cooperation with the legal officers of the institution.

We intend that the spirit and content of this textbook promote a better understanding of the law and its resources for the ethical issues and problems that clinicians and patients face. Chapter 14 specifically discusses how leaders of ethics committees can take steps when they discover, as so many have, that the legal officers for the institution or its retained attorneys have *de facto* control of the ethics process.

We hope that our readers, especially clinicians, become less fearful of the law as they learn that it is one of several resources for clinical ethics and not among the "enemies of patients."[7] Also, knowing when legal advice is needed, and when it is not; is very important for the work of ethics committees in healthcare institutions and programs. Learning to work conjointly on ethical problems, alongside and in cooperation with the appointed legal officers of the institution when necessary, is a special task and talent for leaders in clinical ethics. The legal editor of this text, Paul A. Lombardo, has paid special attention to these questions throughout the text.

IV. Audiences and Educational Objectives

The editors and authors have collaborated for 10 years at the University of Virginia (UVa) School of Medicine; teaching clinical ethics. Our backgrounds are in medicine, nursing, law, history, philosophy, journalism, and religious studies. Since 1987, we have used earlier versions of this textbook with three audiences: students entering healthcare professions, clinicians, and members of ethics committees focused on patient care.[8]

A. Students in Healthcare Professions: Educational Objectives

The educational objectives for students preparing for the healthcare professions, presented below, reflect needs identified by students themselves and other teachers of clinical ethics.[9] Students and teachers state that they need to identify the moral aspects of clinical practice, to study and prepare for the ethical problems faced by clinicians and patients, and to discuss the special ethical concerns that arise for students in their role as clinician-trainee.[10] Students who complete a course using this text are expected to accomplish the following objectives:

1. to identify clearly clinicians' ethical obligations in each case and the ethical problems involving patients (Chapters 3 through 13) that clinicians face most frequently in training and practice;

2. to understand the history of these obligations and problems and see them as opportunities to provide the best possible care for patients and families whose lives have been disrupted by illness, pain, and suffering;

3. to be able to use a case method (Chapter 2) that is designed:

a. to prevent ethical problems through planning for the optimal care of patients;
b. to be a process of practical deliberation about ethical problems, when they do arise, that brings major ethical considerations and principles to bear upon the decisions to be made;
4. to be familiar with the services of a clinical ethics program and how to access these resources; and
5. to discuss their ethical concerns as clinician-trainees in relation to their supervisors and patients.

On completion of this course, with effective teaching and leadership of small-group discussion, students should be able to demonstrate knowledge of ethical concepts and certain skills, especially using the case method discussed in Chapter 2. They should be familiar with the history of ethical problems, as well as some landmark legal cases that have helped clarify norms in clinical ethics.

B. Clinicians and Ethics Committee Members: Educational Objectives

The second audience, clinicians and members of ethics committees, can use the text for orientation and for basic education in clinical ethics. The centrality of clinical ethics for clinicians has already been discussed. The first four educational objectives listed above will help to meet clinicians' needs. The choice of these objectives is supported by several studies of clinicians' needs for education in clinical ethics, as well as other literature about these needs.[11]

Ethics committee members are physicians, nurses, and colleagues from other disciplines (such as, law, social work, pastoral care, administration, patient education, and others). Committee membership is inadequate without community members who represent disciplines beyond the healthcare professions, and who are familiar with the values and moral beliefs of the communities served by the institution. These community members should be able to promote open and fair discussion of issues and cases. Section III, especially Chapter 14, discusses how institutions can best develop their resources for a program of ethics services.

In addition to the first four educational objectives above, which are adequate for a course to introduce clinical ethics to clinicians, a fifth objective is needed to meet the needs of ethics committee members:

5. to enable members of ethics committees, especially those involved in education and consultation for ethical problems involving patients, to understand their role and the knowledge and skills required for their tasks.

Members of ethics committees have common needs: to gain insight into their mission and tasks, to develop an overall plan for their activities, and to educate themselves about approaches to the most frequent ethical problems for which they will be asked for advice and help. This textbook can help to meet these needs, but study must be supplemented by discussion and planning in concert with key leaders in the HCO.

Rules of the Joint Commission on Accreditation of Healthcare Organizations (JCAHO), found in Appendix 1, now require a member institution to have "a functioning process to address ethical issues . . . based on a framework that recognizes the interdependence of patient care and organizational ethical issues."[12] In addition, A federal law, the Patient Self-Determination Act of 1990, requires all institutions receiving Medicaid and Medicare funds to provide education to staff and community for ethical issues that underlie advance directives and refusal of treatment.[13] This textbook can be used in such an educational program.

The appendices contain additional resources for strengthening ethics committees, developing a course in clinical ethics, educating an ethics committee, or planning library resources.

- Appendix 2 has guidelines of the Virginia Bioethics Network, designed to develop stronger ethics services in HCOs.
- Appendix 3 has two course outlines designed to use this textbook. One is for medical, nursing, and other students. The second is for ethics committees. Supplemental readings are suggested for each outline.
- Appendix 4 lists basic resources for an institution's library in clinical ethics. This list can be consulted by those planning for acquisitions.

This textbook can be used as a semester course for students or as an orientation and study guide for members of ethics committees. Appendix 3 has course outlines and additional readings for both options. Also, individuals who are training to provide a process for ethics consultation can benefit from knowledge of the problems discussed in this textbook as well as experience in the clinical setting.[14] Chapter 14 presents recommendations for education and training of ethics committee members and consultants.

To teach clinical ethics, we recommend a small-group format, with plenary sessions for students to meet patients, family members, and clinicians who can speak from experience about the ethical problems they have faced. Group leaders (preferably two leaders in a group of no more than 10 students) need to be familiar with the clinical and ethical content in the chapters. Ideally, the teachers will be members of disciplines involved in clinical ethics.

To use the text with an ethics committee, it is perhaps best to begin with a retreat or conference. In this setting, ample time can be given to address questions about the role and tasks of the committee. Such a group almost always faces early resistance--from others and from its own members--to involvement in ethical problems concerning patients. Taking the time to understand this resistance and to meet it by clarifying the committee's role and tasks will go a long way toward reducing resistance. Ethics committees can establish their value by patiently educating themselves and extending educational services to clinicians, as well as developing the ability to assist with consultation on policy issues and difficult cases. After the committee's initial retreat, the text can be used for education in each committee meeting.

The text can be used beyond the healthcare setting--for example, in the curriculum of a community college.[15] Also the text, or parts of it, can be adapted for civic, religious, or other community groups.

Notes

1. We use the term *clinician* to include all members of professions whose goal is clinical care of patients (for example, physicians, nurses, allied health professionals, and so on).

2. For an excellent example of the frustrations of a physician after a one-year fellowship to study medical ethics in the 1970s, see C.B. Moore, "This Is Medical Ethics?" *Hastings Center Report* 4, no. 5 (November 1974): 1-3. For a response to this physician and questions about the overly academic nature of his fellowship experience, see J.C. Fletcher, "A Physician on Ethics" (letter), *Hastings Center Report* 5, no. 1 (February 1975): 4. For a broader view of the "backlash to bioethics," see D. Callahan, "The Ethics Backlash," *Hastings Center Report* 5, no. 4 (August 1975): 18. For two sharp critiques of the influence of analytical philosophers in biomedical ethics, see R.C. Fox and J.P. Swazey, "Medical Morality Is Not Bioethics--Medical Ethics in China and the United States," *Perspectives in Biology and Medicine* 27, no. 3 (1984): 336-60; R.C. Sider and C.D. Clements, "The New Medical Ethics: A Second Opinion," *Archives of Internal Medicine* 145 (1985): 2169-71. For the most comprehensive and balanced overview of the "backlash," see S. Gorovitz, "Baiting Bioethics," *Ethics* 96 (January 1986): 356-74.

3. Bioethics can possibly best be understood as one of a number of social movements that began in the 1960s, in the cultural context of other movements in civil rights, women's rights, and consumer issues. A new academic field arose from this movement's interaction with the disciplines, and it is known as either *bioethics* or *biomedical ethics*. We understand these terms to be interchangeable, but we understand bioethics to be a movement much broader than an academic discipline. Two texts that are useful introductions to biomedical ethics are T.L. Beauchamp and J.F. Childress, *Principles of Biomedical Ethics*, 4th ed. (New York: Oxford University Press, 1994); J. Arras and B. Steinbock, *Ethical Issues in Modern Medicine*, 4th ed. (Mountain View, Calif.: Mayfield, 1995).

4. Chapter 2 of Beauchamp's and Childress's fourth edition (see note 3 above) is a comprehensive and clear discussion of seven perspectives in ethics today. These authors examine the strengths and weaknesses of these perspectives in the context of a discussion of a case in which the father of a five-year-old girl with end-stage kidney disease asks the nephrologist to lie to his family about his suitability as a kidney donor when, in fact, he does not want to be a donor. A well-selected anthology of readings and discussion in ethical theory is P. Singer, ed., *Companion to Ethics* (Colchester, Vt.: Blackwell, 1993).

5. H. Brody, *The Healer's Power* (New Haven, Conn.: Yale University Press, 1992); E. Cassell, *The Nature of Suffering and the Goals of Medicine* (New York: Oxford University Press, 1991); E.J. Emmanuel, *The Ends of Human Life: Medical Ethics in a Liberal Polity* (Cambridge, Mass.: Harvard University Press, 1991); T. Pence and J. Cantrall, *Ethics in Nursing: An Anthology* (New York: National League for Nursing, 1990).

6. A. Baier, "Alternative Offerings to Asclepius,"

Medical Humanities Review 6 (January 1992): 9.

7. R. Macklin, *Enemies of Patients* (New York: Oxford University Press, 1993). Chapter 2 of this book, "Law as an Advocate for Patients: A Case Study of DNR," embodies the same approach to law and ethics that we wish to take. This book is very critical of the biased way that some risk managers, in the author's experience, react to ethical problems in patient care.

8. Twice a year we offer a one-semester course, "Introduction to Clinical Ethics," which meets once a week for two hours. Fall-semester students include nursing students; various graduate and undergraduate students in biomedical ethics, law, and other fields; physicians and nurses; laypersons from the community; and trainees in the Ethics Consultation Service of the UVa Hospital Ethics Committee. In the spring semester, the course is required for 140 first-year medical students. The textbook has also been used widely in "Developing Hospital Ethics Programs," an outreach program of the UVa School of Medicine to prepare resource persons in clinical ethics in hospitals in and beyond Virginia. The graduates of this program, known as "Fellows in Biomedical Ethics," also use the text in the orientation and education of ethics committee members in their hospitals and elsewhere.

9. C.M. Culver et al., "Basic Curricular Goals in Medical Ethics," *New England Journal of Medicine* 312 (1985): 253-56; E.D. Pellegrino et al., "Relevance and Utility of Courses in Medical Ethics," *Journal of the American Medical Association* 253 (1985): 49-53; E.H. Loewy, "Teaching Medical Ethics to Medical Students," *Journal of Medical Education* 61 (1986): 661-65; K.R. Howe, "Medical Students' Evaluations of Different Levels of Medical Ethics Teaching: Implications for Curricula," *Medical Education* 21 (1987): 340-49; S.H. Miles et al., "Medical Ethics Education: Coming of Age," *Academic Medicine* 64 (1989): 705-14.

10. Association of American Medical Colleges, *Promoting Medical Students' Ethical Development: A Resource Guide* (Washington, D.C.: AAMC, 1993).

11. Authors of this text have been involved in two studies regarding the need for clinical ethics education and program evaluation. See R.F. Wilson et al., "Hospital Ethics Committees: Are They Evaluating Their Performance?" *HEC Forum* 5, no. 1 (1993): 1-34; E.M. Spencer et al., "Ethics Programs at Community Hospitals in Virginia," *Virginia Medical Quarterly* 119 (1992): 178-79. The findings in these studies about the needs for education among ethics committee members strongly confirm results of a survey by D.E. Hoffman, "Does Legislating Hospital Ethics Committees Make a Difference? A Study of Hospital Ethics Committees in Maryland, District of Columbia, and Virginia," *Law, Medicine, & Health Care*, 19 (1991): 105-19. Several studies conducted among institutions and ethics committees, clinicians, house staff officers, as well as evaluations of the efficacy of ethics courses in medical and nursing schools also focus on needs embodied in the objectives for students. See, for example, J.A. Jacobson, et al., "Internal Medicine Residents' Preferences Regarding Medical Ethics Education," *Academic Medicine* 64 (1989): 760-64; H. Perkins, "Teaching Medical Ethics during Residency," *Academic Medicine* 64 (1989): 262-66; J.E. Connelly and S. DalleMura, "Ethical Problems in the Medical Office," *Journal of the American Medical Association* 260 (1988): 812-15; S.H. Miles et al., "Medical Ethics Education: Coming of Age," *Academic Medicine* 64 (1989): 705-14.

12. Joint Commission on Accreditation of Healthcare Organizations, *1995 AMH Standards, Rights, Responsibilities and Ethics*, Pre-publication copy. (Chicago, Ill.)

13. The Omnibus Budget Reconciliation Act of 1990; Pub. L. No. 101-508, 104 Stat. 1388.

14. At the University of Virginia, trainees for the Hospital Ethics Committee's Ethics Consultation Service are required to take two courses: (1) the course for students using this text and (2) a course entitled "Principles and Practice of Bioethics Services in Healthcare Organizations." If the trainee is not a physician or a nurse, a third course is required--"Pathophysiology and Clinical Knowledge." Trainees also must attend a weekly meeting of the Ethics Consultation Service where cases are reviewed. Chapter 14 outlines this training process and how it can be adapted by an institution or a regional bioethics network.

15. A course at Piedmont Community College in Charlottesville, Virginia, was inaugurated in 1992 by the Reverend W.B. Arnason, who completed a fellowship in biomedical ethics at UVa. The course continues today under the leadership of C.A. Wise, R.N., a doctoral candidate in nursing at UVa.

SECTION I

UNDERSTANDING THE FIELD

1

CLINICAL ETHICS: HISTORY, CONTENT, AND RESOURCES

John C. Fletcher, Ph.D., Franklin G. Miller, Ph.D., and Edward M. Spencer, M.D.

I. "Doing Clinical Ethics" and the Needs of Readers

Ethics is a practical discipline that deals with real-world problems and practices. The term *clinical* derives from the Greek word *klinikos* or "bedside." Clinical ethics concerns problems and practices in the care of patients in different settings: acute care (in hospitals), long-term care, rehabilitation, home care, and hospice care.

The strategy of this text is pragmatic and problem-centered. We believe that the best way to study clinical ethics is via the most frequent and difficult ethical problems that confront clinicians, patients, and their families at or nearby the bedside--the arena of illness and healing. In these situations, decisions need to be made and actions must be taken. We call this "doing ethics" or moral problem solving.

We emphasize that it is unwise to "do ethics" by waiting for such problems to arise and addressing them only after they fester and become crises. Clinicians and the healthcare organization's (HCO's) ethics program need ways to address current cases and to cope with the occasional "ethics emergency." True ethics emergencies, like the JP case in Chapter 2, cannot be anticipated. A preventive approach clearly is better than a crisis-management approach to recurrent ethical problems. "Preventive ethics" is a significant feature of clinical ethics.[1] Preventive ethics, discussed in Chapter 14, is much more feasible in HCOs that strongly support their ethics programs and reward clinicians for taking the time to develop a plan of care.

Our readers come to the study of clinical ethics with differing motives. Some are students of medicine or nursing who are preparing to deal with ethical problems and legal concerns. Others are practicing clinicians who aim to be current on what is ethically and legally expected. Others are new or continuing members of ethics committees who seek clarity about their role and tasks.

Our experience in teaching is that, despite differing motives, our readers share five needs:

1. the need to learn to lead or participate in a process of practical moral problem solving;
2. the need to study the major ethical obligations and responsibilities of clinicians, and the accepted approaches to the most frequent ethical problems in the care of patients;
3. the need to use the resources of ethics and its concepts: (a) major ethical principles; (b) specific ethical considerations that carry great weight in the relations between clinicians, patients, and society; and (c) some virtues of clinicians in working through ethical problems;
4. the need to learn how to contribute to and use the resources of a program of clinical ethics in a HCO;
5. the need to learn enough about the history of clinical ethics to locate its place in the culture of HCOs and American society.

In trying to meet these needs with this textbook, we avoid giving "ready" answers for complex ethical problems. In real life, no prefabricated solutions to particular ethical problems are available. We do point out where a reasonable degree of consensus exists on a particular problem. In some problem areas, such as forgoing life-sustaining treatment for incapacitated and terminally ill patients, a consensus exists among clinicians, ethicists, and attorneys. Ethical and legal challenges to this consensus, as in the *Baby K* case (Chapter 9) and two recent court of appeals decisions on laws respecting physician-assisted suicide (Chapter 8) are ever present. There is wide variation, less consensus, or no consensus at all on other problems, such as reproductive choices, physician-assisted death, or how basic healthcare ought to be equitably distributed in the United States. However, reasoned positions have been advanced, with which students and clinicians should be familiar.

The text appeals to ethical considerations and principles, but these are not self-explanatory. Rigid formulas are no more appropriate in clinical ethics than in clinical medicine. Ethical judgments, guided by ethical principles and by practices that promote good relations between clinicians and patients, must be weighed in specific situations with particular patients. In the end, studying ethics does not deliver anyone from the burdens and risks of decision making.

Different ethical perspectives, as discussed by Thomas L. Beauchamp and James F. Childress,[2] set forth very different claims and arguments about the moral life and decision making. We introduce a perspective of "clinical pragmatism" in Chapter 2 with roots in the work of philosophers William James and John Dewey. A pragmatic perspective can also serve to integrate three views on ethics that share some common ground: (1) an ethics of principles, (2) casuistry (case-based ethics), and (3) an ethics of care. Elements from these three perspectives figure in the case method explained in Chapter 2 and in the discussions in each successive chapter.

In the present chapter, we trace the emergence of clinical ethics and the community of persons who "do ethics" in clinical settings. We then discuss some key terms and concepts in ethics, followed by a description of the content and conceptual resources for doing clinical ethics. These resources include an understanding of the basic ethical obligations of clinicians, knowledge about approaches to ethical problems that clinicians face, key ethical considerations in clinical ethics, and identification of the virtues of clinicians.

The chapter closes with a section on the relation between law and ethics.

II. The Emergence of Clinical Ethics in Teaching, Research, and Service

In an important review[3] of the evolution of clinical ethics, Siegler, Pellegrino, and Singer argue that it developed in response to two perceived needs: (1) the need for bedside teaching of ethics, in the tradition of William Osler,[4] a 19th-century physician famous for his bedside teaching of medicine; and (2) the need for a method of ethical inquiry especially suitable to individual cases in clinical settings.[5] Implicit within both developments was the belief that ethics, properly understood, is an integral component of the practice of good clinical medicine. We would add a third perceived need--the need to create a bridge between the academic world of bioethics and medical humanities and the world of clinicians and patients.

Bioethics and medical humanities began in the 1960s as intellectual and social movements.[6] The earliest bioethicists were concerned with novel moral dilemmas and violations of the autonomy of persons --especially in settings of research and innovative therapy, such as hemodialysis and transplantation for end-stage kidney disease. Coming as it did at the time of the civil rights movement, the birth of bioethics exposed great imbalances of power and authority that endangered research subjects and patients.[7]

Medical humanities is primarily concerned with enlarging the scope of education and socialization of healthcare professionals by studying the arts, literature, social sciences, and law, including critiques of the dominant scientific model in the basic and applied sciences.[8] Medical humanities seeks cooperation and complementarity between the sciences and humanities, rather than subordination of one to the other.

From the origins of bioethics and medical humanities to the present, the concerns of individuals who work in these fields have been largely with teaching, research, and social change. Bioethics became a new arena for interdisciplinary work within the larger field of ethics. Medical humanities was introduced in many of the larger academic medical centers in the United States and Canada. The early focus of social and institutional change was to prevent abuses and enhance the values that cluster around and guide decision making with human subjects of research and patients. Deliberate social change in the research setting, such as prior group review of research in institutional review boards, began in the 1960s and 1970s, well before similar changes were made in patient care settings (such as the use of ethics committees to work on ethical issues in patient care).

As these currents of change influenced clinicians and their practices, their responses (and criticisms) demanded changes and adaptation by clinicians, bioethicists, and medical humanists who desired to teach, do research, and serve in clinical settings.

In particular, clinicians identified three shortcomings of the early bioethics movement.

1. the need for a contextual approach to ethical inquiry;
2. the need to emphasize the relevance of clinical experience when doing clinical ethics; and
3. the need for an orientation toward service in clinical ethics.

The first concern was the need to develop modes of ethical inquiry that take more careful account of the variety of contexts in clinical care and the special needs of ill and suffering patients. The prevailing approach to bioethical inquiry[9] used systematic reflection on moral principles and resolving ethical problems in biomedicine by weighing and balancing the claims of competing principles. Although valuable work was achieved by this mainstream approach, clinicians indicated the need to give more attention to the clinical context within which ethical problems are faced. Some clinicians[10] and philosophers[11] viewed this method as mechanical and one that appeared to deduce ethical conclusions for concrete problematic situations from fixed moral principles or rules. Some identified a need to supply additional resources for ethical inquiry beyond moral principles that are highly abstract and general.

An additional resource for ethical inquiry appeared in the renewal of interest in casuistry, a time-honored art of ethical analysis using cases.[12] Clinical decision making is case-specific: it is directed at the care of a particular patient faced with a particular illness or injury. Each case has a history encompassing the facts leading up to the problems that need medical attention, what the medical problems are, and what needs to be done to resolve these problems.

Accordingly, casuistry is an important method of inquiry in clinical ethics. We weave cases into the discussion in each chapter in this text. Several anthologies and texts have been published with rich collections of cases,[13] including two with cases in ethics consultation[14] and one with cases for the allied health professions.[15] Like the practice of clinical medicine, casuistry builds on the accumulated experience, both individual and collective, of dealing with a variety of cases. Comparing and contrasting somewhat similar cases can help to identify important ethical considerations that may not be apparent when we focus on a particular case in isolation.

An ethics of caring is a prominent new mode of ethical inquiry in clinical ethics. Drawing on the writings of psychologist and educational theorist Carol Gilligan,[16] this view finds that the dominant approach of "principlism" tends to neglect crucial relationships and may fail to recognize the human needs and interests that also underlie the conflicts of principles. In this light, clinical ethics is concerned less with dramatic confrontations of ethical dilemmas and more with restoring and strengthening bonds between professionals, patients, and families. We discuss this perspective below in a section on the virtues of clinicians.

Clinicians' second criticism of the bioethics movement focused on the need to deepen and enrich the study of larger issues and themes in clinical practice, and on the lack of empirical research on important ethical issues such as decision making in critical care and at the end of life. In closing the gap between bioethics and clinical practice, clinician-ethicists or ethicists who had adapted to the clinical setting made progress by using cases and by drawing on knowledge available only through the intimacy of the clinician-patient encounter. Five exemplary studies among many are informative discussions of informed consent,[17] decision making about life and death,[18] pain and suffering,[19] the use of power by clinicians,[20] and helping patients with the trauma and tasks of dying.[21] These studies draw on a variety of disciplines and experiential data obtained in clinical settings. As such, they contribute toward ethical scrutiny and inform understandings and practices in the entire clinical encounter between patients and clinicians.[22] In this way, clinical ethics strengthens the conceptual arm of the bioethics movement with experiential data and helps to motivate clinicians to reform practices.

Recently, clinical ethics has also been informed by a significant increase in empirical research on issues of concern to clinicians, patients, and our society. Here we do not give an exhaustive review but point to the steadily growing knowledge base from empirical research on patients' capacity for healthcare decision making (Chapter 5), outcomes of the informed consent process (Chapter 7), and uses of advance directives and patterns of decision making in care of critically ill and dying patients (Chapter 9).

In the past decade, many more clinicians skilled in research methodology have entered the arena of clinical ethics. Their research results are published regularly in leading medical and professional journals. A noteworthy example is the Study to Understand Prognoses and Preferences for Outcomes and Risks of Treatments (SUPPORT),[23] a five-year effort that accrued 9,105 adult patients in a controlled, multi-institutional assessment and trial of an intervention to improve quality of decision making in the care of seriously ill, hospitalized adults. SUPPORT's findings were largely disappointing in terms of the ideals of shared decision making and the usefulness of advance directives, but it provides a clear baseline for new research and efforts to improve palliative care in acute-care settings.

The third criticism of the early bioethics movement was that; in addition to teaching and research, there should be clinical ethics services for clinicians and their patients. The next section is devoted to this concern.

A. The Clinical Ethics Community and Its Services

Community is meant here in a general sense--that is a body of people sharing a common characteristic or interest living and working in a larger society that does not have that characteristic or interest.[24] Members of the clinical ethics community today have a mission to teach and do research, but their most broadly shared common interest[25] is to provide services to address ethical issues in the care of patients. Those who are served are key decision makers who need to be able to identify, analyze, and resolve ethical problems in patient care.

There are four types of services of clinical ethics in well-developed programs:

1. providing education in clinical ethics for clinicians, patients, surrogates, and the larger community;
2. doing policy studies and making recommendations for institutional and community guidelines to address various ethical issues in patient care;
3. providing a process for case consultation at the bedside or the conference room; and
4. doing targeted research on ethical problems and participating in planning for prevention of such problems, where possible.

Each service involves a complex and difficult set of tasks discussed in more detail in Chapter 14. The fourth task is the most complex, as it requires the expertise of research methodology and preventive planning. To provide any of these services requires education and training. In order to flourish, clinical ethics and its services must become more widely recognized within HCOs, the academic community, and the larger society.

Who belongs to the clinical ethics community? A sociological account of the most to the least visible would include the following:

1. the many thousands of members of ethics committees in patient care, including community members, and those in regional or statewide networks to support these efforts;
2. the faculties, staffs, postgraduate fellows, and graduate students in a few centers or academic departments[26] where study and training in clinical ethics is possible;
3. the members of professional societies[27] concerned directly with clinical ethics; and
4. educators within the nation's schools of medicine, law, and religious life with significant interests in clinical ethics.

B. The Place of Clinical Ethics in Society

If this sketch of a clinical ethics community is reasonably accurate, what is its place and role in society? To whom is a clinical ethics program finally accountable? Whom do clinical ethicists and their colleagues serve? Differing visions of the place of clinical ethics compete in the literature: as a subspeciality of medicine,[28] as an arena for a "new breed" of healthcare consultants with academic backgrounds,[29] or as a multidisciplinary activity largely serving physicians.[30] None of these visions is finally satisfactory, because each locates the source of legitimation in a field or culture external to clinical ethics--that is in medicine or in academics. For clinical ethics to survive and prosper, it must become a more unified multidisciplinary field and elevate its standards, especially for education and training for those who provide its services. Exhibit 1-1 describes the place of clinical ethics, as we see it, in society.

We use the analogy of a bridge to describe the place of clinical ethics between academic and clinical cultures, two larger and more powerful cultures. Another analogy is that of an isthmus between two large land areas (as Panama and Central America are to North and South America).

These larger cultures need more interaction between their different practices, languages, and standards. Bioethics and medical humanities are located in academic culture. Their ways of life are guided by patterns and norms forged in graduate education, by scholarly guilds, and by the political and economic arrangements of universities. The clinical world is deeply influenced by the human experience of disease and suffering, long-standing traditions of medicine and nursing, the special settings of widely varying HCOs, as well as the social and economic arrangements that structure these settings. Above these entities, however, are the larger community, region, and society that support, recognize, and legitimate each of these entities' activities. Society can govern and exercise some degree of control through law, regulation, and encouragement of the tradition of professional self-regulation.

Whom does clinical ethics serve and where is its locus of accountability? In our view, clinical ethics earns its place by serving both academic and clinical cultures; as well as the larger community, region, and society that have encouraged the development of this small territory.

For the word *ethics* in its name to ring true, clinical ethics must authentically bridge between the clinical world and the theoretical disciplines of bioethics and medical humanities in the academic world. Clinical ethics can contribute to a body of knowledge and useful practices for clinicians and patients in different clinical settings. Clinical ethics can also contribute in several ways to bioethics and medical humanities: by empirical and descriptive research on ethical problems; by case narratives and stories of patients and clinicians; and by translation and transmission of the ideas, concepts, and perspectives of theoretical ethics for those who interact within clinical culture. Clinical ethics must not allow its discourse to become dominated by overly academic and theoretical concerns or to permit untrained academic professionals to attempt to provide services. By introducing the members of academic culture to the world of clinicians and patients, clinical ethics is providing a great service to the academic world.

To validate the *clinical* in clinical ethics, those who do clinical ethics must interact professionally and, at times, intimately with clinicians and patients in their world and know their language, practices, and beliefs. To this end, those who do clinical ethics but are not clinicians must become sufficiently educated in medicine and clinical reasoning to understand the language of diagnosis and treatment of disease, the process of medical decision making, and the social structure of a clinical culture. Because most clinical ethics programs are located in and supported by HCOs, the danger is that the interests of the clinical culture will dominate and overwhelm clinical ethics. Wherever this danger exists, it must be overcome by the clinical ethics community's confidence and independence to challenge particular practices and characteristics of clinical culture.

The community, region, and the larger society are ultimate sources of recognition and legitimacy for academic and clinical cultures. Likewise, the clinical ethics community needs to seek recognition for its services. It will do so not by self-proclamation but by completing the growth process to be, by analogy, a more recognized and self-governing territory. The clinical ethics community must help its members, especially those on ethics committees, to pass milestones of education and training that these two cultures and the larger society recognize. Chapter 14 contains practical recommendations, as well as a strategy for accreditation of education and training programs in clinical ethics.

Exhibit 1-1 The Place of Clinical Ethics in Society

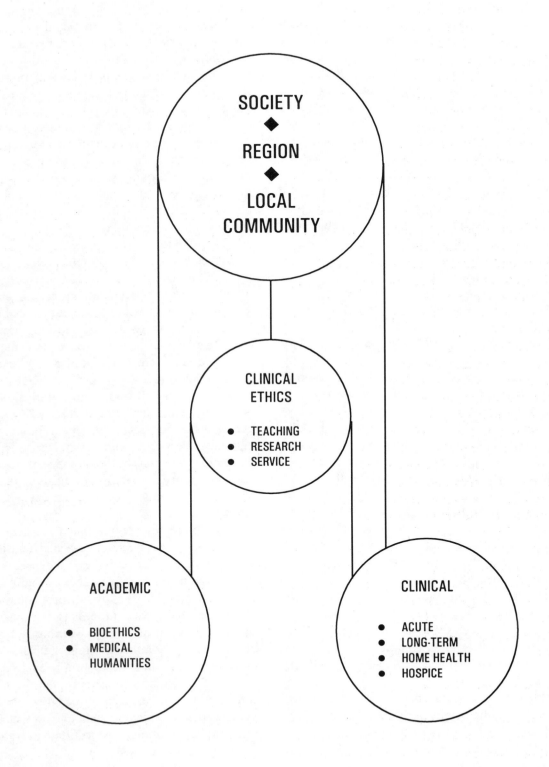

C. Organizational Ethics

In its short lifetime, clinical ethics has mainly addressed issues in patient care and patients' rights. There is a significant need to balance attention to individual cases with ethical analysis of organizational and economic issues.[31] This need has been sharpened by rules of the Joint Commission on Accreditation of Healthcare Organizations (JCAHO) about organizational ethics--issues of institutional integrity for HCOs (see Appendix 1). These rules state that members must have "a functioning process to address ethical issues" that is "based on a framework that recognizes the interdependence of patient care and organizational ethical issues."[32] The JCAHO rules specifically require a process to examine ethical issues in marketing, admissions, discharge, billing, relationships with third-party payers and managed-care plans, as well as a "code of organizational ethics" that addresses each of these areas. Chapter 14 describes how these and other JCAHO rules regarding patients' rights can be met by a HCO's ethics program.

Clinical ethics is a useful resource for clinicians, administrators, and patients involved in managed care and other large, rapidly developing healthcare systems. Iglehart defined managed care as "a system that in varying degrees integrates the financing and delivery of medical care through contracts with selected physicians and hospitals that provide comprehensive health care services to enrolled members for a predetermined monthly premium."[33] He observed, "All forms of managed care represent attempts to control costs by modifying the behavior of doctors, although they do it in different ways."[34] Ethical analysis of healthcare systems draws upon some of the ethical concepts used in this text but requires a different set of skills in describing the context of ethical problems that arise for healthcare and managed-care organizations as such. Chapter 13 examines the ethics of healthcare systems and recommends methods focusing on the behavior of HCOs as systems.

III. *Ethics* and Other Terms

How the word *ethics* is understood makes a real difference to the climate in which moral problem solving can be done effectively. For some clinicians, the word *ethics* refers only to issues of character. Believ-ing that they are already "ethical,"--that is, that their character traits are well formed--they misunderstand, and they resist an ethics committee. They fear that such a group will judge individual physicians or be one more source of interference with the way they practice medicine.

Other clinicians link the term *ethics* only to specific issues in the professional relationship between themselves, patients, and other clinicians. Examples are sexual behavior, unfair fee setting, or self-serving referrals. Such issues and conflicts of interest are within the scope of professional ethics and the self-regulation that clinicians are supposed to exercise. Understanding ethics only within a professional framework creates questions about why "another" ethics committee is needed, when local, regional, and national medical societies already have them.

We recommend the use of the terms *clinical ethics committee* or *ethics services* to reduce misunderstanding. For such reasons, at the outset of studying clinical ethics, some important terms (such as *ethics, morality, moral dilemmas,* and *ethical problems*) need clarification.

A. Ethics and Morality

Although the terms *ethics* and *morality* are often used interchangeably, it is useful to distinguish between them. In the ancient past, the words had similar meanings. *Ethics* stems from the Greek word *ethos,* meaning character. *Morality* is from the Latin word *mores,* meaning character, custom, or habit.[35] In the past, both terms referred to "manners, character, or custom."

We now understand *morality* to mean *customary morality,* or widely shared beliefs about the moral life and norms of right and wrong conduct that prevail in a particular culture or subculture. Anthropologists have found great differences among cultures with respect to such beliefs and norms. Such moral beliefs influence how people habitually respond, without deeper reflection, to everyday moral problems.

The word *ethics* has many meanings. Congress and the media use it to refer to conflicts of interest, as when elected or appointed officials abuse their offices to give special favors. Philosophers, on the other hand, use the word *ethics* to mean *systematic ethics,* or a perspective from which to evaluate and live the requirements of the moral life. In this vein, Beauchamp and Childress define *ethics* as "a generic term for various ways of understanding and examining the moral life."[36]

To some it is distressing that no single unifying ethical theory or vision of the moral life prevails in this society. A pluralistic society has divergent moralities, as amply illustrated by controversy over elective abortion.[37] In the midst of heated moral controversies, a tendency can exist to impose group morality on others who differ. This urge to impose can become extreme among groups with powerful beliefs, such as when a revealed religion is an absolute foundation for all of morality. Although our presentation of clinical ethics does not depend on particular religious commitments, it respects the contribution that religious traditions and thought have made to bioethics and medical humanities.

At another extreme, one can make an absolute of tolerance of cultural differences and noninterference in the moral lives of others. In this view, right and wrong are absolutely relative to culture. This type of ethical relativism empties morality of all content. Its greatest danger is to abdicate any moral standpoint in the face of great and blatant evil (for example; unspeakable crimes such as those perpetrated by the Nazis or the cruel practice of female circumcision). The word *ethics* assumes some reflective and critical judgments about acts and beliefs. The word means both to understand and to critique particular moralities when necessary.

Following Beauchamp and Childress, we use the word *ethics* to mean *systematic ethics*, or the examination of morality, conduct, and social practices. A practical way to distinguish between positive morality and systematic ethics is to regard positive morality as normative or prescriptive, responding to questions about "What ought I (or we) to do in this situation and similar situations?" Systematic ethics is regarded as justificatory, interpretive, and analytical, and responds to questions of "Why should I (or we) do *X* or *Y*? What reasons would justify such action and why?"

B. Moral Dilemmas[38]

A *practical dilemma* (from the Greek, *dilemmatos*--"involving two assumptions") poses a choice between two or more alternatives, both of which appear to be obligatory or desirable. The decision maker is in a bind, or caught between alternatives, because circumstances prevent her or him from doing both. One kind of dilemma for busy, overcommitted people is to find that they have promised to be at two places at the same time. New information may resolve what appears at first to be a dilemma. For example, one date may have been wrongly recorded or can easily be changed. Then the dilemma dissolves. If one horn of the dilemma involves a matter of self-interest (a golf or tennis game) versus a moral obligation (a board meeting of a charitable organization), there is a personal dilemma but no moral dilemma.

A *moral dilemma* occurs when (1) moral obligations to others exist on both sides of the choice to perform or refrain from performing the actions involved, and (2) ethical reasons support choosing both alternatives. What causes moral dilemmas? One frequently reads or hears that "new medical technology causes moral dilemmas." Uses of technologies (such as life supports or tests for genetic conditions) are indeed frequent occasions for moral dilemmas, but the technologies do not cause dilemmas. Moral dilemmas arise in circumstances when moral appeals based on principles and values cross one another, and one cannot act without infringing upon one or more principles or values.

Beauchamp and Childress describe two forms of moral dilemmas. The difference between them is in where the sharpest point of conflict lies: within the society or within an individual. An example of the first form is that within the larger society some communities hold that to do act *X* (for example, an elective abortion) is morally right and other communities hold that it is morally wrong, but the evidence on both sides is inconclusive and debatable. Women looking at abortion in this way and who seek moral consensus in terms of community values can be confronted by a severe dilemma posed from outside themselves. In the second form, a person can morally believe that she or he both ought and ought not to do a specific act. In this situation, a person feels the dilemma acutely from within. Some clinicians and family members feel this kind of dilemma in cases where a dying patient has clear wishes to stop nutrition and hydration, but their own moral tradition has opposed or cautioned against such a choice.

C. Moral Dilemmas: Dynamics and Emotions

Moral dilemmas can also be described by tracing their personal and interpersonal dynamics. In this sense, a dilemma can occur (1) within a single person (intrapersonal) or (2) between two or more persons (interpersonal).

Intrapersonal ethical dilemmas arouse powerful emotions, such as anxiety, fear of social criticism, or anger. In interpersonal conflicts, differences in status and power of decision makers can strongly influence the dynamics of the case. Some patients and family members feel powerless in front of clinicians and may not speak at all. They may fear alienating doctors on whom their care depends. Knowledge and skill is required to promote trust and open dialogue in such situations.[39]

One needs to heed one's feelings to engage in moral problem solving. Without a capacity to feel conflicting emotions and obligations, we fail to recognize that moral dilemmas exist at all. Stress and exhaustion can depress emotions and desensitize clinicians to the ethical dimension of clinical care. Emotions are a key element of the moral life. The capacity to empathize with another person, or to put oneself in the other's place, is needed to be moral at all.

To allow oneself to feel conflicting emotions and conflicting obligations invites a state of moral ambiguity or uncertainty. Moral ambiguity is a "normal" stage in the process of responding to a genuine ethical problem. However, emotional responses in ethical conflicts--"shooting from the hip" or mere reactions--cut off the process of ethical deliberation. The main lesson of Chapter 2 is that moral problem solving requires practical deliberation about the facts--about what the ethical problems are, what needs to be done, how it should be done and by whom, and why such actions are justified. Clinical ethics requires careful deliberation about ethical problems that arise in patient care.

D. Problematic Responses to Moral Dilemmas

One can identify three problematic ways that clinicians often respond to moral dilemmas. Each short-circuits serious ethical deliberation. These include:

1. collapsing moral dilemmas into medical or legal questions;
2. generalizing expertise in medicine to ethics;
3. divorcing ethical and clinical reasoning.

As an example of collapsing moral dilemmas into medical or legal questions, George Annas[40] identifies Nuland's decision to perform surgery on a 92-year-old patient who suffered intensely afterward. Reflecting on his mistake in pressing his patient to concede to surgery, Nuland wrote: "Viewed by a surgeon, mine was strictly a clinical decision, and ethics should not have been a consideration."[41] Physicians habituated to such one-sided reasoning can be blind to abuse of the healer's power.[42] Another frequent response in moral dilemmas is to ask: "What does the law say?" or "Can we be sued?" Neither one of these responses is adequate to the task, although medical and legal information is certainly relevant at key points in moral problem solving.

A second problematic response is to commit the fallacy of "generalization of expertise," described long ago by Robert M. Veatch,[43]--that is, assuming that expertise about the technical facts of an area of medicine gives the physician expertise in the ethical aspects of decision making in that area. This fallacy was probably at work in the early stages of the *Baby K* case,[44] discussed in Chapter 9. Why did physicians of a patient carrying a fetus with anencephaly fail to develop a plan to address the ethical issues raised by her strong demands for "full treatment" at birth? They fell back on their experience and expertise and predicted that she would change her mind upon seeing the infant's head at birth. In short, they had never seen another pregnant woman make such a choice. By this fallacious reasoning, they delayed and then found themselves in a terrible and costly dilemma.

A third problematic response, influenced by theoretical ethics and probably transmitted in medical school courses, is to divorce ethical and clinical reasoning. The two modes of reasoning are learned at different times and remain unintegrated. In a third edition of their widely used text, Beauchamp and Childress wrote self-critically: "We believe one of the major defects in contemporary theory in biomedical ethics is its distance from clinical practice. . . .

But this defect cannot be corrected here."[45] This problem can be corrected by real collaboration between the field's theoreticians, medical and nursing school educators, and clinical ethics programs. Chapter 2 is directly relevant to the integration of clinical and ethical reasoning.

E. Learning to Frame Moral Dilemmas as Ethical Problems

How can these problematic responses be overcome? What must one know to "do" clinical ethics? What is the content of clinical ethics? A major portion of the field's content is information about types of ethical problems frequently faced by clinicians, patients, and surrogates. Learning how to frame frequent moral dilemmas in clinical care of patients as ethical problems, prior to moral problem solving, is the primary skill and area of knowledge involved in clinical ethics.

The word *problem* has two meanings in the Greek language. Originating from the word *problema*, "obstacle" is one meaning of a problem, like a boulder in our path. Dilemmas stop us in our paths and disrupt patient care. Richard Zaner discusses this meaning in a text on clinical ethics.[46] A second meaning, less well known but important for this discussion, comes from the verb from which the word *problema* derived-- *proballein*, meaning "projection" or "to throw forward." This meaning points to a human ability to take a step beyond (or to go deeper than) the initial experience of a dilemma as an obstacle. In facing the dilemma or obstacle, we can "throw forward" or hypothesize ideas about it and how we can move through or around it. Namely, we can externalize dilemmas and place them in a larger context of problems with a history. This meaning of the word is inherent in the activity of planning. We can also anticipate problems before they arise by exercising intuition, imagination, and planning.

Working through dilemmas to identify and frame them as ethical problems is a skill that can be learned. The most frequently recurring moral dilemmas faced by clinicians today arise in (1) cases with circumstances that require, or seem to require, clinicians' infringements of basic obligations to patients; or (2) other particular disputes that arise in choices in diagnosis or treatment at various stages and circumstances of the life cycle.

This text presents and discusses these frequent dilemmas in the framework of ethical problems. Each ethical problem has a different history, and clinicians' approaches to these problems are constantly evolving. Because law and ethics evolve together, the development of health law is also involved in this story.

IV. Basic Ethical Obligations and Ethical Problems

Broad ethical principles shape clinicians' basic obligations to patients. These principles govern not only clinical ethics but also other areas of social and community life. Specifically, four ethical principles are relevant sources of general ethical guidance:

1. *beneficence*, which creates an obligation to benefit patients and other persons and to further their welfare and interests;
2. *respect for patients' autonomy*, which obliges clinicians to protect and defend the informed choices of capable patients;
3. *nonmaleficence*, which asserts an obligation to prevent harm or, if risks of harm must be taken, to minimize those risks; and
4. *justice*, which is relevant to fairness of access to health care and to issues of rationing at the bedside (see Chapter 13).[47]

Later in this chapter, we discuss several ethical considerations that bridge between ethical principles, an ethics of caring, and specific clinical situations.

After the clinician-patient relationship is established, the following obligations are morally binding in each case:

- respecting the patient's privacy and maintaining a process that protects confidentiality;
- communicating honestly about all aspects of the patient's diagnosis, treatment, and prognosis;
- determining whether the patient is capable of sharing in decision making; and
- conducting an ethically valid process of informed consent throughout the relationship.

An ethical problem can arise when circumstances require, or appear to require, clinicians to infringe on one or more of these basic obligations. Such circumstances occur frequently. In managed-care settings, physicians' traditional obligations to the patient and policies of the managed-care organization can conflict, especially if "gag rules" restrict physicians' disclosure of company policy to patients. These obligations, the ethical problems that stem from the need to infringe on them, and exceptions to the obligations are discussed in Section II, Part A, of the text. Nurses and other clinicians share--with physicians--the moral responsibility to fulfill these obligations.

Section II, Part B, presents a second cluster of ethical problems in the clinical setting. These problems probably occur less frequently than those presented in Part A, but they are complex and difficult to resolve when they do occur. Part B discusses six substantive ethical problems of clinical ethics:

1. refusal of medically indicated tests or treatment by competent patients, which can be based on religious, cultural, or personal reasons;
2. problems in care of suffering patients who are terminally ill, including patients' requests for assisted suicide and euthanasia, and the determination that death has occurred;
3. decisions about forgoing life-sustaining treatment for incapacitated patients, including assessments of "medical futility";
4. disputes about treatment of newborns, infants, and children;
5. reproductive choices, including abortion, sterilization, prenatal diagnosis, and other uses of new reproductive technology; and
6. bedside rationing of scarce resources, such as beds in an intensive care unit, organs, blood, and so forth.

Being familiar with these two categories of problems can enable students, clinicians, and ethics committee members to identify ethical problems in cases and engage in moral deliberation about them.

V. Ethically Relevant Considerations and Virtues: Caring for Patients

Ethics involves making judgments about what to do in particular situations and giving reasons in support of these judgments. Judgment and justification are typically preceded by a deliberative process. In this process, identifying the ethical problem(s) is advisable. However, to identify an ethical problem is

only to begin the exploration of its significance. One then needs to ask the question, "What is ethically at stake in this case?" At this point, we recommend a review of those considerations that are most relevant to the problem(s). Ethically relevant considerations consist of the factors that help in focusing our moral judgments.

A. Eight Ethically Relevant Considerations

Below is a brief overview of eight ethical considerations that have the greatest weight and relevance in the care of patients. These considerations bridge between ethical principles, an ethics of caring, and the clinical situation. They are:

1. the balance between benefits and harms in the care of patients;
2. disclosure, informed consent, and shared decision making;
3. the norms of family life;
4. the responsibilities of physicians and nurses in the context of relationships with patients;
5. professional integrity;
6. societal norms of cost-effectiveness and allocation;
7. cultural and religious variations; and
8. considerations of power.

These considerations are examined in greater depth in later chapters. Other works present more broadly systematic and theoretical discussions of ethics and healthcare and the clinician-patient relationship.[48]

1. Balancing benefits and harms in the care of patients is the paramount traditional ethical consideration in the practice of clinical medicine. It carries out the claims of the ethical principles of beneficence, which aims at maximizing benefits to persons, and of nonmaleficence, which aims to minimize harm or avoid it altogether. The responsibility of all clinicians is to use their professional medical knowledge to determine what treatments maximize benefits and minimize harms to their patients. Clinicians are obligated to benefit patients or prevent harm to patients in pursuing the goals of medicine: preserving life, curing (where possible), healing, restoring or maintaining bodily functions and mental capacities, preventing disease or injury, and relieving suffering. Although patients are at the center of ethical focus in this traditional normative orientation, in contemporary medicine the interests of other parties may also be relevant to the assessment of benefits and risks (for example, the health of fetuses or live organ donors).

2. Disclosure, informed consent, and shared decision making have motivated the bioethics movement and legal thought in the past 30 years to challenge whether clinicians should have the unilateral authority to determine what medical treatment is in the best interest of patients. This threefold consideration does the work of an ethical principle of respect for autonomy. Healthcare, particularly when alternative treatments are possible, inevitably involves issues of values, which do not lie within the domain of medical knowledge. How can clinicians determine, in all cases, what is in the best interest of patients without consulting them and adequately disclosing what they need to know to make decisions? (see Chapter 4).

The right of adult, competent patients to determine for themselves whether they will accept treatment is recognized in the legal and ethical doctrine of informed consent (see Chapter 6). In order to exercise voluntary consent, patients need at least to receive truthful disclosure from their clinicians concerning their condition, the benefits and risks of alternative treatments, and their prognosis with and without these treatments. Informed consent requires ongoing dialogue between clinicians and patients. This dialogue and its requirements is often referred to as a shared decision-making process between patients, family members or companions, and clinicians, and in 1982, the President's Commission for the Study of Ethical Problems in Medicine and Biomedical and Behavioral Research specifically endorsed this model.[49]

3. Norms of family life are almost always are at stake, since patients typically face major medical decisions as members of a family rather than as isolated individuals. Familial relationships give rise to moral responsibilities. These norms and responsibilities are nurtured by an ethics of caring. Spouses, children, and other family members provide support, help, and care for patients whose lives are disrupted by illness. Parents are intimately involved in the healthcare of their children, and family members generally have the right

and the responsibility to speak for patients who are no longer capable to make decisions for themselves. Accordingly, the ethics of clinical practice must take into consideration the moral dimension of family life.

4. The relationships between clinicians and patients lie at the heart of clinical ethics, strongly informed by an ethics of caring for others. Professional healthcare providers have a fiduciary responsibility to care for sick and injured patients. The process of healing depends on the trust of patients and the trustworthiness of clinicians. Although patients are vulnerable and dependent, they are entitled to be treated with respect and as partners in the process of making healthcare decisions. In addition to being competent in the technical aspects of healthcare, clinicians are responsible for communicating with patients to enlist their participation in healthcare and for maintaining a caring presence with patients suffering from illness. To treat patients solely as diseased bodies in need of repair amounts to psychological abandonment. The ethics of clinical practice involves the way in which clinicians relate to patients in addition to the process of determining what is the right thing to do in problematic cases.

5. The professional integrity of clinicians plays an important role in determining whether treatment or care requested by patients or surrogates is ethically appropriate. The norms of professional integrity are formed and reformed, over time, and do the work of an ethics of caring for one's companions in the moral struggles to be a good clinician. The right of patients to self-determination means that no treatments can be imposed on competent patients without their consent. Although patients are free to refuse treatment, they are not entitled to receive whatever treatment they demand. Clinicians have no responsibility to offer or provide treatments that are medically inappropriate; for otherwise, clinicians' integrity as professionals would be undermined.[50] Whether physicians should have the unilateral power to withhold or withdraw life-sustaining treatment on grounds of futility is a matter of current controversy. When clinicians and patients or family disagree about the appropriateness of life-sustaining treatment, ethics consultation may be indicated. In any case, clinicians are not obligated to provide treatment that they oppose for reasons of conscience.

6. Cost-effectiveness and allocation are increasingly at stake in questions of the distribution of medical resources and efforts to contain the spiraling costs of healthcare. This consideration carries out claims of the ethical principle of justice. In practice, clinicians are increasingly expected to be familiar with the costs of particular treatments and to consider costs among the outcomes when making decisions about treatment. Practice guidelines and managed care are attempts to combine studies of the outcomes of particular treatments for large groups of patients with efforts to control costs.

On the policy level, two tools for studying outcomes are widely used to frame policy decisions. Cost-effectiveness analysis is a tool that provides information about outcomes in nonmonetary terms, such as years of life, quality-adjusted life years, or cases of disease treated. In cost-benefit analysis, the bottom line is stated in monetary terms.[51]

Even with these efforts, the boundaries between public policy and clinical decision making are still unclear. Managed care and other cost-containment efforts are the occasion for many ethical conflicts between patients, clinicians, and third-party payers (see chapter 13). At times, clinicians cannot avoid the need to select which patients receive scarce medical resources (see chapter 12). Equitable procedures must be applied in order to make ethically acceptable decisions about the allocation of medical care. The clinician is the patient's main advocate for access to medically indicated healthcare and entitlements to coverage under private or public insurance plans.

7. Issues of cultural and/or religious variation often face clinicians who provide healthcare to patients of diverse backgrounds. Traditional cultural norms of family life may place healthcare decisions and access to information in the control of family members rather than the patient. Patient self-determination and truthful disclosure may be foreign to the cultural practices and values of some patients. Clinicians need to apply sensitivity and tact, and perhaps religious and cultural consultation along with ethics consultation, to respond appropriately to the potentially difficult problems posed by such cases.

8. Considerations of power often shape or underlie ethical problems in the clinical setting and deserve special attention in furthering the principle of respect for persons and their autonomy. It is almost always the case that clinicians are in a greater position of power in relation to patients and family members. Sickness and disease render patients more vulnerable and in a dependent position. Howard Brody examines the clinician-patient relationship from the perspective of ways that the power of the clinician is, and should be, exercised.[52] For Brody, the responsible use of therapeutic power is the standard of clinical ethics. Shared decision making requires sharing power. Shared power involves recognizing the patient's moral standing and right to participate in decisions (or the proxy decision maker's right, for an incompetent patient). The major vehicle of shared power is conversation between clinician and patient. Brody writes: "The patient ideally has a right to a relationship that assures that he will be treated with respect and that medical knowledge will be used to further his own life plans and values. Both to show respect and to find out how medicine can be applied to his specific life issues, a particular sort of sustained, reasonable conversation is necessary."[53] Clinicians are obliged to examine the differentials of power among persons and groups involved in a case when ethical problems arise, to be prepared to prevent unnecessary power struggles that can end in needless lawsuits. Power considerations are also important in the interpersonal and interprofessional relationships of physicians, nurses, students, and allied healthcare professionals.

B. The Virtues of Clinicians

The topic of clinical virtues has received less attention in the literature of bioethics than moral rules and principles.[54] Virtues are dispositions of character and conduct that motivate and enable clinicians to provide good care to patients. The clinical virtues function as habits conducive to good practice and as guides to healing and caring interactions with patients.

Faced with ethically problematic situations, clinicians can (and should) appeal to understanding of good practice in addition to relevant moral rules and principles. Some of the principal clinical virtues are described below, with emphasis on the virtue of caring. Clinical excellence, including the ability to respond appropriately to ethical problems in the care of patients, depends on cultivating these virtues. Clinicians who have cultivated these virtues will integrate ethics into their clinical practice and approach the care of patients in ways that minimize ethical conflicts.

1. Technical competence: The good physician or nurse has mastered the requisite knowledge and techniques for practicing the arts of medicine or nursing. Because biomedical knowledge and techniques undergo rapid development, owing to clinical research, the good clinician must be committed to continuing education to maintain competence.

2. Objectivity and detachment: The clinician must learn to become sufficiently distanced emotionally from the gore, pain, and invasiveness that medical treatment entails in order to do what is needed to help the patient, while still maintaining a compassionate, empathetic approach.

3. Caring: Caring is a complex perceptive and emotive disposition to relate to persons with the aim of helping them satisfy their needs. Caring individualizes and personalizes interactions with patients. It mitigates the depersonalization inherent in scientific medicine and institutional healthcare. Caring also counterbalances the impersonality of ethical principles and the "detachment" necessary for maintaining objectivity. By their very nature, principles consist of generalizations: they point to characteristics shared by a variety of situations. Caring gives insight into what is fitting for particular patients in particular problematic situations. Principles specify impersonal moral norms relevant to classes of cases. But each case has unique features, because it involves an individual patient in a particular network of relations with others. To interact ethically with patients, clinicians must attend with care to the situations each case presents. The psychic needs of the patient as a suffering person deserves attention by clinicians in addition to the medical needs of the patient's diseased or injured body. Caring for the patient as a person should be seen as integral to the plan of care. Caring helps the patient get better or make the best of his or her situation by relieving the distress caused by illness and its consequences--dependence, loss of control, vulnerability, and the threat of death. Lack of attention to the suffering of patients amounts to psychological abandonment. Included within caring are the virtues of respect for patients as persons and therapeutic attentiveness. The good clinician respects patients as persons by responding to patients as individuals with life histories and inner worlds rather than merely as bearers of disease. Therapeutic attentiveness is the disposition of the good clinician to appreciate and use the relationship with the patient as a means of promoting healing and relief of suffering. This involves an empathetic presence with patients manifested by listening to them, acknowledging their concerns, explaining their medical situation in understandable terms, and providing reassurance.[55]

4. Clinical benevolence: The clinician is committed to promoting the welfare of his or her patient. This is the preeminent traditional virtue of medicine and nursing.

5. Subordination of self-interest to patient care: This virtue is a necessary condition of benevolence and caring.

6. Reflective intelligence: The good clinician is ready to anticipate problems, set reasonable goals, regard interventions as experimental, and adjust interventions in the light of experience.

7. Humility: The virtuous clinician understands the limits of medical knowledge and technique and recognizes her or his fallibility.

8. Practical wisdom: The good clinician develops the art of clinical judgment under conditions of uncertainty and risk that characterize medicine. In the present context, the good clinician develops the ability to discern his or her appropriate role within large healthcare systems.

9. Courage: The good clinician has the mental and moral strength to venture, persevere, and withstand danger, fear, or difficulty firmly and resolutely. He or she has the courage to maintain bonds of fidelity to patients, regardless of their condition and degree of handicap. Courage is needed in taking the risks to act ethically when it may be contrary to what is legal and be the subject of legal action. Clinicians are often exposed to dangers and hazards in the care of patients, such as exposure to human immunodeficiency virus (HIV) and other infectious diseases and the possibility of physical abuse from patients or relatives. A final point is that courage is required to meet and cope with the costs of caring and empathy. When one is open to the often turbulent feelings and fears of others in the stress of illness, there are dangers to selfhood and even to sanity.

What is the source of authority of these ethical considerations and clinical virtues? They arise out of the practices and institutions of society in its interaction with clinical medicine. They operate as norms and standards recognized as authoritative with respect to family life, routine social interactions, religious communities, professional practices and associations, the law, and the state. The social origins of these ethical considerations and clinical virtues reflect the root meanings of ethics and morality as ethos and mores--the socially instituted norms of human conduct. The discipline of ethics, however, seeks to go beyond the "taken-for-granted" quality of everyday morality to validate these considerations on deeper grounds of ethical principles and ethical theory.

VI. Ethical and Legal Problems

Ethics and law are related. Each field is concerned to identify norms of conduct. However, the domains of these disciplines do not entirely overlap. Law seeks to educate and to regulate by announcing a minimal standard of conduct and establishing disincentives for ignoring that standard. Ethics endorses many basic norms of behavior that are required by law; however, ethics extends beyond the law to prescribe desirable conduct and articulate ideals and virtues to which we should aspire.

Law and ethics have different goals and different sanctions. In law, negative sanctions (punishments such as suspension of license to practice, fines, or even imprisonment) are imposed by society and carried out by actions of the government. Ethical sanctions are generally noncoercive and include the praise or blame of our colleagues or others. Law has the power of official coercion that ethics lacks. Like law, the practice of ethics depends upon analytical precision and forceful argumentation; however, the power of ethics resides primarily in the strength of reason unaccompanied by state endorsement.

Ethical problems arise from conflicts between moral principles, rules, or values that are embedded in society's institutions. These institutions include the courts, the legislatures, and administrative agencies. Legal problems arise from a variety of causes: (1) conflicting interpretations of what the law requires in a specific situation; (2) a threat by a patient or family member to sue; (3) a court ruling that has already been issued (as in the JP case in Chapter 2); or (4) when the law is silent or lacks adequate guidance on a specific legal question in a case having an ethical problem (as in the *Linares* or *Baby K* cases discussed in Chapter 9).

Laws influence the shaping of institutional policies with ethical content. The courts may look to hospital and nursing home policies as the standard of care for clinical behavior, and clinicians are expected to comply with these policies. For example, policies exist for writing do-not-resuscitate-orders or for HIV testing with patients and employees. These policies may include interpretations of the demands of federal or state laws as they circumscribe practice in the clinical setting. In large hospitals, there may be literally dozens of such policy statements, which need to be updated when laws are adopted or amended.

Because respecting the law and its officers is an important moral duty, the legal concerns that arise in clinical cases have ethical relevance. However, what is legally permitted may not be ethically justifiable in a particular case. For example, it would be legally permissible to test a pregnancy and pursue an abortion solely on the basis of fetal gender. Yet, most would agree--including an important President's Commission[56] and a recent Institute of Medicine committee[57]--that there are strong ethical reasons to avoid such a practice and not to cooperate with those who would desire it.

Ethical and legal problems are often entangled in cases presented to an ethics committee. A large and evolving body of law (court cases, statutes, regulations, and so on) is applicable to many of the problems described in this text. Some landmark legal cases have also engendered original ethical debate and deliberation. At times, the issues before a court go to the heart of a moral question (for example, in *Quinlan*,[58] "Is the removal of a ventilator the moral equivalent of killing a patient?"). For this reason, the court's findings in such cases have had an important impact on the evolution of clinical ethics. Court opinions have clarified some of the norms that are expected of clinicians in addressing the problems presented in Section II, Parts A and B. Some of these problems--such as requests for assistance with suicide and euthanasia--await further legal clarification.

The chapters in Section II refer to many legal cases, how they contributed to biomedical ethics, and their relevance for clinical ethics. The relationship between ethics and law in the clinical setting is complex. At times, the law yields to professional experience and/or ethical analysis, looking for norms that are commonly accepted as features of clinical practice. The *Cruzan*[59] case exemplifies such a response, where a court followed the lead of medical professionals and the literature of biomedical ethics. At other times, the law runs ahead of medical practice and ethical deliberation. The case of *Helling v. Carey*,[60] in which a court refused to adopt the received wisdom of the medical community on the proper standard of care for ophthalmological testing and devised a new rule for measuring professional negligence, represents that tendency of the law. The relationship between law and ethics can be thought of as a conversation. Ethicists borrow from legal reasoning, and lawyers build upon an analysis that may have begun in the ethical context.

Despite the similarities between the disciplines, and with attention to the conversation that goes on between them, the main focus of this textbook is on clinical ethics and not on law, its institutions, or legal reasoning. However, those who seek to practice clinical ethics must be familiar with health law in their states and at the federal level. Every state has laws to clarify norms governing most of the problems discussed in Section II. Chapter 14 presents some practical suggestions about how clinicians, ethics committees with an attorney member, and the legal officers of an institution can cooperate on specific cases. Major court cases with which readers should be familiar are included within or at the end of each chapter in Section II.

Notes

1. For an excellent discussion of "prevention" in ethics, see L. Forrow, R.M. Arnold, and L.S. Parker, "Preventive Ethics: Expanding the Horizons of Clinical Ethics," *The Journal of Clinical Ethics* 4, no. 4 (Winter 1993): 287-94.

2. T.L. Beauchamp and J.F. Childress, *Principles of Biomedical Ethics*, 4th ed. (New York: Oxford Uni-

versity Press, 1994), 44. These theories are: utilitarianism, Kantianism, character ethics, liberal individualism, communitarianism, the ethics of care, casuistry, and common-morality accounts.

3. M. Siegler, E.D. Pellegrino, and P.A. Singer, "Clinical Medical Ethics," *The Journal of Clinical Ethics* 1, no. 1 (Spring 1990): 5-9.

4. M. Siegler, "A Legacy of Osler: Teaching Clinical Ethics at the Bedside," *Journal of the American Medical Association* 239 (1978): 951-56.

5. M. Siegler, "Decision Making Strategy for Clinical-Ethical Problems in Medicine," *Archives of Internal Medicine* 142 (1982): 2178-79; A.R. Jonsen, M. Siegler, and W. Winslade, *Clinical Ethics: A Practical Approach to Ethical Decisions in Clinical Medicine*, 3rd ed. (New York: McGraw-Hill, 1992).

6. R.C. Fox, "Advanced Medical Technology: Social and Ethical Implications," *Annual Review of Sociology* 2 (1976): 231-68; J.C. Fletcher, "The Bioethics Movement and Hospital Ethics Committees," *Maryland Law Review* 50 (1991): 859-88.

7. D. Rothman, *Strangers at the Bedside* (New York: Basic Books, 1991); A.R. Jonsen, ed., "The Birth of Bioethics," Special Supplement, *Hastings Center Report* 23, no. 6 (1993): S1-15.

8. E.D. Pellegrino, "Medical Practice and the New Curriculum," *Journal of the American Medical Association* 213 (1970): 748-52; K.D. Clouser, "Humanities in Medical Education: Some Contributions," *Journal of Medicine and Philosophy* 15 (1990): 289-301.

9. See note 2 above.

10. R. Sider and C.D. Clements, "The New Medical Ethics: A Second Opinion," *Archives of Internal Medicine* 145 (1985): 2169-73.

11. K.D. Clouser and B. Gert, "A Critique of Principlism," *Journal of Medicine and Philosophy* 15 (1990): 219-36.

12. A.R. Jonsen and S. Toulmin, *The Abuse of Casuistry*, (Berkeley, Calif.: University of California Press, 1989); J.D. Arras, "Getting Down to Cases: The Revival of Casuistry in Bioethics," *Journal of Medicine and Philosophy* 16 (1991): 29-52.

13. R.M. Veatch and S.T. Fry, *Case Studies in Nursing Ethics* (Philadelphia: J.B. Lippincott Company, 1987); C. Levine, *Cases in Bioethics* (New York: St. Martin's Press, 1989); G. Pence, *Classic Cases in Medical Ethics*, 2nd ed. (New York: McGraw-Hill, 1993); J.C. Ahronheim, J.D. Moreno, C. Zuckerman, *Ethics in Clinical Practice* (Boston: Little, Brown, 1994).

14. C.M. Culver, *Ethics at the Bedside* (Hanover, N.H.: University Press of New England, 1991); N.

Dubler, *Ethics on Call* (New York: Harmony Books, 1992).

15. R.M Veatch and H.E. Flack, *Case Studies in Allied Health Ethics* (Upper Saddle River, N.J.: Prentice-Hall, 1997).

16. C. Gilligan, *In a Different Voice* (Cambridge, Mass.: Harvard University Press, 1992).

17. J. Katz, *The Silent World of Doctor and Patient* (New York: Free Press, 1984).

18. B. Brody, *Life and Death Decision Making* (New York: Oxford University Press, 1988).

19. E. Cassell, *The Nature of Suffering and the Goals of Medicine* (New York: Oxford University Press, 1991).

20. H. Brody, *The Healer's Power* (New Haven, Conn.: Yale University Press, 1992).

21. T.E. Quill, *Death and Dignity: Making Choices and Taking Charge* (New York: W.W. Norton, 1993).

22. R.M. Zaner, *Ethics and the Clinical Encounter* (Englewood Cliffs, N.J.: Prentice-Hall, 1988).

23. A.F. Connors et al., "A Controlled Trial to Improve Care of Seriously Ill Hospitalized Patients," *Journal of the American Medical Association* 274, no. 20 (1995): 1591-98.

24. *Webster's Third New International Dictionary* (Chicago: Encyclopedia Britannica, Inc., 1981), 1: 460.

25. J.C. Fletcher and H. Brody, "Clinical Ethics," in W.T. Reich, ed. *Encyclopedia of Bioethics*, 2nd ed. (New York: MacMillan, 1995): 399-404.

26. There are one-year, postgraduate fellowship programs in clinical ethics at University of Chicago, Cleveland Clinic Foundation, Clinical Center of the National Institutes of Health, Harvard School of Medicine, and the University of Virginia. Some universities offer an M.A. degree program that focuses fully or in part on clinical ethics: Brown, Case-Western Reserve, Georgetown, Pittsburgh, Minnesota, Tennessee, Virginia, Washington, and Wisconsin (Milwaukee). Seven universities now offer a Ph.D. program in biomedical ethics or bioethics, with wide variance in terms of clinical requirements: Baylor-Rice, Georgetown, Loyola (Chicago), Tennessee (Knoxville), Texas (Houston), Virginia, and Washington. See *International Directory of Bioethics Organizations* (Washington, D.C.: Kennedy Institute of Ethics, Georgetown University, 1994).

27. There are four professional societies in which clinical ethics is of interest, although it is most prominently studied in the first: the Society for Bioethics Consultation; the Society for Health and Human Values (medical humanities); the American Association of Bioethics (bioethics); and the American Society of Law, Medicine, and Ethics (health law and ethics). The first three societies have begun to discuss cooperation and eventual unification.

28. J. LaPuma and D. Schiedermeyer, *Ethics Consultation: A Practical Guide* (Boston: Jones and Bartlett, 1994), 58-61.

29. F.E. Baylis, ed., *The Health Care Ethics Consultant* (Totowa, N.J.: Humana Press, 1994).

30. A.R. Jonsen, M. Siegler, and W.J. Winslade, *Clinical Ethics*, 3rd ed. (New York: McGraw-Hill, 1992).

31. S.M. Wolf, "Health Care Reform and the Future of Physician Ethics," *Hastings Center Report* 24, no. 2 (1994): 28-41.

32. Joint Commission on Accreditation of Healthcare Organizations, "Patient Rights and Organizational Ethics," in *Accreditation Manual for Hospitals* (Oakbrook Terrace, Ill.: JCAHO, 1995).

33. J.K. Iglehart, "Physicians and the Growth of Managed Care," *New England Journal of Medicine* 331 (1994): 1167.

34. Ibid.

35. "Ethics and Morality," in *Encyclopedia of Ethics*, ed. L.M. Becker and C.B. Becker (New York: Garland Publishing, 1992), 329.

36. See note 2 above, p. 4.

37. K. Luker, *Abortion and the Politics of Motherhood* (Berkeley, Calif.: University of California Press, 1984); L. Tribe, *Abortion: The Clash of Absolutes* (New York: Norton, 1991); R. Dworkin, *Life's Dominion* (New York: Alfred A. Knopf, 1993).

38. This section draws upon a discussion of dilemmas by Beauchamp and Childress. See note 2 above, pp. 11-13.

39. See R.M. Zaner, "Medicine and Dialogue," *Journal of Philosophy and Medicine* 15 (1990): 303-25. In arguing against the prevailing view of medicine as "applied biology," Zaner reconceives it essentially as "dialogue."

40. G.J. Annas, "How We Lie," *Hastings Center Report* 25 (November-December 1995): S12-14.

41. S.B. Nuland, *How We Die* (New York: Alfred A. Knopf, 1994), 250-253, at 253.

42. See note 20 above.

43. R.M. Veatch, "Medical Ethics: Professional or Universal," *Harvard Theological Review* 65 (1972): 531-59.

44. G.J. Annas, "Asking the Courts to Set the Standard of Emergency Care," *New England Journal of Medicine* 330 (1994): 1542-45.

45. T.L. Beauchamp and J.F. Childress, *Principles of Biomedical Ethics*, 3rd ed. (New York: Oxford Uni-

versity Press, 1989), 21.

46. R.M. Zaner, Troubled Voices (Cleveland, Ohio: Pilgrim Press, 1993), 138.

47. These principles are most clearly discussed and defended by Beauchamp and Childress, see note 2 above.

48. In addition to the Beauchamp and Childress volume already cited, we recommend the following texts: B. Brody, *Life and Death Decision Making* (New York: Oxford University Press, 1988); H. Brody, *The Healer's Power* (New Haven, Conn.:, Yale University Press, 1992); E.J. Cassell, *The Nature of Suffering and the Goals of Medicine* (New York: Oxford University Press, 1991); H.T. Englehardt, Jr., *Foundations of Bioethics*, 2nd ed. (New York: Oxford University Press, 1994); H.B. Holmes and L.M. Purdy, ed., *Feminist Perspectives in Medical Ethics* (Bloomington, Ind.: Indiana University Press, 1992); E.D. Pellegrino and D.C. Thomasma, *For the Patient's Good* (New York: Oxford University Press, 1988); R.M. Veatch, *A Theory of Medical Ethics* (New York: Basic Books, 1981); R.M. Zaner, *Ethics and the Clinical Encounter* (Englewood Cliffs, N.J.: Prentice-Hall, 1988); R. Macklin, *Enemies of Patients* (New York: Oxford University Press, 1993); J.C. Ahronheim, J. Moreno, and C. Zuckerman, *Ethics in Clinical Practice* (Boston: Little, Brown, 1994). Some texts in clinical ethics are also annotated in Appendix 4 of this volume.

49. President's Commission for the Study of Ethical Problems in Medicine and Biomedical and Behavioral Research, *Making Health Care Decisions*, vol. 1 (Washington, D.C.: U.S. Government Printing Office, 1982), 17-18.

50. The Virginia Health Care Decisions Act of 1992 (*Virginia Code, Annotated*, Sec. 54.1-2990 [Michie 1994]) was amended to read: "Nothing in this article shall be construed to require a physician to prescribe or render medical treatment to a patient that the physician determines to be medically or ethically inappropriate.

However, in such a case, if the physician's determination is contrary to the terms of an advance directive of a qualified patient or the treatment decision of a person designated to make the decision under this article, the physician shall make a reasonable effort to transfer the patient to another physician. Nothing in this article shall be construed to condone, authorize or approve mercy killing or euthanasia, or to permit any affirmative or deliberate act or omission to end life other than to permit the natural process of dying." This provision was the first in the nation to affirm the physician's authority in the face of requests for "futile" treatment. This provision is further discussed in Chapter 9.

51. See note 2 above, p. 293.

52. See note 20 above.

53. Ibid., 109.

54. Discussions of clinical virtues and virtue theory do, however, appear in the literature. See Beauchamp and Childress, note 2 above p. 366-99; W.F. May, "The Virtues in a Professional Setting," *Soundings* 68 (Fall 1984): 245-66; C.L. Bosk, *Forgive and Remember: Managing Medical Failure* (Chicago: University of Chicago Press, 1979); J.L. Drane, *Becoming a Good Doctor: The Place of Virtue and Character in Medical Ethics* (Kansas City, Mo.: Sheed & Ward, 1988).

55. H. Zinn, "The Empathetic Physician," *Archives of Internal Medicine* 153 (1993): 306-12.

56. President's Commission for the Study of Ethical Problems in Medicine and Biomedical and Behavioral Research, *Counseling and Screening for Genetic Conditions* (Washington, D.C.: U.S. Government Printing Office, 1983): 6-7, 56-59.

57. Committee on Assessing Genetic Risks, Institute of Medicine, *Assessing Genetic Risks* (Washington, D.C.: National Academy Press, 1994), 105, 85-86.

58. *In Re Quinlan*, 70 N.J. 10, 355 A.2d 647 (1976).

59. *Cruzan v. Director, Missouri Department of Health*, 497 U.S. 261 (1990).

60. *Helling v. Carey*, 519 P.2D 981 (Wash. 1974).

2

CLINICAL PRAGMATISM: A CASE METHOD OF MORAL PROBLEM SOLVING

Franklin G. Miller, Ph.D., John C. Fletcher, Ph.D., and Joseph J. Fins, M.D.

I. Introduction

A standard feature of bioethics has been the appeal to general moral principles, particularly the four principles of respect for autonomy, nonmaleficence, beneficence, and justice discussed in Thomas Beauchamp and James Childress's influential textbook, *Principles of Biomedical Ethics*.[1] Beauchamp and Childress have developed and revised a sophisticated theory of bioethics, in which general principles operate in a "dialectical," mutually supporting relationship with particular moral judgments concerning concrete cases. We have found their analytical work concerning these four principles and other moral considerations to be highly valuable, and we have appealed to aspects of it at various points in this text. The sustained attention to abstract issues of theory, however, makes their book unsuitable as a practical text for introducing clinical ethics. Clinicians need a workable method of moral problem solving and practical guidance on the major ethical issues that are likely to be encountered in various areas of clinical practice.

Moral problems in clinical practice arise in the context of particular cases of patient care. Clinicians faced with morally problematic situations need to know how to assess the morally relevant details of the case and apply general moral considerations, rules, principles, standards, and virtues, in order to arrive at a satisfactory resolution. In this book, we adopt a method of moral problem solving that we call *clinical pragmatism*, which is inspired by the thought of the American philosopher John Dewey.[2]

According to Dewey, there is a generic method of intelligent problem solving adaptable to problematic situations in daily living, professional practice, and the sciences. Dewey argued that this method, which is employed most rigorously in the experimental sciences, should also be applied to the resolution of moral problems. This method proceeds by logical steps. Recognition of a problematic situation prompts empirical inquiry to explain the causes of the problem by observation or diagnostic testing. Hypothetical ideas for how the problem might be resolved are considered. A plan of action, understood as an experimental trial, is decided and implemented. Finally, the observed results are evaluated.

We have developed our formulation of clinical pragmatism in the spirit of Dewey's pragmatic philosophy.[3] The method is *clinical* because it is focused on the circumstances of particular cases of patient care and attentive to the norms and virtues of clinical practice. It is *pragmatic* because it aims to guide the development, implementation, and evaluation of ethically appropriate and effective plans of action by means of a collaborative process of problem solving involving all those concerned with the case.

It is important to understand the scope and limits of the case method of moral problem solving. First, it is meant as a tool for inquiry and problem solving. Its efficacy depends crucially on the experience, skill, and character of those who adopt it. No method of clinical ethics can substitute for the cultivation of competence, insight, and virtue. Second, because it is a case-specific method of moral problem solving, it is not designed to guide either systematic reform of clinical practice or policy analysis and decision making. These tasks can be informed by detailed case studies, but they require other methods of inquiry and intervention (such as field observations, survey research, and controlled experimental trials). Finally, there is no guarantee that the use of this, or any other, method of moral problem solving will generate a satisfactory resolution of a problem. In some cases, moral conflict may remain intractable and, in spite of the dedicated efforts of skilled and caring clinicians, appeal for judicial review may be required.

II. The Method of Clinical Pragmatism

We describe and illustrate in this chapter a four-step method for clinicians to use in moral problem solving. What should clinicians do when faced with a moral problem that threatens to disrupt the planning or provision of care for a patient, or with a case that poses a novel and perplexing moral issue? The clinicians' task, in such cases, is to try to resolve the moral problem(s) effectively so that the care of the patient can be continued or altered appropriately. The four steps in the case method involve the following tasks:

1. *Assessment* of medical facts, contextual factors, the patient's capacity, the patient's preferences and needs, surrogate decision makers, competing interests, institutional factors, and issues of power;
2. *Moral diagnosis* of the problems posed by the case and options for resolution;
3. *Goal setting, decision making, and implementation* of a plan of action by means of a shared, deliberative process;
4. *Evaluation* of results.

This method of moral problem solving parallels the process of clinical problem solving, which proceeds by means of (1) data collection (history and physical exam), (2) differential diagnosis, (3) therapeutic trial, and (4) follow-up.

Under the principle of respect for patient autonomy and the doctrine of informed consent, clinical problem solving should take the form of shared decision making.[4] Moreover, because moral issues are not within the realm of technical expertise, participatory dialogue, negotiation, and consensus building are essential features of the process of moral problem solving in clinical practice.

Clinical pragmatism adopts a democratic model of moral problem solving. Clinicians and ethics consultants facilitate and guide the process of moral problem solving without dictating or engineering the outcome. Instead, in clinical pragmatism, this process is understood as located within a context of reciprocity, in which all concerned parties to a case are entitled to be heard and work together to arrive at a mutually satisfactory resolution.

Moral problem solving should be understood as an integral part of clinical practice. To the extent possible, clinicians working with patients and family members should strive to resolve moral problems as they arise. When such efforts fail, owing to interpersonal conflict or perplexity about the right thing to do in a morally complex situation, ethics consultation may be desirable to facilitate resolution.

Exhibit 2-1 contains a detailed outline of the method of clinical pragmatism, illustrated by the case presentation in Section IV of this chapter. Not every item will be relevant in every morally problematic case. Although the method is presented as a linear progression, in practice these steps may occur simultaneously or in a different sequence. The outline should be treated as a flexible guide, rather than a rigid checklist, because the process of problem solving should be tailored to the particular features of a case as they emerge in clinical practice.

This method is meant for use both prospectively by clinicians who face moral problems in the care of patients and retrospectively for the education of clinicians and ethics committee members. It may also be used to assess the quality of efforts at moral problem solving. Ethics committee members and ethicists who use this method in the context of ethics consultation should function as facilitators of moral problem solving by the clinicians, patients, and family members involved in the case. Ethics consultants should not act as moral arbiters called on to render authoritative judgment on what to do. Rather, they should promote careful consideration of the range of reasonable options that are available, ensure that all concerned parties have an opportunity to be heard, and endeavor to mediate conflicts.

III. The Use of Principles in Clinical Ethics

Principles play a vital role in clinical ethics, but it is important to understand the pitfalls that may occur with a simplistic use of principles. Unfortunately,

Exhibit 2-1
Clinical Pragmatism:
A Case Method of Moral Problem Solving

1. Assessment
   a. What is the patient's medical condition?
      i.   Identification of medical problems and history
      ii. Diagnosis/diagnostic hypotheses
      iii. Predictions and uncertainties regarding progno-sis (What are the prospects for full or partial recovery? Is the patient terminally ill?)
      iv. Provisional formulation of goals of treatment and care
      v.   Treatment recommendations and reasonable al-ternatives
   b. What are the relevant contextual factors?
      i.   Demographic factors (age, gender, education)
      ii.   Life situation and lifestyle of patient
      iii. Family relationships
      iv.   Setting of care (home or institution)
      v.   Socioeconomic factors (such as insurance cov-erage)
      vi.   Language spoken
      vii. Cultural factors
      viii. Religion
   c. Is the patient capable of decision making?
      i.   Legally incompetent (for example, the patient is a child or a court has determined the patient to be incompetent)
      ii. Clearly incapacitated (for example, patient is un-conscious)
      iii. Diminished capacity (for example, patient is di-agnosed with depression or other mental disor-der interfering with understanding or judgment)
      iv. Fluctuating capacity
      v.   Prospects for enhancing capacity
   d. What are the patient's preferences?
      i.   Understanding of condition
      ii. Views on quality of life
      iii. Values relevant to decision making about treat-ment
      iv. Current wishes for treatment
      v.   Advance directives
      vi. Reasons for seeking treatment that is regarded as medically inappropriate or refusing treatment that is regarded as medically indicated

   e. What are the needs of the patient as a person?
      i.   Psychic suffering and possible interventions for relief
      ii. Interpersonal dynamics
      iii. Resources and strategies for helping patient cope
      iv. Adequacy of home environment for care of pa-tient
      v.   Preparation for dying
   f. What are the preferences of family/surrogate decision makers?
      i.   Competence as surrogate decision maker
      ii. Judgment and evidence of relevant patient pref-erences
      iii. Opinions on quality of life of patient
      iv. Opinions on best interest of patient
      v.   Reasons for seeking treatment that is regarded as medically inappropriate or refusing treatment that is regarded as medically indicated
   g. Are there interests other than, and potentially com-peting with, those of the patient?
      i.   Interests of family (for example, concerns about burdens of caring for patient or disagreements with preferences of patient)
      ii. Interest of fetus
      iii. Scarce resources and competing needs for their use
      iv. Interests of healthcare providers (for example, professional integrity)
      v.   Interests of healthcare organization
   h. Are there issues of power or conflict in the interac-tions of the key actors in the case that need to be addressed?
      i.   Between clinicians and patient/family
      ii. Between patient and family members
      iii. Among family members/surrogates
      iv. Between members of the healthcare team (for example, between attending physicians and house staff, between physicians and nurses)
   i. Have all the parties involved in the case had an oppor-tunity to be heard?
   j. Are there institutional factors contributing to moral

Exhibit 2-1, continued

problems posed by the case?
i.   Work routines
ii. Fears of malpractice/defensive medicine/legal problems
iii. Biases favoring disproportionately aggressive treatment or neglect of treatable conditions
iv. Cost constraints/economic incentives

2. Moral diagnosis
   a. Examine how the moral problems in this case are being framed by the participants. Determine whether this framing should be reconsidered and replaced by an alternative understanding.
   b. Identify and rank the range of relevant moral considerations.
   c. Identify any relevant institutional policies pertaining to the case.
   d. Consider ethical standards and guidelines, drawing on consensus statements of commissions or interdisciplinary or specialty groups.
   e. Consider similar cases and discussions in the literature that might shed light on the analysis and resolution of moral problems in the case.
   f. Identify the morally acceptable options for resolving the moral problems posed by the case.

3. Goal setting, decision making, and implementation
   a. Consider or reconsider and negotiate the goals of treatment and care for the patient.
   b. Consider ideas (hypotheses) for possible interventions to meet the needs of the patient and resolve moral problems.
   c. Deliberate regarding merits of alternative options for resolving the moral problems.
   d. Endeavor to resolve conflicts.
   e. Assess whether ethics consultation is necessary or desirable.
      i. Is there persistent conflict between clinicians and patients/surrogates or among clinicians regarding how to resolve the moral problems posed by the case?

ii. Would ethics advice be helpful in understanding or providing guidance on moral issues presented by the case?
   f. Negotiate acceptable plan of action.
   g. If negotiations, including ethics consultation, fail to achieve satisfactory resolution, consider judicial review.
   h. implement plan of action.

4. Evaluation
   a. Current evaluation
      i.   Is the plan of action working? If not, why not?
      ii. Do the observed results of implementing the plan indicate the need for a modification of the plan?
      iii. Have conditions changed in a way that suggests the need to rethink the plan?
      iv. Are interactions between clinicians and the patient or surrogate helping to meet the needs of the patient, to respect the patient as a person, and to serve the goals of the plan of care?
      v.   Are there relevant interests, institutional factors, or normative considerations that have not been adequately addressed in planning for the care of the patient?
   b. Retrospective evaluation
      i.   What opportunities for resolving the moral problem were missed?
      ii. How did the care received by the patient match up to standards of good practice?
      iii. What factors contributed to a less than optimal resolution of the problems posed by the case?
      iv. Was the process of problem solving satisfactory in this case?
      v.   What might have been done to improve the care of the patient?
      vi. Are there desirable changes in institutional policy, feasible changes in the clinical environment, or educational interventions that might help to prevent or resolve the moral problems posed by similar cases?

clinical ethicists who use principles in clinical practice tend to adopt a mechanical approach to moral problem solving, which often leads to premature moral judgment. To jump to a conclusion about which principle is relevant in a specific case is akin to reaching a medical diagnosis before all the clinical facts are known and weighed. Dewey aptly described this problem of premature judgment as follows:

> Imagine a doctor called in to prescribe for a patient. The patient tells him some things that are wrong; his experienced eye at a glance takes in other signs of a certain disease. But if he permits the suggestion of this special disease to take possession prematurely of his mind, to become an accepted conclusion, his scientific thinking is by that much cut short. A large part of his technique, as a skilled practitioner, is to prevent the acceptance of the first suggestions that arise; even, indeed, to postpone the occurrence of any definite suggestion till the trouble, the nature of the problem, has been thoroughly explored. In the case of a physician this proceeding is known as diagnosis, but a similar inspection is required in every novel and complicated situation to prevent rushing to a conclusion. The essence of critical thinking is suspended judgment; and the essence of this suspense is inquiry to determine the nature of the problem before proceeding to attempts at its solution.[5]

The diagnosis and resolution of moral problems in the care of patients also requires such a disciplined process of inquiry. Although invoking one ethical principle or rule (such as respecting the patient's autonomy or "doing no harm," may seem to provide structure to a case analysis, this move can constrict the emerging ethical discourse necessary for moral problem solving, especially at the outset, when it needs to be most open and inclusive. At its worst, such a mechanical approach could lead to orchestrated outcomes, in which the selected ethical principle or rule predetermines an inappropriate approach to resolving the moral problem.

The method of clinical pragmatism, in contrast, deploys principles and other moral considerations as "working hypotheses," to provide orientation and guidance in moral problem solving. It aims to arrive at carefully considered, principled judgments about what to do in morally problematic cases; however,

clinical pragmatism is attentive to the details of the clinical situation and in the context of a collaborative process of inquiry, negotiation, and decision making.

IV. Illustration of Clinical Pragmatism: The Case of JP

The case of JP is used to demonstrate a four-part case method of moral problem solving. The facts have not been changed to protect privacy and confidentiality, as one would normally do when writing a teaching case that occurred locally. The case is used with the permission of those involved, including patient, family, and clinicians. The case analysis is in italics. When working on other cases, readers can refer to the nonitalicized sections of this chapter to review the tasks of the case method.

A. Case Report

In October 1987, JP, a 36-year-old single male, suffered a traumatic injury while repairing a fence at the Blacksburg, Virginia, airport. He was working with a mechanically driven posthole digger and accidentally caught the sleeve of his jacket in the machine. As his jacket, shirt, and pants were torn from his body, both of his arms were also torn off. Incredibly, no harm was done to his head or other parts of his body.

JP was a member of a Jehovah's Witness congregation. His wallet, which was in his car, contained a signed and witnessed document widely used by Jehovah's Witnesses stating that he would refuse blood transfusions under any and all circumstances.

The local rescue squad arrived at the scene shortly after the accident. Recognizing the gravity of JP's injury, they summoned The University of Virginia's (UVa's) emergency air transport service, Pegasus, which was dispatched immediately. JP had lost consciousness for a short period after the accident. However, he was awake and alert when the flight team arrived on the scene.

JP was immediately transported by helicopter to UVa Hospital. His severed arms were also transported in the hope of possible reattachment. On the flight, JP made clear to the members of the response team that he was a Jehovah's Witness, and he refused any blood products.

On admission to the emergency room at UVa, he reiterated his refusal of blood products to members of the treatment team, stating, "I would rather die first." A standardized statement used by the emergency room for Jehovah's Witness cases (signed by a nurse who acted as a proxy), which indicated his refusal of blood products, was put into his medical record.

JP was taken to the operating room, where a plastic surgeon attempted microsurgical reattachment of his least damaged arm. The surgical procedure lasted for several hours, during which time JP's intravascular volume losses were replaced with artificial volume expanders. Following his surgery, JP was admitted to the surgical intensive care unit (SICU) in critical condition. He had been intubated before surgery and remained intubated and on mechanical ventilation in the SICU.

The SICU medical and nursing staff realized that, without blood products, surgical reattachment of JP's arm would be unsuccessful. Worse, his very survival was tenuous. JP was informed of these problems. The staff was unsure if he would live through the night without an increase in the oxygen-carrying capacity of his blood. On admission to the SICU, JP's hematocrit (an indicator of the amount of hemoglobin available to carry oxygen to cells) was 16 percent (normal is 35 to 47 percent). During the next few hours, his hematocrit dropped to 10 percent. The SICU resident and nurses were able to communicate with JP during this period and explained his dire situation. JP continued to refuse transfusions, and his hematocrit dropped to 8 percent.

Alarmed by JP's refusal of blood transfusions, and seeking to save his life, JP's father (a physician who was a retired member of the UVa medical faculty) and the plastic surgeon sought and obtained a judge's authorization that allowed them, but did not order them, to give blood products to JP. The judicial ruling was obtained by phone between 1:00 a.m. and 2:00 a.m. The judge did not come to the hospital to speak to or observe JP. Later, hospital staff would learn that JP had significant conflicts with his parents over his choice to join a Jehovah's Witness congregation.

The surgeon called the SICU and ordered that blood be given to JP. The SICU resident and nurses giving care to JP were distressed. Although the patient was critically ill, they believed that he was a capable decision maker who clearly understood that he might not live through the night without blood prod-

ucts. They did not want to give blood to JP against his will, even in the light of the court order. (They were also relatively uninformed about the law on such cases.) After intense discussion with JP regarding the possibility of his death (JP at this point was indicating assent or dissent by gesturing and by nodding his head), the resident and nurses decided not to give blood, even though a court order permitting it had been issued.

The resident telephoned the surgeon and informed him of the staff's decision not to order or give blood products to JP. The senior physician responded angrily, "I'll come in and hang the blood myself! I'm on my way!"

The chief resident in medicine, who had been consulted by the SICU resident on alternative methods of intravascular volume management that might increase oxygen delivery, was at JP's bedside during this interchange. Observing the treatment team's immediate dilemma, he suggested that the resident ask for ethics consultation. The resident then called an ethics consultant.

B. Four-Part Case Method

I. Assessment

a. Patient's Medical Condition

The first step in case method is to assess the patient's medical condition and set some provisional goals for treatment and care. The initial tasks for which all clinicians are trained are to identify the patient's basic medical problems, to make a diagnosis, and to predict prognosis. If choices about tests or treatment must be made, the empirical risks and benefits of each procedure for the health of the patient must be described.

A basic ethical issue concerns whether needed tests or treatments are *medically indicated* (that is, recommended by physicians on the basis of proven benefit for the patient's condition) or *experimental* or unproven. The standard of care in medicine is strongly influenced by what is empirically proven or unproven. Refusal of an experimental treatment is not an ethical problem, because the results are still unproved and problematic. However, when JP refused a proven treatment that would save his life, a real ethical conflict existed for clinicians between preserving life and respecting the patient's refusal of treatment. The case also has implications for professional integrity.

The grave concern of SICU staff was based on the fact that they had never seen a patient survive such massive blood loss and such a low hematocrit. JP's prognosis was almost certain death. His potential for surgical reattachment was nil without transfusion. The consequence of further attempts to reattach without transfusion was certain death, although the surgeon believed that with transfusion, he had a good chance to reattach one arm. Clearly, blood transfusion was medically indicated in JP's case. No experimental treatment was involved.

The quest for medical facts is always tempered by clinical uncertainty. All medical tests and statements of prognosis have a margin of error. Also, presentations of facts are influenced by values and perceptions. Facts are always being interpreted and evaluated and are never completely "pure" and unbiased.

b. Contextual Factors

The next step, admittedly difficult in emergencies, is to assemble the best set of facts about the patient and his or her life situation. In a hospital, a special effort is needed to discover the patient as a person. Who was he or she before this illness? What do we know about his or her life plans? This information is related to the diagnosis and treatment plan. The illness disrupts a life story to which clinicians aim to restore the patient. With a thorough history and good information about the patient's family and values, clinicians will have done much to accomplish this step.

Each case has a context, a set of interrelated conditions in which the ethical problems arise. Beauchamp and Childress emphasize understanding the context of a case, "which always has unique features."[6] These features involve demographic facts (age, education), the life situation and lifestyle of the patient, family relationships, the institutional setting, socioeconomic facts, insurance coverage, language spoken by the patient and family, cultural factors, and religious issues. (Religious and cultural influences on healthcare decisions have been discussed in recent years.)[7]

At the time of his accident, JP was a 36-year-old, single adult man, a college graduate with a degree in engineering, who was employed by the airport authority in Blacksburg, Virginia. He was self-supporting and independent. He was also a licensed pilot. JP, of Cuban descent, had been raised in Charlottesville, Virginia, as one of seven children in a prominent family. The other key family member in the case was JP's father, a retired physician. He and JP had sharply differed over JP's decision to become a Jehovah's Witness, which JP did after deliberating and studying the Witnesses' teachings for one year.

The overriding interest of JP's father was to save his son's life. JP's mother agreed with her husband, but she was not directly involved in decisions about JP's care or in the effort to obtain a court order.

Important cultural factors included the Cuban and Roman Catholic heritage of this family, headed by a strong father. Dr. P was a widely admired physician who had also been a member of the faculty at the UVa Medical Center. Trained as a surgeon, he had immigrated to the United States prior to the revolution that brought Castro to power.

The hospital to which JP was flown is a tertiary-care university medical center, which at the time had 550 beds, with a surgical intensive care unit (SICU) of 16 beds. The hospital's ethics committee, founded in 1982, had recently decided to form an ethics consultation service. The hospital did not have a specific policy on refusals of blood transfusion by Jehovah's Witnesses. The department of emergency services had developed a form for Jehovah's Witnesses to sign, indicating their refusal. Because JP could not sign it, a nurse signed it as a proxy.

JP had a strong network of social support in his congregation and in his family if he were to survive. He had private health insurance related to his job, which covered the majority of costs connected with surgery, hospitalization, and rehabilitation. The costs of care or allocation of resources were not factors influencing decisions in this case.

In this case, the Jehovah's Witness position on transfusion of blood products is a central element. The Witnesses believe that the present world is impossibly corrupt and about to be destroyed. Only those who strictly obey the eternally valid commands of God in the Bible will be rescued. Blood transfusions are strictly forbidden, based on Witnesses' interpretation of biblical texts (Gen. 9:3-4; Lev. 17:13-14; Deut. 12:33; Acts 15:28-29). Except for blood product transfusions, Witnesses readily use the services of modern medicine.

The patient's parents and family of origin were Roman Catholic.

c. Capacity of the Patient

JP was a capable decision maker and remained so in the emergency room and throughout the episode in the SICU. He was aware of his surroundings, although he was too weak to communicate. He was intubated in the operating room prior to surgery and remained intubated postoperatively in the SICU to maximize oxygenation. His ability to talk was inhibited by the endotracheal tube, although he communicated throughout by nodding or shaking his head. His capacity to make decisions was evaluated by the emergency rescue team and by those who first received him at the hospital. The team never determined JP to be incapable of making healthcare decisions, although they expressed concern that the trauma and postaccident shock could have affected his reasoning.

d. The Patient's Preferences

JP made his preferences for no transfusions clear as soon as he regained consciousness after the accident. He had also recorded this preference in a document in his wallet. There was no doubt about his moral position as a Jehovah's Witness to avoid transfusion. He understood his condition and that the consequence of refusing transfusion could be death. In terms of quality of life, JP clearly believed that he would be better off, even without arms or dead, than if he were to violate his religious convictions. He made it clear that the integrity of his religious beliefs hung in the balance. His preference was noted on the medical record in the emergency room by use of a special form.

e. Needs of the Patient as a Person

JP's greatest need as a person, in addition to the immediate relief of his suffering and pain, was for his religious beliefs to be respected. He would later make a reference to forced transfusion as the "moral equivalent of rape," although at the time, he could not speak for himself except by nodding or shaking his head. He was receiving medication for pain and intensive care. He was prepared to die for his beliefs, and members of his congregation came to the hospital to be near him.

f. Preferences of Family

There was no need to appoint a surrogate decision maker, because JP remained capable of understanding throughout the early part of the case. The preferences of his parents were directly opposed to his preferences. They, like his surgeon, believed that blood transfusions would save his life, and they preferred this treatment to his death.

g. Competing Interests

The major interests competing with the interests of JP were those of his father and family. They disagreed with JP's preferences and did not share his religious beliefs. His father and mother believed that they should do everything possible to save his life. There were no questions about scarce resources. In addition, the plastic surgeon's professional integrity was competing with the patient's interest, as the surgeon was thoroughly committed to saving JP's life.

h. Issues of Power or Conflict

There were clearly issues of power and status in this case. The surgeon caring for JP was in the role of attending physician. The resident was lower in the clinical hierarchy, as were the nurses in the SICU. Yet, the resident and nurses made their preferences clear, taking some risks because of their status. There was also a power issue at work in the ease with which the surgeon and JP's father obtained a court order permitting a transfusion.

i. Opportunity for All Parties to Be Heard

As the case unfolded, all parties had opportunities to express their views, but the ethics consultation left a great deal to be desired along these lines. The ethics case consultation in the JP case will be discussed in the final section.

j. Institutional and Legal Factors

Institutional factors include a pattern of behavior among physicians in the hospital where JP was treated. Prior to the 1980s, physicians had routinely overridden the refusals of adult Jehovah's Witnesses to receive blood transfusions. The physicians justified their actions by arguing that the "physician can be blamed for the spiritual transgression" and that the patient would later be grateful to be alive. An-

other institutional factor was that a significant conflict broke out between SICU clinicians (resident and nurses) and a powerful, influential surgeon who was allied with JP's father.

Legal factors include possible violations of specific statutes or findings of court cases that would be relevant to conflicts or disputes within a case. Legal concerns also include threats to sue or appeals for legal advice made by anyone involved in a case.

The most immediate legal factor was a local judge's authorization, which allowed but did not order blood transfusion, that was issued to JP's father and the surgeon. Those who opposed the blood transfusion were concerned about acting contrary to the wishes of the father and the attending physician, which had the legal backing of a judge. However, many court cases, as indicated below, support the right of a competent Jehovah's Witness to refuse blood transfusion, unless there are major overriding circumstances such as pregnancy or a number of dependent children. Courts have differed on cases with overriding circumstances. The U.S. Supreme Court, in the Cruzan decision (see Chapter 9), strongly upheld the right of competent adults to refuse any medical treatment. The recent assisted suicide cases have repeated the language from Cruzan. The appeal of JP's father and the surgeon clearly swayed the judge. However, it is questionable whether an order to authorize treatment over the objection of a patient would be legal in 1987 or today. The fact that JP was capable of voicing his objections, religious or otherwise, would not have put him in the category of "unable to give informed consent." If he had been in this category, he would have been entitled to an attorney to advocate on his behalf in a proceeding.

There were no issues regarding cost constraints or economic incentives. The JP case occurred in a period before the advent of managed care in this part of the nation. Because JP was an insured person, there was never any question about his access to care or to the kind of care he received during hospitalization and rehabilitation.

2. Moral Diagnosis

a. Framing the Moral Problems

When faced with a moral problem, each participant identifies and frames the problem. The clinician or ethics consultant must simultaneously discern how participants frame the problem(s) and decide whether their views need to be reconsidered and replaced by an alternative understanding. The greatest skills and uses of authority in clinical ethics are in accurate moral diagnosis and teaching. There is always a possibility of a faulty diagnosis of the ethical problems in the case. Further, there is usually a rush to judgment by virtually everyone in the early stages of a problem, rather than exercise of the art of suspended judgment in deliberation, or waiting until all options have been fairly considered. These missteps can lead to an ethics disaster, like the one that occured in the case of Angie Carder, discussed in Chapter 7. Faulty diagnosis can arise from bias, lack of education, anxiety, anger, or a "shoot-from-the-hip" labeling of ethical problems in the case. Such a reaction can distort the situation and lead to mistakes that have serious and adverse consequences for the institution, its professionals, and the patient.[8]

JP's father and the surgeon framed the moral problem only in terms of beneficently saving the patient's life. They never met directly with the staff of the SICU. The resident and nurses framed the problem only in terms of respecting JP's religious convictions and refusal of transfusions. They did not have an opportunity to hear the option of treatment with transfusion clearly presented and defended. JP himself framed the problem in a very similar way. Given his religious commitments and his condition, it was unlikely that he could give the option of transfusion an authentic hearing.

How can moral problems be framed clearly and accurately? It is not helpful to define a problem initially as a conflict between ethical principles (for example, "there is a conflict in this case between autonomy and beneficence"). Such framing is too abstract and mechanical to be of much help at this early stage of deliberation. Further, it is a premature use of principles in moral problem solving, as explained above.

Ethics is a practical discipline. Failure to assess the facts and understand the ethical problems within the context of the case defeats ethical analysis. Ethical principles are best employed at the third step of deliberation, as sources of appeals and justification for the alternatives and options for choices. A more practical approach than resorting to principles is to identify ethical problems within the two general types discussed in this text (Chapter 1, pp. 11-12) and then to follow the four-step method explained in this chapter as a guide to problem solving. This approach has safeguards against premature judgment and, if followed, will give all morally acceptable options a fair hearing and defense. An approach to framing ethical problems is to begin by identifying the types of ethical problems found in the case, in order of priority.

In this case, the primary ethical problem is the validity of JP's refusal of medically indicated treatment deemed necessary to save his life. A second problem is the possibility that JP's capacity to refuse treatment may have been diminished, as he was in a state of shock and medicated for pain. A third problem is the court order, since an important moral duty is to obey the law and respect officers of the law such as a judge. (The third problem is qualified by the nature of the court order; it permitted but did not order a transfusion.)

One can further enrich the description of moral problems by identifying them as intrapersonal (within a person) conflicts and interpersonal (between persons) conflicts.

JP cared for his family and was also a faithful member of his congregation. He must have experienced a painful moral dilemma within himself between a duty to respect the teachings of his religion and a duty to respect his father and cooperate with clinicians who were intent upon saving his life.

Each clinician in the case also had an intrapersonal conflict: each wanted to benefit JP by blood transfusion and save his life. However, there is a strong duty not to coerce a competent adult into treatment without powerful and overriding ethical reasons, such as the harm that might be done to innocent third parties. If clinicians gave him blood against his religious principles, it would be a form of coercion that some have called "religious rape."

The case also had interpersonal conflicts. First, there was conflict between JP and his father, extending back to his choice to become a Jehovah's Witness. Second, the SICU team had a significant conflict with the surgeon. The resident was caught in the middle. Jehovah's Witnesses are in significant conflict with the ethical beliefs and practices of the ma- jority of Americans. In cases of Jehovah's Witness children who need transfusion, courts routinely resolve the conflict by ordering blood.[9] The courts' reasoning is that children cannot make mature religious commitments; thus if their parents avoid proven medical treatments in the name of religion, the state can intervene on behalf of children. Alternately, the courts have reasoned that parental rights do not extend to forcing children to die for the parents' religious beliefs.

b. Identifying and Ranking the Range of Relevant Moral Considerations

After identifying the ethical problems in the case, one ought to ask, "What are the morally relevant considerations? What is going on here morally?"

The JP case is more complex than it seems at first impression. A measure of complexity is that seven of the eight ethical considerations discussed in Chapter 1 are directly implicated and in conflict in this case:

1. *the need to balance benefits and harms in the care of patients;*
2. *disclosure, informed consent, and shared decision making;*
3. *the norms of family life;*
4. *the responsibilities of physicians and nurses in the context of relationships with patients;*
5. *professional integrity;*
6. *cultural and religious variations; and*
7. *considerations of power differences between the surgeon, the resident, and the nurses.*

Of the eight ethical considerations, only cost-effectiveness and allocation which carry out claims of the ethical principle of justice, do not seem to be directly implicated in this case.

c. Identifying Institutional Policies

There was no institutional policy in the hospital where JP was treated regarding refusal of medically indicated treatment.

At a minimum, a healthcare organization (HCO) should follow a guideline stating: "A formal institutional policy should encourage documentation of patient refusals in a patient statement about choice of care."

d. Identifying Guidelines for Clinicians on Models of Good Practice

Are there ethical guidelines or recommendations for clinicians in this type of case? This step involves a search for respected authorities' visions of good practice for such situations. Clinicians are not alone or without sources of advice concerning many of the most frequent or difficult ethical problems.

Many groups (such as professional societies, interdisciplinary task forces, national commissions, and teams of scholars) have shaped guidelines for problems in clinical ethics. These guidelines include codes of ethics and recommendations adopted by national and international assemblies of physicians and nurses, as well as by specialty societies. The recommendations of the President's Commission for the Study of Ethical Problems in Medicine and Biomedical and Behavioral Research (1978 - 1983) have been very influential, especially for issues of informed consent and determining capacity, as well as problems of refusal, forgoing life-sustaining treatment, and securing access to healthcare.[10] The commission's work has influenced important court decisions and guidelines for nurses and physicians on specific problems.

Chapters 3 through 13 briefly summarize ethical guidelines for clinicians about specific issues or problems discussed in each chapter. These guidelines and recommendations distill the moral experience--learned to date--of clinicians, assisted by scholars in law, ethics, and the humanities in response to ethical problems in several types of cases. We enter a note of caution here. Although the ethical reflection that undergirds such guidelines is very influential, such guidelines alone will not be sufficient to resolve ethical problems in a case. Guidelines bring the best thinking at the time to bear on types of problems but not upon specific cases. To use guidelines rigidly or as a "cookbook" defeats ethical deliberation and reasoning. In consulting such guidelines, we stand in the company of others who have examined a class of ethical problems in clinical care. However, they have not examined the cases at hand.

Chapter 7 summarizes ethical guidelines for clinicians on refusal of treatment cases (like the JP case) as follows:

1. The capable patient has the right to refuse any treatment, including that which sustains life, when the elements of informed consent have been met.

2. The capable patient has a duty implied within the context of shared decision making . . . to articulate as clearly as possible what motivates a decision to refuse treatment. Such a decision may be motivated by coherent personal reasons, religious beliefs, social or political ideology, or emotions.

3. A formal institutional policy should encourage documentation of the patient's refusal in a statement regarding the patient's choice of care.

Chapter 7 goes on to say that treatment refusals by capable patients are valid when the elements of informed consent have been satisfied. The patient must demonstrate the following:

1. understanding of his/her medical condition;
2. understanding of the consequences of his/her decision; and
3. voluntariness.

JP was a capable patient. He clearly expressed his reasons, which were religious in nature. He understood his medical condition and that he might die without a transfusion. There was no evidence of coercion or other pressure on his voluntary choice. On the basis of JP's understanding of these factors, guidance for clinicians strongly suggests that his refusal should be accepted. However, this suggestion or hypothesis needs to be tested by ethical argument.

On the basis of data about the case and the guidelines that are binding on clinicians, the ultimate outcome of the JP case seemed clear to the SICU staff. They were willing to permit JP to die without blood transfusions, rather than override his objections. However, his father and the surgeon strenuously disagreed, also on ethical grounds, and they sought the aid of a court. An important ethical dispute occurred, for which help was sought in an ethics consultation.

e. Considering Similar Cases

There are few truly novel moral problems. Clinicians who believe that they are facing a situation for the first time may be unaware of other, similar cases. New moral problems are found mostly in the context of research, experimental treatment, and reproductive choices.

After framing the ethical problems in a case, one ought to ask: "What cases are most similar, factually and morally, to my case?" Cases can be found in the legal realm, in the ethics literature,[11] or in clinicians' own experience. Comparing similar and different cases helps with decisions about whether the case fits with other well-settled cases or whether a unique facet or circumstance of the case makes it truly different from others. Also, when reviewing past cases, the question should arise: "What principles or other sources of appeal were used to resolve the case?"

A long line of Jehovah's Witnesses cases exists within a class of cases on refusal of medically indicated treatment by single, competent adults. The J.P. case is clearly in this line of cases. In 1976, in re Melideo,[12] *a hospital asked a court to give blood to a 23-year-old, childless woman of the Witness faith, arguing that it was needed to save her life. The court held that an adult of sound mind cannot be forced to submit to medical treatment unless the state can show an overriding interest.*

As early as 1964, the Bernice Brooks *case[13] upheld the right of competent Jehovah's Witness adults to refuse blood transfusions. Brooks, a Witness who was married with grown children, suffered a hemorrhage due to stomach ulcers and refused a blood transfusion. She was forced by her physician, who was armed with a court order, to undergo transfusion. She survived and sued the physician for violating her constitutional rights, a claim that was later upheld. The court emphasized that her choice was the result of a competent mind. A similar case, entitled "I'd rather live with God than live in sin," is discussed by Baruch Brody.[14]*

An important factor in the JP case is that he is single with no dependents. The prediction of harmful consequences of a parent's refusal of life-sustaining treatment, leaving dependent children and subsequent burdens on society, influences some judges to order a transfusion over the objections of the parent.[15] In In re Osborne, *a court permitted a Jehovah's Witness parent to refuse blood transfusion, because prior planning had taken place for the care of dependent children.[16]*

May a "mature minor" who is a Jehovah's Witness ethically and legally refuse transfusion? In a Georgia case, Novak v. Cobb County, *a U.S. District Court upheld a judge's order to give blood over 16-year-old Gregory Novak's objection, after he had been seriously injured in an auto accident.[17]*

3. Goal Setting, Decision Making, and Implementation

a. Reconsider the Goals of Treatment

The third step begins with the recognition that moral and ethical problems often disrupt the plan of care for the patient. Reconsideration about and negotiation of the goals of treatment and the plan of care cannot be divorced from the task of considering various options to resolve the moral problems in the case. Moral problem solving and planning for the care of patients go hand in hand. For this reason, moral problem solving should not take place "behind closed doors"[18] in an ethics committee but at or near the bedside.

It is worth recalling that ethics is not an alien force, outside of clinical practice, but an integral part of the competent practice of medicine and nursing. Clinical medicine involves planning throughout. Medicine is a consulting profession in which patients bring bodily or mental problems (or potential problems) to the attention of clinicians. The diagnosis and therapy for such problems call for systematic and continuous planning in the light of medical knowledge and clinical experience. The plan of care encompasses the entire encounter between clinicians and patients, even if such an encounter spans years or decades, as it often does in private practice.

b. Consider Ideas for Intervention

At this stage, the discussion of the problems in the case should refocus on the needs of the patient and on ideas (hypotheses) for possible interventions to resolve moral problems. If disputants in the case have taken sides and are still defending their positions strongly, it is crucial to attempt to reframe the debate by focusing on the patient and the possibilities.

c. Weigh the Merits of the Options

Deliberating the merits of alternative options to resolve the moral problem involves:

1. stating and ranking morally acceptable options to resolve the problems;
2. weighing the merits of alternative options, giving justification (the best ethical reasons) for the preferred resolution of the problems (drawing on ethical principles and other re-

sources from ethical theory for this step is clearly appropriate);

3. making a decision (a judgment) about which option is best, under the circumstances.

Each of these points needs further discussion.

i. State and Rank the Ethically Acceptable Options

Participants may offer options that are clearly unacceptable or intolerable in this society. These options ought not to be included for decision making, although they are useful for teaching purposes, in order to frame the parameters within which society permits choices about the problem at hand. For example, doing nothing, euthanizing JP, or not treating his pain were not morally acceptable options. A controversial option is not the same as a morally indefensible option. JP's physician and his father posed a controversial but not patently immoral option.

Stating options is not the same as ranking them. By ranking options, decision makers open themselves to challenge from different ethical claims needing to be further heard for their persuasiveness and relevance. To decide to rank the options evokes specific ethical commitments of decision makers and also considerations of the needs and relationships of the persons in the case. One can always re-rank options, if arguments to do so prevail.

What are the options in the JP case? How should they be ranked? There are only two options: (1) to respect JP's refusal; (2) to transfuse the patient over his objections.

If decision makers are predisposed to rank one option higher than another, more openness to competing ethical claims may occur if arguments for the less preferred option are examined first.

ii. Weigh and Justify the Options

- **Option 2: To transfuse the patient over his objections.** What ethical reasons can be given to override JP's refusal? Some ethical perspectives could support this argument. In a view that bases its supreme claim on consequences for society, one could argue to save the patient's life to benefit society, despite violating his "rights." In this view, society will be better off if JP lives to make his contribution to it, despite his handicap. A dead

person can neither enjoy rights nor contribute to society. One could also argue to override JP's refusal from a view that, without exception, the supreme goal of medicine and a physician's duty is saving human life under any and all conditions. To do so would be paternalistic ("the overriding of a person's wishes or intentional actions for beneficent reasons"[19]). But saving JP's life would be in accord with this goal. The surgeon clearly embraced this second reason until he was confronted by the SICU staff. Yet a third reason might be based on a tradition of religious ethics placing absolute value on the sanctity of human life. JP's religious beliefs would have to give way to another religious belief. From one of these three views, one might rank the second option higher.

- **Option 1: To respect JP's refusal.** Should the surgeon change his mind? Should he, along with other clinicians, respect JP's wishes? An argument for ranking this option highest has at least three reasons to support it: (1) the cogency of the prevailing guidance for clinicians in terms of the facts of this case; (2) less infringement on and violation of important ethical principles than option 1; (3) the harmful consequences of overriding JP's wishes.

Although the case is difficult for several reasons, it can be shown that the prevailing ethical guidance for clinicians in such cases is sound--that is, that capable patients have a right to refuse any treatment when the elements of informed consent have been met. The case is difficult because of (1) the dramatic and devastating injury; (2) the emotional complications of JP's father's intervention; (3) the power differential between a resident, nurses, and an attending surgeon; and (4) the existence of a court order.

However, the first and second reasons are not ethical in nature and do not count against the guidelines that healthcare professionals use in just such cases.[20] The third reason, the power differential; is ethically relevant (as Howard Brody would note) because it could have been used to force action or to close off debate and discussion. The fourth reason, the court order, is ethically significant due to a general moral duty to obey the law and to encourage respect for the court system. The court order permitted but did not order blood transfusions. It left the option to transfuse open and made further dialogue necessary between the parties. The clinicians could have used the court order as a refuge to treat JP, but they did not. It is possible that the judge, in this case, made a legal mistake. Current law would demand a hearing with representation and a certification that the patient was incapable of forming an informed consent.[21] The law at the time of the *J.P.* case also included those requirements. Clinicians must be willing to confront such mistakes on ethical grounds. They ought not abandon their patients or passively acquiesce while others (even relatives) infringe upon their patients' rights.

A strong ethical reason to support option 1 is that JP gave an informed refusal of treatment; he was capable to choose, he was fully informed of the consequences, and he chose voluntarily to risk death.

A second evaluative question is to ask which option will least violate ethical principles or considerations. Either option infringes on one or more principles. Option 1 respects the patient's autonomy and religious liberty; but from the surgeon's perspective, it infringes on the principle of beneficence, which requires that doctors actively try to help patients. In this view, option 1 would also potentially (not actually) infringe on the principle of nonmaleficence, since there was a risk of JP's death.

In option 2, from the patient's perspective, coercion would violate JP's autonomy and continued life. JP would also see imposition of treatment as harm and a violation of the principle of nonmaleficence and not as a benefit in any sense. Beauchamp and Childress caution that in situations where a principle must be overridden, it "does not simply disappear or evaporate. It leaves what Robert Nozick calls 'moral traces.' "[22]

Beauchamp and Childress outline a process for justifying infringements of an ethical principle or moral rule.[23] An examination by this process will show that option 1 involves less infringement on ethical principles than does option 2.

1. The moral objective justifying the infringement must have a realistic prospect of achievement. (The objectives of options 1 and 2 do have a realistic chance of achievement.)
2. Infringement of a principle must be necessary in the circumstances. (Either option necessitates violating one or more principles.)
3. The form of infringement selected must constitute the least infringement possible, commensu-

rate with achieving the primary goal of the action. (On this point, assuming that option 1 is selected, it will infringe on the principle of beneficence as understood by the surgeon; however, the infringement does not have to cancel out beneficence totally. Withholding blood transfusions is the least infringement possible in this case. Clinicians can give other medical care fully, and if the patient begins to die, they can give comfort care.)
4. The agent must seek to minimize the effects of the infringement. (As mentioned above, optimal treatment with other measures can minimize the harms of withholding blood transfusions. It is difficult to minimize coercion, and if one is willing to generalize from one's actions in one case to similar cases, as the ethical perspective of principlism encourages us to do, then one ought to be willing to coerce others in similar situations.)

A third strong reason for option 1 is that to coerce JP and violate his religious principles would severely harm him and his most significant relationships in the Jehovah's Witness community. To respect JP's wishes is to care for him as a person and for the relationships with his congregation and the object of his loyalty that he esteems more than any others. The psychological effect on him, in his current condition, could be disastrous, possibly provoking a crisis in which his condition would worsen. In his theological view, around which his life centers, he would have suffered a grievous violation. If he were coerced and lived, his congregation would not punish or shun him. However, they would be unable to forget the violation that occurred. The continuing memory of the event would place a strain on relationships, whereas were he to die for his principles, only positive feelings and respect for him would endure. The consequences, in terms of violating the rights of individuals and breaching strong traditions of respect for religious liberty of adults, are too harmful to make an exception to the prevailing guidance.

In summary, respect for JP's wishes is the ethically preferable option, although a court order gave approval to option 2. What can be legally acceptable is at times not morally preferable.

d. Endeavor to Resolve Conflicts
Once a decision has been made about the ethically preferable option, clinicians need to discuss how

the resolution is to be effected and who will be involved in attempting it. They should discuss what dialogue and meetings between themselves, patient, and surrogates (family or others) are needed to resolve the ethical and/or legal problems and to implement a satisfactory plan of care for the patient.

In the JP case, the two options were being pursued by separate groups. The SICU staff clearly felt that option 1 was preferable, and the surgeon and JP's father felt that option 2 was preferable. They did not meet to discuss the options prior to the surgeon's seeking the court order at the father's request.

Readers should note that the involved clinicians, working with patients or surrogate decision makers, can accomplish all the steps of moral problem solving. Clinical ethics is part of clinical practice. At times, however, the level of conflict about ethical problems may require ethics case consultation and/or judicial review. If there is persistent conflict regarding how to resolve the ethical problems posed in the case, the responsible clinicians should ask whether ethics consultation would be helpful. The HCO (see Chapter 14) should have the resources available to help with such problems. In addition to the question of appropriate ethics consultation, the case may pose questions that require judicial review, which should be sought by the legal officers of the institution, rather than by the clinicians themselves.

e. Assess Whether Ethics Consultation Is Necessary or Desirable

If consultation is sought from a hospital ethics committee or its consultants, their work can build upon the earlier efforts of clinicians to analyze and resolve the ethical problems in the case. If clinicians have thoroughly covered the first three parts of the four-step method, the consultants can build upon their work. The role of the consultant is to facilitate meetings, to ensure (if needed) participation of all parties with vital interests in the outcome and moral standing in the case, and to encourage dialogue open to different ethical views. The goal of consultation is to continue to educate the key decision makers in the case, and to assist their process in resolving ethical and legal problems. It is not to impose a decision on them.

Ethics consultation in the JP case was requested and proceeded as follows:

The chief resident in medicine called the consultant (C) at 3:00 a.m. and introduced the SICU resident (R), who described the problem and defined the situation as an emergency. The surgeon was on his way to give blood to the patient, and a judge had issued a court order to permit transfusion.

After listening, C asked R if the patient was capable of making decisions and understanding the consequences. R answered positively. C recalled several Jehovah's Witness cases to orient R to the ethical problem. C said that if the facts were as R said, the judge's action could be challenged from an ethical point of view. C asked R how he understood his duty to the patient. R answered, "To respect his wishes, even though he might die. He is awake. He has made his choice." C explored options (and consequences) with R, ranking them as: (1) to respect the patient's wishes and risk his death; or (2) to acquiesce to JP's father's wishes, save the patient's life, and risk adverse legal action brought by JP and the Jehovah's Witnesses for violating the patient's constitutional rights. There were no other options for the patient. R's preference was for a plan of care for the patient that included keeping him in intensive care, medicating for pain, keeping him fully hydrated and fed, but not providing blood transfusions under any circumstances. R's personal options included attempting to prevent coercion of the patient and, if this was impossible, withdrawing from the case in protest.

C readied R for a discussion and possible confrontation with the surgeon. C proposed that, if the surgeon was resolute in his intent, R should place his body between JP and the surgeon. C instructed R that he should tell the surgeon that if the surgeon touched R, it would be a case of assault and battery. Further, if the surgeon touched the patient against his will, it would be a more serious case of assault and battery, even with the court order. C predicted that if the surgeon proceeded to give a transfusion, another court order would void the present court order because the judge did not come to the hospital to see the patient firsthand.

C urged R to have the surgeon telephone C as soon as possible. C also suggested that if an agreement were reached, both physicians should cosign a note in the chart with instructions. Shortly, the surgeon called C and a three-way discussion began.

It was clear that the surgeon had already begun to reframe the issues. The surgeon said that he appreciated having a chance to rethink a position he had taken earlier under considerable emotional stress. He said, "I may have gone too far, but I do not know if I can live with myself if the patient dies and I could have prevented it." He also noted the strong influence that JP's grieving father had in the case.

In this discussion, the surgeon reluctantly reversed his position, seeing that the patient's wishes were clear and his right to refuse was protected by society. Both physicians signed a chart note to the effect that transfusions would not be given, out of respect for JP's informed refusal of blood transfusions, based on religious principles. C asked if he could accompany the surgeon the next morning on his rounds at the bedside. C stated, "We can try to make sure that JP understands the complete situation." The surgeon and R agreed.

The next morning, C attended work rounds with the SICU staff in order to evaluate the intervention of the previous evening. The patient was awake but too weak to speak. By the bedside, assured by JP that he could hear but not speak, C reviewed the case step by step with the SICU team, asking the patient at each point if he understood. At each point the patient nodded. C asked the patient, "Do you agree with what has happened?" He nodded with even more vigor.

C wrote a chart note describing the case as one involving the right to refuse treatment by a capable patient, widely supported in the ethics of clinicians. He noted the disagreement and its resolution, along with JP's continued informed refusal.

Although the ethical imperative to respect JP's wishes was clear, the strong feelings of JP's father still needed to be heard and addressed. C called JP's father to discuss the rationale for the decision. His father expressed the view that he may have gone too far in his desire to save his son's life and asked the consultant for understanding. It was also evident that JP's father had been informed of all of the previous night's events.

JP survived his ordeal, largely due to his good state of health prior to the accident, and he continues to live in Blacksburg. He is very active in his congregation. He has learned to drive an automobile, and he regularly returns to UVa with an elder in the congregation to discuss the case with students and others in a course on clinical ethics.

f. Assess Whether Judicial Review Is Necessary or Desirable

Clearly, judicial review is necessary in cases involving incapacitated patients who have no surrogate decision makers, when the welfare of children and their parents' interests conflict, or when there are novel legal questions posed by the case. Courts should also be consulted if the disputes are serious and cannot be resolved by ethics consultation or other good-faith efforts.

In retrospect, it was not necessary or desirable, from JP's point of view, to seek judicial review or a court order. True judicial review did not occur.

4. Evaluation

Evaluation, the fourth part of the case method, is most directly linked to the plan-of-care approach. Evaluation in such cases begins from two different points in time: (1) evaluation of the plan for intervention in the ethical and/or legal problems(s) that arise within the plan of care, and (2) retrospective evaluation of opportunities that were missed early in the case or in the institution itself to prevent such problems.

a. Current Evaluation

When evaluating the current plan of action to resolve the ethical and/or legal problems, these questions need should be asked: Is the plan working? If not, why not? Do the observed results indicate a need to modify the plan? Have conditions changed in a way that suggests a need to rethink the plan? Are interactions between clinicians and the patient meeting the needs of the patient, respecting the patient as a person, and serving the therapeutic goals of the plan of care?

When the ethics consultant (C) attended rounds on the morning following the joint discussion with the surgeon and resident, he evaluated the decision made to respect the patient's wishes with JP and the clinicians present. All agreed that it was the best course of action under the circumstances. Nothing had changed in the situation to create a need to rethink the plan to withhold blood transfusion. JP was pleased with the outcome. The consultant also called JP's father to be sure that he was aware of the decision. The discussion between them gave his father an opportunity to be heard and to be informed about the plan of action.

b. Retrospective Evaluation

In this evaluative step, decision makers should look back to the origins of the case and to the setting of the institution and its policies. The following questions then can be asked: What opportunities were missed? How did the care received by the patient match up to standards of good practice? What factors contributed to a less than optimal resolution of the case? What might have been done to improve the care of the patient? Are there desirable changes in institutional policy, feasible changes in the clinical environment, or educational interventions that might help to prevent or better resolve the ethical problems posed by similar cases?

In retrospect, the major problem in the resolution stage of the case was with the domineering, paternalistic posture of the ethics consultant. Admittedly, ethics consultation was at an early stage of development in 1987. However, several weaknesses are apparent. First, the consultant readily fell into the framing of the consultation as an "emergency" that had to be dealt with on the telephone. It would have been possible and in keeping with the principles of ethics consultation to have asked R to tell the surgeon that he had requested a meeting with C and that C was "on the way himself" to meet with them before they made a decision. It would also have been possible, under the circumstances, to have involved JP in the meeting. His condition the next morning was similar to his condition during the night.

Education about the options should have taken place. C's influence on the outcome of the case was strong. The surgeon clearly withdrew from his position because of opposition from R, backed by C. C clearly did more to advocate option 1 than to explain and treat option 2 with fairness. Chapter 14 explains the principles and practice of ethics consultation in more detail, but the most important principle is that the consultant's role is confined to educator and mediator.

Shortly after JP was discharged for rehabilitation, the case was the subject of a grand rounds in anesthesiology, led by C. This conference revealed a pressing need to educate clinicians on the Jehovah's Witness position and on the differences between cases of single adults, adults with dependent children, and children. There was little that could have been done to prevent the ethical problem that arose in this case, given the circumstances and personalities in the case. It is possible that, if JP's father had been brought to his bedside with the surgeon to discuss the option of blood transfusion, they would have been persuaded earlier to respect JP's wishes. (His father suffered from emphysema and it was difficult for him to move about.) JP's availability for education twice a year has played a significant role in keeping the issue before clinicians and students. The UVa Hospital still has no specific policy or protocol regarding patient's refusal of treatment, although it is routine practice to document such refusals in the patient's chart.

[Source: Ethics Consultation Service, University of Virginia.]

Notes

1. T.L. Beauchamp and J.F. Childress, *Principles of Biomedical Ethics*, 4th ed, (New York: Oxford University Press, 1994).

2. J.J. Fins and M.D. Bacchetta, "Framing the Physician-Assisted Suicide and Voluntary Active Euthanasia Debate: The Role of Deontology, Consequentialism, and Clinical Pragmatism," *Journal of the American Geriatrics Society* 43 (1995): 563-68. Some of the material for this chapter was drawn from J.J. Fins, M.D. Bacchetta, and F.G. Miller, "Clinical Pragmatism: A Method of Moral Problem Solving," *Kennedy Institute of Ethics Journal* 7 (1997): 129-45.

3. Dewey's moral philosophy and its relevance for clinical ethics is discussed in F.G. Miller, J.J. Fins, and M.D. Bacchetta, "Clinical Pragmatism: John Dewey and Clinical Ethics," *Journal of Contemporary Health Law and Policy*, 3 (1996): 27-51; and J.J. Fins, "From Indifference to Goodness," *Religion and Health* 35 (1996): 245-54.

4. President's Commission for the Study of Ethical Problems in Medicine and Biomedical and Behavioral Research, *Making Health Care Decisions*, vol. 1 (Washington, D.C.: U.S. Government Printing Office, 1982).

5. J. Dewey, *How We Think* (Buffalo, N.Y.: Prometheus Books, 1991).

6. T.L. Beauchamp and J.F. Childress, *Principles*

of Biomedical Ethics, 3rd ed. (New York: Oxford University Press, 1989), 51.

7. For discussions of particular faith traditions and health issues, see entries in W.T. Reich, ed., *Encyclopedia of Bioethics* (New York: Free Press, 1978); also see M.E. Marty and K.L. Vaux, ed., *Health, Medicine, and the Faith Traditions* (Philadelphia: Fortress Press, 1982). A series on 10 faith traditions and healthcare ethics has been published as a project of the Park Ridge Center (676 St. Clair, Suite 450, Chicago, Ill. 60611), by Crossroads, New York. The Park Ridge Center publishes *Second Opinion*, a journal on religion, bioethics, and health care.

8. The Angela Carder case (used as a discussion case at the end of Chapter 7) stands out as an example of the unfortunate consequences of misidentifying ethical problems. In this case, legal and ethical problems were confused as well. For more discussion of this case, see M.L. White, "Reflections on The Case of Angela Carder: A Tragedy of Decision Making," *BioLaw* 2 (1990): S433-42; G.J. Annas, "She's Going to Die: The Case of Angela C," *Hastings Center Report* 18 (February-March 1988): 23-25; G.J. Annas, "Foreclosing the Use of Force: A.C. Reversed," *Hastings Center Report* 20 (July-August 1990): 27-29. An article by D.B. Mishkin and G.J. Povar, "Decision Making with Pregnant Patients," *The Joint Commission Journal on Quality Improvement* 19 (1993): 291-302, comprehensively describes how the ethics committee at George Washington University Hospital responded to the Carder case by developing a policy regarding decision making with pregnant patients. This article is a model for good policy studies by an ethics committee. The Linares case, discussed in Chapter 9, is also widely regarded as a disaster for the institution in which it occurred. For several articles about this case, see "Family Privacy and Persistent Vegetative State: A Symposium on the Linares Case," *Law, Medicine, & Health Care* 17 (1989): 295-346.

9. Many court cases reason along these lines in the United States, especially with life-threatening illnesses in children when parents refuse *proven* medical treatments. For these cases, see A. Holder, *Legal Issues in Pediatrics and Adolescent Medicine*, 2nd ed. (New Haven, Conn.: Yale University Press, 1985).

10. A.M. Capron, J.P. Bunker, and M.S. Yesley, "Assessing the President's Commission," *Hastings Center Report* 13 (October 1983): 7-12.

11. A good collection of cases in clinical ethics is in G.E. Pence, *Classic Cases in Medical Ethics: Accounts of the Cases That Have Shaped Medical Ethics, with Philosophical, Legal, and Historical Backgrounds* (New York: McGraw-Hill, 1990). Other case anthologies include C. Levine, *Cases in Bioethics* (New York: St. Martin's Press, 1989); R.M. Veatch and S.T. Fry, *Case Studies in Nursing Ethics* (Philadelphia: J.B. Lippincott, 1987). The following textbooks have rich case reports and analyses: B. Brody, *Life and Death Decision Making* (New York, Oxford University Press, 1989); R.M. Zaner, *Ethics and the Clinical Encounter* (Englewood Cliffs, N.J.: Prentice-Hall, 1988); R.M. Zaner, *Troubled Voices: Stories of Ethics and Illness* (Cleveland, Ohio: Pilgrim Press, 1993); C.M. Culver, *Ethics at the Bedside* (Hanover, N.H.: University Press of New England, 1991); B.J. Crigger ed., *Cases in Bioethics* 2nd ed. (New York: St. Martin's Press, 1992); J.C. Ahronheim, J. Mareno, and C. Zuckerman, *Ethics in Clinical Practice* (Boston: Little, Brown, 1994).

12. *In re Melideo* 88 Misc.2d 974, 390 N.Y.S.2d 523 (1976).

13. *In re Estate of Brooks*, 32 Ill.2d 361, 205 N.E.2d 435 (1965).

14. B. Brody, *Life and Death Decision Making* (New York: Oxford University Press, 1988), 128-32.

15. *In re President and Directors of Georgetown College, Inc.*, 331 F.2d 1000 (D.C. Cir. 1964); the cases in this section are discussed in A.J. Rosoff, *Informed Consent*, (Rockville, Md.: Aspen Publishers, 1981), 265-67.

16. *In re Osborne*, 294 A.2d 372 (D.C. Ct. App. 1972).

17. *Novak v. Cobb County*, 849 F.Supp. 1559 (N.D. Ga. 1994).

18. B. Lo, "Behind Closed Doors: Promise and Pitfalls of Ethics Committees," *New England Journal of Medicine* 317 (1987): 46-50.

19. See note 6 above at 214.

20. Also see A.M. Capron, "Right to Refuse Medical Care," in *Encyclopedia of Bioethics*, W.T. Reich, ed., (New York: Free Press, 1978), 1501.

21. *Virginia Code Annotated*, sec. 37.1-134.5 (Michie Supp. 1995).

22. R. Nozick, "Moral Complications and Moral Structures," *Natural Law Forum* 12 (1968): 1-50.

23. See note 6 above at 53, including the reference to Nozick.

SECTION II

ETHICAL OBLIGATIONS
AND PROBLEMS IN CLINICAL CARE

A. ETHICAL OBLIGATIONS IN EACH CASE

3

RESPECTING PRIVACY AND CONFIDENTIALITY

Mary Faith Marshall, Ph.D.

I. Introduction

The right to privacy is one of the most basic of human rights. At a fundamental level, privacy is integrally connected with personal integrity. Our inner worlds of thoughts and feelings, prejudices and aspirations, mental vices and virtues define us as individuals. What information we share and with whom we share it is a continually selective process that defines our relationships with others. Most, if not all of us have certain self-knowledge that remains secret. Loss of control over our private thoughts would deprive us of one of our most basic freedoms.

Privacy, as a characteristic of the human condition, involves both negative and positive rights. The negative right comprises the right to noninterference, or the right to be left alone. It is a basic prerequisite of self-determination and thus of moral agency. As a positive right, privacy involves a person's prerogative to control access to and distribution of information about himself or herself. Included in these negative and positive rights might be visual or physical access to one's person, auditory access to one's conversation, or access to written information about one.

Confidentiality is one of the mechanisms by which a person's right to privacy is recognized and honored. It reflects the premise that individuals should exercise control over certain information that pertains to them--that it is their moral property. It is a form of promise, and is based on a trusting (fiduciary) relationship. Without the presumption of confidentiality and its underlying foundation of trust, true intimacy between persons would be impossible. We could not form lasting, intimate relationships with significant others--be they friends, lovers, and family members, or professionals such as healthcare providers, clergy, or attorneys--without the expectation of confidentiality.

Recent technological developments in the areas of genetic, infectious disease, and drug screening pose new challenges to the appropriate use of information that was formerly available only in the clinical setting. Test kits for illicit substances such as cocaine or marijuana as well as for legal substances such as alcohol and tobacco are now available to the general public. Tests for infectious diseases such as the human immunodeficiency virus (HIV) can be completed at home with over-the-counter test kits. Although these new opportunities clearly enhance certain privacy protections (women can test for pregnancy at home, adults can test their HIV status in private), they may also allow for serious incursions into privacy. Even though these test kits are available on the mass market, such questions as whether parents have the right to perform drug screens on their children, or whether employers should perform tobacco screens on employees remain to be answered.

Patient confidentiality has become a serious marketing concern of healthcare institutions that compete for managed-care contracts. Many large hospitals and medical centers would like to attract their own employees (and employees' families) and the employees of regional businesses as patients. Historically, concerns about privacy have driven many employees away from receiving healthcare in their employing institutions. Unless these institutions implement explicit policies that govern the confidentiality of patient information (including security audits and meaningful sanctions for confidentiality violations), their employees will seek care elsewhere.

II. History of the Concept of Confidentiality

The clinician's duty to protect his or her patient's privacy and to honor the constraints of confidentiality can be traced back to the oath of Hippocrates. Early in the fourth century B.C., the authors of the Hippocratic corpus wrote, "And whatsoever I shall see or hear in the course of my profession, as well as outside my profession in my intercourse with men, it is be what should not be published abroad, I will never divulge, holding such things to be holy secrets."[1] The oath requires a broad spectrum of allegiance from physicians, mandating that any information regarding the patient to which the physician might be privy falls under the umbrella of protected confidence. While broad in scope, however, the oath has not historically been interpreted as absolute. The proscription against "noising things abroad" pertains only to those things "which ought not to be noised abroad," ostensibly leaving room for judgment about what constitutes a holy secret.

The Code of Medical Ethics for Physicians, written by the British physician Thomas Percival in 1803, was the first modern attempt to regulate physician's behavior. The code stated: "Patients should be interrogated concerning their complaint in a tone of voice which cannot be overheard."[2]

III. Contemporary Sources of Authority

Sources of authority binding contemporary clinicians to maintain their patients' confidentiality include the American Hospital Association's Patient's Bill of Rights, codes of ethics adopted by the various clinical disciplines, state statutes and case law, review and accreditation organizations such as the Joint Commission on Accreditation of Health Care Organizations, federal regulations, and hospital or organizational policies. Principle 4 of the American Medical Association's *Principles of Medical Ethics* states: "A physician shall respect the rights of patients, of colleagues, and of other health care professionals, and shall safeguard patient confidences within the constraints of the law."[3]

The International Council of Nurses' Code for Nurses provides that "the nurse holds in confidence personal information and uses judgement in sharing this information."[4] The Code of the American Nurses Association is more stringent, stating: "The nurse safeguards the client's right to privacy by judiciously protecting information of a confidential nature."[5] The accompanying interpretive statement dictates the following:

> When knowledge gained in confidence is relevant or essential to others involved in planning or implementing the client's care, professional judgement is used in sharing it. Only information pertinent to a client's treatment and welfare is disclosed and only to those directly concerned with the client's care . . . the nurse-client relationship is built on trust. This relationship could be destroyed and the client's welfare and reputation jeopardized by injudicious disclosure of information provided in confidence.[6]

The American Hospital Association's Patient Bill of Rights, which has been adopted or adapted by most hospitals as policy, guarantees the patient that "you have the right to have all information about your illness and care treated as confidential."[7]

Many states have enacted statutes that define the confidentiality constraints of the patient-clinician relationship. Such statutes often invoke the legal concept of "privileged communication." A privileged communication may not be disclosed by a clinician in a court proceeding without the consent of the patient who provided it. According to George Annas, "Privilege, sometimes called 'testimonial privilege,' is a legal rule of evidence, applying only in the judicial context."[8] The privilege belongs to the patient, not to the clinician. The clinician is bound to honor and exercise this privilege on behalf of the patient. (There are some legal exceptions to privilege, such as when information shared with a physician also has been disclosed publicly.)

Confidentiality of information is just as important in the area of human subjects research as it is in the therapeutic setting. Federal regulations govern the protection of privacy of human research subjects.[9] In their research proposals, investigators must discuss their methods for maintaining the privacy and confidentiality of information pertaining to their research subjects. This includes the use of institutional data bases, storage of research records, access of affiliated researchers to research records, and a statement in the informed consent document elucidating confidentiality mechanisms. Especially important are safeguards to vulnerable populations such as children, psychiatric patients, and substance abusers. How, for example, would a researcher maintain the privacy of an adolescent who is a potential research subject when exclusion criteria might include pregnancy or substance abuse, and when informed consent must be provided by the subject's parents or legal guardian?

IV. Realities within the Current Healthcare Environment

In a classic article in the *New England Journal of Medicine*, physician-ethicist Mark Siegler argued: "Medical confidentiality as it has traditionally been understood by patients and doctors no longer exists. This ancient medical principle, which has been included in every physician's oath and code of ethics since Hippocratic times, has become old, worn out, and useless; it is a decrepit concept."[10] Siegler justified his position by describing his contemporary clinical practice, which involves teams of healthcare providers caring for individual patients as well as complex systems of information sharing, including computerized data banks. The notion that information about the patient could possibly be confined to the physician-patient relationship is outdated. After one of his patients complained about a respiratory therapist reading his chart, Siegler conducted an informal survey and determined that more than 75 clinicians or hospital employees had legitimate access to his patient's medical record.

The modern medical environment easily lends itself to breaches of patient confidentiality. The more persons who have access to information, the greater the possibility that it will be shared. Effective safeguards against such breaches are possible, however. Siegler maintains that a high degree of patient privacy can be achieved in private physicians' offices if staff members adhere judiciously to their professional duty of maintaining confidentiality.

Large institutions, in which access to information about patients is exponentially greater, should institute safeguards that limit access to only the particular information that a certain category of clinician might need. For example, a clinical laboratory technician should only be able to access that portion of the patient's data base dealing specifically with the technician's type of laboratory data. The patient's record can be compartmentalized with access limita-

tions by user category. Denise Nagel, president of the National Coalition of Patient Rights, advocates strongly for such limitations. She states: "Guarantees that health information is protected are no longer a value-added option. Any company that ignores the need for medical record privacy in their health plan will be at a serious competitive disadvantage."[11] Nagel suggests that comprehensive privacy policies should do the following:

1. preserve and enhance the ability of patients to communicate in confidence with their physicians or other healthcare professionals;
2. recognize and protect the right to privacy of personally identifiable medical information;
3. provide that this right cannot be waived in the absence of meaningful consent; and
4. provide that the right of meaningful notice and consent not be eroded or eliminated in the absence of a specific waiver, except in rare instances of a countervailing public interest.[12]

Healthcare providers are responsible for implementing effective confidentiality safeguards such as those just mentioned. At a minimum, healthcare institutions and providers should have formal policies and procedures regarding:

1. release of patient information;
2. confidentiality of patient information;
3. access to computerized medical records;
4. access to institutional data bases;
5. use of access/sign-on codes to medical information systems;
6. security measures such as computer audits or information safety officers;
7. mechanisms for reporting alleged, apparent, or potential breaches of confidentiality; and
8. disciplinary measures for noncompliance with institutional confidentiality policies.

Many institutions now state that employment is conditional on compliance with confidentiality policies via their employment contracts for staff and faculty. Violations of confidentiality policies could lead to formal reprimand, loss of clinical privileges, or loss of employment given the nature of the offense. The matriculation of student clinicians should also be contingent on compliance with institutional policies on confidentiality and privacy.

Patients, who often have naive expectations regarding information management in the healthcare setting should be informed about what confidentiality means in the current healthcare environment. Although the concept of patient privacy differs not at all in spirit from its historical antecedents, the realities of modern healthcare delivery and the process of medical record keeping have changed the patient care milieu dramatically. Patients should be aware that, in certain environments and circumstances, numerous clinicians and professional personnel are involved in their care and thus have a legitimate need for certain information about them. Patients have the right to expect, however, that each of these healthcare professionals will maintain the same degree of confidentiality that inheres in the traditional clinician-patient relationship, and that affiliated institutions will do the same.

V. Indiscretions

Siegler accurately observes that the violation of privacy most feared by patients is the inadvertent or wanton indiscretion. He says:

> Somehow, privacy is violated and a sense of shame is heightened when intimate secrets are revealed to people one knows or is close to--friends, neighbors, acquaintances, or hospital roommates--rather than when they are disclosed to an anonymous bureaucrat sitting at a computer terminal in a distant city or to a health professional who is acting in an official capacity. . . . I suspect that the principles of medical confidentiality, particularly those reflected in most medical codes of ethics, were designed principally to prevent just this sort of embarrassing personal indiscretion rather than to maintain (for social, political, or economic reasons) the absolute secrecy of doctor-patient communications.[13]

Clinicians' behaviors such as conversing about patients in hospital elevators, halls, and cafeterias; entertaining friends with clinical "war stories"; or dictating case notes with portable voice recorders while traversing public corridors are all breaches of patient confidentiality and heedless indiscretions.

VI. Legitimate Breaches of Confidentiality

As stated in the discussion of the Hippocratic oath, the duty to honor patient confidentiality is not absolute. Modern professional codes of ethics recognize that such breaches may be necessary when in the public interest, or when the patient or a third party is at risk of harm. For example, public reporting statutes require clinicians to report certain information (such as vital statistics, contagious and dangerous diseases, child abuse and neglect, and criminally inflicted injuries) to public authorities. Also, when a patient makes his or her condition a pertinent issue in a lawsuit (such as in a personal injury trial) or when a patient sues a clinician, the defendant is generally allowed to testify about that patient's medical condition.

In 1974, the duty to warn third parties who are at risk of injury by the patient was established in *Tarasoff v. Regents of the University of California*.[14] This case involved a young man who, while undergoing psychotherapy, threatened to kill a former girlfriend. The therapist tried to have the patient detained in temporary psychiatric custody. His initial efforts were unsuccessful, and his medical director ordered him to drop the case. Months later, when the patient carried out his threat and killed the young woman, her family sued the therapist. The California Supreme Court, in two separate opinions, clearly established the duty to warn as a responsibility of a psychotherapist. Beauchamp and Childress summarize the details of the case as follows:

> On August 20, 1969, Prosenjit Poddar was a voluntary outpatient receiving therapy at Cowell Memorial Hospital. Poddar informed his therapist, Dr. Lawrence Moore, that he was going to kill an unnamed girl (readily identifiable as his former girlfriend, Tatiana Tarasoff) when she returned home from spending the summer in Brazil. Moore, with the concurrence of two colleagues, Dr. Gold, who had originally examined Poddar, and Dr. Yandell, assistant to the director of the department of psychiatry, decided that Poddar should be committed for observation in a psychiatric hospital. Moore called the campus police and spoke with officers Atkinson and Teel, notifying them that he was requesting commitment. Moore then sent a letter to Police Chief

William Beall requesting the assistance of the police department in securing Poddar's confinement.

Officers Atkinson, Brownrigg and Halleran took Poddar into custody, but, satisfied that Poddar was rational, released him on his promise to stay away from Tatiana. Dr. Powelson, director of the department of psychiatry at Cowell Memorial Hospital (where Poddar had seen Dr. Moore for therapy), then asked the police to return Dr. Moore's letter, directed that all copies of the letter and notes that Moore had taken as a therapist be destroyed, and ordered "no action to place Prosenjit Poddar in a 72-hour treatment evaluation facility."

Poddar subsequently befriended Tatiana Tarasoff's brother, moving in with him as his roommate. On October 27, 1969, Poddar killed Tatiana Tarasoff.[15]

Upon hearing this case in 1974, the California Supreme Court ruled: "When a doctor or psychotherapist, in the exercise of his professional skill and knowledge, determines or should determine, that a warning is essential to avert danger arising from the medical or psychological condition of his patient, he incurs a legal obligation to give that warning."[16]

The court discussed the history of medical confidentiality at length and emphasized that protecting private information was a primary duty of a mental health professional. Nevertheless, the court found that an exception to the usual rule was justified when a specifically articulated threat concerning an identifiable third party was communicated by a patient to a therapist. In that unusual instance, the court concluded: "The protective privilege ends where the public peril begins."

The California Supreme Court considered a second aspect of the case in 1976 and, in a second opinion, expanded the therapist's duty not only to warn the patient, but to exercise professional judgment regarding the necessary course of action to protect potential victims:

When a therapist determines or pursuant to the standard of this profession should determine, that his patient presents a serious danger of violence to another, he incurs an obligation to use reasonable care to protect the intended victim

against such danger. The discharge of this duty may require the therapist to take one or more of various steps depending on the nature of the case. Thus, it may call for him to warn the intended victim or others likely to apprise the intended victim of danger, to notify police, or take whatever steps are reasonably necessary under the circumstances.[17]

Since *Tarasoff*, courts in a number of other states have held that the duty of a psychotherapist to protect people who are not patients applies under two primary conditions: (1) when the violence is foreseeable; and (2) when the therapist has enough control over the patient to prevent the violence (that is, the patient is in an institutional setting).

Foreseeability is determined by three factors:

1. a history of violence;
2. a threat to a named or clearly identifiable victim; and
3. a plausible motive.

If at least two of these factors are present, courts have generally found a duty to warn. If only one is present, courts have gone either way. If none of these factors is present, the courts have rarely held that violence was foreseeable.[18]

Although the duty to warn is generally acknowledged within the medical bioethics communities,[19] some psychotherapists disagree with the finding in the *Tarasoff* case. They argue that civil commitment of a potentially violent patient is preferable to warning an identifiable victim, because commitment maintains confidentiality while simultaneously preventing harm. With only a warning, the onus is on the potential victim to protect himself or herself. In *Ethics and Psychiatry: Toward Professional Definition*, psychiatrist Allen Dyer argues against the *Tarasoff* finding:

The Tarasoff decision is widely discussed as a threat to confidentiality. An alarming decision by the California Supreme Court, Tarasoff involves the state's willingness to use the therapist as its own agent when the patient/client appears likely to harm an identifiable third party. It is argued that protecting public safety is the rationale for overriding confidentiality . . . . The Tarasoff decision is particularly bad because it weakens the legal protection of confidentiality for reasons that will probably accomplish very little. The real issue in the Tarasoff case is not confidentiality or even the prediction of violence, but the extreme emphasis on individual liberties and the difficulty in utilizing civil commitment procedures. Although most therapists would probably compromise confidentiality in the likely event of imminent physical danger--as did Poddar's therapist--the disclosure of the threat in itself does little to protect the would-be victim. The real issue is the taking away of one person's civil liberties through involuntary hospitalization when those liberties threaten the existence of something else. The Tarasoff decision does not address these crucial issues. Warning potential victims then gives them the responsibility of protecting themselves, a responsibility that the state has abdicated. Indeed, the Tarasoff decision is really a testimony to social indifference and anonymity in an urban community. Tatiana Tarasoff's murder was tragic; the Tarasoff decision reduces the situation to melodrama.[20]

VII. HIV-Positive Patients

There is something which does not displease us in the misfortunes of a good friend . . .
                                   La Rochefoucauld

Nonconsensual disclosures of the diagnoses of HIV-positive patients or patients with acquired immunodeficiency syndrome (AIDS) are especially troublesome given the personal, social, and professional sequelae that may follow such indiscretions. The judge's decision in *Doe v. Barrington*, a New Jersey breach-of-confidentiality case involving a patient with AIDS, acknowledges these dangers:

The sensitive nature of medical information about AIDS makes a compelling argument for keeping this information confidential. Society's moral judgements about the high-risk activities associated with the disease, including sexual relations and drug use, make the information of the most personal kind. Also, the privacy interest in one's exposure to the AIDS virus is even greater than one's privacy interest in ordinary medical records because of the stigma that attaches with the disease. The potential for harm in the event of a nonconsensual disclosure is substantial.[21]

In his decision, Judge Brotman cited several unfortunate examples of public persecution of persons with AIDS based on fear and ignorance. These included removing a teacher with AIDS from teaching duties; refusing to rent an apartment to male homosexuals for fear of AIDS; firebombing the home of hemophiliac children who tested positive for AIDS; healthcare workers' refusing to treat people with or suspected of having AIDS; co-workers' refusing to use a truck used by a person with AIDS; filing a charge of attempted murder against a person with AIDS who spat at police; requiring a person with AIDS to wear a mask in a courtroom; denying access to schools for children with AIDS; threatening to evict a physician who treated homosexuals; firing homosexuals who displayed cold symptoms or rashes; paramedics' refusing to treat a heart attack patient for fear that he had AIDS; police officers' refusing to drive a patient with AIDS to the hospital; police officers' demanding rubber masks and gloves when dealing with homosexuals; refusing to hire Haitians; and funeral directors' refusing to embalm the bodies of persons with AIDS.[22]

Although many of these events reflect early, hysterical reactions to AIDS based on unfounded fears, tragic sequelae of nonconsensual disclosures continue to occur. These actions often come at a time of crisis for a newly diagnosed patient, and they undermine the medical plan of care as well as the patient's ability to cope with the disease.

A case in point is that of otolaryngologist and plastic surgeon William Behringer (*Estate of Behringer v. The Medical Center at Princeton*).[23] In June 1987, Behringer was admitted as a patient to the Medical Center at Princeton, where he was employed as a surgeon. He had an acute pulmonary illness, which was subsequently diagnosed as *Pneumocystis carinii* pneumonia (PCP). Because this type of pneumonia is frequently a complication of HIV infection virus or of AIDS, Behringer's physicians tested him for the virus. Prior to the test, Behringer had signed a general consent form for HIV testing that stated: "I, William Behringer, hereby give my consent to the Medical Center at Princeton to have my blood tested for antibodies to HTLV III Virus as ordered by my physician. The results of the test will be reported only to the ordering physician."[24]

No pretest counseling occurred, and the test results ultimately made their way into Behringer's medical record, where they were readily available to anyone reading the chart. The test result was positive. When informed of his diagnosis, Behringer was shocked. His companion, who had accompanied him to the hospital, asked the treating physician who else knew about the diagnosis. The physician replied that he had told his wife, as the couple were close friends of Behringer and his companion.

Recognizing the imminent possibility of a breach of confidentiality within the medical center, Behringer's treating physician suggested that Behringer be transferred to another hospital where he was not well known. Unfortunately, no beds were available in other regional hospitals. Driven by a concern for maintaining his privacy, Behringer and his treating physician opted for immediate discharge from the hospital. Behringer would be treated at home, where his companion would care for him. Upon discharge, Behringer opted to forgo traditional wheelchair transportation and walk out of the hospital unassisted, in order to downplay the appearance of a serious medical condition. Deviating from protocol, Behringer's treating physician directed that his laboratory results not be placed in his medical record until immediately before his discharge.

Unfortunately, these privacy safeguards were ineffective. Shortly after he got home, Behringer began receiving sympathy calls from physicians who practiced with him at the medical center and who obviously knew his diagnosis. Although these physicians were professional colleagues as well as social friends, none of them was directly involved in Behringer's care. Some of the callers queried Behringer's companion as to whether she had been "tested." Later that evening, Behringer received sympathy calls from nonmedical social friends.

Soon, Behringer's office staff began receiving calls from patients and referring physicians asking about Behringer's diagnosis. Appointments were canceled, the number of referrals diminished, and patients had their records transferred to other physicians. Three of Behringer's office employees resigned. One temporary employee resigned the day after being hired, having learned of Behringer's diagnosis. Within weeks, Behringer's surgical privileges at the medical center were suspended. Although he maintained an office practice until his death in July 1989, Behringer never performed surgery again. During the two years following his diagnosis, Behringer developed an ulcer, was hospitalized for one week with a virus, and lost his sight in one eye.

As a result of his loss of surgical privileges, Behringer sued the Medical Center at Princeton for a breach of the medical center's and certain individual employees' "duty to maintain the confidentiality of his diagnosis and test results" (included was Dr. Leung Lee, director of the medical center laboratories) and for a violation of the New Jersey Law Against Discrimination. On 25 April 1991, Judge Carchman found in Behringer's favor. He eloquently stated:

> The confidentiality breached in the present case is simply grist for a gossip mill with little concern for the impact of disclosure on the patient. While one can legitimately question the good judgement of a practicing physician choosing to undergo HIV testing or a bronchoscopy procedure at the same hospital where he practices, this apparent error in judgement does not relieve the medical center of its underlying obligation to protect its patients against the dissemination of confidential information. It makes little difference to identify those who "spread the news." The information was too easily available, too titillating to disregard. All that was required was a glance at the chart, and the written words became whispers, and the whispers became roars. And common sense told all that this would happen.
>
> This court holds that the failure of the medical center and Lee as director of the department of laboratories, who were together responsible for developing the misstated informed consent form, the counseling procedure and implementation of the charting protocol, to take reasonable steps to maintain the confidentiality of plaintiff's medical records, while plaintiff was a patient, was a breach of the medical center's duty and obliga-

tion to keep such records confidential. The medical center is liable for damages caused by this breach.[25]

Judge Carchman admonished the medical center for failing to enact a policy on privacy and confidentiality that would have limited access to Behringer's medical record and would have made sensitive patient information available on a "need-to-know" basis only:

> The medical center's disregard for the importance of preserving the confidentiality of plaintiff's patient medical records was evident even before the charting of the HIV test results. A review of plaintiff's hospital chart reveals not only the HIV test results, but the results of the bronchoscopy--PCP--which all concede was a definitive diagnosis of AIDS. While the medical center argues that the decision regarding charting is one for the physicians to make, the medical center cannot avoid liability on that basis. It is not the charting per se that generates the issue; it is the easy accessibility to the charts and the lack of any meaningful medical center policy or procedure to limit access that causes the breach to occur. Where the impact of such accessibility is so clearly foreseeable, it is incumbent on the medical center, as the custodian of the charts, to take such reasonable measures as are necessary to insure that confidentiality. Failure to take such steps is negligence.[26]

In addition to raising the issues of a patient's privacy and confidentiality and the hospital's obligation to protect the confidentiality of a clinician's AIDS diagnosis, the *Behringer* case raises the issue of the hospital's right to restrict the surgical or other invasive activities of an HIV-positive clinician. This aspect of the case pits the competing privacy interests of the infected clinician against the patient's right to adequate disclosure as a prerequisite for informed consent. This same sort of tension exists when clinicians are aware that their HIV-positive patient is placing friends, family members, or others at risk because of nondisclosure and high-risk behavior. To explore adequately the competing interests in these sorts of cases, we must return to the *Tarasoff* case.

Although the *Tarasoff* case arose in the mental health context, the principle it yielded is often seen as pertinent to the general medical setting as well. Most recently, commentators have debated application of the duty to warn to the situation that clinicians may face with HIV-positive patients who persist in risky behavior.

Because of the serious nature of the risks involved in both disclosing and not disclosing the status of an HIV-positive patient, the guidance from professional associations regarding this issue is controverted, and is often in clear conflict with statutes and case law. The "Policy Statement on Confidentiality, Disclosure, and Protection of Others" of the American Psychiatric Association directs that if "a psychiatrist has received convincing clinical information that the patient is infected with HIV and is engaging in behavior that places others at risk of infection, the psychiatrist should seek the patient's agreement either to cease that behavior or to inform the individual(s). In some circumstances, the psychiatrist may be able to help a reluctant patient make such a notification. Alternatively, patients may prefer that the psychiatrist, another clinician, or public health authorities make such notification,"[27] However, "any breach of confidentiality should be undertaken only after all other efforts to work with the patient have failed. Before deciding to inform third parties, the psychiatrist should consider the potential profound impact of such notification and the problems it may generate."[28]

The Council on Ethical and Judicial Affairs of the American Medical Association has taken a much stronger position establishing a duty to warn. It states:

> Where there is not a statute that mandates or prohibits the reporting of seropositive individuals to public health authorities and a physician knows that a seropositive individual is endangering a third party, the physician should:
>
> 1. attempt to persuade the infected patient to cease endangering the third party;
> 2. if persuasion fails, notify authorities; and
> 3. if the authorities take no action, notify the endangered third party.[29]

The position taken in a joint position paper of the American College of Physicians and the Infectious Diseases Society of America is not as direct: "The confidentiality of patients infected with HIV should be protected to the greatest extent possible, consistent with the duty to protect others and to protect the public health."[30]

Statutory guidance regarding reporting of HIV status is developing quickly in many states. However, state statutes and case law conflict in this area. Some statutes impose only broad limits on confidentiality while others impose narrow, strict limits. In some states, unauthorized disclosure of HIV status constitutes a civil penalty; in others it constitutes grounds for a misdemeanor. One state allows disclosure to applicants for marriage licenses after mandatory testing (Illinois).

Case law has tended to follow the *Tarasoff* precedent, which limits the duty to warn to cases with identifiable third parties. Included in this category have been the patient's spouse, fiancee, and healthcare workers whose duties place them at risk.

The duty to maintain patients' confidentiality, standing alongside the perceived ethical obligation to warn those at risk and the lack of a clear legal duty to do so, can create a difficult dilemma for clinicians. The ethical impetus toward a duty to warn often seems a more compelling directive than the norm of confidentiality. Clinicians should not lose sight, however, of the primary ethical and legal obligation of maintaining patient confidentiality. Breaches of that obligation should not be undertaken lightly.

VII. Confidentiality and Psychotherapists

A recent U.S. Supreme Court ruling (*Jaffee v. Redmond*) held that relations between a patient and his or her psychotherapist are confidential and thus protected from disclosure in federal trials.[31] Prior to this ruling, only communications between spouses or between attorneys and their clients were privileged in federal courts. In the case of *Jaffee v. Redmond*, a police officer was sued by the family of a suspect whom the officer had shot and killed. The family attempted to gain legal access to the records of the psychotherapist who treated the police officer after the shooting occurred. In writing for the majority, Justice Stevens stated: "The psychotherapist-patient privilege is rooted in the imperative need for confidence and trust. . . . [A patient] must be willing to

make a frank and complete disclosure of facts, emotions, memories, and fears. . . . The mere possibility of disclosure of confidential communications may impede development of the relationship necessary for successful treatment.[32] This ruling applies only to communications between patients and mental health professionals, and does not speak to the nature of other clinician-patient communications.

IX. Guidance

A. Incorporating privacy and confidentiality concerns into the plan of care is an integral component of healthcare delivery. Ensuring that patients are aware of their rights to privacy should be a component of the admissions process. Ascertaining whether patients understand the realities of the clinical environment or hold false expectations in terms of the number and types of clinicians with access to information about them is the responsibility of the primary clinicians caring for the patient.

B. In the patient-clinician relationship, the patient has the right to expect, either by implied or express agreement, that the clinician will not disclose information regarding the patient to anyone not directly involved in the patient's care and treatment. Patients should be informed in advance of any limits placed on confidentiality by the clinician.

C. In addition, according to George Annas, the following rights are encompassed by the patient's right to privacy:

1. To refuse to see any or all visitors.
2. To refuse to see anyone not officially connected with the hospital.
3. To refuse to see persons officially connected with the hospital who are not directly involved in the patient's care and treatment.
4. To refuse to see social workers, chaplains, and others not directly involved in the patient's care and to forbid them to view the patient's records.
5. To wear his or her own bedclothes, so long as they do not interfere with the patient's treatment.

6. To wear religious medals.
7. To have a person of the patient's own sex present during a physical examination by a medical professional.
8. Not to remain disrobed any longer than is necessary for accomplishing the medical purpose for which the patient is asked to disrobe.
9. Not to have the patient's case discussed openly in the hospital.
10. To have the patient's medical records read only by those directly involved in treatment or the monitoring of its quality.
11. To insist on being transferred to another room if the person sharing it with the patient will not let the patient alone or is unreasonably disturbing the patient.[33]

D. Exceptions to the clinician's duty to maintain the patient's privacy and confidentiality may include situations when the interests of the public, an identified third party, or the patient himself or herself outweigh the consequences of a breach of confidentiality. Also included are situations where the patient has made his or her medical condition pertinent to a lawsuit. These exceptions are situational and depend on the good judgment of the clinician. A foundational tenet applies in cases involving breaches of confidentiality: Any person who would breach medical confidentiality must always overcome the presumption in favor of the patient's expectation; the onus is on the clinician to defend the grounds for privacy invasion or breach of confidentiality.

X. Cases for Further Study

Case 1. Cocaine Use and Patient Self-Reporting

In the 26 February 1992 issue of the *Journal of the American Medical Association*, a study entitled "High Prevalence of Recent Cocaine Use and the Unreliability of Patient Self-Report in an Inner-City Walk-In Clinic" was reported.[34] The study's objective was to determine the prevalence of recent cocaine use and the reliability of patients' self-reported cocaine use. The investigators compared individual patient self-reported cocaine use with urine screening results when the patients were unaware that their urine was being

tested for illicit drugs. The patients were asked to participate in a study about asymptomatic carriage of sexually transmitted diseases (STDs). The study population included male patients who presented to the emergency ambulatory care triage desk of Grady Memorial Hospital in Atlanta, Georgia. Inclusion criteria included an age range of 18 to 39 years, and participants must have been sexually active within the previous six months. Exclusion criteria included presenting with a urogenital complaint, history of kidney disease, any antibiotic use in the prior three weeks, or illness too severe to delay medical care. Of the 415 eligible men who participated in the study, the average age was 29.5 years; 91.6 percent of the participants were black, and 89 percent were uninsured.

Subjects who agreed to participate in the study were paid $10 for participation. Informed consent was obtained for the STD study. Both the STD study and the study that anonymously tested urine for cocaine metabolites were approved by the Emory University School of Medicine Human Investigations Committee. Patients were told that their urine would be tested for STDs. They were not told that their urine would be tested for cocaine metabolites. The investigators state in their report that the patients were never told that their urine would *not* be tested for drugs.

The consent forms were the only source linking the subjects' names with the study subjects' identity numbers. Prior to urine drug testing, the unique identity number was permanently removed from each consent form.

Consider the merits of the study from the perspective of the Human Investigations Committee. If you were a member of this committee, would you have voted to allow this study to proceed?

[Source: Adapted from S.E. McNagny and R.M. Parker, "High Prevalence of Recent Cocaine Use and the Unreliability of Patient Self-Report in an Inner-City Walk-In Clinic," in *Journal of the American Medical Association* 267, no. 8 (1992): 1106-08.]

Case 2: Dear Ann Landers

Dear Ann Landers:

I'm 18 and I have a problem that involves my doctor. He happens to be a good friend of my parents and they insist that I go to him whenever I'm sick.

The minute I get to his office, he sends me to the examining room to take off my clothes, no matter what I'm seeing him for, even if it's a sore throat.

When he comes in to see me I have to stand there with nothing on and tell him what is bothering me.

After a complete physical exam (every visit) he wants to have a conversation with me while I'm undressed. He always has a lot of questions about school and boyfriends.

Last time I asked him if it was okay for me to put my clothes back on, and he said, "No, it's healthy for a girl to be relaxed about nudity. This is good for you."

When he finally let me get dressed, he stayed in the room and watched me put everything on. I felt very self-conscious.

I told my mother that I want to go to another doctor and why. She said, "Absolutely not. Dr. X is wonderful. Get over our false modesty."

Ann, I want to be fair. He really hasn't done or said any thing that could be considered "fresh," but I still feel uncomfortable about my visits to his office. Am I being foolish? The only other doctor I ever went to was my pediatrician, I saw her until I was 16. Can you help me?

--L.W., New Britain, Conn.

How should Ann Landers respond to this request for help? Begin with, "Dear New Britain . . ."

[Source: Permisson to reprint granted by Ann Landers/Creators Syndicate.]

Case 3: *Knecht v. Vandalia Medical Center, Inc.*

Ms. X, a minor, had, for many years, been a patient at the Vandalia Medical Center where Mrs. Frances Gillespie was employed as a secretary/receptionist. In May 1980, Ms. X was treated at the outpatient clinic of the medical center for a sexually transmitted disease (venereal disease, or "VD"). Through her employment at the medical center, Mrs. Gillespie became aware of this treatment.

A short time before 9 September 1980, Mrs. Gillespie's son, John, a high school senior, had been employed by Thrifty Rent-A-Car, (along with two other young men and two young women, one of whom was Ms. X), to drive cars from Vandalia to Kansas City. These five returned in the same car, and the trip took longer than Thrifty management thought it should have taken. On 9 September 1980, when Mrs. Gillespie came home for lunch, her son told her that Thrifty said that John and his coworkers could never drive for them again because of the unwarranted length of time for car delivery. Thrifty thought that the reason for the time length was because the young men were "messing around" with the "girls." Mrs. Gillespie inquired as to who the "girls" were, and when she found out that one of them was Ms. X, she told her son, "Well, if this is true, then you'd better get yourself checked at the doctor's office," and she told him that Ms. X had been treated for VD.

Thereafter, John told Phil Sisk, one of the young men on the Kansas City trip about Ms. X's history of treatment for VD. Ms. X subsequently brought action against the medical center and Mrs. Gillespie for damages arising from the secretary's disclosure to her son that Ms. X had received medical treatment for venereal disease. [*Note*: Although Ms. X has been identified in the public domain, we have chosen not to disclose this information in respect for her right to privacy.]

What would you advise Mrs. Gillespie to do if she had called you prior to disclosing to her son?

[Source: 14 Ohio App.3d 129, 470 N.E. 2d 230 (1984)]

Case 4: Violence Begets Violence--The Case of the Abused Wife

For the past six months, a 43-year-old woman with a diagnosis of dysthymic disorder (morbid anxiety and depression accompanied by obsession) and dependent personality disorder has been seen in twice-per-week psychotherapy. The patient is a very successful accountant. No medications have been prescribed. A central theme in the treatment has been the suppression and denial of her rage. The psychiatrist has a good working relationship with the patient.

The patient has been married for six years and has a 3-year-old daughter. During the past year and a half, her alcoholic corporate executive husband has become increasingly physically abusive. On one occasion, he knocked two of his wife's teeth loose and on another struck her on the side of the head with a baseball bat, causing a laceration and a mild concussion. The patient confided this history of abuse to a number of her close friends who have been of considerable support to her. While the patient has long suffered because of marked dependency needs and a history of physical abuse as a child, she has increasingly harbored fantasies of revenge toward her husband. After the last episode of physical abuse two weeks ago, when the husband injured her shoulder by twisting her arm, she threatened to kill him. She spoke with a favorite uncle, who is a sportsman, about purchasing one of his guns. The husband refused all requests by the psychiatrist to come to an interview either individually or with his wife. When the husband inadvertently learned about his wife's request to purchase a gun, he threatened to strangle her.

The patient now fears for her own life. Though never violent in the past, she is determined to protect herself if her husband abuses her again. She has sent her daughter temporarily to stay with an aunt. The patient is increasingly beset by unbidden murderous impulses toward her husband and frightening nightmares involving his dismemberment. There is no evidence of psychosis. She reluctantly purchases a gun from her uncle.

The psychiatrist determines that the patient requires immediate psychiatric intervention; the patient refuses psychiatric hospitalization. The psychiatrist calls the ethics consultation service to discuss the issue of patient confidentiality versus the duty to protect a third party. What options should the case participants consider?

[Source: R.I. Simon, "The Duty to Protect in Private Practice," *Confidentiality versus the Duty to Protect: Foreseeable Harm in the Practice of Psychiatry,* James C. Beck, ed. (Washington, D.C.: American Psychiatric Press, 1990): 37.]

XI. Study Questions

1. What is a "privileged communication" within the healthcare context?
2. What is your opinion of Mark Siegler's argument that medical confidentiality is a "decrepit concept"?
3. In considering your future medical practice, what will your personal policy be regarding discussing cases/patients with your spouse or significant other (assuming that such a relationship exists)?
4. How comfortable would you be, from a privacy and confidentiality perspective, being a patient in the hospital where you practice as a clinician. Would you anticipate that your feelings about this would change as you progress from first-year medical student to medical resident, to attending physician (or a similar professional progression for other clinicians)? How do your feelings about this relate to Siegler's observation that the most feared privacy violation is the wanton indiscretion?
5. Do you think that Dr. Moore had a duty to warn Tatiana Tarasoff of Prosenjit Poddar's threat to kill her? Why do you think Dr. Powelson asked the campus police to return Dr. Moore's letter and subsequently ordered that all of the records that Dr. Moore had taken as a therapist be destroyed? Would you have complied with this order if you were Dr. Moore?
6. What action would you take if one of your HIV-positive patients was having unprotected sex with an unknowing third party and refused to notify him or her?
7. In Case 2, "Dear Ann Landers," what would you do if you were the young woman's former pediatrician and she came to you with her story?

8. Consider Case 3, *Knecht v. Vandalia Medical Center, Inc.* What if this scenario were to happen to you in your role as a clinician (that is, you learn that your son or daughter has had sex with a partner/patient who is infected with a sexually transmitted disease)?

Notes

1. S.J. Reiser, "Selections from the Hippocratic Corpus: 'Oath,' 'Precepts,' 'The Art,' 'Epidemics I,' 'The Physician,' 'Decorum,' and 'Law',' in *Ethics in Medicine: Historical Perspectives and Contemporary Concerns,* S.J. Reiser, A.J. Dyck, W.J. Curran, ed. (Cambridge, Mass.: Massachusetts Institute of Technology Press, 1977): 5-9.
2. See note 1 above, pp. 18-25.
3. American Medical Association, "Principles of Medical Ethics," *Code of Medical Ethics: Current Opinions with Annotations* (Chicago: AMA, 1997), p. *xiv.*
4. W.T. Reich, "Code for Nurses," in *Encyclopedia of Bioethics,* 2nd Edition, ed. W.T. Reich, ed. (Washington, D.C.: Georgetown University Press, 1995), 2710.
5. American Nurses Association, "Code for Nurses," *Code for Nurses with Interpretive Statements* (Washington, D.C.: American Nurses Publishing, 1985), 1.
6. Ibid., pp. 4-5.
7. See note 1 above, pp. 148-49.
8. G. Annas, *The Rights of Patients,* 2nd ed. (Carbondale and Edwardsville, Ill.: Southern Illinois University Press, 1989), 176.
9. 45 *Code of Federal Regulations* Part 46.
10. M. Siegler, "Confidentiality in Medicine: A Decrepit Concept," *New England Journal of Medicine* 307, no. 24 (1982): 1518-21.
11. C. Marwick quotes Denise Nagel on this point: C. Marwick, "Medical Records Privacy a Patient Rights Issue," *Journal of the American Medical Association* 276, no. 23 (1996): 1861-62.
12. Ibid.
13. See note 10 above, p. 1520.
14. *Tarasoff v. Regents of the University of California,* 118 Cal.Rptr. 129, 529 P.2d 553 (Cal. 1974).
15. T.L. Beauchamp and J.F. Childress, *Principles of Biomedical Ethics,* 4th ed. (New York: Oxford University Press, 1994), 509-12.
16. See note 14 above.
17. *Tarasoff v. Regents of the University of California,* 131 Cal.Rptr. 14, 551 P.2d 334 (Cal. 1976) (*en*

banc).

18. J.C. Beck, "Current Status of the Duty to Protect," in *Confidentiality versus the Duty to Protect: Foreseeable Harm in the Practice of Psychiatry*, J.C. Beck, ed., (Washington, D.C.: American Psychiatric Press, 1990): 10.

19. For example, Beauchamp and Childress assert: "The court correctly held in *Tarasoff* that therapists have a duty, not an option, to warn third parties of their patient's serious intention to kill or harm them" (see note 15 above, p. 424). Annas concurs: "The broader we as a society make the health care professional's mandate to report the patient's condition to others, the more like a policeman the professional becomes. Nevertheless, the California Supreme Court's decision that health care providers have an obligation to society as well as to their patients is correct in life-and-death situations and has been followed by other courts" (see note 8 above, p. 184).

20. A.R. Dyer, *Ethics and Psychiatry: Toward Professional Definition* (Washington, D.C.: American Psychiatric Press, 1988), 61-62.

21. *Doe v. Barrington*, 729 F.Supp. 376, at 384 (D. N.J. 1990).

22. Ibid, n8.

23. *Estate of Behringer v. The Medical Center at Princeton*, 249 N.J. Super. 597, 592 A.2d. 1251 (1991).

24. *Estate of Behringer v. The Medical Center at Princeton*, 592 A.2d 1251 at 1261.

25. *Estate of Behringer v. The Medical Center at Princeton*, 592 A.2d 1251 at 1273.

26. *Estate of Behringer v. The Medical Center at Princeton*, 592 A.2d 1251 at 1272.

27. American Psychiatric Association, "Policy Statement on Confidentiality, Disclosure, and Protection of Others," *Policy Statements and Guidelines on AIDS and HIV Disease* (Washington, D.C.: APA, 1997), 1-2.

28. Ibid.

29. See note 3 above, pp. 61-62.

30. Health and Public Policy Committee, American College of Physicians and the Infectious Diseases Society of America, "The Acquired Immunodeficiency Syndrome (AIDS) and Infection with the Human Immunodeficiency Virus (HIV)," *Annals of Internal Medicine* 108, no. 3 (1988): 466.

31. J. Roberts, "U.S. Court Rules on Confidentiality," *British Medical Journal* 312, no. 7047 (1996): 1629-30.

32. *Jaffee v. Redmond*, 116 S.Ct. 1923, at 1928 (1996).

33. The list in item C is from Annas, *The Rights of Patients*, see note 8 above, pp. 190-91.

34. S.E. McNagny and R.M. Parker, "High Prevalence of Recent Cocaine Use and the Unreliability of Patient Self-Report in an Inner-City Walk-In Clinic," *Journal of the American Medical Association* 267, no. 8 (1992): 1106-08.

4

COMMUNICATION, TRUTHTELLING, AND DISCLOSURE

Robert J. Boyle, M.D.

Cases

AB was informed by her gynecologist that she had an ovarian tumor and needed immediate surgery. Naturally, she was upset and, as a former cancer researcher with special knowledge of the subject, she began to ask questions. The questions and answers became prolonged, and the physician became progressively annoyed with the time the consultation was taking. He abruptly ended the session.

CD is a 40-year-old patient who was admitted for severe back pain. Admitted initially to the neurology service, he saw a neurosurgical resident and attending physician in consultation, had a physical therapy evaluation, had a psychiatric evaluation for the possibility of a nonorganic cause for the pain, and finally is seeing you in the pain clinic. What is your role in communicating with this patient? How much should you tell him? Should you leave this to his primary physician? What does the patient know/not know about the results of other studies and consultations?

Mr. and Mrs. E were referred for genetic counseling due to Mrs. E's age of 41. She has recently learned that she is pregnant. The couple wants the child, but they are concerned about the risk of Down syndrome, (trisomy 21). After counseling, the couple agrees to proceed with amniocentesis. The results show 47 chromosomes with no evidence of Down syndrome. However, the child is XYY. Some research has suggested that XYY individuals have an increased tendency toward violence, sexual offenses, and criminal behavior. Because the couple expressed interest only in the risk of Down syndrome, and because the research on XYY is not conclusive, the genetics team is considering whether to disclose this result.

FG is a 75-year-old widower whose wife died with cancer several years ago after a long illness. He is admitted to the hospital for evaluation of weight loss. Tests reveal a mass in his lung. You are aware of the diagnosis. As you are about to enter his room, his two sons meet you and insist that their father not be told that he has cancer, since it will upset him terribly and they are not sure what he might do.

HK is a 70-year-old widow admitted for myocardial infarction. Evaluation reveals extremely poor myocardial function and an extremely poor prognosis. She is currently quite stable, alert, and conversant. Her physician believes that it would be inappropriate to discuss her prognosis with her or to recommend a do-not-resuscitate (DNR) order, since it may upset her and "kill her." The patient is asking her bedside nurse many questions. The nurse believes the patient needs to hear the prognosis and begin making some decisions and arrangements.

LM is a 55-year-old woman who has just completed her annual checkup. You inform her that a screening mammogram would be in her best interest. She replies that her health insurance would not pay for the test unless there is a mass or other objective evidence of a tumor. She requests that you submit the request for payment using the latter criteria.

NP has recently been diagnosed with metastatic breast cancer. She subscribes to a managed-care plan that will not cover bone marrow transplants for breast cancer. The physician believes this is the only option for her disease, but is reluctant to discuss the financial details of why the managed-care plan has made this choice. He knows that he would have to invest a lot of time and effort in challenging the policy.

RS was admitted to the hospital with a hypertensive crisis. The physician elects to treat the patient with diazoxide. She administers the usual dose of 100 milligrams. Shortly after, RS's blood pressure falls and she does not respond to resuscitation. The patient dies. The nurse notices that the vial actually contained 1,000 milligrams of medication, a fatal dose.

I. Introduction

A patient comes to a clinician with a problem or potential problem. The evaluation, diagnosis, and resolution of these problems call for collaboration that is characterized by mutual acceptance, trust, and respect between patient and clinician and among clinicians from a variety of professions. The goal of this interaction should be to develop a plan of care, with the patient or surrogate as full partner, for this evaluation and treatment. Development of this plan begins as soon as the patient-clinician relationship is established. It should be a systematic and continuous plan, constantly reevaluated and adjusted in light of medical information, changes in the patient's condition, changes in the contextual framework of the situation, and so forth. None of this planning can be accomplished without effective communication among all of the parties involved.

Clinicians must recognize that they are members of a team involved in developing a plan of care for the patient: nurse, physician, chaplain, social worker, physical therapist, consultant, medical student, dialysis technician, and so forth. Communication among all of these members is critical to the process.

With regard to the specific content of communication with a patient, anxieties and conflicts often develop around several questions: What should the patient be told? What should the family be told? Who should be told first? Who should inform the patient? When? How? Where? Can actual truth be disclosed without destroying hope? Is lying ever ethically justifiable--especially to protect the patient from harm?

In this chapter, we focus on a range of issues dealing with communication, realizing that good communication is necessary for all of the issues discussed in this text, from confidentiality to reproductive choices. The cases above introduce the more general issue of communication (Cases AB and CD) and proceed to more specific problems with truthtelling and disclosure (Cases E, LM, and NP), the conflict engendered by a disclosure that the clinician or others believe may be harmful to the patient (Cases FG and HK), and the fear of retribution for disclosing mistakes (Case RS). Disclosure as it pertains specifically to the process of informed consent is discussed in Chapter 6.

II. History

Communication and disclosure are not mentioned in the Hippocratic oath, which states that the physician's duty is to act for the benefit of the patient. Other Hippocratic writings, in fact, speak against disclosure: "Perform [these duties] calmly and adroitly, concealing most things from the patient while you are attending to him. Give necessary orders with cheerfulness and serenity, turning his attention away from what is being done to him; sometimes reprove sharply and emphatically, and sometimes comfort . . . revealing nothing of the patient's future or present condition."[1]

Early Christian moralists, prompted by puzzling scriptural episodes of lying, began to wonder whether it is ever right to lie. According to Jonsen and Toulmin, "Although the wrongness of deception was widely recognized, the practice of deception was not uniformly condemned in the early Christian community."[2]

Yet Augustine (fourth century A.D.) argued powerfully for an absolute prohibition of any lie. He discussed what was to become the "classic case" through the Middle Ages until the 18th century: An innocent person, unjustly condemned, is hidden in your house. May you lie to the police officers who come to arrest him? Augustine asserted that even good consequences could never justify a deliberate lie. Centuries later, Kant held that a lie is wrong even when based on benevolent motives, because it degrades the person who lies and violates the universal social duty to tell truth.

Medieval "casuists" gradually relaxed Augustine's radical position: an immense literature developed on ambiguity, mental reservation, "white lies," and equivocation. The genuine moral insight driving this literature was that, on occasion, part of the truth may be withheld. Concealing the truth was considered permissible when a person was questioned unjustly or when revealing it could cause great harm to another person.

The physician's conversation with a patient was intended to comfort and induce the patient to take the cure. The patient's role was one of obedience to the physician, although medicine and science had little to offer the patient at that point in history.

The 19th-century English physician Thomas Percival's code of medical ethics[3] and the first code of the American Medical Association (AMA) that was based on it were oblivious to the issue of disclosure and informed consent. These codes focused on words or behaviors of the physician that might upset the patient and be a detriment to the patient's recovery. According to the AMA code: "The life of a sick person can be shortened not only by the acts, but also by the words or manner of a physician. It is, therefore, a sacred duty to guard himself carefully in this respect, and to avoid all things which have a tendency to discourage the patient and depress his spirits."[4]

By 1980, the AMA code, now named "Principles," had changed minimally. However, the *Current Opinions of the Judicial Council of the AMA* did address disclosure and truthtelling: "The patient's right of self-decision can be effectively exercised only if the patient possesses enough information to enable an intelligent choice. . . . Social policy does not accept the paternalistic view that the physician may re-

main silent because divulgence might prompt the patient to forgo needed therapy."[5]

III. Shifting Attitudes about Diagnostic Disclosures

During the past 30 years, there has been a remarkable change in physicians' attitudes about whether to tell the patient bad news, specifically a diagnosis of cancer:

- In 1953, 69 percent of physicians favored not telling.[6]
- In 1961, 88 percent favored not telling.[7]
- In 1979, 90 percent favored telling.[8]

The following reasons have been offered to account for the obvious evolution: availability of more treatment options for cancer (including experimental treatments); improved rates of survival from some forms of cancer; fear of malpractice suits; involvement of other disciplines/professions in healthcare; altered societal attitudes about cancer; and increased attention to patients' rights, including the right to information.[9]

Yet troubling conflicts persist, and clinical reality is often fraught with tensions that prompt less than complete disclosure. For example, in the 1979 study that reported that 97 percent of physicians approved of telling the diagnosis of cancer (Novack et al.), the authors also reported significant ambiguity about whether the obligation of disclosure is focused on the patient or the family. Respondents identified "a relative's wishes regarding disclosure to the patient" as one of the four most frequent factors considered in the decision whether to tell the patient the truth.[10]

Another example of the disparity between what people say and what they do comes from a 1982 survey of medical and nursing staff caring for elderly patients who died. The authors of the study reported that only 18 percent of the respondents had discussed the diagnosis with patients, and even fewer had discussed impending death. The staff had not fully appreciated the communication needs of over half of the dying patients.[11]

The authors of a 1989 study of physicians' attitudes toward the use of deception to resolve ethical problems in clinical practice reported that there was little relationship between the physicians' answers to the case questions and their stated general attitudes toward the use of deception:

- The majority indicated a willingness to misrepresent a diagnostic test to secure an insurance payment.
- The majority would mislead the wife of a gonorrhea patient to ensure her treatment and preserve the marriage.
- One third would offer incomplete or misleading information to a patient's family if a mistake led to a patient's death.

The authors concluded that the respondents justify their decisions in terms of the consequences and place a higher value on their patients' welfare and keeping patients' confidences than truthtelling for its own sake.[12]

Likewise, the author of a 1993 study of oncologists defined three styles that physicians used to inform their patients about the cancer: (1) telling patients what they want to know, (2) telling patients what they need to know, and (3) translating information into terms that patients can take. The styles were supported by the principles of respecting the truth, respecting patients' rights, honoring doctors' duty to inform, preserving hope, and honoring individual contract between physician and patient. There was dramatic variation among physicians as to which style they used and which principles they emphasized. There was much more openness about diagnosis and treatment and much less about prognosis. The author noted "varying degrees of openness, willingness to spend time with the patient, sensitivity to patients' subtle cues and active elicitation of patients' desire to know."[13]

IV. Communication

Emanuel and Dubler have described "the ideal conception of the physician-patient relationship" as choice, competence, compassion, continuity, lack of conflict of interest, and communication.[14] A long-standing relationship between a patient and a primary-care clinician of the patient's choosing has often survived because of the trust that has developed between the parties. Predecessors of today's physicians rec-

ognized the therapeutic value of communication, albeit one-sided. Much of the aid a clinician gives a patient appears to depend upon the clinician's ability to mobilize the patient's positive expectations and faith within an emotionally supportive relationship.[15] As physicians' relationship with patients has evolved, physicians have come to recognize that this communication is a two-way street. The clinician and the patient each come to the relationship with a common goal, but each brings different, often overlapping, agendas. Patients bring to the relationship their perceived problems, all of their life values and goals, their family background--a history both medical and personal. Clinicians bring their training and expertise, values and goals, and so forth. How these agendas are shared is critical to the therapeutic process.

Emanuel and Dubler define good communication as follows:

> Good communication means that physicians listen to and understand the patient and communicate their understanding. This entails understanding the patient's symptoms, the patient's values, the effect of the disease on the patient's life, family, job and other pursuits and any other health related concerns the patient deems important. In addition, patients should be able to tell their physicians what kind of information they want and do not want to know.
>
> When communication is good, patients are less likely to misinterpret the information they receive, more willing to ask for clarification when information is unclear, quicker to call if symptoms fail to resolve.[16]

This communication includes not only verbal data but also verbal style, choice of words, demeanor, attitude, body language, etc. As one scholar of the nature of patient-clinician communication has asserted: "The spoken language is the basic tool of doctor-patient communication, the more one knows about it, the more effective is the tool. [Clinicians need to know] how the spoken language works in medicine: how words do their work and can have meanings and impact at many different levels, affecting even the body itself; how the attentive listener can know not only what speakers mean but what kind of people they are by their word choice; how all normal speech is logical, and what that knowledge can do for the physician."[17]

In a review of the doctor-patient relationship, Jensen concludes: "Through our verbal and nonverbal communication, we affect our patients for good or bad. The doctor-patient rapport is indeed our most universally applicable therapeutic tool; like any potent medication, it must be used judiciously, with an understanding of the variables involved and with close scrutiny to monitor possible side effects. Even a simple word of advice may have widely varying results, depending on the doctor, the patient, and the relationship between them."[18]

Unfortunately, this communication is often inadequate. Korsch and colleagues reported that while only 6.75 percent of patients questioned the technical competence of the physician, 24 percent expressed dissatisfaction with their contact with the physician. Reasons included the physician's lack of warmth and friendliness, failure to consider the patient's concerns and expectations, use of unfamiliar terms, and lack of adequate explanations concerning the diagnosis and cause of illness.[19] Although some medical education curricula have begun to include training in interpersonal skills and humanistic care, the relative lack of emphasis in these areas in the face of overemphasis on specialization and technical expertise will continue to produce physicians who are limited in communication skills.[20]

Other researchers have found that physicians commonly underestimate patients' desire to communicate information and their interest in receiving it. Patients routinely fail to communicate their frustrations in not being asked and their desire for increased information.[21]

What patients want most from a doctor's appointment is, first, a chance to tell their story and, second, information about their problem and how to solve it. Unfortunately, the traditional approach to history-taking and patient evaluation often does not allow patients the opportunity to tell their story and does not allow the clinician truly to understand who the patient is. The clinician begins to acquire information and quickly fits it into the traditional model. The patient, on the other hand, may present information in a free-association, random-thought manner. Information that the patient feels is important may be neglected. The data from the history and physical are then written into the traditional format that may, in the end, not reflect what really concerns the patient and what the patient understands. Donnelly recommends recording the "story" and the patient's feelings about his or her situation in the patient's words as part of the history.[22]

Likewise, the social history reflects very little of who patients really are; where and how they live; how they function on a daily basis; what their life goals, values, and preferences are; whom they want involved in decision making, and so forth. What ethnic or cultural issues are important to the patient during this illness? Clinicians are legally required to inquire about advance directives, but is this inquiry *pro forma* or in the face of a broader discussion of issues with the patient? Researchers who conducted a recent study at Baylor University reported that many patients felt their physicians were not interested in dialogue about "life-or-death" choices.[23] If one goal of clinicians is to develop a plan of care, prospectively identifying potential ethical concerns rather than waiting for a crisis to develop, then this information is important. Forrow et al. use the term *preventive ethics*.[24]

V. Barriers to Communication

There are institutional and economic barriers to good clinical interaction between clinicians and patients. Physicians who perform high-tech procedures and surgery earn proportionately far more per minute spent with patients than do primary-care physicians. A history and an interview with a new patient in a primary-care practice may take as long as 90 minutes, for which the physician might be paid $100. A physician who spends 10 minutes reading a nuclear magnetic resonance scan might be paid $400 for those 10 minutes. Thus, we reward action, not communication. With new attention to primary-care services, this phenomenon may be gradually improving. However, the rapid emergence of managed care--with pressure for shorter office visits, reduced physician utilization, termination of long-standing clinician-patient relationships, and frequent changes in contracts and options--may undermine continuity and communication still more. In addition, some managed-care contracts limit clinicians' disclosures about options for treatment, financial incentives, or negative incentives for subspecialist referral.[25] Such "gag rules" have come under recent federal and state legislative control.

The effectiveness of communication and adequate disclosure are often compromised by the complexity of the modern healthcare system. The patient who has a relationship with a single clinician or small group of clinicians and is referred to a tertiary-care center or a subspecialist may be interviewed (often briefly) and examined by multiple attending physicians, residents, nurses, and students. The patient may not feel able to relate to any of these individuals in their brief encounters. One clinician may assume that the other has provided the patient the necessary information (case CD). The importance of a primary-care team that is responsible for communication and coordination cannot be overlooked.

From another point of view, the clinician has a professional responsibility to communicate information about the patient, the patient's condition, potential treatment plans, and so forth, to other members of the healthcare team. Failure to communicate with other personnel may jeopardize the welfare and safety of the patient. As stated in the American Nurses Association (ANA) Code for Nurses: "The complexity of healthcare delivery systems requires a multidisciplinary approach to delivery of services that has the strong support and active participation of all health professions."[26]

Communication among care providers is not always encouraged or fostered. In their traditional paternalistic role, physicians have not wanted input from others involved in the patient's care. In addition, different professions fail to or are unwilling to recognize that each profession may have a different style, technique, or focus in regard to the information they have acquired about a situation or possible solutions to a problem. The classic conflict is between the physician and the nurse; other conflicts include those between critical care nurse and general ward nurse, nurse and physical therapist, and physician and social worker.

Many of the "ethical dilemmas" that lead to ethics consultation are, in fact, problems resulting from lack of effective communication within the healthcare team. How should the clinician respond when he or she feels strongly that the patient is not getting the information needed to participate as fully as possible in decision making? (case HK). How does the bedside nurse respond to the patient's questions about test results, when the tradition on that unit places this responsibility in the hands of the attending physician?

Effective planning of the patient's overall care and communication among caregivers should facilitate resolution of these issues.

VI. Culture and Language

Communication also suffers when cultural differences or language barriers exist. What may be very important in one culture may be insignificant in another. For example, the dynamic of the family; the role of the elderly; the importance of intellectual achievement; the value of life, however impaired; the belief in an afterlife--all may place the patient and the clinician on different planes with little effective communication about a particular situation. For example, Pellegrino suggests that in many cultures the patient implicitly delegates authority for decision making to the family, thereby enabling the patient to avoid bad news.[27] Authors of a recent study of ethnicity and patient autonomy reported that Korean-American and Mexican-American subjects were less likely than African-American and European-American subjects to believe that the patient should be told about a terminal prognosis and more likely to believe that the patient's family rather than the patient should make decisions about life support.[28]

When language barriers are present or when the clinician must rely on translation, much of the feeling, spontaneity, and true meaning of the communication may be lost.

VII. Truthtelling, Lying, and Deception

Effective communication and the patient's participation in decision making about healthcare require that the communication be truthful. The information that the patient processes must be honest and as complete as necessary for valid decision making. If important information has been withheld or purposely inaccurate information given, the patient's self-determination is frustrated. There is a strong negative duty not to lie that is owed to all persons. The ordinary business of life depends on the expectation of truthtelling. Our society expects clinicians to manifest the highest standards of professional integrity. If that integrity is undermined, the individual patient's and the public's trust in the clinician and in medicine in general is undermined. There is also a positive duty to tell the truth--to inform others about what one knows, believes, or thinks, if the other person has a right to that knowledge. According to Higgs:

> The temptations to lie are common. . . . Everyday, if a meticulous health professional examines his work, there are demands that the truth be bent, folded, redirected or simply screwed up and binned. Mostly, he accepts that this is part of the job, sometimes to the point that the deception is no longer seen. It is actually part of a larger and more disreputable truth, that we all have to get by, somehow, someway, until the challenge becomes clear--an angry patient, a desperate relative, a complaint, a case in law. All of a sudden, our personal and professional standards are on the line, and we have to decide: what, and how important, is telling the truth.[29]

Referring back to the cases that open this chapter, should LM's physician falsify the insurance claim to enable a screening mammogram to be done? Should RS's nurse or physician inform the family of a mistake in dosage or tell them that the patient died as a complication of his disease?

VIII. Deception

The overriding ethical assumption is that truthfulness normally best serves the patient; the empirical evidence indicates that virtually all patients want the truth even though many may ask the clinician to choose the best approach.

Some clinicians and many family members believe that disclosure of a terminal diagnosis is detrimental and may lead to acute decompensation, depression, or suicide. In fact, the chance is very remote. In a 17-year review of deaths by suicide, researchers found that only one could be attributed to transmission of the diagnosis of cancer.[30]

According to the President's Commission for the study of Ethical Problems in Medicine and Biomedical and Behavioral Research:

> There is a very little empirical evidence to indicate whether and in what ways information can be harmful.

> Not only is there no evidence of significant negative psychological consequences of receiving information, but on the contrary some strong evidence indicates that disclosure is beneficial. Several studies have focused upon the effects of giving patients information about their surgery and its recovery period. Preoperative counseling appears to reduce anxiety and complications during convalescence. Fewer analgesic medicines and days in hospital are required by those who are counseled than by those who are not. Providing information has also proved useful in burn treatment, in stress experienced by blood donors, in childbirth, and in sigmoidoscopy examinations.[31]

In a study of discussion of advance directives with patients suffering from early dementia, some family members initially predicted that patients would be upset by discussing end-of-life issues. However, at the conclusion of the study, researchers found no measurable adverse effects immediately following the discussion or after five days. All patients denied feeling worried, sad, or letdown by their doctor.[32] Likewise, an English study of geriatric patients' attitudes about resuscitation reported that 67 percent welcomed inquiry about their preferences, 78 percent wanted to participate in decisions, and 43 percent wanted to be the sole decision maker.[33]

Moreover, we know that identifying the cause of the patient's illness will help mobilize family support and cohesion. Patients desire to have a "name for their disease" as a way of contending with the unknown, which is often the source of greatest fear. Researchers who studied with children and adolescents reported that both the patient and parents were relieved when they were informed of the diagnosis of cancer, because they then knew what the problem was and what to expect.[34] Adequate information allows patients to make not only medical decisions, but also decisions about aspects of their life, finances, final days, and so forth.

Clinicians vary in the detail of their disclosures. Several studies report that although oncologists agree that the patient needs to know the diagnosis and treatment options, many oncologists manage the information, especially about prognosis, in order to "preserve hope" or "instill an optimistic attitude."[35]

Some modern philosophers, such as Bentham and Sidgwick, affirm that consequences should determine the evaluation of a deception. The "utilitarian" defense of occasionally justified lying is that withholding the truth is permissible when doing so will prevent direct harm. Beauchamp and Childress criticize this position in clinical ethics; they argue that it is too complicated, even impossible, in actual experience to balance the benefit of lying against the resulting loss of trust. They add that, even "on utilitarian grounds deception may have long-term negative effects on the patient's self-image and may threaten trust in healthcare professionals."[36] Others have argued, along the same lines, that the practice of "benevolent deception," may actually promote self-deceptive rationalization of more lies than are truly justified, as the "entire history of medicine before about 1960 is the history of routine deception and withholding of information."[37] In the words of the President's Commission: "There is much to suggest that therapeutic privilege has been vastly overused as an excuse for not informing patients of facts they are entitled to know."[38]

Physicians may grant unjustified influence to family members in decisions about disclosure to patients (see case FG). The patient has the primary moral entitlement to the knowledge of his or her condition, and should have decision-making authority over family involvement. However, there may be situations in which the patient, for a variety of reasons, has placed authority in the hands of family members. Pellegrino suggests that such delegation may be a cultural expectation of the sick person that need not be explicit. He believes it is a "harmful misrepresentation of the moral foundations of respect for autonomy" to thrust the truth on the patient in such a situation.[39] He contends that the clinician must get to know the patient well enough through discussion to discern when, and if, the patient wants to contravene the cultural mores. Freedman reaches a very similar conclusion. He suggests "offering truth" by attempting to ascertain from the patient how much he or she wants to know. For example, "Do you have any questions you want to ask? Do you want to talk? Some patients want to know all about their disease, while others do not want to know so much, and some want to leave all of the decisions in the hands of their physician and family. What would you like?"[40] The patient is offered the opportunity to learn the truth, at whatever level of detail the patient desires. This decision should be the patient's.

Deception or flawed disclosure may take many forms:[41]

1. *"Just the facts":* This is a very complete and scientific rendition of the truth, in which medical jargon obscures patient comprehension and prevents the clinician from feeling discomfort or guilt. "True statements" can be deceptive if not authentically communicative.

2. *"There's always hope":* This is the "miracles sometimes happen" dodge that represents an overly optimistic falsification of the best available clinical judgment. The fallibility and probability that are inherently part of medical practice must be honestly acknowledged by the clinician in a temperate manner.

3. *"You can't tell a patient everything":* Although it may be true that "the facts are literally infinite," the ethical obligation of the clinician is not to disclose "everything"; the clinician's duty is to tell the patient what is meaningful, important, and useful to the patient in his or her condition. The inevitable selectivity and interpretive ingredients in each clinician's communication should be affirmed as the personal voice of the clinician.

4. *Omission:* Remaining silent when speech would be ethically appropriate does not change the fact that omission is a form of lying.

5. *Evasion:* Although it is true that hard news is sometimes communicated more effectively in a less blunt and more indirect manner, the language of indirection can become avoidance and self-deception. The alternative to injurious bluntness is not evasive indirection but talk that is gentle, considerate, and open.

Deception in any circumstance in the clinician-patient interaction is problematic. Even when the deception is practiced jointly by the clinician and patient, there are significant risks to the overall relationship. If the patient knows the clinician is willing to lie to the insurance company to obtain payment for a test (case LM), there is a potential to alter the trust that may be critical in future interactions. In addition, the action risks investigation by the insurer and alterations of trust with other patients as well.

IX. Disclosing Uncertainty

Uncertainty in many areas of medicine is an often overlooked problem in full disclosure. This age-old tension between medicine as art or science continues. Katz notes that a great deal of the problem is the natural human fear of uncertainty, especially when persons are facing serious illness and really want a magical cure rather than a scientific analysis of probabilities and statistics.[42] Treatment of breast cancer, surgery versus angioplasty versus medical management for coronary artery disease, routine mammography, myringotomy tubes for children's ear infections--all represent questions that would initiate a lively debate in a gathering of clinicians. However, an individual clinician usually has made a decision about which treatment is best. This decision may have been based consciously or unconsciously on factors including specialty (for example, surgeons operate), previous training, peer pressure, economics, or prestige. At times the uncertainty causes disagreements in the clinical team about which test or treatment is best for a patient. Discussions between clinician and patient may highlight the fact that critical pieces of information are controversial or unknown. Prognosis or potential morbidity may be documented as statistical probabilities, but how those probabilities relate to that specific patient are impossible to predict; it is impossible to know whether a 40 percent cure rate will include a particular patient.

Many clinicians are reluctant to reveal these uncertainties to patients who, clinicians feel, may not have the capacity to understand such complex matters and who may suffer further anxiety and distrust. Conveying the uncertainty may undermine the patient's faith in the ability and knowledge of the clinician, which some believe is an important therapeutic feature in the patient-clinician relationship. Many patients (as well as some clinicians) continue to expect the clinician to be infallible and omniscient. Clinicians themselves may cope with the uncertainty by failing to acknowledge it fully in certain circumstances.

Katz sees potential value in disclosing uncertainty:

1. it would lighten physicians' burdens by absolving them from the responsibility for implicitly having promised more than they or medicine can deliver;
2. it would give patients a greater voice in decision making;
3. it would greatly reduce the exploitation of unwarranted certainty for purposes of control rather than care; and
4. it would significantly reduce the feelings of abandonment that patients experience when-

ever they sense that doctors are withdrawing behind a curtain of silence or evasion.[43]

Brody suggests that both clinicians and patients have a psychological interest in maintaining a mutual charade that medicine is much more certain and powerful than we know it to be; patients think this way so that they can hope in miracles, clinicians so that they can think of themselves as meriting the great faith and trust that patients places in them. Moreover, the more severely ill patient may regress psychologically, so that the relationship is more like a child to parent than an adult-to-adult relationship. (Parents do not usually feel that full disclosure of information to children is necessary or helpful.) As a result of these and similar forces, both clinician and patient may find strategies to dodge or evade real honesty; these strategies, over time, often become embedded in customary medical practice and the usual expectations that patients have of clinicians.[44]

X. Disclosure

During the course of the patient-clinician interaction, the clinician possesses a tremendous amount of information, derived generally from education, training, and experience, and specifically from the history and diagnostic evaluation of a specific patient. It is obviously unrealistic to expect the clinician to share all of this information with the patient, especially when most of it may not be pertinent to the patient's situation at a particular time or may be extremely technical. The issue is how the clinician determines how much the patient needs to know. What information can the patient demand? How much information is too much? The patient--by his or her questions, responses, and actions--guides the decision about how much information is helpful. The clinician must consider the importance of the information to each patient's specific clinical situation, personal needs, future implications of the information, and so forth.

Take, for example, the case of Mr. and Mrs. E. Although the immediate concern about Down syndrome has been answered, the clinician has additional significant information about the pregnancy. Although disclosure may cause initial confusion and require further counseling and disclosure, more harm would be done if the family later heard the result or read of

its implications. This harm would be further com-
pounded by their loss of confidence in the counselor.[45] These situations are not uncommon in everyday
practice involving laboratory data, genetic testing, and
antenatal diagnosis.

XI. Therapeutic Errors

How do clinicians approach truthful disclosure
when doing so may not be to their advantage, when
disclosure may end their relationship with the patient,
or when disclosure may expose them to liability for a
therapeutic mistake? Clinicians feel major pressure
to avoid malpractice litigation. Does admitting error
increase or decrease this risk? (case RS). In a 1989
study, Novack and colleagues reported that one-third
of the physicians responding would not disclose a fatal error to the family. However, the attitude of the
majority of physicians, as noted in this study and others, would be to disclose the error.[46]

Hilfiker begins to define the complexity of dealing with errors: Was there a mistake? What were the
real consequences? Was the mistake avoidable? Does
the profession have a place for discussing mistakes?
How can a clinician vent emotional responses?[47]
Gillon suggests that the tendency of clinicians to close
rank in their own individual and group interests is not
compatible with the principle of medical beneficence.[48] He and others[49] agree with Hilfiker that if a
mistake has been made, the clinicians should "out of
common decency, let alone the principle of medical
beneficence, say we are sorry."[50] This requirement
may, in any case, be of considerable benefit to the
clinician as well as to the victim of his mistake.

There is no uniform legal code demanding disclosure in these circumstances, although some case
law suggests a legal duty to disclose mistakes to patients or their families.[51] Codes of medical ethics do
not discuss the issue. How the disclosure is made, in
what context, and with how much sensitivity, will in
part determine the patient's or family's response to
the disclosure.

Finally, is it necessary to disclose all errors in
clinical practice? There are numerous minor errors.
For instance, a drug may have been incorrectly ordered, incorrectly dispensed by the pharmacist, or
incorrectly administered by the nurse, without causing the patient complications. Should these events be
disclosed at the risk of causing anxiety and loss of
trust in the healthcare system? Or should the disclosure be limited to those events that have an effect on
the patient?

XII. Ethical Grounding for Communication, Truthtelling, and Disclosure

The primary ethical grounding for all of these
interactions with patients is based on the principle of
respect for the patient's autonomy. Adequate communication and truthful information is necessary for
patients' participation in decision making as well as
their self-determination in planning their lives. Without knowing their medical condition, their prognosis,
what to expect from treatment, and so forth, they cannot validly proceed. In addition, this clinical relationship and communication, both verbal and nonverbal,
carry tremendous power to promote good for the patient (beneficence) and avoid harm (nonmaleficence).

The duty not to lie or deceive is similarly based.
Lying violates respect for persons and may cause
harm. It manipulates the patient for another's purpose.
It frustrates the patient's self-determination, because
it leads the patient to proceed with incorrect data.
Lying undermines the trust the patient should have in
the relationship with the clinician involved and in all
past and future relationships.

XIII. Authoritative Statements

The 1992 edition of the American Medical
Association's (AMA's) *Principles of Medical Ethics*
affirms as the second standard of honorable behavior: "A physician shall deal honestly with patients and
colleagues, and strive to expose those physicians deficient in character or competence, or who engage in
fraud or deception."[52]

In "Fundamental Elements of the Patient-Physician Relationship," the AMA Council on Ethical and
Judicial Affairs elaborates on the therapeutic relationship:

The patient-physician relationship is of greatest
benefit to patients when they bring medical problems to the attention of their physicians in a timely

fashion, provide information about their medical condition to the best of their ability, and work with their physicians in a mutually respectful alliance. Physicians can best contribute to this alliance by serving as their patients' advocate and by fostering these rights:

1. The patient has the right to receive information from physicians and to discuss the benefits, risks, and costs of appropriate treatment alternatives. Patients should receive guidance from their physicians as to the optimal course of action. Patients are also entitled to obtain copies or summaries of their medical records, to have their questions answered, to be advised of potential conflicts of interest that their physicians might have, and to receive independent professional opinions.[53]

The American Nurses Association *Code for Nurses with Interpretive Statements* says: "Truthtelling and the process of reaching informed choice underlie the exercise of self-determination, which is basic to respect for persons. . . . Clients have the moral right to determine what will be done with their own person; to be given accurate information, and all the information necessary for making informed judgements."[54]

The official position of the American Hospital Association, as approved by the Board of Trustees and House of Delegates, is contained in *A Patient's Bill of Rights*. The relevant passages are as follows:

The patient has the right to obtain from his physicians and other direct caregivers relevant, current, and understandable information concerning his diagnosis, treatment, and prognosis.

Except in emergencies, when the patient lacks decision-making capacity and the need for treatment is urgent, the patient is entitled to the opportunity to discuss and request information related to the specific procedures and/or treatments, the risks involved, the possible length of recuperation, and the medically reasonable alternatives and their accompanying risks.[55]

The American College of Physicians "Ethics Manual" (1992) states:

Whatever the treatment setting, at the beginning of a relationship the physician must understand the patient's complaints and underlying feelings and expectations. After they agree on the problem before them, the physician presents one or more courses of action. If both parties agree, the patient may then authorize the physician to initiate a course of action, and the physician accepts the responsibility. The relationship has mutual obligations: The physician must be professionally competent, act responsibly and treat the patient with compassion and respect. The patient should understand and consent to the treatment and should participate responsibly in the care. . . .

Physicians and patients may have different concepts of the meaning and resolution of medical problems. The care of the patient and the satisfaction of both parties are best served if the physician and patient discuss their expectations and concerns openly. The physician must be flexible and open to compromise to address the patient's concerns. The physician cannot be required to violate fundamental personal values, standards of scientific or ethical practice, or the law. There are occasions when the patient's beliefs--religious, cultural or otherwise--dictate decisions that run counter to medical advice. The physician is obliged to try to understand clearly the beliefs and viewpoints of the patient.

The patient must be well informed to make healthcare decisions and work intelligently in partnership with the physician. Effective physician-patient communication can dispel uncertainty and fear and enhance healing and patient satisfaction.

Information should be given in terms the patient can understand. The physician should be sensitive to the patient's responses in setting the pace of disclosure, particularly when the illness is very serious. Disclosure should never be a mechanical or perfunctory process. Upsetting news and information should be presented to the patient in a way that minimizes distress. If the patient is unable to comprehend, then the patient's condition should be fully disclosed to an appropriate surrogate.

In general, disclosure to patients is a fundamental ethical requirement. However, society recognizes the "therapeutic privilege," which is an exemption from detailed disclosure when such disclosure has a high likelihood of causing serious and irreversible harm to the patient. On balance, this privilege should be interpreted narrowly; invoking it too broadly can undermine the entire concept of informed consent.

In addition, physicians should disclose to patient information about procedural or judgement errors made in the course of care, if such information significantly affects the care of the patient.[56]

The American Academy of Pediatrics, Committee on Bioethics (1994) states:

There is a strong presumption that all information needed to make an appropriate decision about healthcare . . . should be provided to the patient, parents or surrogates. Experience and study suggest that most patients, family members or other decision makers want to hear the reality of their situation. Open and honest communication reduces tension in the physician-patient relationship.

Information may not be withheld on the grounds that it might cause the patient or surrogate to decline a recommended treatment or choose a treatment that the physician does not want to provide. Nor may information be withheld because its disclosure might upset the patient, parents or other decision maker.

Physicians may withhold information when a competent patient clearly indicates that he or she does not wish to have the information provided, and the physician has previously offered to provide such information. Some commentators believe that parents and other surrogates do not have the same prerogative to refuse information or decline participation in decision making.

Physicians may withhold information if they believe the information would pose an immediate and/or serious threat to a patient's or surro-

gates health or life. These circumstances will occur rarely, if ever. A physician who withholds information assumes the burden of supporting the decision not to make customary disclosures. The physician should withhold only the specific information that might produce a threat.[57]

The American Medical Association Council on Ethical and Judicial Affairs (1995) states:

The duty of patient advocacy is a fundamental element of the physician-patient relationship that should not be altered by the system of healthcare delivery in which physicians practice.

Managed care plans must adhere to the requirements of informed consent that patients be given full disclosure of material information. . . . The physician's obligation to disclose treatment alternatives is not altered by any limitations in the coverage provided by the patient's managed care plan. Full disclosure includes informing patients of all their treatment options, even those that may not be covered. . . . Patients may then determine whether an appeal is appropriate or whether they wish to seek care outside the plan for treatment alternatives that are not covered.[58]

XIV. Guidance

The clinician's goal should be an honest and tactful discussion of the medical facts--sensitive to the needs, capacities, emotions, and basic beliefs and values of the particular patient--so that the patient can participate in the decision-making process. The clinician should respect the right of the patient to obtain complete current medical information concerning diagnosis, alternatives for treatment, and prognosis, in terms the patient can be reasonably expected to understand, and with open discussion of the element of uncertainty involved in the patient's care.

Truthfulness should mark the communication process between clinicians and patients; clinicians should not intentionally lie, deceive, or manipulate patients, through words, actions, or silence. The "therapeutic privilege" (or "benevolent deception") may be exercised validly to withhold information only with documentation and a second opinion that disclosure would with high probability cause substantial harm to the patient's physical or mental well-being. The therapeutic privilege is intended to prevent direct harm to the patient; however, the moral presumption is that such cases are extremely rare and, therefore, therapeutic privilege should never be used as an excuse to limit the patient's right to be informed.

XV. Cases for Further Study

Case 1: "She'll Be Happier if She Never Knows"

It was the first time the 54-year-old patient had been hospitalized. She was born in Puerto Rico and had lived in Spanish Harlem for the past ten years. She had come to the emergency room two weeks earlier with a severe pain and a mass in her lower right abdomen. The previous December she suffered a severe attack in the same area. Her history revealed that she was past menopause. She had worked in a nursing home and so was familiar with medical procedure.

A third-year medical student obtained the pertinent material in her medical history and talked with her briefly. She told him that she was afraid that she had cancer. When the student assured her that she would have a complete work-up, she replied sadly, "If it was cancer you doctors wouldn't tell me." The student did not comment on the patient's statement, but said that the lab tests and examinations would tell them much more about the possible causes of the pain and the mass. Two days later, after the patient had been examined by the medical students, the resident, the chief resident, and the attending physician, the woman was diagnosed as having a degenerating fibroid, which would explain the severe pain and the mass. It was pointed out, however, that after menopause the most common cause of a painful mass was cancer. The patient went to surgery the next morning. The same day, the medical student spoke to the resident, who reported that she had stage IV cancer of the cervix. They had cleaned out all the tumor they could see, but since it had spread to the pelvic wall, the only alternative was to try chemotherapy and radiation. The five-year survival rate of stage IV cancer at the time was not more than 20 percent.

When the patient awoke from the surgery, the medical student's first reaction was to go to her and explain the findings. He felt he should speak frankly with her, attempt to share her grief, and be there to support her. However, since he had not had much experience with cancer and this was his first patient "who had been given a death notice," he decided to speak first to the chief resident about how best to approach

telling this woman. The medical student explained that she had cancer, and that he felt close enough to share some of the process. The chief resident's action was agitated. "Never use the word 'cancer' with a patient," he said, "because then they give up hope." He suggested using other words or medical jargon.

The student was in turmoil. He felt it was important to convey to the patient what he knew himself: that, according to the best medical understanding of her condition, she had a limited time to live; that new biomedical technology and medical discoveries meant that there were possible treatments, which could be tried; that new discoveries are continually being made. But he wanted to convey to her that the chances were that she would not live out her normal life span--in fact, she would not survive more than a few years.

The discussion got more heated. The resident angrily asked, "I'd like to know how you'll feel when the patient jumps out the window." The student's response was that he felt he had to evaluate the patient's desire to know and that this woman had given a clear message that she wished to know.

The resident told the young student a story about a distinguished internist, the senior attending physician on the service and internationally known as author of a major medical textbook, who while on grand rounds asked if there was anyone present who would tell the patient they had just seen that he had cancer. When one medical student raised his hand, the internist said, "You march down to the dean's office and tell him that I said you are to be kicked out of medical school." Since an authoritarian and often hostile relation between master and student still exists in the clinical teaching setting, the student took him very seriously and turned toward the door. At that point the internist said, "Now you know what it's like to be told you have cancer. Tell a patient that, and it will destroy the last years of her life."

The student left the meeting with the resident wondering what the patient should be told and who should do the telling. He had a good idea what would be said by the senior attending physician, by the resident, and by himself. How would you advise the student?

[Source: R.M. Veatch, *Death, Dying, and the Biological Revolution* (New Haven, Conn.: Yale University Press, 1989), 166-67.]

Case 2: "Can Complicity in Deception Be Sometimes Justified?"

A five-year-old girl had been a patient in a medical center for three years because of progressive renal failure secondary to glomerulonephritis. She had been on chronic renal dialysis, and the possibility of a renal transplantation was considered. The effectiveness of this procedure in her case was questionable. On the other hand, it was the feeling of the professional staff that there was a clear possibility that a transplanted kidney would not undergo the same disease process. After discussion with the parents, it was decided to proceed with plans for transplantation.

Tissue typing was performed on the patient; it was noted that she would be difficult to match. Two siblings, age two and four, were thought to be too young to serve as donors. The girl's mother turned out not to be histocompatible. The father, however, was found to be quite compatible with his daughter. He underwent an arteriogram, and it was discovered that he had anatomically favorable circulation for transplantation.

The nephrologist met alone with the father and gave him these results. He informed the father that the prognosis for his daughter was quite uncertain. After some thought, the girl's father decided that he did not wish to donate a kidney to his daughter. He admitted that he did not have the courage and that, particularly in view of the uncertain prognosis, the very slight possibility of a cadaver kidney, and the degree of suffering his daughter had already sustained, he would prefer not to donate. The father asked the physician to tell everyone else in the family that he was not histocompatible. He was afraid that if they knew the truth, they would accuse him of allowing his daughter to die. He felt that this would "wreck the family." The physician felt very uncomfortable about this request. How would you advise him to respond?

[Source: M.D. Levine, L. Scott, and W.J. Curran, "Ethics Rounds in a Children's Medical Center: Evaluation of a Hospital-Based Program for Continuing Education in Medical Ethics," *Pediatrics* 60 (August 1977): 205.]

Case 3: "Will the Truth Spoil the Vacation in Australia?"

A 69-year-old male, estranged from his children and with no other living relatives, underwent a routine physical examination in preparation for a brief and much anticipated trip to Australia. The physician suspected a serious problem and ordered more extensive testing, including further blood analysis, a bone scan, and a prostate biopsy. The results were quite conclusive: The man had an inoperable, incurable carcinoma--a small prostate nodule commonly referred to as cancer of the prostate. The carcinoma was not yet advanced and was relatively slow growing. Later, after the disease had progressed, it would be pos-

sible to provide good palliative treatment. Blood tests and X-rays showed the patient's renal function to be normal.

The physician had treated this patient for many years and knew that he was fragile in several respects. The man was quite neurotic and had an established history of psychiatric disease, although he functioned well in society and was clearly capable of rational thought and decision making. He had recently suffered a severe depressive reaction, during which he had behaved irrationally and attempted suicide. This episode immediately followed the death of his wife, who had died after a difficult and protracted battle with cancer. It was clear that he had not been equipped to deal with his wife's death, and he had been hospitalized for a short period before the suicide attempt.

Just as he was getting back on his feet, the opportunity to go to Australia materialized, and it was the first excitement he had experienced in several years. The patient also had a history of suffering prolonged and serious depression whenever informed of serious health problems. He worried excessively and often could not exercise rational control over his deliberations and decisions. His physician therefore thought that disclosure of the carcinoma under his present fragile state would almost certainly cause further irrational behavior and render the patient incapable of thinking clearly about his medical situation.

When the testing had been completed and the results were known, the patient returned to his physician. He asked nervously, "Am I OK?" Without waiting for a response, he asked, "I don't have cancer, do I?" How would you advise the physician to respond?

[Source: From *Principles of Biomedical Ethics* by Beauchamp and Childress. Copyright © 1994 by Beauchamp and Childress. Used by permission of Oxford University Press, Inc.]

XVI. Study Questions

1. If, during a patient interview, you as a medical student were erroneously introduced to a patient as "Dr. So-and-So," would you correct the error or let it go? What motivates your response? Would you challenge an authority figure who misled or engaged in dysfunctional communication with a patient? Why or why not? Consider Case 1, "She'll Be Happier if She Never Knows." Do the data support the resident and attending physicians' arguments in this case? What would you do if you were the medical student in the case?

2. All clinicians inevitably make mistakes in their clinical practice. You will make mistakes too. These can range from simple and uneventful medication

errors, to misdiagnoses, to lethal mistakes. Consider the probability of your committing a clinical error that causes a patient moderate to severe harm. Suppose that you give a patient an intrathecal injection (into the spinal cavity) of the wrong chemotherapeutic drug, which results in your patient's paraplegia. How will you handle this in terms of your personal feelings? Will you disclose your error? Will you say you are sorry? How will you feel about yourself?

3. Consider Case 2, "Can Complicity in Deception Be Sometimes Justified?" How would you handle the situation if you were the nephrologist? What procedural safeguards could be put in place to avoid this situation happening again?

4. In Case 3, "Will the Truth Spoil the Vacation in Australia?" is the therapeutic privilege the best option in this case? What are the risks and benefits of such a course of action?

Notes

1. Hippocrates, *Decorum*, W. Jones, tran. (Cambridge, Mass.: Harvard University Press, 1967), 297

2. A.R. Jonsen and S. Toulmin, *The Abuse of Casuistry: A History of Moral Reasoning* (Berkeley: University of California Press, 1988).

3. T. Percival, *Medical Ethics; or A Code of Institutes and Precepts, Adapted to the Professional Conduct of Physicians and Surgeons* (Manchester, England: S. Russell, 1803).

4. American Medical Association, *Code of Medical Ethics* (adopted May 1847), Chapter 1, Article 1, Section 4 in J. Katz, *The Silent World of Doctor and Patient* (New York: Free Press, 1984), 20.

5. American Medical Association, *Current Opinions of the Judicial Council of the AMA* (Chicago: AMA, 1981), ¶ 8.07.

6. W.T. Fitts and I.S. Ravdin, "What Philadelphia Physicians Tell Patients about Cancer," *Journal of the American Medical Association* 15 (1953): 901.

7. D. Oken, "What to Tell Cancer Patients: A Study of Medical Attitudes," *Journal of the American Medical Association* 175 (1961): 1120.

8. D.H. Novack et al., "Changes in Physicians' Attitudes Toward Telling the Cancer Patient," *Journal of the American Medical Association* 241 (1979): 897.

9. R. Veatch and E. Tai, "Talking about Death: Patterns of Lay and Professional Change," *Annals of the American Academy of Political and Social Science* 447 (1980): 29-45.

10. See note 7 above.

11. H. Graham and B. Livesley, "Dying as a Diagnosis: Difficulties of Communication and Management in Elderly Patients, " *Lancet* 2 (1982): 670-72.

12. D.H. Novack et al., "Physicians' Attitudes toward Using Deception to Resolve Difficult Ethical Problems," *Journal of the American Medical Association* 261 (1989): 2980.

13. N.T. Miyaji, "The Power of Compassion: Truthtelling Among American Doctors in the Care of Dying Patients," *Social Science and Medicine* 36 (1993): 249-64.

14. E.J. Emanuel and N.N. Dubler, "Preserving the Physician-Patient Relationship in the Era of Managed Care," *Journal of the American Medical Association* 273 (1995): 323.

15. J.D. Frank, "The Faith That Heals," *Johns Hopkins Medical Journal* 137 (1975): 127-31.

16. See note 13 above, p. 323.

17. E.J. Cassell, *Talking with Patients* (Boston: Massachusetts Institute of Technology Press, 1985).

18. P.S. Jensen, "The Doctor-Patient Relationship: Headed for Impasse or Improvement?" *Annals of Internal Medicine* 95 (1981): 769-71.

19. B.M. Korsch, E.K. Gozzi, and V. Francis, "Gaps in Doctor-Patient Communication," *Pediatrics* 42 (1968): 855-71.

20. See note 13 above, p. 325.

21. H.L. Hirsch, "The Physician's Duty to Stop, Look, Listen and Communicate," *Medicine and Law* 5 (1986): 449-61.

22. W.J. Donnelly, "Righting the Medical Record: Transforming Chronicle into Story," *Journal of the American Medical Association* 260 (1988): 823-25.

23. R.L. Fine, "Personal Choices: Communication between Physicians and Patients When Confronting Critical Illness," *The Journal of Clinical Ethics* 2 (1991): 57-58.

24. L. Forrow, R.M. Arnold, and L.S. Parker, "Preventive Ethics: Expanding the Horizons of Clinical Ethics," *The Journal of Clinical Ethics* 4 (1993): 287-93.

25. J. Firshein, "US Doctors Fight Gag Clauses in Contracts," *Lancet* 347 (1996): 113.

26. American Nurses Association Committee on Ethics, *Code for Nurses with Interpretive Statements* (Washington, D.C.: ANA, 1983), 16, ¶ 11.3.

27. E.D. Pellegrino, "Is Truthtelling to the Patient a Cultural Artifact?" *Journal of the American Medical Association* 268 (1992): 1734-35.

28. L.J. Blackhall et al., "Ethnicity and Attitudes toward Patient Autonomy," *Journal of the American*

Medical Association 274 (1995): 820-25.

29. R. Higgs, "Truthtelling, Lying and the Doctor-Patient Relationship," in *Principles of Health Care Ethics*, R. Gillon, ed. (Chichester, England: John Wiley & Sons, 1994), 501.

30. M. Elian and G. Dean, "To Tell or Not to Tell the Diagnosis of Multiple Sclerosis," *Lancet* 2 (1985): 27.

31. "President's Commission for the Study of Ethical Problems in Medicine and Biomedical and Behavioral Research," *Making Health Care Decisions*, vol. 1 (Washington, D.C.: U.S. Government Printing Office, 1982), 99-100.

32. T.E. Finucane et al., "Establishing Advance Medical Directives with Demented Patients: A Pilot Study," *The Journal of Clinical Ethics* 4 (1993): 51-54.

33. P. Bruce-Jones et al., "Resuscitating the Elderly: What Do the Patients Want?" *Journal of Medical Ethics* 22 (1996): 154-59.

34. J. Vernick and M. Karon, "Who's Afraid of Death on a Leukemia Ward?" *American Journal of Disease of Childhood* 109 (1965): 393-97; G. Koocher, "Psychosocial Issues During the Acute Treatment of Pediatric Cancer," *Cancer* 58 (1986): 468-72.

35. See note 12 above; M. Delvecchio et al., "American Oncology and the Disclosure of Hope," *Culture and Medical Psychology* 14 (1990): 59-79.

36. T.L. Beauchamp and J.F. Childress, *Principles of Biomedical Ethics*, 3rd ed. (New York: Oxford University Press, 1989), 313.

37. H. Brody, "The Physician/Patient Relationship," in *Medical Ethics*, R.M. Veatch, ed. (Boston: Jones and Bartlett, 1989), 78-79.

38. See note 31 above.

39. See note 27 above, p. 1734.

40. B. Freedman, "Offering Truth: One Ethical Approach to the Uninformed Cancer Patient," *Archives of Internal Medicine* 153 (1993): 572-76.

41. Adapted from R.M. Veatch *Death, Dying and the Biologic Revolution*, (New Haven, Conn.: Yale University Press, 1976), 222-29.

42. J. Katz, *The Silent World of Doctor and Patient* (New York: Free Press, 1984), 165-206.

43. Ibid., 206.

44. See note 37 above, p. 79.

45. R.M. Veatch *The Patient-Physician Relation: The Patient as Partner, Part 2* (Bloomington: Ind.: Indiana University Press, 1991), 123.

46. See note 11 above.

47. D. Hilfiker, "Facing Our mistakes," *New England Journal of Medicine* 310 (1984): 118-22.

48. R. Gillon, "Doctors and Patients," *British Medical Journal* 292 (1986): 466-69.

49. L.M. Peterson and T. Brennan, "Medical Ethics and Medical Injuries: Taking Our Duties Seriously," *The Journal of Clinical Ethics* 1 (1990): 207-11.

50. See note 48 above, p. 468.

51. J. Vogel and R. Delgado, "To Tell the Truth: Physicians' Duty to Disclose Medical Mistakes," *UCLA Law Review* 28 (1980): 52-94.

52. American Medical Association, *Principles of Medical Ethics* (Chicago, AMA, 1992), xii.

53. Council on Ethical and Judicial Affairs, American Medical Association, *Code of Medical Ethics, Annotated Current Opinions* (Chicago, AMA, 1992), xxv.

54. See note 26 above, p. 2, ¶ 1.1.

55. American Hospital Association, *A Patient's Bill of Rights* (Chicago: AHA, 1992), 1.

56. "American College of Physicians Ethics Manual," *Annals of Internal Medicine* 117 (1992): 947-60.

57. Committee on Bioethics, American Academy of Pediatrics, "Guidelines on Forgoing Life-Sustaining Medical Treatment," *Pediatrics* 93 (1994): 532-36.

58. Council on Ethical and Judicial Affairs, American Medical Association, "Ethical Issues in Managed Care," *Journal of the American Medical Association* 273 (1995): 330.

5

DETERMINING PATIENTS' CAPACITY TO SHARE IN DECISION MAKING

Robert J. Boyle, M.D.

Cases

AB, a 90-year-old woman living alone and independently, is described as very spry and mentally "with it." She presents to the emergency room with gastrointestinal bleeding. Her surgeon advises her that, without surgery for what is presumed to be colon cancer, she will bleed to death. She refuses, stating she realizes that her "time has come." The surgeon is alarmed that this very active person is refusing the proposed treatment. He is concerned that she is "too old" to decide for herself.[1]

CD is a 15-year-old high school student with aplastic anemia that will require a bone marrow transplant. His parents have been fully informed, but they believe that their son is too young to participate in the decision on whether to proceed.[2]

EF is a 35-year-old construction worker who has been injured on the job. He is bleeding profusely. When brought to the emergency room, he is still alert and oriented, and informs the staff that he is a Jehovah's Witness. He refuses all blood products. His surgeon informs him that he will die without a transfusion. He understands and again refuses. The surgeon begins the process to obtain a court order to transfuse because the patient's religious beliefs are not "rational."[3]

GH is a 40-year-old man who is unemployed and very unsophisticated. He is admitted to the hospital with severe dehydration and impending shock following 36 hours of vomiting. Evaluation reveals a possible small bowel obstruction. After intravenous rehydration, he feels much improved and wants to leave. His family agrees with his wishes. His physician, who is concerned that the patient may still have a bowel obstruction, obtains a court order to treat on the grounds that the patient is "retarded."[4]

JK is a 70-year-old retired attorney who has been treated for the past two years for lymphoma. He has a previous history of moderately severe depression following the death of his wife five years ago. Over the past three weeks he has become more withdrawn, has missed several medical appointments, and has missed his usual visits to his son. He is now admitted with fever and low white blood cell count, with a probable diagnosis of septicemia. The patient refuses antibiotic therapy, saying he wants to die rather than continue treatment for his primary disease.[5]

LM is a 78-year-old woman with progressive Alzheimer's disease who is admitted with pneumonia and other medical problems. She recognizes no one and has been incontinent for more than a year. Despite aggressive therapy the pneumonia fails to resolve, and it is probable that she will not survive to discharge. The patient's husband has begun requesting that the physicians be less aggressive in her treatment and, in fact, decrease the intensity of her treatment. Discussion with the husband reveals that he recently proposed marriage to the couple's housekeeper. The medical staff is concerned that the husband is no longer a valid surrogate.[6]

NP is an 18-year-old high school athlete who was injured in a motorcycle accident. His left foot was crushed, and attempts to save the limb have been unsuccessful. Infection in the foot now threatens the boy's life. However, he refuses the surgery saying, "If I cannot play sports, my life is meaningless."[7]

I. Introduction

As noted in the previous chapter, patients' interests and well-being are best served when they understand their situation and participate in deciding on care and treatment. This is the ethical basis for informed consent (to be discussed in the following chapter). Participation in decision making implies an ability (capacity) to do so.

All would agree that a patient in a coma, an infant, a severely retarded adult, a severely mentally ill patient, and a heavily intoxicated adult are not capable of decision making. But less obvious situations similar to those presented in the examples above are encountered frequently in the clinical setting. For example: (1) Our aging society includes increasing numbers of elderly individuals--living alone, with family, or in nursing homes--whose decision-making abilities may be questionable. (2) Following the release of many psychiatric inpatients from state mental hospitals in the 1970s, many individuals with mental illness, who are able to function to varying degrees, now live on the street, in group homes, or with family. (3) Advances in medical technology have resulted in frequent major life-and-death dilemmas for patients who are no longer fully conscious or able to make decisions.

How does one determine whether a patient is capable or incapable of medical decision making? If the patient is not capable, who then makes the decision? How is the decision made?

II. Background

Society has long recognized that some of its members are unable to make decisions for themselves.

Under English common law, the king had the authority and obligation to protect individuals who were incapable of protecting their own interests. This duty extended to appointing guardians to take custody of children and administer any estates with which they may have been left.

III. Competence versus Capacity

The terms *capacity/incapacity* and *competence/incompetence* have different meanings in the legal context than in the medical context. Unfortunately, many writers use the terms interchangeably.

Incompetence is the legal term used when a person has been judged by a court to be completely unable to take care of himself and manage his property. The judge will base such a determination on testimony of psychologists, psychiatrists, neurologists, other clinicians, officers of the law, or social workers. A declaration of incompetence completely negates a person's legal rights. The person who is declared incompetent may not vote, enter a contract, hold a license, or make any other legally significant decision. Traditionally, definitions of *incompetence* have also included people whose mental capabilities might not be at issue (for example, children). People who are declared incompetent by a court usually are cared for by a court-appointed guardian.

The related but distinct term *incapacity* is used in the legal context to designate those whose individual limitations--mental or physical--do not globally restrict their cognitive abilities or life activities. Capacity is usually considered a functional matter that refers to specific functional deficits. A person may be declared incapacitated for purposes of handling financial affairs (and may have a limited guardian appointed for this purpose) while retaining the legal right to make all other decisions for himself or herself.

Only since the turn of the 20th century has the use of these terms raised questions in the medical realm. For example, who may give consent for surgery upon a person who is *non compos mentis* (of unsound mind)?

The terms *capacity* and *incapacity* share certain similarities in the medical and legal spheres. However, in the medical setting, the terms are used to describe the functioning of sensory and mental powers to process data and draw conclusions. Incapacity can be developmental or pathological. Developmental incapacity would include the immature mental processes of infants, children, and the developmentally retarded. Pathologic incapacity might result from some temporary or permanent deficit in psychophysiologic processes, such as encephalopathy, senile dementia, acute psychosis, or depression.[2] In this and following chapters, the term *capacity* is used not in its strict legal sense, but from the perspective of a clinician who must make a functional analysis about a patient's decision-making ability.

IV. The Concept of Capacity

Capacity is essentially the ability to make a decision. It is an absolutely basic element in the process of informed consent. Clinicians are, in simple terms, asking the question, "Should we allow this person to make this decision under these circumstances?" The consent of a person who is incapable does not validly authorize a clinician to perform medical treatment. Conversely, a clinician who withholds treatment from an incapable patient who refuses treatment may be held liable to that patient if the clinician does not take reasonable steps to obtain some other legally valid authorization for treatment.[3]

Any determination of capacity must relate to the following:

- the individual abilities of the patient;
- the requirement of the task at hand; and
- the consequences likely to flow from the decision.[4]

A. Capacity Standards

There is no "classic" definition of *capacity to make medical decisions*, nor is there a universally accepted legal definition for the term. In fact, there is considerable debate about clinical definitions of *capacity*, which is beyond the scope of this chapter.[5] A variety of often-used definitions or standards have evolved.

1. Outcome

A patient is judged capable based on the outcome of his/her decision. If the decision reflects values not widely held or rejects conventional wisdom, capacity may be called into question. This situation often arises when the patient's decision goes against the clinician's

values. Patients are less likely to have their capacity questioned if they agree with the clinician. For example, clinicians questioned the decision of EF, the Jehovah's Witness patient who would allow himself to bleed to death rather than be transfused. In the case of GH, who wished to leave the hospital after rehydration, the patient reached a decision that clinicians opposed. They then questioned his capacity on the grounds that he was "retarded."

In the case of William Bartling, (*Bartling v. Superior Court*),[6] hospital attorneys and the court redefined the legal issue of competence into a medical issue; they judged that the patient's prognosis was "optimistic" and the patient's responses were "ambivalent."

Bartling was a 70-year-old man with complex medical problems including inoperable lung cancer. Following a lung biopsy, he required intubation and mechanical ventilation in the intensive care unit (ICU). Bartling found the process of mechanical ventilation to be extremely uncomfortable and repeatedly asked that it be discontinued. He frequently removed himself from the ventilator and required hand restraints. Bartling consulted his attorney about forgoing mechanical ventilation. Bartling's physicians agreed to the plan, as long as the hospital administrator agreed. The latter also agreed but wanted the approval of the hospital's attorney. The attorney refused permission, stating that Bartling was not terminally ill, in a persistent vegetative state, brain dead. In a hearing, Bartling stated that he "did not wish to die," but did not "want to live on the respirator." The judge upheld the hospital attorney's position and refused to order the clinicians to discontinue mechanical ventilation or to allow Bartling's hands to be untied so that he could disconnect himself. No one questioned Bartling's competence. The patient died four months later. The case was reversed on appeal two months later.

Attorney/ethicist George Annas refers to Bartling as "Prisoner in the ICU."[7] Annas suggests that those involved may have seen themselves as responsible for the actions of a competent patient and were more concerned with their own suffering and discomfort following the patient's death than with the suffering of the competent patient.

The outcome standard is rejected by most. Capacity does not necessarily mean "what is rational to me, the clinician."

2. Category

A patient is judged capable based on his/her category or status. The patient is said to be incapable because he/she is mentally ill or mentally retarded (even mildly), or aged, or an adolescent minor, or critically ill (the "patient is too sick to decide"). However, many of these individuals are able to participate in decision making. There is a spectrum of ability to function in any group. This outcome standard is rejected by most.

For example, AB, the 90-year-old woman who is independently living and mentally spry, is capable. She is not depressed. She understands her situation and the consequences of refusal. Her decision is understandable. It is based on logic and fact. She is 90 and ready to die. If she had refused surgery because she does not make decisions on Tuesdays in July, it is not likely that she would be considered capable. In the latter case, she may understand that she will die, but her decision is not based on a rational process of decision making.

CD, the 15-year-old bone marrow transplant candidate is capable of participating with his family in deciding on this highly invasive therapy. His status as a minor should not negate this.

3. Functional

The functional standard is the most widely accepted standard in determining the patients' capacity. It recognizes the patient's functional ability as a decision maker. There are a variety of definitions of this standard that help to clarify specific aspects of capacity. For example, the President's Commission for the Study of Ethical Problems in Medicine and Biomedical and Behavioral Research suggested that capacity is determined by whether a patient can do the following:

- *Understand information relevant to the decision.* How the information is presented is critical [see Chapter 6, which discusses informed consent]. Does the patient understand the problem and the proposed therapy? Is the patient alert? Is his/her attention span long enough to allow adequate intake?
- *Communicate with caregivers about the decision.* Does the patient respond? Can the patient explain the decision, or is there ambiguity, indecision or vacillation? Does the pa-

tient have a thought disorder, short-term memory problem, depression, waxing/waning consciousness?
- *Reason about relevant alternatives, against a background of reasonably stable personal goals and values.* Is the patient affected by psychosis, dementia, extreme phobia/panic, anxiety/euphoria, depression or anger?[8]

Appelbaum and Grisso use similar terminology:

- *Ability to communicate choices.* The patient has to maintain and communicate stable choices. Thought disorders, problems with short-term memory, or ambivalence resulting in alternating choices would affect this element. It can be tested simply by asking for a response. If there is doubt, the question can be repeated a few minutes later.
- *Ability to understand relevant information.* Deficits in attention span, intelligence and memory may interfere. Testing might include asking the patient to paraphrase the disclosure.
- *Ability to appreciate the situation and its consequences.* Pathologic distortion, denial or delusion would alter this element. The patient should be able to define the illness, the need for treatment, and the likely outcome.
- *Ability to rationally manipulate information.* Here the coherence and logic of one's reasoning is in question, not the outcome. Rational manipulation involves the ability to reach conclusions that are logically consistent with the starting premises. Psychosis, delirium, dementia, phobia, euphoria, depression, or anger may interfere. Patients should be able to indicate the major factors in their decisions and the importance assigned to them.[9]

White defines four broad categories of criteria for capacity:

- *Informability*: involves the ability to (1) receive information; (2) recognize relevant information as information; and (3) remember information.
- *Cognitive and affective capability*: includes the ability to (1) relate situations to oneself; (2) rea-

son about alternatives; and (3) rank alternatives ("construct personalized burden to benefit ratios for each option . . . assess the probability that each will occur . . . foresee how one's life would be variously changed").[11] "These faculties enable patients to consider the wisdom of pursuing different alternatives, and to correlate past, present and future aspects of their lives, and to organize their lives in terms of their value structures."[12]

- *Resolution and resignation*: incorporates the ability to (1) select an option; and (2) resign oneself to the choice. The patient reaches a conclusion, sets aside his or her uncertainties, and proceeds, even in the face of doubt.
- *Recounting one's decision-making process*: the ability to explain, by recognizable reasons, how one came to a particular decision.[10]

Multiple authors in psychiatry, ethics, and law have expressed concern that currently applied standards for capacity may place excess emphasis on the patient's alertness and ability to reason, while the patient may in fact have significant distortion in logic, cognitive errors, and distorted perception of his or her situation.[13] for example, NP refused surgery because he felt that without sports his life was meaningless.

B. Determining Capacity

In most clinical situations, determining capacity is not a complicated process. It is a common-sense judgment. Clinicians do it every time they interact with a patient. However, in many situations determination of capacity may be quite problematic. Many clinical disease processes are often associated with altered mental status (such as meningitis, alcohol withdrawal, multiple sclerosis, and stroke). The presence of these or other conditions does not in itself justify a determination of incapacity, but it should raise the clinician's suspicions. Likewise, a serious or life-threatening illness may lead to maladaptive behavior with resultant post-traumatic stress disorder or depressive responses. Denial of life-sustaining therapy in this situation may reflect altered capacity.[14]

Because depriving patients of decision-making rights is a serious infringement on their autonomy, every effort should be made to help patients perform at their best. For example, clinicians should minimize psychoactive drugs; try to evaluate and involve the patient when he or she is "up" and not exhausted or medicated; involve family members or other clinicians who know and can communicate well with the patient and who have the patient's trust. Patients with communication disorders (such as deafness, aphasia, or dysarthria) may require a great deal of time, skill, and attention to determine capacity.

It is important to reevaluate patients as their situations change for better or worse. Someone who is poorly responsive today due to anxiety, depression, psychosis, or medical illness may be much improved tomorrow.

Capacity should be determined, in part, by the importance of the decision at hand. Decisions about taking a laxative and about cardiac transplant are on different levels of a "sliding scale." Drane's model defines three categories of medical situations where, as the consequences potentially resulting from the decisions become more serious, the capacity standards for consent or refusal become more stringent: (1) For easy, effective treatments that are not dangerous and are in the patient's best interest, awareness and assent may be all that is required; (2) for less certain treatments--when the diagnosis is doubtful, the condition is chronic, or the treatment is more dangerous or less effective--the patient must be able to understand the risks and benefits of the options and make a decision; (3) For dangerous treatments and treatments that run counter to professional and public rationality, the patient is required to show the highest standards of understanding and judgment.[15]

Roth and colleagues describe a hierarchy of competency tests, which include the following:

- evidencing a choice--a very low-level test, most respectful of autonomy, looking only for consent or denial;
- reasonable outcome of choice;
- choice based on rational reasons;
- ability to understand; and
- actual understanding, the highest test.[16]

These authors conclude that, in most situations, the test applied combines elements of all the tests and that the tests are chosen based on the risk-benefit ratio of the treatment and whether the patient consents or refuses. Therefore, with a consent to a high-benefit and low-risk treatment, a low-level test of capacity would be applied, while a refusal may require a higher capacity standard.

When there is doubt--due to the patient's clinical situation, the significance of the decision at hand, or dispute among care providers (clinicians, family, or potential surrogates)--psychiatric/psychologic or neurologic consultation may be extremely important and helpful. This will allow evaluation for depression or organic brain disease. But also, in most situations, it falls to these professionals to make formal determinations of capacity. In most cases, a complete mental status examination should be performed. The Mini-Mental Status Examination (MMSE), the Mattis Dementia Rating Scale, the Short Portable Mental Status Questionnaire, and the Cognitive Capacity Screening Examination are the more commonly used instruments. But again, they measure traits of mental status and are not specifically measures of decision-making capacity.[17] For example, the MMSE measures orientation in time and place, immediate recall, short-term memory, calculation, language, and constructive ability. According to Finucane et al., "It can be affected by anxiety, depression, intelligence, education and the patient's sociocultural background. People with high scores may actually be [incapable] while those with relatively low scores may retain the ability to make some rational decisions. It is best to regard the MMSE as a useful but limited screening test."[18]

According to one well-known authority:

"There is no international clinical, legal, philosophical or ethical consensus about competence criteria . . . there is no agreement about the threshold of decision-making or functional capacity necessary to consider a person legally or morally competent. In a given case, there may be wide consensus among clinicians, legal professionals, and ethicists that a particular person is, or is not, competent. . . . However, disagreement is likely in many cases. In part, this derives from the fact that competence determinations are not essentially factual, objective, or empirical matters but rather are value-laden judgments about the relative importance of autonomy and beneficence to the person, as assessed by the clinician or others."[19]

Numerous studies have identified the problem of application of standards by clinicians in a variety of settings, with wide variations in "accuracy" of determinations of capacity.[20]

Freedman[21] and colleagues have suggested guidelines for assessing capacity in patients with cognitive deficits due to neurologic disorders:

- Does the patient have an adequate level of attention, or is there wandering or drifting attention?
- Is the patient able to comprehend relevant instructions; retain information long enough to evaluate it in relation to relevant, recent, and remote experiences; and express his/her wishes? Assessment might include spontaneous speech, auditory comprehension, writing, and reading comprehension, as well as recent and remote memory. Recent memory is important to retain information long enough to take all relevant facts into consideration. Remote memory is important for integration of current issues with past knowledge.
- Does the patient have sufficiently intact judgment? Frontal lobe dysfunction may affect ability to select goals, plan to achieve the goals, monitor performance, and evaluate consequences.

Janofsky and colleagues[22] have proposed an instrument that uses a standarized essay that would be read to patients, followed by a series of questions that correlated well with formal psychiatric determination of capacity. Using a similar technique (a series of vignettes read to the patient followed by a series of questions), Fitten et al.[23] in a nursing home population and Marson et al.[24] in a population with different stages of Alzheimer's disease found that standard, indirect, cognitive screening assessment by the primary physician significantly underestimated the prevalence of impaired capacity. These authors concluded that with populations at risk for altered capacity, clinicians should more systematically and directly probe the patient's decision-making capacity when significant clinical decisions approach.

C. Depression

Depression can alter the patient's capacity for decision making. In the cases of JK and NP, clinicians might ask if these patients' refusal is rationally based on their primary disease and the discomfort they are experiencing. Or is the refusal entirely or in part due to depression? Isn't a patient in this situation entitled to be depressed? Howe et al. note that the depressed patient may have capacity for clear thought and be able to express those thoughts, but have altered decision-making abilities due to mood and affect derangement and distorted logic.[25] Depression is relatively common; in one study, 25 percent of hospitalized cancer patients met criteria for depression, while 15 percent of elderly patients living at home met the criteria.[26] Depression in the elderly may be difficult to distinguish from dementia and, in some cases, the only means of making this differentiation may be to try antidepressant therapy. Depressed patients may feel hopeless and refuse treatment or food and water. They selectively perceive the more depressing or negative aspects of their environment. They tend to focus on negative feedback. They have no hope and give "logical reasons" why no therapeutic intervention can succeed. Suicidal ideation is not uncommon.

In patients with terminal illness, it is very difficult to distinguish realistic from pathological hopelessness. Depression may be a "reasonable" response to serious medical illness and may produce subtle distortions of decision making. Its diagnosis is neither necessary nor sufficient for determining that a patient is not a capable decision maker.[27]

Mild to moderate depression has little predictive value in determining preferences toward life-sustaining treatment of elderly, medical patients, and these patients appear to experience no increase in desire for medical therapy after recovery from depression.[28] However, with severely depressed psychiatric inpatients, recovery from depression is associated with an increased desire for lifesaving medical therapy in patients who initially believed their situation to be hopeless and underestimated the benefit of treatment.[29] Gerety et al. noted similar findings in depressed nursing home patients.[30] The prognosis for depression in older individuals is worse compared to adults who are under the age of 65. In addition, prognosis is worse when acute or chronic illness is also present. Lee concludes a review of the issue, stating: "For the older patient with life-threatening illness, the literature supports vigorous treatment of depression, because the likelihood of a favorable response is high, and the risk of increased mortality for medically ill depressed, older patients is substantial. Therefore, in general, life-sustaining therapy should not be withheld until efforts have been made to reverse depression. However, this recommendation is not absolute. In some cases an older patient, although depressed, may have the capacity to refuse."[31]

In a review of depression and refusal of treatment, Sullivan and Youngner note: "It is essential for psychiatrists to accept that a seriously ill person's choice to die may be rational, especially in situations where the medical prognosis is very poor."[32] When depression compromises capacity, the authors recommend treating the depression. But they also recognize that there are times when psychiatric treatment is not appropriate, when it may intensify suicidal ideas, when the depression is absolutely treatment-resistant, or when the patient refuses treatment. They conclude:

> Psychiatrists need to recognize that some treatment refusals that result in death are legitimate, even if they are accompanied by suicidal intent. Evaluating the role of depression in these refusals and determining the effect of depression on competence are difficult tasks. They are best accomplished on the basis of a clear distinction between diagnosis of depression and assessment of competence. We must not overestimate or underestimate the value of treatment of depression for patients with severe medical illness. It is often valuable to diagnose and treat depression in the seriously ill patient, but sometimes it is valuable to accept the patient's decision to die.[33]

D. Capacity in Older Children and Adolescents

Most children would not be considered legally or ethically fully capable of making healthcare decisions. However, recent developments in the understanding of the cognitive development of the child, the desire to enhance the child's autonomy and skill as a decision maker, and the recognition of the need of the minor patient to know the diagnosis and proposed treatment have led to an increased role in decision making for the child-patient.[34] In the cases at the beginning of this chapter, should patient CD be included in the decision-making process about a bone marrow transplant completely, in part, or not at all?

Children begin life able to understand little about their illness; proceed to feel they caused the illness; then externalize causes, and by age 12, manifest formal logical thinking. Their cognitive development evolves from the concrete to the ability to think abstractly, reason deductively, consider multiple factors, and understand future consequences. Many factors may influence these abilities: intelligence, experience, maturity, emotional stability, or family situation. For example, the child with a chronic disease has dealt with the problems associated with the disease; has seen other patients with the disease improve or die; and, therefore, may be much better equipped to take part in decision making than a child of the same age just hearing of her diagnosis. Likewise, the child whose parents have encouraged participation in other decisions relating to family or personal matters may be better prepared to make decisions. On the other hand, even the older adolescent may have trouble anticipating the future, which may cause difficulty when that adolescent attempts to weigh the effect of decisions on her future.

Researchers have found that children as young as age seven have developed many of the capacities needed to make good decisions. They may not yet be ready for full, independent consent but are capable of participation.[35] Researchers have found that most adolescents beyond the age of 14 have full decisional capacity.[36] The clinician must individually evaluate each child and adolescent's capacity. Other professionals (nurse, child psychiatrist/psychologist, social worker) may provide important insight into a particular child's developmental level and ability to comprehend the information presented. As with older individuals, capacity should be judged based on the decision at hand.

Several Canadian provinces have enacted legislation that entitles children to make their own healthcare decisions. In British Columbia, the clinician must be convinced that the child understands the risks and benefits of healthcare and has taken reasonable steps to conclude that the care is in the child's best interest; New Brunswick requires two physicians to make a similar assessment.[37] Public policy in Great Britain is also moving in this direction; children have been granted the right to receive appropriate information, to express their views, and to grant or withhold consent--provided that they are considered to be capable by the clinician who is acting in good faith. British policy makers assert that the assessment of capacity should be based on functional ability, not on age. All children of school age should be presumed capable.[38]

Others have suggested caution in evaluating and accepting capacity in the adolescent.[39] Some studies indicate that younger adolescents tend to think in terms of short-term and hedonistic needs, and that until they develop a higher cognitive maturity level, they will be disinclined to comply with an uncomfortable course of treatment.[40] Chronically or acutely ill adolescents demonstrate high rates of illness-related emotional distress. Striving to become autonomous with their own identities apart from family, they face impediments to these goals of normal adolescent development. Hospitalized and isolated from peers, they may regress to earlier stages.[41] They suffer from depression, family problems, anxiety, and other emotional disorders at rates exceeding peers and younger children or adults with similar disorders.[42] A study of adolescents in a pediatric renal clinic reported that 49 percent of the subjects suffered from a major emotional disorder related to their illness.[43]

Several specific categories of minors who are assumed to be capable, unless other circumstances are involved, are defined below:

- *Emancipated minor*: This category includes minors who are married or not subject to parental control. They may be self-supporting and living on their own. Definitions vary from state to state. In most states this category includes college students and military personnel. Pregnant or parent minors are usually considered emancipated and able to consent for themselves and their children.
- *Mature minor*: Adolescents have a right to participate to varying degrees appropriate to their age and maturity in decisions about their healthcare. This definition also varies according to jurisdiction. Courts have occasionally absolved clinicians and hospitals from liability and accepted the older minor's consent when medical care was rendered without parental consent.
- *Statutory adult*: In some states, a minor can give consent for medical or mental health services involving diagnosis or treatment of venereal or other contagious disease, birth control or pregnancy, or substance abuse or outpatient mental health treatment.

E. Decision Making for the Incapacitated Patient

The prospective, plan-of-care approach would recommend anticipating when a patient may become incapable in the future, discussing the patient's values and preferences, and possibly suggesting formal written directives or appointment of a healthcare proxy. This discussion is appropriate for outpatient, primary-care clinicians as well as clinicians in the acute-care hospital setting. It is appropriate for inclusion in the standard medical history interview.

1. Who Makes the Decision?

Surrogate or proxy decision makers must be moral as well as legal representatives of the incapacitated patient's interests. They fall into four major groups:

- *Designated proxies*: The patient may have previously, voluntarily designated a proxy, in a living will or durable power of attorney for healthcare.
- *Family members*: The family is usually very concerned with the patient's interests, is aware of the patient's values and goals, and generally has the "highest and most loving" motives.[44] Most people would prefer to have decisions made on their behalf by a relative rather than a stranger. All surrogates, including clinicians and judges, may be biased by their own values and interests. Family members motivated by love may be better able to compensate for such biases. The New Jersey Supreme Court suggests that family members "provide for the patient's comfort, care and best interest" and "treat the patient as a person, rather than a symbol of a cause."[45]
- *Institutional committees*: Committees have been established in a variety of circumstances, both formal and informal, as decision makers or advisors to decision makers. New York State has a system of volunteer committees for the mentally ill who have no family.[46] Infant bioethical review boards were suggested for decisions regarding neonates during the 1980s. Some institutional ethics committees require routine review of some categories of surrogate decisions (such as withholding/withdrawing life-sustaining therapy). Committees may be cumbersome, of variable quality, and unaware of the patient's specific values and goals.
- *The courts*: The courts are often cumbersome, adversarial, unfamiliar with the patient's goals, and usually strongly dependent on the physician's viewpoint. According to the New Jersey Supreme Court: "Courts are not the proper place to resolve the agonizing personal problems that underlie these cases. Our legal system cannot replace the more intimate struggle that must be borne by the patient, those caring for the patient, and those who care about the patient."[47] However, they may be useful as a last resort when other modes fail to resolve a conflict--for instance, when surrogates are not acting in good faith, or when decisions of the surrogates cannot be considered by a reasonable person to be consistent with the patient's wishes or best interest. In these sorts of situations, the courts may be better suited to choose appropriate surrogates than to make decisions about patient care.[48] For patients who have no identifiable surrogate (either family member or previously appointed), it will probably be necessary, in most situations, to apply through the courts for a guardian to make decisions for the patient. This process may be very time-consuming. The guardian often has no prior knowledge of the patient or the patient's values.

Most states have defined a hierarchy of decision makers for the incapacitated patient. The Virginia Health Care Decisions Act[49] recognizes the following surrogates in order of priority when the patient has not made an advance directive for a surrogate:

1. a guardian or committee for the patient;
2. the patient's spouse;
3. an adult child of the patient;
4. a parent of the patient;
5. an adult brother or sister of the patient; and
6. any other relative of the patient in descending order of blood relationship.

Problems may arise when the legally determined proxy has a potential conflict of interest, (for example, the separated but not yet divorced spouse) or when the ethically more suitable proxy has no legal standing, (such as a long-term significant other or partner). In many cases, the proxy can amicably be transferred by mutual agreement to a more appropriate party.

2. How Is the Decision Made?

Several standards have evolved legally and ethically:

- *Substituted-judgment standard*: This standard allows the patient's own values and definition of well-being to shape healthcare decisions. In some cases, the patient has previously expressed a prior directive or an opinion about the situation he or she is now in. This may be verbal or, preferably, written. The living will defines what the patient wants done if he or she becomes incompetent and critically/terminally ill. Ideally, the proxy decision maker arrives at the same decision the patient would if competent.
- *Best-interests standard*: English common law gave the government the authority and obligation to protect the incapacitated. In addition, a long history of medical paternalism ("what I think is best for you") evolved into the concept of the proxy decision maker who considers what will be best for the patient and who avoids doing the patient harm (benefits versus burdens). The proxy decision maker should consider relief of suffering, preservation and restoration of function, and the quality and extent of the life sustained. This standard is intended to be applied to patients who have never been competent (such as patients with severe retardation or children) or when the patient has never expressed a specific opinion or his or her opinion is not known. The proxy decision maker should promote the welfare of the "average" patient. In the courts, the application of the best-interest and substituted-judgment standards has not always been clearly defined, and scholars debate terminology.
- *Other standards*: The professional standard (where the physician decides) may subject patients to decisions that conflict with their own values. Or, if there are no clear standards, patients may be subjected to over- or undertreatment.

Although proxy decision making is becoming more recognized and endorsed, it has also become apparent through a number of empiric studies that there are limitations in the day-to-day application. Proxies and patients often have not discussed in meaningful detail the issues and values that the proxy would need to make a decision as the patient expected. Families are often quite unreliable at assessing the patient's quality of life, and such assessments often include biases (for example, biases about elderly patients' functional status). Finally, proxies are not accurate in predicting patients' preferences for life-sustaining treatment. In fact, some researchers have found that a proxy's selection of therapy is not much better than a random chance.[50] Emanuel and Emanuel have proposed several options to improve decision making: revision of the justification for and expectations of proxies to honor families' "good-faith" decisions based on patients' best interests, use of more comprehensive documentation of advance-care planning, or development of community-based standards for terminating care of incapable patients.[51]

F. The Questionable Surrogate

The clinician should take reasonable care to ensure that the surrogate's decisions are motivated by respect for the patient's interests and values. The clinician is the patient's advocate and has a duty to the patient and to no other person in the interim.[52] Families or other surrogates may have other agendas that do not include the best interest of the patient. Take, for example, the Philip Backer case.[53] Philip was a mildly retarded 12-year-old with Down syndrome. He could communicate verbally, was educable, could dress himself, had good motor and manual skills, and took part in school and Boy Scout activities. At age 12, he was diagnosed with a cardiac defect, which, if corrected, was compatible with a normal life span and quality of life. If uncorrected, he would suffer progressive distress and eventual death. Although Philip had never lived at home, his parents refused the surgery. They were concerned with the care that would be available to him as he aged and did not want him to be a burden on the other children in the family. The court upheld the family's refusal.

The surrogate's role may be shaded by issues of inconvenience to themselves, financial obligations, prior emotional conflicts or guilt, religious beliefs, or disinterest. Is LM's husband's role as surrogate invalidated by his relationship with another woman? Is he no longer able to make reasonable decisions for his wife? In many situations, property or large inheritances are at stake. How much of a role might these factors play in the surrogate's decision? Do they automatically call the surrogate's validity into question? Some surrogates have standing under law, but in fact may not be the best surrogate for the patient. The husband who has been estranged from his wife for 10 years but not divorced is still the legal surrogate; however, an adult child of the patient may be much closer to the patient. Just as the patient may be an incapable decision maker, surrogates also, for exactly the same reasons, may be incapable.[54]

When the clinician has cause to question the surrogate's capacity, believes a decision is not consistent with the patient's wishes or best interest, or believes that the surrogate has a major conflict of interest, that clinician has an obligation to pursue the matter. This might involve further discussions with the surrogate; participation of other professionals; consultation; legal counsel; or, if the concern is not resolved, intervention by the court. In the question of whether a surrogate is impaired, most agree that the burden of proof rests with those who question the surrogate's decision.[55]

G. Ethical and Legal Dimensions of Landmark Cases

In Re Quinlan, 1976 (New Jersey). The parents of Karen Quinlan, a young woman in a persistent vegetative state due to barbiturate-alcohol intoxication, petitioned the court to allow withdrawal of mechanical ventilation, based on the patient's previous statements about life-prolonging therapy.[56]

Supt. of Belchertown State School v. Saikewicz, 1977 (Massachusetts). The court allowed the withholding of chemotherapy from Mr. Saikewicz, a severely mentally retarded, 76-year-old, with leukemia, based on the best interest of the patient (although the court used *substituted-judgment* terminology).[57]

Rogers v. Okin, 1979 (Massachusetts) The court allowed mental patients committed to a state institution to refuse psychotropic medications. The court was persuaded that "although mental patients do suffer at least some impairment of their relationship to reality, most are able to appreciate the benefits, risks, and discomfort that may reasonably be expected from receiving psychotropic medication."[58]

Cruzan v. Director, Missouri Department of Health, 1990 (U.S. Supreme Court). Nancy Cruzan was in a persistent vegetative state following an auto accident. Her parents petitioned to have her feeding tube removed based on her values and general lifestyle. The patient had never made explicit statements about a situation similar to hers at the time. Her roommate remembered a conversation in which Nancy indicated that "if sick or injured she would not want to continue her life unless she could live 'halfway normally.'" Missouri courts had ruled that there was no "clear and convincing evidence" to prove Nancy's desires. The U.S. Supreme Court upheld the Missouri decision, holding that states may establish safeguards to protect against abuses as well as sustain the person's own previously established values and preferences.[59]

In re A.C., 1990 (District of Columbia). Angela Carder, a 27-year-old, married woman with terminal cancer, was delivered by cesarean section at 26 weeks' gestation under a court order, in spite of the objections of her family, physicians, and her court-appointed attorney. There was some confusion and conflict as to whether the patient was capable of making her own decision. In overturning the original decision for surgery, the court ruled that substituted judgment should have been used to determine what the patient's own wishes would have been. The court held that "[The] right of bodily integrity belongs equally to persons who are competent and persons who are not. . . . To protect that right against intrusion by others . . . we hold that a court must determine the patient's wishes by any means available, and must abide by those wishes unless there are truly extraordinary or compelling reasons to override them. When the patient is incompetent, or when the court is unable to determine competency, the substituted judgment procedure must be followed."[60]

Florida Department of Health and Rehabilitative Services v. Benito Agrelo, 1995 (Florida). Benny, a 15-year-old boy who had undergone two liver transplants (the first five years previously) began to experience side effects from his immunosuppression and other medications, resulting in hallucinations and severe headaches. He stopped taking his medications against the advice of his physicians but with his family's support. A team of police and social workers carried him from his home strapped to a stretcher to the hospital for treatment. In the hospital, he continued to refuse treatment. Three days later, a circuit court judge ruled in favor of Benny, saying that quality of life was a personal decision.[61]

V. Ethics Grounding

The guidelines on capacity are based on the principle of respect for persons. The capable patient's right to participate actively in medical decision making is based on the principle of autonomy--the right to be self-governing. However, when the patient is no longer or has never been capable, his or her personhood still must be respected. When others must make decisions for the incapacitated patient, the principles of beneficence (provision of benefits and the balancing of benefits and harms) and nonmaleficence (not inflicting harm) should prevail.

VI. Statements by Authoritative Bodies

The President's Commission for the Study of Ethical Problems in Medicine and Biomedical and Behavioral Research states: "For patients to participate effectively in making decisions about their health care, they must possess the mental, emotional and legal capacity to do so. . . . Decision-making capacity is specific to a particular decision and depends not on a person's status or on the decision reached, but on the person's actual functioning in situations in which a decision about health care is to be made."[62]

According to the American College of Physicians:

All adult patients are considered competent to make decisions about medical care unless a court declares them incompetent. In clinical practice, however, physicians and family members usually make decisions for patients who lack decision making capacity, without a formal competency hearing in the courts. This clinical approach can be ethically justified if the physician has carefully determined that the patient is incapable of understanding the nature of the proposed treatment, the alternatives, the risks and benefits, and the consequences.

When a patient lacks decision making capacity, an appropriate surrogate should make decisions with the physician. Ideally, surrogate decision-makers should know the patient's choices

and values and act in the best interests of the patient. If the patient has designated a proxy, as through a durable power of attorney for health care, that choice should be respected. When patients have not selected surrogates, standard clinical practice is for family members to serve as surrogates. Some states designate the order in which family members will serve as surrogates, and physicians should be aware of legal requirements in their state for surrogate appointment and decision making. In some cases, all parties may agree that a close friend is a more appropriate surrogate than a relative.

Physicians should take reasonable care to assure that the surrogate's decisions are consistent with the patient's preferences and best interests. When possible, these decisions should be reached in the medical setting by physicians, appropriate surrogates, and other caregivers. Physicians should emphasize that decisions be based on what the patient would want and not on what the surrogates would choose for themselves. If disagreements cannot be resolved, hospital ethics committees may be helpful. Courts should be used as a last resort, when other processes fail or as required by state law.[63]

With regard to decision-making capacity in children, the Council on Judicial and Ethical Affairs of the American Medical Association has concluded:

Determination of . . . [decision making capacity] must be based on an evaluation of the patient's ability to understand, reason and communicate. In general, adolescents 14 and above appear mature enough to make decisions about their medical care, but [capacity] must be evaluated on a case by case basis.[64]

Parents and physicians are in the best position to demonstrate a child's ability to understand, reason and communicate. They are most familiar with the child's maturity level and reasoning skills. Moreover, a physician may have a history with the child and be able to judge the child's present ability to participate in decisions affecting his or her health as well as the child's independence of thought and freedom from family pressure.[65]

VII. Guidelines for Healthcare Professionals

A. Determining Capacity

A patient is functionally able to make a particular healthcare decision when he or she can do the following:

- understand the information relevant to the decision;
- communicate with caregivers about the decision;
- reason about relevant alternatives and consequences against a background of personal values and goals.

B. Prior Directives

Capable persons should strongly consider defining prior directives for their care should they become incapacitated and/or terminally ill. Clinicians, families, attorneys, and others should encourage this process. Clinicians should inquire about such directives when the patient is competent.

C. Decision Making for the Incapacitated Patient

Clinicians have an obligation to implement healthcare decisions for the incapacitated patient that:

- are consistent with the values and goals of a patient who has lost decision making capacity (substituted judgment); and
- Best reflect the interests of a patient who has never been decisionally capable (best interest).

VIII. Cases for Further Study

Case 1: "What's the Difference? He's Still Going to be a Drug Addict"

HD is a 28-year-old man who presented to the office of his internist with complaints of back pain, secondary to Hodgkin's disease. His history dated back five years, when he had been evaluated for fever, weight loss, and an enlarged lymph node. He was diagnosed with Hodgkin's disease and received mantle irradiation. Two years later, he again developed fever and sweats, at which time the relapse was treated with chemotherapy. His medical records that he brought to his first office visit with this internist indicated that his oncologist believed he had gone into a complete remission after the chemotherapy.

He had remained well until six months prior to presentation, when he first developed back pain. Lumbar disk involvement was suspected. A myelogram revealed an epidural mass. Recurrent lymphoma in the spine was found at surgery. His oncologist recommended local radiation therapy and chemotherapy. The patient's old records revealed very poor compliance with the radiation therapy, with frequently missed appointments. At the time of his initial visit to the internist, the patient explained that this was because of his extreme ambivalence about the therapy. He further indicated that he had decided to forgo further treatments and that he wished only symptomatic relief. He preferred to "live out my time" comfortably without any further treatment. He stated he had been receiving the narcotic hydromorphone (Dilaudid), which provided good pain relief, and wished only to have this continued. The physician discussed the patient's wishes with him at great length, with particular emphasis on the likelihood of paraplegia from the spine lesion. The patient demonstrated clear understanding of this risk, but stood firm in his position. The internist prescribed additional Dilaudid and referred the patient to a hospice program.

The physician was subsequently contacted by a narcotics agent with the state health department, who provided copies of numerous prescriptions for Dilaudid from a large number of physicians in the area. He explained how the patient was well known to the agency because he had made similar contacts with several physicians, obtaining Dilaudid from each. The agent, patient, and the physician subsequently met in the physician's office, where the patient promised to get his prescriptions from only one physician in the future. Over the next several months, the internist provided a few more prescriptions for the drug.

The physician subsequently received a phone call from the patient's mother who explained that her son had been an intravenous narcotics user for several years predating his Hodgkin's Disease. He crushed the Dilaudid tablets, dissolved them, and injected the drug intravenously. She was distraught about this, noting that he often locked himself in the bathroom and lost consciousness after injecting the drug. She had recently removed the bathroom door from its hinges.

Before the patient could be confronted with these revelations, he was admitted to the hospital complaining that he had back pain and had run out of Dilaudid. He revealed that he had experienced left-eyelid droop for four weeks, as well as increased weakness in the lower extremities. He further admitted to some fecal incontinence. On examination, he was noted to be febrile and lethargic, and he demonstrated mild to moderate weakness of both legs. His left pupil was larger than the right, with abnormal eye movements (nystagmus) noted. Rectal sphincter tone was diminished, and bladder catherization revealed urinary retention. Urinary tract infection and/or endocarditis were suspected, as well as some intracranial process, probably recurrent tumor. His mental status deteriorated rapidly, and computed tomography (CT scan) of his head was consistent with obstructive hydrocephalus. The neurosurgeons placed a ventriculoperitoneal shunt to decompress the intracranial pressure. Although this procedure provided some temporary improvement in the patient's mental status, he remained delirious and disoriented. When he again began to deteriorate, the neurosurgeons indicated that the shunt was probably obstructed. They agreed to do a shunt revision, but only if the procedure was done in conjunction with radiation and/or chemotherapy to improve the shunt's chance of remaining unobstructed.

The clinicians discussed the therapeutic alternatives with the patient's mother. She was aware of his previous statements refusing radiation and chemotherapy, which at face value seemed clear, relevant; and durable. However, the clinicians and his mother were concerned about the authenticity of the patient's directives. The hypothesis that the patient's directives presented a goal-directed maneuver to obtain drugs could disqualify his pronouncements. However, now that he was incapacitated, the question could not be evaluated.

The patient's mother, his only relative, had enormous difficulty separating the patient's addiction and the turmoil it caused her from the patient's oncologic problems. "What's the difference what we do? He's still going to be a drug addict if he gets better and goes home."

As the internist caring for this patient, how would you proceed?

[Source: Adapted from J.P. Freer, "Decision Making in an Incapacitated Patient," *The Journal of Clinical Ethics* 4 (1993): 55-58.]

Case 2: The Case of Arlene A

Arlene A (AA) is a 38-year-old woman who was admitted to the emergency department of the University of Virginia Medical Center following an overdose of tricyclic antidepressants on 16 November 1990. She had checked into the Charlottesville Quality Inn on November 15 and was discovered by a housekeeper at 13:00 the following afternoon. She was unconscious,

and lying in a prone position with a suicide note dated November 15. The note asked her family to forgive her for any inconvenience that she might have caused, stated that she loved them all, and requested that they please take care of her cat. While conducting a room search, rescue personnel discovered a partially full bottle of imipramine (a tricyclic antidepressant).

Rescue personnel noted that AA was unresponsive to verbal and painful stimuli. She was transported to the emergency room at the University of Virginia. On admission, she presented with a blood pressure of 140/70 and pulse of 114. She was dusky, and had dried vomit on her face. The cardiac monitor revealed a sustained sinus tachycardia (rapid cardiac rhythm) with a wide QRS complex (indicating some ventricular dysfunction). She was intubated and placed on mechanical ventilation; a nasogastric tube was placed and gastric lavage was performed. Her extremities were warm. Neurological exam revealed intact gag and corneal reflexes, marked clonus, and unresponsiveness to verbal or painful stimuli. She had one generalized tonic/clonic seizure while in the emergency room. This was treated with 5 milligrams of diazepam (Valium) administered intravenously. Her cardiac rhythm progressed to sustained ventricular tachycardia. She was started on intravenous lidocaine and norepinephrine infusions and transferred to the medical intensive care unit.

The patient's head CT scan was normal. A Swan-Ganz catheter and radial artery line were placed without event to allow direct measurement of cardiac and pulmonary status and blood pressure. AA's condition stabilized until November 18, when she suffered a pneumothorax (collapsed lung) during replacement of the Swan-Ganz catheter. This was successfully treated with the placement of a chest tube. AA subsequently developed persistent fevers, and her chest X-ray showed pulmonary infiltrates. She was diagnosed with an aspiration pneumonia, probably resulting from the inhalation of vomit. Blood cultures were positive for *Staphylococcus aureus*. All invasive catheters were replaced, and a course of antibiotic therapy was begun. When she remained persistently febrile despite the antibiotics, her diagnosis was amended to fever of unknown origin.

AA's condition worsened. She developed adult respiratory distress syndrome, leading to progressive difficulties in maintaining adequate ventilation and oxygenation. Her lungs became increasingly stiff, requiring high-pressure mechanical ventilation. She developed subcutaneous emphysema and bilateral pneumothoraxes, which required additional chest tube placement. Because she was becoming increasingly difficult to ventilate, she was pharmacologically paralyzed with vercuronium, sedated with Versed, and placed on a pressure-control mechanical ventilator. The pulmonologists gave her a grim prognosis. They considered it doubtful that she would survive to discharge, or ever be weaned from the ventilator.

AA's prior medical history is significant for schizoaffective disorder, borderline personality anxiety disorder, and four suicide attempts.

AA's father visits daily. He lives near Roanoke, Virginia. where he cares for his wife, who is bedridden and suffers from advanced Alzheimer's disease. He tells the staff that AA lives alone in Richmond, and is unemployed. She has been in psychotherapy for many years and has battled emotional problems for most of her adult life, with little benefit from therapy or medications. He says, "She has tried so hard, but nothing has helped." AA's two brothers live in New York and California. They call frequently to inquire about their sister.

AA's physicians have discussed her grim prognosis with her father and brothers. Dr. Smith, the attending physician, and Dr. Jones, the medical resident, have had detailed discussions with the family members. AA's father and brothers have requested that no further chest tubes be placed, and that no resuscitative efforts be made in the event of cardiac arrest. The family and healthcare team agree that a do-not-resuscitate (DNR) order is medically indicated, and DNR is written in AA's chart.

Because the treatment team and family members would like AA's input if possible, they decide to discontinue paralysis and sedation in hopes that AA will regain consciousness. On December 4, AA slowly awakens and is found to be neurologically intact. She is oriented to person and place and recognizes her father. At first, she indicates no memory of the recent suicide attempt. Later that day, she expresses alarm and dismay at being alive and demands (by mouthing words) that the ventilator be turned off. Dr. Jones develops a good rapport with her over the next two days and discusses her situation with her in depth. She firmly maintains her wish to die. She pleads with Dr. Jones to "let her go" and specifically requests that the ventilator be turned off. She refuses any further psychiatric treatment or medications. She offers to be an organ donor.

The psychiatric consultant who is following the case has learned from AA's previous treating psychiatrist that she is suffering from borderline personalty disorder rather than a severe depressive episode. She has a history of schizoaffective disorder and has had only marginal response to antidepressants in the past. The psychiatric consultant finds no evidence of current psychosis or delirium. AA is alert and oriented, and capable of answering questions by indicating "yes" or "no" with a nod of the head and by mouthing words. The consulting psychiatrist writes the following note in the chart: "Answers 'yes' when asked if she is feeling depressed. Answers 'yes' if asked if she wants ventilator disconnected. Says 'yes' she understands she will probably die if this happens. She states that she wants to die no matter what her physical condition. Denies hallucinations and strange thoughts. Able to pick month, year, season, hospital from multiple choice." The consulting psychiatrist suggests (but does not write in the chart) electroconvulsive therapy followed by a course of antidepressants.

The treatment team believes that AA is competent and capable of making her own decisions. Discussions with her and her family members yield the consensus that she has rejected a future on the ventilator and that the most humane course is to respect her wishes and let her die as comfortably as possible. The consulting psychiatrist believes that she is clearly aware of what she is requesting and of the consequences; that the humane course is probably to withdraw treatment; but that because she has been suicidal, she cannot be allowed to make this decision. Furthermore, because of her suicide attempt, to allow the ventilator to be turned off would be tantamount to assisted suicide.

AA's brothers, John and Richard, have made arrangements to travel to Charlottesville. John is in complete agreement with his father's desire to respect AA's wishes, even though he does not want AA to die. He states that he knows what she has been through most of her life, and he wants her to be at peace. Richard understands AA's desire to be taken off of the ventilator, but he now states that he does not agree with suicide. He wants to see his sister and knows that she may die soon, even with continued mechanical ventilation. Both brothers agree, however, to respect AA's wishes. They will both be arriving within a few days.

On December 6, AA's father and Dr. Jones jointly request an ethics consultation. AA's father wants more people involved in the decision-making process. He wants to honor his daughter's request, but does not want the burden of being the sole decision maker. As the ethics consultant, how would you proceed?

[Source: Ethics Consultation Service, University of Virginia]

Case 3: You Can't Go Home

JT is a 49-year-old male admitted to the emergency room after vomiting for several days. He presented with moderately severe dehydration and shock.

His blood pressure was low. He was resuscitated with large volumes of intravenous fluids. His urine output was quite low, and a Foley catheter was placed in his bladder to monitor urine output. A nasogastric tube (NG tube) was inserted to drain gastrointestinal secretions. Abdominal X-ray suggested a small bowel obstruction. He was transferred to a surgical ward where vigorous fluid therapy was continued. His diagnosis was recorded as "severe dehydration, shock, and probable small bowel obstruction, for observation and possible laparotomy." He was not allowed to receive any food or liquid by mouth.

Within 24 hours, JT was feeling much better. He was making adequate amounts of urine, suggesting that there had been no insult to his kidneys from his dehydration and shock. His vomiting had stopped, although he still had the NG tube draining his stomach. The volume of drainage was relatively small. He still had not taken anything to eat or drink. He wanted to leave the hospital because he felt better.

The surgical resident was called and discussed the patient's situation with him. There was still the possibility that JT had a partial bowel obstruction, he had not had a trial without the NG tube, he had not taken liquids, and he still needed to have his renal function monitored to ensure complete recovery. JT still demanded to leave. The intern discussed the situation with the patient's wife, who agreed with the patient.

The couple was moderately unsophisticated and of lower socioeconomic status. The physician appraised the patient as "mildly retarded" and noted that he did not feel the patient was able to make appropriate decisions for his care. The physician contacted the psychiatric liaison service who suggested obtaining a temporary detaining order from the court to require continued hospitalization for the patient. The hospital administrator was called. The special justice was contacted, who issued the order. The hospital administrator, however, felt uncomfortable with the situation and called the ethics consultation service. The ethics consultants--a pediatrician and social worker--and the sheriff with detaining order in hand arrived on the ward at the same time.

After initial discussion with the resident, the consultants, the resident, and the patient's nurse met with JT and his family (his wife, his married son, and his daughter-in-law). The resident explained again the medical problems and the risks of leaving the hospital at that time (recurrence of vomiting, dehydration, and shock--possibly with life-threatening consequences). JT said he understood all of this information, but he felt much better. He explained that he must get home

that evening to be with his elderly mother, who was afraid to be alone and would be angry with him if he was not there. Various alternative arrangements were suggested for the mother's care, but none of the family members believed that the alternatives were acceptable. The ethics consultants' impression was that JT was unsophisticated but clearly understood the issues at hand. In addition, his wife and son also understood and agreed completely with the patient.

The patient and family agreed that if the patient left that evening he would be in contact with his private physician immediately if the symptoms recurred.

As the ethics consultant involved in this case, what would you recommend at this point?

[Source: Ethics Consultation Service, University of Virginia]

IX. Study Questions

1. What is the difference between decisional capacity in the medical context versus legal competence?
2. How does a "sliding-scale" determination of capacity relate to risk-benefit assessment? How does one apply the sliding scale in patient decision making?
3. Differentiate between substituted judgment and best interest as standards for surrogate decision making. Which one takes precedence logically and ethically?
4. What would you do if you believed that an incapacitated patient's surrogate decision maker:
   a. was not using substituted judgment as the criterion for decision making and was in clear conflict with the patient's known values?
   b. was not acting in the patient's best interest, given the inability to apply the substituted-judgment standard?
5. Consider Case 2, "The Case of Arlene A." What do you think of the consulting psychiatrist's opinion that because the patient had been suicidal, she should not be allowed to make the decision to disconnect the mechanical ventilator? What do you think about the psychiatrist's subsequent opinion that to withdraw the ventilator would be assisted suicide?

Notes

1. J.F. Drane, *Clinical Bioethics: Theory and Practice in Medical-Ethical Decision Making* (Kansas City, Mo.: Sheed & Ward, 1994), 155.

2. A.R. Jonsen, M. Seigler, and W.J. Winslade, *Clinical Ethics: A Practical Approach to Ethical Decision in Clinical Medicine*, (New York: MacMillan, 1982), 57-58.

3. L.H. Roth, A. Meisel, and C.W. Lidz, "Tests of Competency to Consent to Treatment," *American Journal of Psychiatry* 134 (1977): 279- 84.

4. President's Commission for the Study of Ethical Problems in Medicine and Biomedical and Behavioral Research, *Making Health Care Decisions*, vol. 1 (Washington, D.C.: U.S. Government Printing Office, 1982), 57.

5. C. Elliott, "Competence as Accountability," *The Journal of Clinical Ethics* 2 (1991): 167-71; E.H. Morreim, "Impairments and Impediments in Patients' Decision Making: Reframing the Competence Question," *The Journal of Clinical Ethics* 4 (1993): 294-307; B.C. White, *Competence to Consent* (Washington, D.C.: Georgetown University Press, 1994).

6. *Bartling v. Superior Court*, 163 Cal. App.3d 186, 209 Cal. Rptr. 220 (1984).

7. G.J. Annas, *Judging Medicine* (Clifton, N.J.: Humana Press, 1988), 317-22.

8. See note 4 above, pp. 57-62.

9. P.S. Appelbaum and T. Grisso, "Assessing Patients' Capacities to Consent to Treatment," *New England Journal of Medicine* 319 (1988): 1635-38.

10. See White, note 5 above, pp. 154-83.

11. Ibid., 174.

12. Ibid., 167.

13. E.G. Howe, D.S. Gordon, and M. Valentin, "Medical Determination (and Preservation) of Decision-making Capacity," *Law, Medicine & Health Care* 19 (1991): 27-33; L. Ganzini et al., "Depression, Suicide, and the Right to Refuse Life-Sustaining Treatment," *The Journal of Clinical Ethics* 4 (1993): 337-40; M.A. Lee, "Depression and Refusal of Life Support in Older People: An Ethical Dilemma," *Journal of the American Geriatric Society* 38 (1990): 710-14; H.J. Bursztajn, "From PSDA to PTSD: The Patient Self-Determination Act and Post-Traumatic Stress Disorder," *The Journal of Clinical Ethics* 4 (1993): 71-74; L. Ganzini et al., "Is the Patient Self-Determination Act Appropriate for Elderly Persons Hospitalized for Depression?" *The Journal of Clinical Ethics* 4 (1993): 46-50.

14. See Bursztajn, note 13 above.

15. See note 1 above, pp. 152-54.

16. See note 3 above.

17. D.M. High, "Surrogate Decision Making: Who Will Make Decisions For Me When I Can't?" *Clinics in Geriatric Medicine* 10 (1994): 445-62.

18. P. Finucane, C. Myser, and S. Ticehurst, "Is She Fit to Sign, Doctor?: Practical Issues in Assessing the Competence of Elderly Patients," *Medical Journal of Australia* 159 (1993): 400-03.

19. B.A. Lustig, "Competence," in *Encyclopedia of Bioethics*, ed. W.T. Reich (New York: Simon & Schuster MacMillan, 1995), 447.

20. L.J. Markson et al., "Physician Assessment of Patient Competence," *Journal of the American Geriatric Society* 42 (1994): 1074-80; T. Grisso and P.S. Appelbaum, "Comparison of Standards for Assessing Patients' Capacities to Make Treatment Decisions," *American Journal of Psychiatry* 152 (1995): 1033-37.

21. M. Freedman, D.T. Stuss, and M. Gordon, "Assessment of Competency: The Role of Neurobehavioral Deficits," *Annals of Internal Medicine* 115 (1991): 203-08.

22. J.S. Janofsky, R.J. McCarthy, and M.F. Folstein, "The Hopkins Competency Assessment Test: A Brief Method for Evaluating Patients' Capacity to Give Informed Consent," *Hospital and Community Psychiatry* 43 (1992): 132-36.

23. L.J. Fitten, R. Lusky, and C. Hamann, "Assessing Treatment Decision-Making Capacity in Elderly Nursing Home Residents," *Journal of the American Geriatric Society* 38 (1990): 1097-1104.

24. C.C. Marson et al., "Assessing the Competency of Patients with Alzheimer's Disease under Different Legal Standards: A Prototype Instrument," *Archives of Neurology* 52 (1995): 949-54.

25. See Howe et al., note 13 above.

26. M. Plumb and J. Holland, "Comparative Studies of Psychological Function in Patients with Advanced Cancer," *Psychosomatic Medicine* 39 (1997): 264-76.

27. M.D. Sullivan and S.J. Youngner, "Depression, Competence, and the Right to Refuse Lifesaving Medical Treatment," *American Journal of Psychiatry* 151 (1994): 971-78.

28. M. Lee and L. Ganzini, "Depression in the Elderly: Effect on Patient Attitudes toward Life-sustaining Therapy," *Journal of the American Geriatric Society* 40 (1992): 983-88.

29. Ibid.

30. M.B. Gerety et al., "Medical Treatment Preferences of Nursing Home Residents: Relationship to Function and Concordance with Surrogate Decision-Makers," *Journal of the American Geriatric Society* 41 (1993): 953-60.

31. See Lee, note 13 above, p. 713.

32. See note 27 above, p. 977.

33. Ibid.

34. J.C. Fletcher et al., "Ethical Considerations in Pediatric Oncology", in *Principles and Practice of Pediatric Oncology*, ed. P.A. Pizzo and D.G. Poplack (Philadelphia: J.B. Lippincott, 1989), 309-20; N.M.P. King and A.W. Cross, "Children as Decisionmakers: Guidelines for Pediatricians," *Journal of Pediatrics* 115 (1989): 10-16; S.L. Leikin, "Minors' Assent or Dissent to Medical Treatment," *Journal of Pediatrics* 102 (1983): 169-76; S. Leikin, "The Role of Adolescents in Decisions Concerning Their Cancer Therapy," *Cancer* 71 (1993): 3342-46.

35. W.G. Bartholome, "Care of the Dying Child: The Demands of Ethics," *Second Opinion* 18 (April 1993): 25-38.

36. D. Brock, "Children's Competence for Health Care Decision-making," in *Children and Health Care: Moral and Social Issues*, ed. L. Kopelman and J. Moskop (Boston: Kluwer Academic, 1989); R.H. Nicholson, "Can Children Permit Research?" *Medical Research with Children: Ethics, Law and Practice* (New York: Oxford University Press, 1986).

37. E. Kluge, "Informed Consent by Children: The New Reality," *Canadian Medical Association Journal* 152 (1995): 1495-97.

38. P. Alderson and J. Montgomery, *Health Care Choices: Making Decisions with Children* (London: Institute for Public Policy Research, 1996).

39. M. Oberman, "Minor Rights and Wrongs," *Journal of Law, Medicine & Ethics* 24 (1996): 127-38.

40. G.M. Ingersoll et al., "Cognitive Maturity, Stressful Events and Metabolic Control Among Diabetic Adolescents," in *Emotion, Cognition, Health and Development in Children and Adolescents*, E.J. Susman, L.V. Feagans, and W.J. Ray, ed. (Hillsdale, N.J.: Erlbaum, 1992), 121-32.

41. See note 39 above, pp. 134-35.

42. Ibid., 135.

43. B.M. Korsh et al., "Non-compliance in Children with Renal Transplants," *Pediatrics* 61 (1978): 874.

44. *In re O'Connor*, 72 N.Y.2d 517, at 533, 531 N.E.2d 607 at 615 (1988).

45. *In re Jobes*, 108 N.S. 394, at 415, 529 A.2d 434 at 445 (1987).

46. S.S. Herr and B.L. Hopkins, "Health Care Decision Making for Persons with Disabilities: An Alternative to Guardianship," *Journal of the American Medical Association* 271 (1994): 1017-22.

47. *Jobes*, 529 A.2d at 451.

48. B. Lo, F. Rouse, and L. Dornband, "Family Decision Making on Trial: Who Decides for Incompetent Patients? *New England Journal of Medicine* 322 (1990): 1228-32.

49. *Code of Virginia*, sec. 54.1-2986.

50. E.J. Emanuel and L.L. Emanuel, "Proxy Decision Making for Incompetent Patients: An Ethical and Empirical Analysis," *Journal of the American Medical Association* 267 (1992): 2067-71.

51. Ibid., 2069-70.

52. "American College of Physicians Ethics Manual. Part 2: The Physician and Society, Research, Life-Sustaining Treatment, Other Issues," *Annals of Internal Medicine* 111 (1989): 327-35.

53. *In re Phillip B*, 92 Cal. App. 3d 796, 156 Cal. Rptr. 48 (1979).

54. S. Van McCrary, W.L. Allen, and C.L. Young, "Questionable Competency of a Surrogate Decision Maker under a Durable Power of Attorney," *The Journal of Clinical Ethics* 4 (1993): 166-68.

55. B. Lo, "Caring for Incompetent Patients: Is There a Physician on the Case?" *Law, Medicine & Health Care* 17 (1989): 214-20.

56. *In Re Karen Quinlan, an Alleged Incompetence*, 70 N.J. 10, 355 A.2d 647 (1976).

57. *Supt. of Belchertown State School v. Saikewicz*, 370 N.E. 2d 417 (Mass. 1977).

58. *Rogers v. Okin*, 478 F. Supp. 1342 (1979), 643 F.2d 650 (1st Cir. 1980).

59. *Cruzan v. Director, Missouri Dept. of Health*, 573 A.2d 1235, at 1246 (D.C. Ct. App. 1990).

60. *In re A.C.*, 497 U.S. 261 (1990).

61. *Florida Dept. of Health and Rehabilitative Services v. Benito Agrelo*, as reported by A. Driscoll, "Teen Shunned Medication," *Miami Herald* 21 August 1994, 1A.

62. See note 4 above, p. 55.

63. "American College of Physicians Ethics Manual," *Annals of Internal Medicine* 117 (1992): 947-60.

64. American Medical Association, Council on Ethical and Judicial Affairs, "Confidential Care of Minors," in *Code of Medical Ethics: Current Opinions with Annotations*, (Chicago: AMA, 1997), ¶ 5.055, 86-87.

65. American Medical Association, Council on Ethical and Judicial Affairs, "The Use of Minors as Organ and Tissue Donors," *Code of Medical Ethics Reports*, vol. 1 (Chicago: AMA, 1994), 231.

6

THE PROCESS OF INFORMED CONSENT

Robert J. Boyle, M.D.

Case Histories

AB is a 35-year-old woman who seeks a surgeon's advice about a mass in her breast. Physical exam and mammography are compatible with carcinoma of the breast. During the initial office visit, the physician presents the patient with this information and discusses with her the current controversy about surgical management of breast cancer--including questions about whether to perform radical mastectomy, modified radical mastectomy, lumpectomy, with or without chemotherapy and with or without radiation therapy. He presents to her his recommendation based on his clinical experience and his interpretation of the literature. He provides her with patient education materials about breast cancer and the various options. He recommends that she discuss the matter with her husband and family and return in one week.

The patient returns with her husband, and they and the surgeon decide to have a lumpectomy performed as soon as possible. The patient's concerns center on the risk of recurrent disease and the disfigurement of the more invasive procedures. The patient is referred to the breast clinic, where the nurse coordinator provides her with additional information about the disease, the planned procedure, what will be done, what the scar will look like, how she will feel after the sur-

gery, what concerns other patients have, and so forth.

AB is admitted to the hospital the morning of the procedure, is interviewed and examined by an anesthesiologist, and is asked to sign a consent for the surgery by the surgical resident.

CD is a 65-year-old man who is transferred from his local hospital to the University Medical Center for evaluation and treatment of a possible cerebral aneurysm. He is seen immediately by a neurosurgeon, whom he has never met before, who states that the patient requires a cerebral arteriogram. The radiologist who is to do the procedure follows along quickly; he discusses the procedure, the risks, and alternatives --all in moderate detail--and asks the patient if he has any questions. The patient at this point is overwhelmed and asks no questions. Shortly before the procedure, a resident asks the patient to read and sign the standard consent form.

I. Introduction

In an observational study of physician-patient interactions in a university medical center, Lidz et al. noted:

1. There was a great variety in what doctors told patients, what patients learned from other

sources, what patients understood, and how decisions were made.

2. The ways in which decisions were made varied from rather close conformity with the legal model in a few situations to a type of decision making that bore almost no resemblance to the legal model. There were a variety of intermediate patterns, some involving a lesser degree of "disclosure" than legally required and some involving a different temporal order of events than contemplated by the legal model.

3. To the extent that actual decision making processes approximated the legally contemplated model, they included one important variable --time--of which the legal model does not take account. Informing and consenting often took place over time, and the greater the degree of patient participation in the process, the more this was so.

4. In general the physician was clearly the dominant actor in terms of making decisions about what treatments, if any, a patient was to have.

    a. The doctor's ordinary role, in practice, was to decide what was to be done and to inform the patient of that decision. Ordinarily that information came in the form of a recommendation; though ... it might be better characterized along a spectrum running from an "order" at one end to a neutral disclosure of alternatives at the other end.

    b. The patient's ordinary role, in practice, was to acquiesce in the physician's recommendation.

5. The decision making process was influenced by the medical setting (surgical outpatient vs. inpatient, medical vs. surgical patient), the type of procedure in question (routine blood drawing vs. a surgical procedure), and the nature of the patient's disorder (acute vs. chronic).[1]

Lidz and colleagues concluded that "disclosure" does not typically occur. Rather, patients learn various bits of information--some relevant to decision making, some not--from doctors' and nurses' efforts

to obtain compliance and from "situational-etiquette" conversations held because "that's what humans do." Patients do not make "decisions"; instead doctors make "recommendations" to patients. "Consent" does not exist. Instead, these authors found "acquiescence," the absence of "objection," or occasionally a "veto."[2]

Lidz and colleagues found in the study discussed above and in an earlier study[3] that when patients are given information about their treatment and treated as if they had decision-making authority, they act in a passive manner. When asked, most patients are happy with the amount of information that they receive. When they said they wanted information to make treatment decisions, they often acted as if they would rather have the doctors decide because of doctors' technical expertise and commitment to the best interest of the patients. Patients felt they were unequal to the task of making medical decisions.

In response to a survey conducted by Harris and Associates, only 10 percent of the patients interviewed saw themselves as having an active role in decision making, 43 percent of the public and 58 percent of physicians described informed consent as informing patients about their condition and recommended treatment. However, while 43 percent of the public closely associated the term with permission or consent to treatment, only 26 percent of physicians interpreted it in that manner. Of physicians, 47 percent described informed consent in terms of explaining treatment risks, while only 8 percent of the public mentioned this aspect. Even fewer physicians (14 percent) included the discussion of alternative treatments in informed consent.[4]

In actual practice, there is a wide variation in what is understood and carried out as "informed consent." Many surgeons believe that the process of informed consent is an externally imposed requirement that is necessary to protect them from lawsuits. Others resent the pressures to describe in detail the possible complications or alternative methods of therapy when evidence exists that patients forget most of what they are told, they often ask no questions, and most accept the surgeon's recommendations. Still others consider informed consent as no more than a hospital form to be signed.[5]

This chapter continues the discussions of disclosure (Chapter 4) and capacity (Chapter 5) as a foundation for the shared decision-making process that is expected in contemporary clinical encounters. Prior to initiating medical or surgical treatment or enrolling subjects into research protocols, clinicians are required ethically and legally to seek consent and to ensure that the consent is informed. As a legal requirement, the burden of ensuring informed consent lies with the physician. However, the ethical standard must recognize informed consent as shared decision making involving the patient, physician, nurse, family, and all those with an ethical interest in the patient. The informed-consent process is typically recognized in the patient's signature of the consent document prior to surgery. However, it must be recognized that this, in fact, represents only one segment of a much broader process. Decision making involves not only high-risk surgical procedures, but also low-risk diagnostic testing in the physician's office and prescribing medication. Decision making may involve a one-time discussion between clinician and patient, a series of discussions in the office prior to hospital admission, or a long-term relationship between clinician and patient.

The mechanics of informed consent for human research protocols have been carefully defined and detailed by governmental and institutional regulation. This area of informed consent is not discussed specifically in this chapter.

II. History of the Concept of Informed Consent

Informed consent is a relatively new concept in medicine. As noted in Chapter 4, the Hippocratic oath does not mention a physician's obligation to converse with patients. The duty was to "follow that system of regimen which according to my ability and judgement I consider for the benefit of my patients." Other Hippocratic writings, in fact, spoke against disclosure. In the ancient Greeks' view, cooperation between physician and patient was important, not for the sake of sharing decision-making burdens, but for the sake of friendship that, in turn, led to trust, obedience, and then to cure.

In the Middle Ages, conversation with patients was intended to comfort, reassure, and induce patients to take the cure. Obviously with what was available to medicine at that time, the choices and results were limited.

By the 18th century, physicians were advocating that the public become more enlightened about medi-

cal matters. However, this enlightenment did not extend to involving parties in shared decision making. Rather, the intent was to bring patients into common cause with the physician against disease and suffering and foster acceptance of the physician's authority.

Nineteenth-century English physician Thomas Percival, in his treatise *Medical Ethics; or A Code of Institutes and Precepts, Adapted to the Professional Conduct of Physicians and Surgeons*, urged physicians to be attentive to the patient's welfare, treating the patient with "attention, steadiness and humanity." However, he did not mention the patient's right to liberty of choice. He recommended care when the patient opposed treatment, not because of concern for the patient's rights, but because of the potential medical complications of using force. He wrote "the prejudices of the sick are not to be condemned or opposed with harshness" because such physician behavior might create "fear, anxiety and watchfulness," which could be a detriment to the patient's recovery.[6]

Percival's *Medical Ethics* later became the basis for the first code of ethics of the American Medical Association (AMA) in 1847.[7] Oblivious to the issue of informed patients, the code asserted that doctors "have a right to expect and require that their patients should entertain a sense of the duties which they owe to their medical attendants." Patients' "obedience . . . should be prompt and implicit."[8]

The doctrine of informed consent began to evolve in the courts after the turn of the 20th century. In 1914, Justice Benjamin Cardozo wrote, "Every human being of adult years and sound mind has a right to determine what shall be done with his own body."[9] The case involved a patient with a uterine growth. She gave consent for an examination under anesthesia, but specifically refused to authorize any additional surgery. When the physician found a tumor, he removed it without the patient's consent. Infection followed the surgery, gangrene set in, and the patient eventually suffered serious long-term morbidity.

In 1957, the courts began to define the legal requirement for consent. In *Salgo v. Leland Stanford, Jr., University Board of Trustees*, the court declared that uninformed consent is not true consent. "A physician violates his duty to his patient and subjects himself to liability if he withholds any facts necessary to form the basis of an intelligent consent by the patient to the proposed treatment."[10] The ruling emphasized disclosure, however, and not the right of the patient to make the decision.

The AMA's code evolved into shorter statements that provided little insight into the respect required of physician-patient interactions. The 1957 code, now called *Principles*, stated, "The prime objective of the medical profession is to render service to humanity with full respect for both the dignity of man and the rights of patients."[11]

The accompanying *Opinions* of the AMA's Judicial Council provided three specific instructions with respect to disclosure and consent:

1. a surgeon is obligated to disclose all facts relevant to the need and performance of the operation;
2. an experimenter is obligated, when using new drugs or treatments, to obtain the "voluntary consent" of the person; and
3. investigators involved in clinical investigations primarily for treatment must "make relevant disclosure and obtain the voluntary consent of patients."[12]

The first provision was added to comply with malpractice law and the other two to comply with congressional legislation on the conduct of research.[13]

By 1980, the *Principles* had changed minimally. However, the *Current Opinions of the Judicial Council* did address the issue of informed consent:

> The patient's right of self-decision can be effectively exercised only if the patient possesses enough information to enable an intelligent choice. The patient should make his own determination on treatment. Informed consent is a basic social policy. . . . Social policy does not accept the paternalistic view that the physician may remain silent because divulgence might prompt the patient to forgo needed therapy. Rational, informed patients should not be expected to act uniformly, even under similar circumstances, in agreeing to or refusing treatment.[14]

The forces and "social policy" that shaped the doctrine of informed consent at this time included the civil liberties revolution, the movement for consumer rights and advocacy, media coverage of medical is-

sues, and consumers who were better informed about treatments and alternatives.

III. Elements of Informed Consent

Valid informed consent requires the presence of multiple, interrelated elements:[15]

- threshold elements (preconditions)
  1. capacity (to understand and decide)
  2. voluntariness (in deciding)
- information elements
  1. disclosure (of material information)
  2. recommendation (of a plan)
  3. understanding (of disclosure and recommendation)
- consent elements
  1. decision (in favor of a plan)
  2. authorization (of the chosen plan)

A. Threshold

1. Capacity

Valid consent requires a capable decision maker, as defined in Chapter 5.

2. Voluntariness

Voluntariness implies exercising choice that is free of coercion or other forms of controlling influences by other persons. Beauchamp and Childress note that "control over another person is necessarily an influence, but not all influences are controlling."[16] In a broad context, influence may include both positive and negative influences: acts of love, threats, education, lies, manipulative suggestions, emotional appeals, bedside vigil, and so forth.

Beauchamp and Childress define three categories of influence: coercion, persuasion, and manipulation. *Coercion* occurs when one person intentionally uses an actual threat of harm or force to influence another (for example, the threat of abandonment or refusal to do procedure X if procedure Y is not agreed to as well). With *persuasion*, a patient is convinced to consent through the merits of reasons advanced by another person. With their recommendation of a plan of care, clinicians almost always persuade the patient to some degree toward one choice based on physicians' knowledge and expertise. If a patient refuses or is uncertain about a procedure or treatment that offers significant benefits to the patient, the clinician has an obligation to continue to inform and work with the patient. How intense the activity becomes determines when it becomes a negative influence. *Manipulation* represents attempts to influence that are neither coercion nor persuasion. Here the influence usually occurs with informational manipulation--playing with the data to change a person's understanding. Here the model begins to overlap with the disclosure element.

In fact, rarely, if ever, is a patient entirely free from various pressures. "Fully voluntary choice" is an ideal. We make decisions in a context of competing needs, familial interests, legal obligations, persuasive arguments, religious beliefs, and so forth. However, if pressure from a clinician, family members, religious groups, or others is difficult for the patient to resist, valid informed consent does not occur. For example, a patient who is pressured by members of his religious group to refuse treatments, or a potential bone marrow or organ donor who is badgered by the potential recipient and his family to proceed with donation, would present challenges to the voluntary element of consent. Consent must be a situation in which there are "no strings attached."

Clinicians have a responsibility to be aware of situations when voluntariness is threatened. Others involved with the patient have a responsibility to refrain from coercion, even subtle coercion, and to allow the patient to make his or her decision freely.

B. Information

1. Disclosure

The clinician is obligated to disclose to the patient or surrogate the information necessary to make an informed judgment. The disclosure should include information on the following:

1. the nature of the therapy;
2. the purpose;
3. the risks and consequences;
4. the benefits;
5. the probability that the therapy will be successful;
6. the feasible alternatives; and
7. the prognosis if the therapy is not given.

The clinician is not required to list every possible risk. Patient CD, in the case history given at the beginning of this chapter, seemed overwhelmed by the amount of information presented to him in a brief period of time.

The legal doctrine of informed consent defines two standards of disclosure: the *professional standard* and the *reasonable-person standard*. These standards have been criticized as either too clinician-centered or too vague to be useful for clinical care. The professional standard requires that the physician disclose only what other physicians would disclose in a similar situation. Although some states still hold this standard, many believe that this paternalistic, physician-centered approach undermines patients' autonomy.[17] Cases such as *Canterbury v. Spence* have led some states to adopt a reasonable-person standard. In *Canterbury*, a surgeon failed to disclose risks of neurologic injury following a laminectomy, describing them as "not any more [risky] than any operation."[18] The court concluded that, although the likelihood of injury was relatively low, the potential severity of harm (paralysis and loss of function) required more elaborate disclosures to be made. The ruling allowed the jury to decide whether the informed consent requirement was violated. If an "average, reasonable person" would decline to proceed with treatment in the face of fully disclosed risks, the physician who fails to make appropriate disclosures can be liable for any injuries that follow the treatment provided.

The reasonable-person standard, while defined in the legal framework in some jurisdictions, has been criticized as impossible to satisfy. What the reasonable person needs to know depends very much on the patient's particular circumstances at the time. It does not provide the clinician much assistance in defining what must be disclosed. From this discussion has evolved the *subjective standard*, which requires the clinician to disclose whatever information is material to the particular patient, in a particular situation or context. If patients have a right to make idiosyncratic choices, they may need information that would not be considered significant by the profession or the average person.[19] The concert pianist might certainly prefer much more information about risks of hand surgery than another patient about to undergo the same procedure. Some patients may require the detail listed in a drug package insert before agreeing to a particular course of medication.

In the usual case, the risks and benefits that most "average reasonable patients" would prefer to have explained should be explained. The clinician is not required to list every possible, extremely rare or theoretical risk. To do so may be counterproductive to the entire decision-making process. The severity of the risk must also be considered. For example, the risk of paralysis associated with a laminectomy (*Canterbury*), although only 1 percent, should be disclosed, whereas it may not be necessary to disclose the risk of a hematoma following venipuncture.

If communication is effective and the patient is truly a partner in the process, then the extent of disclosure should be apparent from the questions and concerns of the patient, the patient's situation, and so forth. The clinician's judgment about what to disclose is still important, but that judgment should be based on his or her interaction with the patient and not a predetermined script.

Brody has proposed a model--*transparency*--for disclosure in informed consent not based on previous standards. The clinician discusses why the proposed treatment is recommended over the alternatives, the patient is allowed to ask questions suggested by the disclosure of the clinician's reasoning, and those questions are answered to the patient's satisfaction. Disclosure is adequate when the clinician's basic thinking has been rendered transparent to the patient. The clinician engages in the typical thought process involved in the management of patients, only he or she does it aloud in language understandable to the patient.[20]

The case of *Moore v. Regents of the University of California*[21] presented a different issue related to disclosure. Mr. Moore was diagnosed with a rare leukemia. His physician recommended a splenectomy, and Moore consented to the procedure. The physician obtained portions of the spleen and eventually established a patented cell line with a potential market value of several billion dollars. The physician requested that Moore continue to see him periodically for checkups, at which time additional blood, skin, bone marrow, and sperm were collected (some of which were to be used for research). The California Supreme Court eventually concluded that Moore had no property interests in his excised spleen, but the court did recognize that the physician had failed to disclose his research interest in the spleen and subsequent samples.

The court concluded that doctors have a duty to inform patients of research interests deriving from treatment, that a person's consent to treatment requires complete information, and the physician has a duty to disclose all information that is relevant to a patient's decision, including research or economic interests.

According to Veatch:

The implications [of this evolution] are enormous. It means that, in principle, no professional can determine what to disclose to a patient by introspecting about what he or she would want to know in that circumstance. It also means that the question cannot be answered by turning to one's colleagues or examining what is normally disclosed in similar circumstances. If the principle of autonomy is the foundation of the informed consent doctrine, then patients will have to be told what ever they reasonably want to know, even if it is not normal practice for that information to be disclosed.[22]

The recent controversy among the Centers for Disease Control and Prevention, Congress, and numerous professional societies about informing patients of clinicians' human immunodeficiency virus (HIV) status adds another element to this discussion. How much is the clinician obligated to tell the patient about personal issues that may place the patient at increased risk? *Behringer v. The Medical Center at Princeton* explored the status of someone who was both an HIV positive patient and a surgeon. As a patient, the individual had the same right to privacy as anyone else, and improper disclosures of his condition led to liability for the hospital. At the same time, the court upheld the hospital policy requiring him, as a condition of surgical privileges, to disclose his HIV-positive status to patients during the informed consent process.[23]

In *Hidding v. Williams*, a malpractice action in which the patient agreed to surgery in the absence of informed consent, the court reached two critical conclusions. First, the fact that the patient signed a form for informed consent did not relieve the doctor of liability when he--and the form--failed to disclose significant risks of surgery to the patient. Second, the surgeon's chronic alcohol abuse should have been revealed to the patient; failure to make this disclosure constituted a violation of the requirement of informed consent.[24]

In the future, will physicians be required to disclose other information--such as a history of substance abuse, mental illness, or performance measures such as infection rates or malpractice history--because this information may be material to a patient's decision?[25]

2. Recommendation

It is important in most circumstances that the clinician, having disclosed the necessary information about the proposed therapy and its alternatives, make a recommendation. This is the clinician's area of education and expertise, and this is why the patient seeks care from the clinician. In fact, disclosure of information is often less important than the clinician's recommendation. Recommendations may be far more meaningful to the patient than results of empirical studies.[26] With the recognition of patient autonomy and the progressive development of the concept of informed consent, it is apparent that at times the message has been exaggerated. Patients are presented with lists of options and told "it's your decision." Patients may feel lost, abandoned, overwhelmed by the issues, and confused by the uncertainty. With a shared approach, the patient seeks the clinician's advice, but is free to reject the recommendation, ask for a second opinion, and investigate other alternatives.

3. Understanding

The information obviously must be disclosed in a manner a particular patient can understand. Huge amounts of technical information and medical jargon may overwhelm or confuse most patients and would not validly inform them. The clinician should recognize that words may have special meaning or no meaning for the patient. Illness, anxiety, or borderline capacity may also influence understanding. The clinician should confirm that patients understand by asking them to describe in their own words the medical problem and the proposed therapies. The question "Do you understand?" may not provide this validation. This emphasis upon patients' understanding may be especially important in pediatric or geriatric patients, those with limitations of intelligence, or those with negative experiences with the medical system.

In the case history at the beginning of this chapter, the validity of CD's consent should be questioned on the basis of his understanding what was disclosed. Time, repetition, and innovative teaching techniques (videotapes or brochures) may also dramatically improve the patient's understanding.

C. Consent

1. Decision

After consideration and discussion, a process that in many cases may occur over time and with one or several clinicians, the patient makes a decision about treatment or a plan of care. The patient may, at any time, change his or her decision. However, the decision must be in the context of what the alternatives are. For example, if a patient is offered a choice of treating mild hypertension or undergoing further observation, the patient cannot choose what specific drug she wants to take; that decision is the physician's.

2. Authorization

The patient must do more than express agreement or comply with a proposal. He or she must authorize a professional to do something through an act of informed and voluntary consent.[27]

IV. Exceptions to the Requirement for Informed Consent

The following exceptions to the requirement for informed consent have been recognized:

1. *Emergency*: When the patient is in a life-threatening situation and unable to consent.
2. *Incapacity*: When the patient is unable to consent; the process must involve the surrogate decision maker.
3. *Patient waiver*: When the patient waives the right to know: "I don't want to know. Just do what you think is best." The physician must be certain that this is, in fact, what the patient wants.
4. *Therapeutic privilege*: When informing poses a significant threat to the patient's well-being, not because it will make the patient feel upset or depressed. Therapeutic privilege should be invoked

only in rare circumstances. (For a discussion of the concept of therapeutic privilege, see Chapter 4.)

5. *National/state waivers*: When the federal or state government waives informed consent for vaccination programs, newborn genetic screening, and so forth.

V. Implementing Informed Consent

Valid informed consent in our medical system may be difficult. This is especially so in a tertiary-care center where care is so specialized. A patient's care may involve many different professionals who have very brief contact with the patient and no opportunity to form a relationship with the patient. (Malpractice studies confirm the problem of lack of patient-clinician relationship.)

Lidz[28] defines two models for informed consent based on different types of medical care:

1. *Event model*, in which the clinician meets the patient, explains the procedure, obtains the patient's consent and signature (for example, the case of CD).
2. *Process model*, in which the patient and clinician establish individual responsibilities (for example, the case of AB). Several questions may arise with this model. What is the clinician's role--primary clinician or consultant? What is the clinician's area of expertise? What is the anticipated duration of care?

In the process model of informed consent, the patient's problem is defined in dialogue (Katz uses the metaphor "conversation"[29]) between clinician and patient. Does the patient agree with what the clinician thinks the problem is? They set goals, (such as curing the disease or treating the symptoms). Finally, they select appropriate therapy using the elements of information and consent discussed above.

VI. Other Considerations

A. Children as Decision Makers: Assent/Dissent

The recognition of the progressive capacity of the older child and adolescent to participate in decision making, the desire to enhance the child's autonomy

and skill as a decision maker, and the recognition of the child's need to know the diagnosis and proposed treatment have led to an increased role in decision making for the child-patient (see Chapter 5). Clinicians and parents have an obligation to involve a child as that specific child is able--from encouraging participation in decisions (the younger child) to granting full decision-making power (the adolescent over 14 years of age).[30]

The term *assent* was suggested in the mid-1970s by a national commission on human research to distinguish a child's agreement to treatment from a legally valid consent, which can only be given by a competent adult.[31] The American Academy of Pediatrics suggests that *assent* should include at least the following elements:

1. Helping the patient achieve a developmentally appropriate awareness of the nature of his or her condition;
2. Telling the patient what he or she can expect with tests and treatments;
3. Making a clinical assessment of the patient's understanding of the situation and the factors influencing how he or she is responding (including whether there is inappropriate pressure to accept testing or therapy);
4. Soliciting an expression of the patient's willingness to accept the proposed care. Regarding this final point . . . no one should solicit a patient's views without intending to weigh them seriously. In situations in which the patient will have to receive medical care despite his or her objection, the patient should be told that fact and should not be deceived.[32]

The child's situation influences each of the elements of consent. The clinician must present information in a manner suited to the child's developmental level. Parents should be able to assist, but in some cases they may be too close to the situation to assess the child's status accurately. Other professionals (such as pediatrician, nurse, child psychiatrist/psychologist, or social worker) may provide important insight into a particular child's developmental level and comprehension of the information presented.

Children render the voluntary consent element problematic. The risk of coercion is much higher in the parent-child relationship. Younger children are less likely to assert themselves against their parents; they tend to acquiesce to and attempt to please those in authority, while adolescents may do the opposite. Intervention by the clinician, an outsider, in situations where the family's influence seems excessive may be very difficult. The clinician's relationship with the family and understanding of the family's values and culture, and the family's previous experience with the child's decision making are important. At times; it may be necessary for the clinician to confront the family with the issue. Chapter 10 discusses in more detail the issues surrounding parents' role and rights in decision making for children of all ages.

Some jurisdictions have given children much broader rights of decision making (see Chapter 5). The American Academy of Pediatrics suggests that clinicians seek the assent of the school-age patient as well as informed permission of the parent for procedures such as venipuncture for diagnostic study in a 9 year old, psychotropic medication for attention-deficit disorder in an 8 year old, or an orthopedic device for scoliosis in an 11 year old. For older children and adolescents, the organization encourages the clinician to seek informed consent from the patient for a pelvic examination in a 16 year old, long-term antibiotics for severe acne in a 15 year old, or diagnostic evaluation for recurrent headache in an 18 year old.[33]

B. The Nurse's Role

The role of the nurse in informed consent is complex and will become progressively more so as nursing and its collegial relationship with physicians evolve. In Lidz's observational study, nurses obtained the patients' signatures on consent forms, a practice that is rapidly changing. However, probably more significantly, nurses provided a major portion of information about treatment.[34] In fact, in many situations the nurse spends more time than the physician talking with the patient, either in a formal educational process or in informal bedside conversation. The paradox is that, in our current environment, physicians and not nurses make decisions about treatment. In this role as patient educator, the potential exists for nurses to appear to challenge the traditional authority of the physician. The discussion of risks, which a physician might not have disclosed, may seem to question the physician's recommendation. There is no doubt, how-

ever, that the active role of nurses in educating patients certainly furthers the goal of informed consent. The nurse's role includes evaluation of the process of informed consent: adequacy of disclosure, the patient's understanding, capacity, and voluntariness. Anyone with concerns about an invalid or questionable informed consent should present those concerns to the individual primarily responsible for the consent.

C. The Consent Form

The consent form is often the focus of the process, but in fact it should only be a written record of a process of disclosure and discussion. A signed form alone does not represent valid consent legally or ethically.

VII. Ethical and Legal Dimensions of Other Landmark Cases

In addition to the cases noted above, a number of others have further expanded the legal doctrine of informed consent.

Natanson v. Kline, in which the physician failed to disclose the risks of radiation therapy, defined the "professional standard."[35] This standard assumes the physician "knows best" about what should be disclosed to the patient.

In *Cobbs v. Grant*, Mr. Cobb suffered from a duodenal ulcer that required surgery. The surgeon, Dr. Grant, explained the nature of the operation with the patient but did not discuss any of the inherent risks. After surgery, Cobb developed abdominal bleeding due to a tear in the splenic artery. He later developed a new ulcer that required further surgery. Finally he required additional surgery for bleeding due to suture failure. All of these complications were identified subsequently as potential risks from the initial and subsequent procedures. The court reasoned that the surgeon's failure to inform may have constituted a violation of the physician's duty. The patient sought disclosure of information about risks and alternatives that the "reasonable" person would find significant in deciding whether to consent to or refuse treatment.[36]

Mohr v. Williams resulted in a plaintiff's judgment against a physician who had obtained consent to operate on the patient's right ear. After the patient was anesthetized, the physician decided to operate instead on the left ear. The court ruled there was no urgent need to proceed without consulting the patient.[37]

In *Arato v. Avedon*, the Supreme Court of California ruled that the physician was not obligated to disclose statistical life-expectancy information to a patient with pancreatic cancer. In recommending a course of chemotherapy and radiation treatment, none of the treating physicians specifically disclosed the high mortality rate for this type of cancer. The patient ultimately died. The physicians justified the nondisclosure on the grounds that it was medically inappropriate given the patient's anxiety, the risk of depriving any hope of cure, and the problem of predictive data when applied to a specific patient.[38] The patient had been informed that the type of cancer he had was usually fatal.

VIII. Ethical Grounding for Informed Consent

As with capacity, the patient's right to participate actively in medical decision making is based on the principle of autonomy. Individual autonomy must be respected as long as the individual's actions do not infringe on the autonomous actions of others. The person has the right to self-governance--personal rule of the self by adequate understanding, while remaining free from controlling interference by others and from personal limitations that prevent choice. To respect an autonomous agent is to recognize that person's capacities and perspective, including his or her right to hold certain views and to take certain actions based on personal values and beliefs. In the realm of informed consent, autonomy requires the patient to do more than yield to, express agreement with, acquiesce in, or comply with an arrangement or a proposal.[39]

In tension with the principle of autonomy in informed consent is the traditional clinician-patient relationship in decision making, in which the clinician makes the decision for the patient. In this traditional relationship, the clinician was acting in the patient's best interest and was committed to "doing no harm." Clinicians' decisions were based in good faith on their training and medical knowledge. Indeed, the doctrine of informed consent should not and does not question the clinician's integrity or dedication. One could argue that the traditional clinician-patient relationship

in decision making was based on the principle of beneficence, "doing good" for the patient. There is still an element of beneficence in this relationship, but it must be balanced to prevent paternalism. Paternalism is defined as "the interference with a person's freedom of action or freedom of information, or the deliberate dissemination of misinformation";[40] "substitution of one person's judgement for another's."[41] Paternalism dictates the view that physicians should assume the entire burden of deciding what treatment any patient in whatever condition should undergo, because only clinicians have the necessary medical information and skill. They are the experts.

The tension between autonomy and beneficence allows us to define the patient's and clinician's roles as compatible with both. The clinician's role is to:

1. determine the patient's problem, in cooperation with the patient;
2. determine how the problem can be treated;
3. determine the risks and benefits of the possible therapy; and
4. communicate this information to the patient.

The clinician's role is primarily cognitive, medical, and technical.

The patient's role is to use the information in the context of his or her own personal values and subjective preferences in order to make a decision. The patient's role is primarily affective, personal, and subjective.[42] The patient brings something to the process that the clinician cannot know: an understanding of his or her individual priorities, needs, concerns, beliefs, and fears. The need for informed consent is an acknowledgment that a medical procedure or act is meant to be done "for" and not "to" a person.[43]

IX. Statements by Authoritative Bodies

According to the President's Commission for the Study of Ethical Problems in Medicine and Biomedical and Behavioral Research:

The ethical foundation of informed consent can be traced to the promotion of two values: personal well-being and self-determination. To ensure that these values are respected and enhanced, the commission finds that patients who have the capacity to make decisions about their care must be permitted to do so voluntarily and must have all relevant information regarding their condition and alternative treatments, including possible benefits, risks, costs, other consequences and significant uncertainties surrounding any of this information.[44]

According to the American Hospital Association's *Patient Bill of Rights*:

The patient has the right to obtain from his physician complete current information concerning his diagnosis, treatment, and prognosis in terms the patient can be reasonably expected to understand. . . .

The patient has the right to receive from his physician information necessary to give informed consent prior to the start of any procedure/treatment. Except in emergencies, such information for informed consent should include but not necessarily be limited to the specific procedure/treatment, the medically significant risks involved, and the probable duration of incapacitation. Where medically significant alternatives for care or treatment exist, or when the patient requests information concerning alternatives, the patient has the right to such information.[45]

According to the American Nurses Association's *Code for Nurses*:

Truthtelling and the process of reaching informed choice underlie the exercise of self-determination, which is basic to respect for persons. Clients should be as fully involved as possible in the planning and implementation of their own health care. Clients have the moral right to determine what will be done with their own person; to be given accurate information and all the information necessary for making informed judgements; to be assisted with weighing the benefits and burdens of options in their treatment; to accept, refuse, or terminate treatment without coercion; and to be given necessary emotional support. Each nurse has an obligation to be knowledgeable about the moral and legal rights of all clients and to protect and support those rights. In situations in which

the client lacks the capacity to make a decision, a surrogate decision maker should be designated.[46]

In its 1992 *Code of Medical Ethics*, the American Medical Association stated: "The patient has the right to make decisions regarding the health care that is recommended by his or her physician. Accordingly, patients may accept or refuse any recommended medical treatment."[47]

The Council on Ethical and Judicial Affairs, of the American Medical Association defines the following statement:

8.08 INFORMED CONSENT. The patient's right of self-decision can be effectively exercised only if the patient possesses enough information to enable an intelligent choice. The patient should make his own determination on treatment. The physician's obligation is to present the medical facts accurately to the patient or to the individual responsible for his care and to make recommendations for management in accordance with good medical practice. The physician has an ethical obligation to help the patient make choices from among the therapeutic alternatives consistent with good medical practice. Informed consent is a basic social policy for which exceptions are permitted (1) where the patient is unconscious or otherwise incapable of consenting and harm from failure to treat is imminent; or (2) when risk-disclosure poses such a serious psychological threat of detriment to the patient as to be medically contraindicated. Social policy does not accept the paternalistic view that the physician may remain silent because divulgence might prompt the patient to forgo needed therapy.

8.12 PATIENT INFORMATION. The physician must properly inform the patient of the diagnosis and of the nature and purpose of the treatment undertaken or prescribed. The physician may not refuse to so inform the patient.[48]

The American College of Physicians issued the following statement in 1992:

The physician is obligated to ensure that the patient or, where appropriate, the surrogate be adequately informed about the nature of the patient's medical condition, the objectives of the proposed treatment, treatment alternatives, possible outcomes, and the risks involved.

The doctrine of informed consent goes beyond the question of whether consent was given for a treatment or intervention. Rather, it focuses on the content of that consent. The physician is required to provide enough information to allow a patient to make an informed judgement about how to proceed. The physician's presentation should be understandable to the patient, should be unbiased, and should include the physician's recommendation. The patient's (or surrogate's) concurrence must be free and uncoerced.

In most medical encounters, when the patient presents to a physician for evaluation and care, consent can be presumed. The underlying condition and treatment options are explained to the patient, and treatment is rendered and not refused. In medical emergencies, consent to treatment necessary to maintain life or restore health can generally be implied, unless it is known that the patient would refuse the intervention.[49]

X. Guidelines for Healthcare Professionals

Decisions in healthcare ultimately rest with capable and informed patients, in a context of shared decision making with clinicians and family. An ethically valid informed consent has seven necessary elements, discussed in Section III of this chapter: (1) capacity, (2) voluntariness, (3) disclosure, (4) recommendation, (5) understanding, (6) decision, and (7) authorization.

XI. Cases for Further Study

Case I: "The Placebo"

Mr. X was a 65-year-old, retired army officer who had been very successful in the military and in teaching and research. He had undergone several abdominal operations for gallstones, postoperative adhesions, and bowel obstructions. He was somewhat depressed because of chronic pain. He had lost weight, had poor hygiene, and had withdrawn socially because it was necessary for him to assume awkward or embarrassing postures in order to control his pain. He had used Talwin six times a day for more than two years to control the pain, but he had so much tissue and muscle damage that he had trouble finding injection sites. And Talwin may itself be addictive.

Stating that his goal was "to get more out of life in spite of my pain," Mr. X voluntarily entered a psychiatric ward, where his treatment included individual behavior therapy programs, daily group therapy, and so forth. Mr. X reduced his Talwin usage to four times a day, and he insisted that this level was necessary to control his pain. After considerable discussion with their colleagues, the therapists decided to withdraw the Talwin over time without the patient's knowledge by diluting it with increasing proportions of normal saline. Although Mr. X experienced nausea, diarrhea, and cramps, he thought that these withdrawal symptoms were actually the result of Elavil (amitriptyline), which the therapists had introduced to relieve the withdrawal symptoms.

Self-control techniques were continued, and the intervals between injections were increased. Although the patient was aware of the changes in intervals, he was not aware that he was receiving only saline. The therapists justified this deceptive use of a placebo on the grounds of its effectiveness: "We felt ethically obliged to use a treatment that had a high probability of success. To withhold the procedure may have protected some standard of openness but may not have been in his best interests. We saw no option without ethical problems." As a member of this team caring for Mr X, do you agree with the treatment approach?

[Source: Adapted from T.L. Beauchamp and J.F. Childress, *Principles of Biomedical Ethics*, 3rd ed. (New York: Oxford University Press, 1989), 406-07. Original source: P. Levendusky and L. Pankratz, "Self Control Techniques as an Alternative to Pain Medication," *Journal of Abnormal Psychology* 84 (1975): 165-68.]

Case 2: "Terry Adolphson"

The physician is a clinician who must make decisions on the basis of probabilities. Most patients, however, have little experience with this method of decisionmaking and are often unwilling to accept the uncertainty of medicine. If I express doubt that a particular diagnosis or treatment is completely reliable, this doubt may seem to my patient that I am not competent, or haven't been thorough, or don't care. Almost all decisions in medicine are made (whether consciously or not) on the basis of probabilities. When I am quite explicit about this process, it can become--even with sophisticated patients--a time-consuming matter, and the pressures of my schedule, if nothing else, often made me want to pull back from such explanations.

Terry Adolphson, for instance, was a 36-year-old friend with a terrible family history of heart disease: all the male family members on his father's side had died with heart attacks before the age of forty. Terry had recently developed pain in the chest, or angina, suggesting that he too had a serious disease of the coronary arteries, the small blood vessels leading to the heart, a disease that could progress to a heart attack and quite possibly death. Recent articles in the medical literature had suggested that certain patients with angina not only had better pain relief but also lived longer if they had coronary-artery bypass surgery than if they were treated only with medicines. On the other hand, these patients had a definite chance of dying during surgery.

To complicate matters further, even the process of examining Terry to discover whether he had disease in the arteries which should be operated upon required a special examination of the coronary arteries (coronary arteriography). There was a small (usually less than 1 percent) chance of heart attack and even death during such an examination.

As I discussed the situation with Terry, I realized that in order to recommend this single test, I had to review with him some very complicated medical studies. There were, at the time, differences of opinion among leading cardiologists about who should receive coronary bypass surgery, since the studies had not yet shown convincingly that such surgery was advantageous. Two studies of which I was aware had followed for five years patients who had symptomatic and arteriographically proven heart disease. In each study, the patients were randomly divided into two groups. One group had surgery, and the other was treated only with medicine. The studies showed that for blockages in certain coronary arteries there was no real difference in survival between the surgical and nonsurgical groups; in some cases the nonsurgical group even did better. However, for blockages in other coronary arteries--the left main artery, for example--a greater number of patients were alive five years later in the subgroup that chose surgery than in the subgroup that was treated with medicine alone.

Terry and I reviewed the reasons for his undergoing the coronary arteriography and the chances of his dying during the examination. Since there was no reason even to consider the arteriography test unless he was interested in surgery, we went over the studies that seemed to show advantage for the surgical treatment of some patients. We examined what the litera-

ture had to say about the statistical chances of dying during the surgery, as well as the chances of surviving with or without the surgery. I realized that I was not merely informing Terry about a complex disease involving complex therapy but also about a method of decision making which, though routine in medical circles, was quite alien to him. Medical science could only report what had happened to groups of other people; these statistical "certainties" could not be translated into an individual certainty--into a reliable prediction for Terry. The discussion was time-consuming and therefore expensive. It took him several days just to absorb the concepts.

My only alternative (on the surface, the easier path) would have been to ignore this reasoning process and tell him: "I, as your physician and friend, recommend that you have this operation. Trust me." But the situation was not at all black and white. It involved not only uncertainties but values. Did Terry wish to take a chance on death resulting from an "unnatural" surgical intervention or on "natural" death as a result of avoiding surgery? Did he wish to risk a smaller chance of dying sooner (with the surgery) or a larger chance of dying in the indefinite future? Although I could interpret the medical information for Terry so that he could understand it, ultimately he had to take responsibility for the decision.

Even so, I did not share with Terry certain more complex uncertainties. I decided not to complicate the discussion further by reminding Terry of the uncertain nature of any statistical analysis. Perhaps even the studies that showed improvement after surgery were the result of coincidence or of some unknown difference between the surgical and nonsurgical groups. A statistical analysis of the studies could tell me there was only a 5 percent chance that the results were due to coincidence, but we could not be 100 percent sure even that the studies were reliable. Nothing seems 100 percent sure in medicine! But Terry had enough uncertainty in his life. I chose to keep my "5 percent probabilities" to myself.

Terry decided, after much thought and consultation, to proceed with the coronary arteriography, and it indeed showed a blockage in those coronary arteries which, the statistics indicated, it would be advantageous to bypass. He had the surgery, but the first nine months after the operation were difficult. Symptoms continued, a repeat coronary angiogram was required, and there was much uncertainty about the wisdom of surgery. Had I initially talked Terry into the surgery by insisting that he trust me, that trust would have been severely threatened by all the unforeseen complications he experienced. Instead, he was able to face his future with some equanimity because he had made a reasonable decision based on adequate, if sometimes frustrating, information.

[Source: Reprinted from D. Hilficker, *Healing the Wounds* (New York: Pantheon Books, 1985), 64-67.]

Case 3: "Whose Choice Really?"

WL is a 22-year-old man who worked as a farm laborer. He is married with one child. The patient first noted a swelling on his left hip about 15 months earlier. It was tender but caused no impairment in his daily work. Approximately five months ago he began to experience pain in his left leg and some restriction in its use. Soon thereafter he noted a swelling in his abdomen. He consulted a general practitioner in a nearby town and was referred to a cancer center 300 miles from his home.

Diagnostic evaluation established that he suffered from a bone cancer arising in the ridge of the left hip. The cancer had extended along the pelvic bone and across the middle of the abdomen. Workup for metastases was negative. The extent of the tumor precluded surgical resection. The patient was placed on a protocol of front-line experimental chemotherapy, but within two months there was documented progression of the tumor. With the failure of this regimen, it was no longer realistic to hope that he could be cured. However, physicians believed that alternative chemotherapy might achieve temporary remission of the disease, and the patient was switched to escalating doses of methotrexate.

At this time, the management of his pain had become a significant problem. He requires very high doses of morphine and Dilaudid, which are often insufficient to provide adequate pain control but cause him to slip in and out of a clouded state of consciousness. The fact that he has not yet developed lung metastases and the observation that the tumor is growing slowly has led the clinicians to suspect that he might survive for as long as a year. Given this prospect, physicians are deeply concerned about long-term pain control. Because WL is in relatively constant and often severe pain, he is pressing the staff for more adequate pain management.

There are three options for improving control of the pain. One is to amputate his left leg by performing a hemipelvectomy. This would remove the leg in which intense pain is occurring and reduce the amount of tumor in the abdomen. Substantial pain relief, after surgical recovery, could be expected, although recurrence of pain would be expected with further spread of the disease. Some rehabilitation would be necessary, such as learning to use crutches.

A neurosurgical consultant has suggested two other options. One is to control pain through nerve-block procedures. This would require a series of procedures in which specific nerve roots are exposed to chemicals that impair their ability to conduct pain impulses. The results of each procedure would be used to determine what additional nerve roots might be blocked to achieve additional pain relief. Completion of this process might require several weeks. Although nerve-block procedures carry less than a 10 percent risk of urinary bladder and bowel incontinence, there may be motor weakness in the affected limb. The neurosurgeon thinks it unlikely that WL's pain could be completely controlled in this way, but it is reasonable to expect a very substantial reduction in WL's need for analgesics.

The other neurosurgical approach involves performing a cordotomy, a procedure that surgically severs nerve tracts responsible for pain conduction. The neurosurgeon believes that the procedure, performed at the level of the 12th thoracic vertebra, is virtually certain to produce complete pain relief. The patient would be able to leave the hospital within a few days after the operation. However, there are side effects. Although sensation of touch, vibration, and position are preserved, sensation of temperature is eliminated. More importantly, the surgeon estimates an 80 percent chance of urinary bladder and bowel incontinence.

As WL's physician, you are faced with how to manage the process of informed consent. There are significant trade-offs among the options for treatment. How the patient might assess these options would depend on his reaction to the specific benefits and problems associated with each treatment. For example, if complete pain relief were his overriding and exclusive concern, the cordotomy would be the obvious choice. By contrast, if he were hesitant to risk impotence and the loss of bladder function willing to accept an extended hospitalization away from his family, he might choose to have the nerve blocks. You could remain neutral, helping the patient compare the alternatives and allow WL to make the final choice. On the other hand, you could be more directive.

WL has shown a clear proclivity toward surgical removal of his tumor. Although his doctors explained the uselessness of surgical resection for curing his disease before they initiated chemotherapy, the patient continues to ask frequently about surgery. He seems to view it as a decisive, one-shot approach to the removal of the tumor and the relief of his pain, which does not carry the chronic suffering (nausea, vomiting, and so forth) associated with chemotherapy. WL also has some difficulty understanding how chemotherapy works. He has a common-sense understanding of cutting a tumor out, but the idea of "melting it away" with drugs is confusing, and he has little confidence in this mode of treatment. In preliminary discussions, he seemed to lean toward the hemipelvectomy for these inappropriate reasons, despite the fact that the procedure would be mutilating and would provide only temporary pain control.

A second concern is that WL's preference seems to vary with the intensity of his pain. On several occasions when his pain was especially severe and had persisted for several hours, he said that cordotomy would probably be the best step to take. However, when he had achieved moderate pain relief, he expressed much deeper concern about being rendered impotent and incontinent by the cordotomy. At these times he was also less inclined to undergo the hemipelvectomy. As a result, he seemed to favor a series of nerve blocks. Thus, there is legitimate concern that his choice might reflect how tolerable his pain is on a given day, rather than a careful weighing of the risks and benefits of each option.

You and your team are also concerned about the patient's needs in the coming months before his death and about WL's ability to genuinely appreciate those needs at this time. You believe that his most serious need will be for pain relief. You expect his pain to worsen with time. Only the cordotomy would ensure complete pain control without heavy use of analgesics. If performed, it would reduce the physical drain of pain-related suffering and allow him more quality time to share with his family. The patient's other need is to be reunited with his family. They have little money, and his wife has been unable to visit during this hospitalization. The remaining period before his death is limited, so spending time at home is quite important. Moreover, the patient's degree of suffering might decline if he could be with his wife, child, and extended family. Again, either alternative to the cordotomy would require an additional hospitalization of several weeks. With the cordotomy, he could return to his family within several days.

You wish to respect the patient's choice, but you are concerned about these various impairments of the patient's capacity to make a decision based on his own values and interests. WL is typically very quiet, cooperative, and deeply respectful of the authority of the nurses and physicians, and he could be easily persuaded to undergo the cordotomy with directive and persuasive recommendations. How should you proceed?

[Source: Adapted from T.F. Ackerman and S. Strong, *A Casebook of Medical Ethics* (New York: Oxford University Press, 1989), 14-17.]

XII. Study Questions

1. What is the difference between the "event" model of informed consent and the "process" model of informed consent? What sorts of medical situations would justify either approach?
2. What do you think of Brody's "transparency" model of informed consent? What are its strengths and/ or weaknesses?
3. Consider again Case 1 in Chapter 3, "Cocaine Use and Patient Self-Report." Evaluate the study described in this case in terms of its compliance with the doctrine of informed consent. Are there different standards for informed consent in the research context than in the general therapeutic context? Should there be?

Notes

1. C.W. Lidz et al., "Informed Consent and the Structure of Medical Care," in President's Commission for the Study of Ethical Problems in Medicine and Biomedical and Behavioral Research, *Making Health Care Decisions*, vol. 2 (Washington, D.C.: U.S. Government Printing Office, 1982), 317-410.

2. C.W. Lidz et al., *Informed Consent: A Study of Decision-making in Psychiatry* (New York: Guilford Press, 1984).

3. C.W. Lidz et al., "Barriers to Informed Consent," *Annals of Internal Medicine* 99 (1983): 539-43.

4. L. Harris & Associates, "Views of Informed Consent and Decision-Making: Parallel surveys of Physicians and the Public," in President's Commission for the Study of Ethical Problems in Medicine and Biomedical and Behavioral Research, *Making Health Care Decisions* (Washington, D.C.: U.S. Government Printing Office, 1982), vol. 1, 17-18.

5. W.S. Edwards and C. Yahne, "Surgical Informed Consent: What It Is and Is Not," *American Journal of Surgery* 154 (1987): 574-78.

6. T. Percival, *Medical Ethics; or A Code of Institutes and Precepts, Adapted to the Professional Conduct of Physicians and Surgeons* (Manchester, England: S. Russell, 1803) as noted in J. Katz, *The Silent World of Doctor and Patient* (New York: Free Press, 1984), 17.

7. J. Katz, *The Silent World of Doctor and Patient,* see note 6 above, pp. 16-22.

8. American Medical Association, "Code of Medical Ethics" (adopted May 1847, Chapter 1, Article 1, Section 4), in J. Katz *The Silent World of Doctor and*

Patient, see note 6 above, p. 21.

9. *Schloendorff v. Society of N.Y. Hospital*, 211 N.Y. 125, 105 N.E. 92 (1914).

10. *Salgo v. Leland Stanford, Jr., University Board of Trustees*, 317 P.2d 170 at 181 (1957).

11. American Medical Association, "Principles of Medical Ethics" (adopted 1957, Section 1), in J. Katz, *The Silent World of Doctor and Patient*, see note 6 above, p. 22.

12. American Medical Association, "Opinions and Reports of the Judicial Council, 1957," in J. Katz, *The Silent World of Doctor and Patient*, see note 6 above, p. 23.

13. See note 7 above, p. 23.

14. American Medical Association, "Current Opinions of the Judicial Council, 1981," in J. Katz, *The Silent World of Doctor and Patient* (New York: Free Press, 1984), 23.

15. T.L. Beauchamp and J.F. Childress, *Principles of Biomedical Ethics* (New York: Oxford University Press, 1994), 145-46.

16. Ibid., 164.

17. R.R. Faden and T.L. Beauchamp, *A History and Theory of Informed Consent* (New York: Oxford University Press, 1986), 30-34, 133-38.

18. *Canterbury v. Spence*, 464 F.2d 772 (D.C. Cir. 1972).

19. See note 17 above.

20. H. Brody, "Transparency: Informed Consent in Primary Care," *Hastings Center Report* 19, no. 5 (1989): 5-9.

21. *Moore v. Regents of the Univ. of California*, 51 Cal.3d 120, 793 P.2d 479 (1990) (*en banc*).

22. R.M. Veatch, *The Patient-Physician Relation: The Patient as Partner, Part 2* (Bloomington, Ind.: Indiana University Press, 1991), 84.

23. *Estate of Behringer v. The Medical Center at Princeton*, 249 N.J.Super. 597, 592 A.2d 1251 (1991).

24. *Hidding v. Williams*, 578 So.2d 1192 (La.Ct.App. 1991).

25. B. Spielman, "Expanding the Boundaries of Informed Consent: Disclosing Alcoholism and HIV Status to Patients," *American Journal of Medicine* 93 (1992): 216-18.

26. See note 15 above, p. 145.

27. Ibid., 143-44.

28. See note 1 above.

29. See note 6 above, p. 130-47.

30. J.C. Fletcher et al., "Ethical Considerations in Pediatric Oncology," in *Principles and Practice of Pediatric Oncology*, P.A. Pizzo and D.G. Poplack, ed.

(Philadelphia: J.B. Lippincott, 1989), 309-20; N.M.P. King and A.W. Cross, "Children as Decisionmakers: Guidelines for Pediatricians," *Journal of Pediatrics* 115 (1989): 10-16; S.L. Leikin, "Minors' Assent or Dissent to Medical Treatment," *Journal of Pediatrics* 102 (1983): 169-76; Committee on Bioethics, American Academy of Pediatrics, "Informed Consent, Parental Permission, and Assent in Pediatric Practice," *Pediatrics* 95 (1995): 314-17.

31. National Commission for the Protection of Human Subjects of Biomedical and Behavioral Research, *Report and Recommendations Concerning Research Involving Children* (Washington, D.C.: Department of Health, Education, and Welfare, 1977, DHEW Publication no. (OS)77-0005).

32. See note 30, Committee on Bioethics, American Academy of Pediatrics, pp. 315-16.

33. Ibid., 317.

34. See note 1 above, pp. 363-73.

35. *Natanson v. Kline*, 186 Kan. 393, 104 Cal.Rptr. 505, 350 P.2d 1093 (1960).

36. *Cobbs v. Grant*, 502 P.2d 1 (1972).

37. *Mohr v. Williams*, 95 Minn. 261, 104 N.W. 12 (1905).

38. *Arato v. Avedon*, 5 Cal.4th 1172, 858 P.2d 598 (Cal. 1993).

39. T.L. Beauchamp, "Informed Consent," in *Medical Ethics*, R.M. Veatch, ed. (Boston: Jones and Bartlett Publishers, 1989), 173-200.

40. A. Buchanan, "Medical Paternalism," *Philosophy and Public Affairs*, 4 (1978): 372.

41. G. Dworkin, "Autonomy and Informed Consent," in President's Commission for the Study of Ethical Problems in Medicine and Biomedical and Behavioral Research, *Making Health Care Decisions* (Washington, D.C.: U.S. Government Printing Office, 1982), volume 3, 70.

42. See note 3 above.

43. E.J. Cassell and J. Katz, "Informed Consent in the Therapeutic Relationship," in *Encyclopedia of Bioethics*, W.T. Reich, ed. (New York: MacMillan Free Press, 1978).

44. President's Commission for the Study of Ethical Problems in Medicine and Biomedical and Behavioral Research, *Making Health Care Decisions* (Washington, D.C.: U.S. Government Printing Office, 1982), 2.

45. American Hospital Association, *A Patient's Bill of Rights* (Chicago: American Hospital Association, 1992).

46. Committee on Ethics, American Nurses Asso-

ciation, *Code for Nurses with Interpretive Statements*, (Washington, D.C.: American Nurses Association, 1983), ¶ 1.1, p. 2.

47. American Medical Association, Council on Ethical and Judical Affairs, "Fundamental Elements of the Patient-Physician Relationship," updated June 1994, in *Code of Medical Ethics* (Chicago: AMA, 1997), *xxxix*.

48. American Medical Association, Council on Ethical and Judical Affairs, "Opinions on Practice Matters," issued March 1981, in *Code of Medical Ethics* (Chicago: AMA, 1997), 120.

49. "American College of Physicians Ethics Manual," *Annals of Internal Medicine* 117 (1992): 947-60.

SECTION II

ETHICAL OBLIGATIONS
AND PROBLEMS IN CLINICAL CARE

B. ETHICAL PROBLEMS IN
PARTICULAR CASES

7

TREATMENT REFUSALS BY PATIENTS AND CLINICIANS

Mary Faith Marshall

Cases

When Dax Cowart was critically burned in a propane gas explosion near Henderson, Texas, he begged a passing farmer for a gun with which to kill himself. On his way to the hospital, he pleaded with medics to let him die. For weeks his life hung by a thread. For more than a year, against his will, he endured excruciating treatment: he underwent tankings in a whirlpool bath to slough his burned skin, his right eye and several fingers were removed, his left eye was sewn shut. His pain and his protests were unrelenting. One night he crawled out of bed to try to throw himself out of a window, but was discovered and prevented. He was incarcerated in the Burn Unit, unable to make telephone calls, unable to contact a lawyer, forbidden to leave the floor.

That was many years ago. Cowart is now a law school graduate living in Texas and managing his investments. Yet to this day he argues that doctors violated his right to choose not to be treated. "It doesn't take a genius to know that when you're in that amount of pain, you can either bear it or you can't," he says. "And I couldn't." He still resents the powerlessness of patients who are forced to live when they beg to die. "The physicians say that when a patient is in that much pain, he is not competent to make judgements about himself. It's the pain talking. And then when narcotics are given to subdue the pain, they say it's the narcotics talking. It's a no-win situation."[1]

In 1985, a motorcycle accident left Larry James McAfee of Fulton County, Georgia, a quadriplegic. He was rendered ventilator dependent, without chance of improvement.

Four years after the accident, Mr. McAfee filed a petition in Fulton County Superior Court seeking authority to disconnect his ventilator via a mouth-operated timer. He also asked the court to approve the administration of a sedative to alleviate any pain or air-hunger that he might experience when the ventilator was disconnected.

The trial court found that his constitutional rights of privacy and liberty (federal and Georgia constitutions), as well as his right to refuse treatment, allowed him, as a competent person, to make this decision. The trial court determined that while it could not order a clinician to administer the requested sedative, no civil or criminal liability would attach to any clinician who did so.

The the case was appealed to the Georgia Supreme Court which, in a unanimous decision, affirmed the trial court's decision. The court stated that competent adults have the right to refuse medical treatment in the absence of conflicting state interests. In this case, the court wrote, the only implicated interest of the state would be the general interest in preserving life, which the state conceded did not outweigh Mr. McAfee's right to make his own decision.

The court also held that Mr. McAfee's right to be free from pain when the ventilator is disconnected is inseparable from his right to refuse medical treatment. It noted that he had made previous attempts at disconnection but had failed because of the severe pain he suffered when deprived of oxygen. His right to have a sedative (which the court defined as "a medication that in no way causes or accelerates death") was described as part of his right to control his medical treatment.[2]

In the case of JP, described in Chapter 2, clinicians who are traditionally less powerful (a resident physician-in-training and a group of nurses) found themselves refusing to provide an unwanted (but potentially lifesaving) blood transfusion to a patient in defiance of a powerful surgeon who was also a department head. Power differentials make it difficult and awkward (but not impossible) for students, allied health professionals, potential research subjects, and patients to voice their reservations or objections regarding a particular therapy or research protocol.

I. Statement of the Problem

The right to informed refusal of treatment is a corollary of the right to informed consent. If one possesses the right to consent to receive treatment or participate in human subjects research, one necessarily possesses the right to refuse it. Without its corollary, the right to informed consent is meaningless.

Deprived of the right to noninterference, individuals are subject to coercive or forceful intrusions by others. Such intrusions in either the context of treatment or research might include physical battery or assault, violation of privacy, or nonvoluntary exposure to information about oneself or others. Forced medical interventions or therapeutic trials may increase suffering, prolong dying, create unwanted medical bills, or impose an unacceptable quality of life upon an unwilling patient. In the worst circumstances, as in the case of Dax Cowart, the patient may become a virtual prisoner of the medical establishment.

II. Ethical Foundation

The ethical foundation for the right to refuse medical treatment or to refuse to participate in a research protocol is grounded in the principle of autonomy, or respect for persons. It connotes respect for the choices of others, not for persons *per se*. The principle embodies both the positive right to self-determination and the negative right to noninterference (to be left alone). Freedom from restraint or coercion is necessary for moral action. Without the freedom of self-determination, individuals lack the capacity for moral behavior, as they cannot choose how to act.

The right to self-determination has been cogently argued by the philosopher Immanuel Kant, a deontologist. Deontology is a theory of ethics that holds that some acts are morally obligatory regardless of their consequences. Kant's argument for the right to self-determination centers on his regard for the unconditional worth of persons. He asserted that all persons must be allowed to control their own destinies. To deny them this right is to use individuals for one's own purposes, to treat them as means to an end rather than as ends in and of themselves. Kant argued that exerting control over others is legitimate only in situations where their choices may cause harm to others.

This sole conditional limitation to freedom of thought and action was also advocated by the utilitarian philosopher John Stuart Mill. Perhaps the most famous espousal of the right to noninterference was made by Mill in his essay *On Liberty*:

> The object of this Essay is to assert one very simple principle, as entitled to govern absolutely the dealings of society with the individual in the way of compulsion and control, whether the means used be physical force in the form of legal penalties, or the moral coercion of public opinion. That principle is, that the sole end for which mankind are warranted, individually or collectively, in interfering with the liberty of action of any of their number, is self-protection. That the only purpose for which power can be rightfully exercised over any member of a civilized community, against his will, is to prevent harm to others. His own good, either physical or moral, is not a sufficient warrant. He cannot rightfully be compelled to do or forbear because it will be better for him to do so, because it will make him happier, because in the opinions of others to do so would be wise, or even right. . . . Neither one person, nor any number of persons is warranted in saying to another human creature of ripe years, that he shall not do with his life for his own benefit what he chooses to do with it. . . . All errors

which the individual is likely to commit against advice and warning are far outweighed by the evil of allowing others to constrain him to what they deem his good.[3]

Bioethicist Gerald Dworkin has provided the following analysis of the structure of Mill's argument:

1. Since restraint is an evil, the burden of proof is on those who propose such restraint.
2. Since the conduct which is being considered is purely self-regarding, the normal appeal to the protection of the interests of others is not available.
3. Therefore, we have to consider whether reasons involving reference to the individual's own good, happiness, welfare, or interests are sufficient to overcome the burden of justification.
4. We cannot advance the interests of the individual by compulsion. The attempt to do so involves evils which outweigh the good done.
5. Hence, the promotion of the individual's own interests does not provide a sufficient warrant for the use of compulsion.

III. Historical Perspective

Historically, many refusals of medical treatment have been made on religious grounds. A variety of theological beliefs proscribe such diverse medical interventions as autopsy, blood transfusion, the use of non-naturalistic medications and therapies, and the treatment of female patients by male physicians. Some religious sects prohibit all professional medical interventions based on a deterministic belief in predestination, (that is, that the outcome of an individual's illness is in the individual's or God's hands). Prohibition against touching another without permission originated with an ancient Germanic tradition forbidding the torture of free men.[5] Its basis in English case law served as a foundation for the development of American legal doctrine on informed consent, also based in common law.

Unlawful touching by a physician was formally established in American law in the 1905 case of *Mohr v. Williams*, when the court ruled that ear surgery that took place without the permission of the patient constituted a tort or wrongful act.[6] The legal premise un-

derlying this decision was more cogently presented the same year in the case of *Pratt v. Davis*. The court argued:

Under a free government at least, the free citizen's first and greatest right, which underlies all others--the right to the inviolability of his person, in other words his right to himself--is the subject of universal acquiescence, and this right necessarily forbids a physician or surgeon, however skillful or eminent, who has been asked to examine, diagnose, advise and prescribe (which are at least necessary first steps in treatment and care), to violate without permission the bodily integrity of his patient by a major or capital operation, placing him under anesthetics for that purpose.[7]

Perhaps the most famous opinion articulating the right of refusal is that of Justice Benjamin Cardozo in the 1914 *Schloendorff v. Society of New York Hospital* case: "Every human being of adult years and sound mind has a right to determine what shall be done with his body, and a surgeon who performs an operation without his patient's consent commits an assault for which he is liable in damages."[8]

In the 1960 precedent-setting case of *Natanson v. Kline*, the Kansas Supreme Court specifically addressed the refusal of life-sustaining treatment. The court opinion stated: "Anglo-American law starts with the premise of a thorough-going self determination. It follows that each man is considered to be master of his own body, and he may, if he be of sound mind, expressly prohibit the performance of life-saving surgery."[9]

More recently, state supreme courts in New York and Missouri have questioned the ability of surrogate decision makers to refuse treatment when acting as agents for incapacitated patients. The conflict of the state's interest in preserving life versus the patient's right to refuse (forgo) treatment has fueled furious debate.

IV. Current Trends

Medical knowledge has advanced exponentially within the past 50 years. From a technologic and scientific standpoint, medical treatment has reached the stage in which the benefits offered may outweigh the burdens imposed. Advances in the arenas of public health and tertiary care have prolonged average life expectancies and have increased survival rates following previously fatal conditions. An attendant irony of modern medical success is the frequency with which patient's refuse treatment based on "quality-of-life" considerations. Unbearable pain and suffering, acknowledged futility of treatment, and unnecessary prolongation of dying are often-cited reasons for refusing treatment.

V. Value Conflicts and Protherapeutic Authoritarianism

According to Robert Veatch, "refusing medical care believed necessary by the physician is nothing more than the patient's expression of what is fitting in his or her system of values."[10] Personal values reflect an individual determination of the relative "good." Treatment choices, including refusals, should be determined and defended by values. Ideally, they should reflect coherent choices based on consistently held personal beliefs. Because the determination of the rationality of another's beliefs is a subjective and value-relative enterprise, an indictment of irrationality may not be used to justify overriding a patient's refusal. Patients' beliefs need not be congruent with the belief systems of healthcare workers, family members, or laypersons. A "wrong" decision is the prerogative of the capable patient.

Limits to respect for persons are justified only in cases of actual or potential harm to innocent third parties. Refusals in such cases are often forbidden by law. Harm to others usually involves children or other dependents who might themselves be deprived of medical treatment, or cases of second-party refusals when a surrogate decision maker opts to forgo life-sustaining treatment for questionable reasons.

Refusal of treatment may signify an underlying value conflict between patient and clinician regarding the goals of therapy or the means by which the therapy is to be provided.[11] Patients' refusals of treatment, especially life-sustaining treatment, frequently result in frustration and inner conflict for clinicians. The desire to ensure respect for persons may directly oppose the felt obligation to provide needed treatment (to do good) or to prevent harm.

Patients' clear and informed refusals sometimes are overridden by zealous healthcare providers, family members, or surrogate decision makers who value life over respect for persons. U.S. Supreme Court Justice Louis Brandeis stated, "The greatest dangers to liberty lurk in insidious encroachment by men of zeal, well-meaning but without understanding."[12]

Bioethicists Susan Braithwaite and David Thomasma have labeled such behavior on the part of clinicians "protherapeutic authoritarianism" and argue that "advocacy or imposition of medical interventions by individuals whose personality, motives, and methods are authoritarian, not only exists but is directed toward other goals than the goals of medicine."[13] The physician as authoritarian is a popular and often accurate characterization. Physicians-in-training are often socialized by role models to acquire an authoritarian demeanor.[14]

In a physician, a fine thread of authoritarianism may be laced through an otherwise admirable personality. The attribute can be observed in the power struggles that occur within academic medicine or group practices, in professional neutralization of bureaucratic authority, in degrading treatment of subordinates, and in the overvaluation of status (my career) at the expense of family, personal and patient welfare. The physician frequently resists efforts by the patient to gain control or understanding of the treatment, dismissing questions as neurotic, not because they are viewed as a challenge to his authority, but precisely because the patient is uncomprehending and ineffectual compared to the physician. This quality--scenting out weakness, then finding oneself goaded to destroy--is characteristically authoritarian. The doctor's suppression of the offending questioner takes the form of irritability, contempt or rejection. . . .

Authoritarian attitudes about healthcare are by no means held only by physicians. Nursing personnel and lay people sometimes seem motivated by zealous adherence to a cause more than by concern for the patient under discussion.[15]

The case of Elizabeth Bouvia is a prime example of how clinicians can force their values about medical treatment on a defenseless patient.

In 1983, Elizabeth Bouvia was a 26-year-old woman afflicted with cerebral palsy. Her disease was severe enough to deprive her of any function of her skeletal muscles or her limbs. She had limited use of her right hand, which enabled her to operate an electric wheelchair, and she could eat when fed by another person. In September 1983, Bouvia was admitted to Riverside County General Hospital, in Riverside, California. While a patient there, she determined that her quality of life was such that she did not want to continue living, and she subsequently refused to eat, planning death by starvation.[16]

The clinicians at Riverside County General Hospital did not honor Bouvia's refusal of feeding. Bouvia then took her case to court, represented by the American Civil Liberties Union (ACLU). The chief of psychiatry at Riverside, Donald Fisher, testified in court that he would force-feed Bouvia with a nasogastric tube even if the court ordered him not to. His position was based on his belief that Bouvia, by virtue of her refusal, was attempting suicide and must, therefore, be mentally ill. Although the judge who heard the case determined Bouvia to be competent, he disallowed her refusal based on the onerous effect it would have on the staff and other patients at Riverside Hospital.

Bouvia then began an odyssey through several hospitals in the United States and Mexico in an attempt to find an institution that would honor her wish not to be fed. In December 1985, she was transferred to High Desert Hospital in California, where she continued to be force-fed. Her physicians there went even further, claiming a "right to rehabilitate" her, and pursued a treatment plan to increase her weight of 70 pounds to an "ideal" weight of 104 to 114 pounds. They stated, "Since she is occupying our space she must accede to the same care which we afford every other patient admitted here, care designed to improve and not detract from chances of recovery and rehabilitation."[17] Bouvia also was forced to socialize with other patients after being threatened that her smoking privileges would otherwise be withdrawn, and that her morphine doses would be lowered.

Bouvia once again took her case to court, with the support of ACLU attorneys. Again, the judge decided in the hospital's favor. The case was appealed, however, and the lower court's decision was overturned. The appeals court reasoned:

A person of adult years and in sound mind has the right, in the exercise of control over his own body, to determine whether or not to submit to lawful medical treatment. . . . It follows that such a patient has the right to refuse any medical treatment, even that which may save or prolong her life. *Bartling v. Superior Court*, 163 Cal. App.3d 186 (1984). . . . The right to refuse medical treatment is basic and fundamental. It is recognized as a part of the right of privacy protected by both the state and federal constitutions. . . . Moreover, as the *Bartling* decision holds, there is no practical or logical reason to limit the exercise of this right to "terminal" patients. The right to refuse treatment does not need the sanction or approval by any legislative act, directing how and when it shall be exercised. . . . It is indisputable that petitioner is mentally competent. She is not comatose. She is quite intelligent, alert, and understands the risks involved. . . . Here Elizabeth Bouvia's decision to forgo medical treatment or life support through a mechanical means belongs to her. It is not a medical decision for her physicians to make. Neither is it a legal question whose soundness is to be resolved by lawyers or judges. It is not a conditional right subject to approval by ethics committees or courts of law. It is a moral and philosophical decision that, being a competent adult, is hers alone. . . . Being competent she has the right to live out the remainder of her natural life in dignity and peace. It is precisely the aim and purpose of the many decisions upholding the withdrawal of life-support systems to accord and provide as large a measure of dignity, respect and comfort as possible to every patient for the remainder of his days, whatever be their number. The goal is not to hasten death, though its earlier arrival may be an expected and understood likelihood. . . . Moreover, if a right exists, it matters not what "motivates" its exercise. We find nothing in the law to suggest the right to refuse medical treatment may be exercised only if the patient's motives meet someone else's approval. It certainly is not illegal or immoral to prefer a natural, albeit sooner, death than a

drugged life attached to a mechanical device.
. . . Personal dignity is a part of one's right to
privacy.[18]

Ironically, it is occasionally the legal system, not
clinicians, that imposes unwanted treatment on patients. Or perhaps, it would be more accurately stated
that clinicians too often allow hospital attorneys or
administrators to dictate their medical practice. Such
unfortunate circumstances lead to celebrated ethical
disasters of the sort found in the Linares case (Chapter 9), the case of AC (case study for this chapter).

VI. Sources of Authority

The right to refuse treatment is stated in the
American Hospital Association's *Patient's Bill of
Rights*, which holds: "The patient has the right to
refuse treatment to the extent permitted by law and to
be informed of the medical consequences of his action."[19]

A patient's right to self-determination is explicitly stated in the report of the President's Commission for the Study of Ethical Problems in Medicine
and Biomedical and Behavioral Research: "In the
context of health care, self-determination overrides
practitioner-determination even if providers were able
to demonstrate that they could (generally or in a specific instance) accurately assess the treatment an informed patient would choose. To permit action on
the basis of a professional's assessment rather than
on a patient's choice would deprive the patient of the
freedom not to be forced to do something--whether
or not that person would agree with the choice."[20]

Legislation allowing advance directives to govern healthcare choices in the event of patient incapacity has been passed more than 40 states and the
District of Columbia. The right to refuse to participate in human subjects research funded by the federal government is clearly articulated in a policy statement that applies to all federal departments and agencies that conduct, support, or regulate research.

VII. Guidance

1. The capable patient has the right to refuse any
    treatment, including that of a life-sustaining na-

ture, when the elements of informed consent have
been met.

2. The capable patient has a duty implied within the
    context of shared decision making for healthcare
    to articulate as clearly as possible what motivates
    a decision to refuse treatment. Such a decision
    may be motivated by coherent personal reasons,
    religious beliefs, social or political ideology, or
    emotions.

3. A formal institutional policy should encourage
    documentation of patients' refusals in a patient
    choice-of-care statement (see Exhibit 7-1) or in
    the progress notes of the medical record.

4. Medical treatment cannot be conditioned on a pro-
    spective subject's refusal to participate in a re-
    search protocol. Research subjects can withdraw
    from a research protocol at any time.

VIII. Discussion

Medical treatment without the consent of the patient should be undertaken by healthcare professionals only in carefully circumscribed situations. Such
an action would be warranted in a life-threatening
emergency when the patient is incapacitated and a
surrogate decision maker or advance directive is not
available. A capable patient's refusal of treatment is
valid when the elements of informed consent have
been met. The patient must demonstrate the following:

1. understanding of his or her medical condition;
2. understanding of the consequences of his or her
    decision; and
3. voluntariness.

Refusals by patients who are not capable decision makers are invalid by the same rationale that dis-
allows them giving valid consent. These invalid refusals include refusals by patients who lack understanding, or who act on misinformation or delusions,
since the necessary elements of informed consent are
lacking. A patient's lack of capacity to consent does
not leave clinicians free to decide in the patient's behalf. Except in emergencies, a proxy for the patient
must be located or appointed by the court, and must
give consent before treatment can proceed. As dem-

Exhibit 7-1
Patient Choice of Care Statement

1. The patient, the family and significant other persons have been properly and adequately informed (to the extent possible) regarding the condition of the patient.
    Patient: Yes _____ No _____
    If not, why? _____
    Family: Yes _____ No _____
    If not, why? _____

2. The patient has a written statement concerning a positive choice of treatment (a negative choice to forgo certain treatments) and wishes to make or has already made that written statement part of the medical record.
    Yes _____ No _____
    If not, why? _____

3. The patient has a living will, power of attorney for health care, or other advance directives which I have discussed with the patient.
    Yes _____ No _____

4. The patient is not competent or cannot communicate. The family or significant other persons have made a treatment decisions, applying the concept of substituted judgment if possible, or best interest.
    Yes _____ No _____
    What decision? _____

5. The patient, family, or significant persons wish to consult with the ethics consultant service or pastoral care service about the choice of care issue.
    Yes _____ No _____
    Consult initiated? _____
    Yes _____ No _____
    If not, why? _____

_____ Physician's Signature   _____ Date

onstrated in the case of Elizabeth Bouvia, clinicians have a direct conflict of interest in acting as their patients' agents. Even when clinicians think that they are acting in their patient's best interest, their judgment is driven by their own value systems.

IX. Religious Values

Establishing the validity of religious beliefs is impossible, because the evaluative criterion is personal faith, which has no empirical basis. Adherence to established religious dogma is not a legitimate criterion for assessing religious validity. Individual beliefs are no less relevant or justifiable because they lack orthodoxy. The law is consistent in this area as demonstrated by the following judicial opinions:

- In *United States v. Ballard* (1944), the court ruled: "Men may believe what they cannot prove. They may not be put to the proof of their religious doctrines or beliefs. Religious experiences which are as real as life to some may be incomprehensible to others."[21]

- In *Thomas v. Review Board*, the court ruled: "Religious beliefs need not be acceptable, logical, consistent, or comprehensible to others in order to merit First Amendment protection."[22]

Consequently, clinicians should not attempt to evaluate the "validity" of a patient's beliefs when religion is invoked as the basis for refusing treatment.

X. Human Subjects Research

The principle of respect for persons that governs the doctrine of informed consent/refusal within the context of medical treatment also governs this doctrine as it applies to research involving human subjects. The first-large scale attempt to apply the doctrine of informed consent and refusal to human subjects research was the development of the Nuremberg Code in 1949. This code was written by the International Military Tribunal that tried the 23 physicians and scientists who performed coerced experiments on concentration camp inmates during World War II. The first principle of the code clearly articulates a requirement of informed consent to research involving human subjects: "The voluntary consent of the human subject is absolutely essential. This means that the person involved should have legal capacity to give consent; should be so situated as to be able to exercise free power of choice without the intervention of any element of force, fraud, deceit, duress, over-reaching, or other ulterior form of constraint or coercion."[23]

This principle informs all of the codes regarding research on human subjects that were subsequently developed in the United States. Until 1991, the various federal agencies that supported or regulated research with human subjects each followed its own guidelines regarding informed consent to participation in research.

In 1991, all federal agencies directly or indirectly involved in human subjects research adopted a common federal policy for protecting research subjects. These regulations require that investigators provide potential subjects with particular information as part of the consent process. This information must include: "A statement that participation is voluntary, refusal to participate will involve no penalty or loss of benefits to which the subject is otherwise entitled, and the subject may discontinue participation at any time without penalty or loss of benefits to which the subject is otherwise entitled, and the subject may discontinue participation at any time without penalty or loss of benefits to which the subject is otherwise entitled."[24]

The federal policy explicitly requires the disclosure of information that may relate to a subject's willingness or continued willingness to participate in a research protocol. Statements regarding the following information must be included in the process of informed consent and should be included in any written consent document:

- Anticipated circumstances under which the subject's participation may be terminated by the investigator without regard to the subject's consent;
- The consequences of the subject's decision to withdraw from the research and procedures for orderly termination of participation by the subject;

- A statement that significant new findings developed during the course of the research which may relate to the subject's willingness to continue participation will be provided to the subject.[25]

XI. Exceptions to the Right to Refuse Medical Treatment

Rarely have competent refusals by patients been overridden in order to protect third parties. Examples of these exceptions are cases involving transfusion for minors, treatment of a pregnant woman carrying a fetus, or situations where the refusal of treatment has serious consequences for a person who is dependent on the patient. These cases are highly controversial, and there is no expert consensus regarding the ethical aspects of their outcomes. The best practical posture is to assume, as a rule of thumb, that the single significant variable that can negate a patient's normal right to refuse is mental capacity.

Clinicians who raise the question of a patient's mental state in the face of a refusal should ask whether a similar question would arise if the patient had acquiesced to the recommended treatment. Clinicians should be no more motivated to challenge the thought process of an uncooperative patient than they are to accept consent from a compliant patient.

Treatment refusals often unleash powerful emotional responses from patients and healthcare providers who feel frustrated and angry with the medical circumstances or lack of cooperation on the part of a patient. When emotional conflicts arise, the source of the problem should be identified and an assessment of the situation from the ethical perspective should be made. Open and honest communication between patients and clinicians is vital to informed decision making. Involving family members and other healthcare professionals may encourage information sharing and improve the patient's ability to make decisions. Too often, the unfortunate combination of dysfunctional communication patterns, unbridled emotions, and ignorance of the law results in costly and often unproductive legal confrontations rather than honest attempts at mediation and compromise.

XII. Refusal to Treat

Clinicians often are faced with personal and professional ethical dilemmas when patients, family members, or peers demand treatment that is, in the clinician's judgment, ethically wrong, medically inappropriate, or futile. This situation frequently arises when a patient is terminally ill or dying, and family members request aggressive treatment, stating that they want "everything done" for the patient, including cardiopulmonary resuscitation. Another example of a dilemma for clinicians might be a couple's request for abortion based on sex selection. A third example is the JP case (Chapter 2), in which a group of critical care doctors and nurses refused to override a Jehovah's Witness patient's refusal of blood products. This refusal to treat occurred in spite of a court order obtained by a powerful attending physician and by the patient's father (also a physician), and with the acknowledgment of the patient's possible death.

Clinicians have the right to refuse to render treatment that violates their personal or professional ethical standards. Fidelity to one's professional ethics is a necessary criterion for professionalism. In cases involving refusal to treat, clinicians may not abandon their patients, but must make every reasonable effort to transfer the patient to the care of another clinician. The Joint Commission for Accreditation of Healthcare Organizations has recognized the need for formal policies governing clinicians' refusals to treat patients based on personal ethical standards in its standards on patients' rights. All employees of a healthcare organization should know the contents of such policies and should recognize their responsibilities to honor a patient's refusal to undergo treatment or a fellow healthcare professional's refusal to render it.

Virginia was one of the first states to include a conscience clause that specifically addressed the issue of professional ethical standards (the Virginia Health Care Decisions Act).[26] A recent, precedent-setting case tested the limits of this statute. Baby K, an anencephalic infant (anencephaly is a congenital malformation in which a large portion of the brain and skull are missing), was born in October 1993 at Fairfax Hospital in Fairfax County, Virginia. Because such children lack any cognitive abilities or awareness, they are generally provided with only comfort care after birth, and most die within days or weeks.

In keeping with her religious beliefs and values, Baby K's mother, Ms. H, demanded full, aggressive support for her child. With supportive hospital and nursing home therapy, Baby K survived for two years. Although she resided in a nursing home, Baby K oc-

casionally suffered respiratory distress and required transportation to the hospital for mechanical ventilation and more aggressive therapy.

Attorneys for Fairfax Hospital sought a declaratory judgment from the courts absolving the institution and its caregivers from the responsibility of providing treatment other than comfort care and nutrition and hydration. The U.S. Court of Appeals for the Fourth Circuit, upholding a lower court ruling, found that the Emergency Medical Treatment and Active Labor Act (EMTALA), a 1985 federal law designed to protect indigent patients from being denied emergency treatment, required Fairfax Hospital to provide emergency and stabilizing treatment for Baby K when she required such treatment for respiratory distress. The appeals court specifically stated that by virtue of being federal legislation, the EMTALA overrode the Virginia Health Care Decisions Act.

The Baby K case is given a more thorough treatment in Chapter 9 in a discussion of medical futility and forgoing life-sustaining treatment. Of interest here are the case's implications for clinicians who refuse to provide what they determine to be medically or ethically inappropriate care.

Formal standards for limiting care are emerging in the medical literature. In its recent "Consensus Statement on the Triage of Critically Ill Patients," the Society of Critical Care Medicine (SCCM) Ethics Committee stated that, while triage policies should be prospectively disclosed to patients and families, "triage decisions may be made without patient or surrogate consent."[27] The triage officer may make unilateral decisions regarding exclusion or discharge of a patient from an intensive care unit (ICU). The SCCM Ethics Committee identified the sorts of patients who could or should be denied access to critical care:

> Examples of terminally ill patients who may be excluded from the ICU, whether beds are available or not, include those with severe, irreversible brain damage or irreversible multiorgan failure and those with metastatic cancer unresponsive to therapy unless the patients are in specialized ICUs or on specific protocols.
>
> Examples of patients who should be excluded from the ICU, whether beds are available or not, include those who competently decline intensive care or request that invasive therapy be withheld, those declared brain dead who are not organ do-

nors, and those in a persistent vegetative or permanently unconscious state.[28]

As in the JP case, an absolute refusal to provide unwanted, medically inappropriate, or unethical care is the clinician's prerogative. An absolute refusal should be made only if more reasonable alternatives are not available or have been pursued unsuccessfully. Refusal to treat should be preceded by an examination and acceptance of the personal and professional consequences of such an act.

XIII. Analysis of a Complex Case

Treatment refusals by adolescents pose their own special problems. Children who are on the threshold of adulthood possess varying levels of maturity and understanding. Testing the limits of authority while simultaneously testing the strength of parental bonds is a rite of passage to young adulthood. It is difficult, if not impossible, to determine the autonomy of an adolescent's beliefs and values and to sort out strength of conviction versus allegiance to parents or other authority figures. The ability to delay gratification, to weigh alternatives in relation to future benefits or burdens, and to consider one's own mortality or life goals is generally less developed in adolescents than in those with more life experience. For this reason, an adolescent's refusal of treatment may be troublesome for clinicians who wish to honor the young patient's autonomy but question the patient's reasoning process.

Special attention to the criteria for decision-making capacity coupled with meticulous application of the tenets of informed consent and refusal should provide some degree of protection against overly restrictive or exceedingly liberal oversight of adolescent decision making. Although most adolescents may be capable of understanding the basic facts of their medical conditions, they may not fully possess the capacity to weigh alternatives against a stable value system for the simple reason that the value system has yet to be formed. Alternatively, a set of stable values may not be projected against competing alternatives, because future morbidity and mortality are consequences that cannot be imagined or appreciated. The safest method of evaluating an adolescent's refusal of treatment is a faithful application of the guidance regarding capacity and informed consent and refusal.

The following case is an exercise in applying these guidelines to the situation of an 11-year-old patient with cancer who refuses potentially lifesaving chemotherapy.

A. The Case of MT

MT, an 11-year-old girl from a neighboring state, was diagnosed in August 1987 with spindle-cell sarcoma (a malignant, solid tumor), which had invaded her left abdominal wall. The following month she had surgery at University Hospital (UH), during which a large (10-centimeter) tumor was removed. Postsurgical bone scan, bone biopsy, and lymph node biopsy showed no spread of the cancer.

MT's mother, a housewife, and her father, a logger, are members of a conservative, Fundamentalist congregation that has provided great support to the family during this difficult time. A devoutly religious person, Mrs. T attends church three times per week.

Following her first surgery, MT had a brief course of chemotherapy that was begun at UH and continued by a local physician when she returned home. Early in the course of her therapeutic regimen, MT stopped her chemotherapy against the advice of the UH team and her local physician because of its noxious side effects (including burning of the skin from an intravenous infiltration, hair loss, and nausea). A person with strong religious convictions, MT told her parents and sister, "God is trying to tell you something; I shouldn't be in all this pain." Her parents, affected by MT's pain and suffering, honored her refusal. They said that they were "trying not to kill her faith," and drew support from their religious beliefs.

Dr. R, MT's pediatric surgeon at UH, considered asking for legal advice regarding her refusal of chemotherapy. However, the pediatric oncology team wanted to wait, in part because the tumor had been excised and they did not know whether it would recur, and because the efficacy of chemotherapy in treating spindle-cell sarcoma was so low. Previous attempts had yielded only a 5 to 10 percent "effective" treatment rate (effective treatment is defined as a one- to two-year period free from cancer).

By the fall of 1988, MT's cancer had reappeared in the form of pulmonary tumors. She underwent surgery again at UH on November 29 and had an uneventful postoperative course. The subsequent pathology report showed the tumors to be a recurrence of the spindle-cell sarcoma. Dr. B, MT's pediatric oncologist, wrote a note in the chart on December 2 stating: "I doubt that cure is possible, but would advise chemotherapy using Vincristine, Actinomycin-D, cisplatin, and Adriamycin since this is the only chance and there has never been an adequate trial of chemotherapy. . . . Chemotherapy was a devastating experience at diagnosis and M is having a hard time accepting the idea again." When MT was discharged on December 5, she and the family had not yet reached a decision regarding chemotherapy.

After the second surgery, the pediatric oncologists once again reviewed the literature and also asked a pathologist to review the slides of the tumor. This pathologist identified the tumor as one of many kinds of "undifferentiated sarcoma" known to be more responsive to chemotherapy than the spindle-cell type. The pediatric oncologists became guardedly more optimistic. They raised their estimate to a 15 to 20 percent chance that combination chemotherapy would effectively treat this type of cancer.

With this report, Dr. R felt even more strongly that MT's parents were irresponsibly aiding an immature minor to refuse potentially lifesaving treatment. Although he had not communicated this to MT's parents, he considered seeking a court order to override the parents' refusal. Dr. R was hesitant about the legal option because neither he nor the pediatric oncology team had been very assertive about trying to reverse the first refusal. Feeling that he should seek help to confront the patient and her parents before acting on a legal option, the surgeon asked for an ethics consultation. He described the issue as "whether we were justified in pushing MT to accept treatment, and what expectation in prognosis we need to justify legal intervention."

A conference was arranged on the occasion of MT's next clinic visit at UH, on 9 January 1989. Dr. R wrote to MT's parents to inform them that a meeting was planned "with members of the ethics committee" to review the problem of MT's refusal and to discuss the options. Dr. R's position going into the meeting was that if they continued to refuse, he would confront them with the option of legally overriding them and say that he was willing to pursue it. The members of the pediatric oncology team were eager for MT to accept treatment but were actively opposed to a court-ordered approach. They emphasized how disruptive it would be for a court to assign someone custody of MT over her parents' objections. The child psychiatrist treating MT and her family had encouraged MT "to make her own decision." Up to the day of the conference MT continued to refuse chemotherapy, saying that she "didn't want to talk about it," and she became increasingly withdrawn. Her parents upheld her refusal, reiterating her bad experience with chemotherapy and stating their belief that "Jesus will heal M."

During this time, MT's 19-year-old married sister, CT, who lived in another state, had been helping out at home. She criticized MT and her parents, believing that they were denying the reality of the cancer and should accept chemotherapy.[29]

B. Analysis

The clinicians in the case must decide whether to honor MT's refusal of treatment or to pursue a legal override. The case contains evidence of a variety of conflicting values:

1. MT and her parents are holding out for divine intervention. They believe that God does not mean for her to suffer this way. Perhaps they are not convinced that the relatively low likelihood of success justifies the pain that chemotherapy will cause.

2. Dr. R, the pediatric surgeon, believes that MT's parents are acting irresponsibly by condoning her refusal. He apparently believes that any possibility of success should be pursued, and does not want to accept the failure that is implied when a patient dies.

3. The pediatric oncologists oppose court-ordered intervention, although they want MT to undergo chemotherapy.
4. The child psychiatrist has encouraged MT to make her own decision.
5. MT's sister believes that MT and her parents are denying the reality of the cancer. She advocates chemotherapy.

Dr. R has requested an ethics consultation, and a multidisciplinary conference with the patient and her family has been arranged. What options are available?

1. Honor MT's religiously grounded refusal. Alternatively, recognize that high-risk, low-yield therapy does not always represent a good choice, even for children.
2. Attempt judicial override of the refusal. Seek the appointment of a legal guardian for MT on the grounds that her parents are not acting in her best interest.
3. During the conference, attempt to convince MT and her parents of the consequences of her refusal. Ensure that they are aware that she will probably die without chemotherapy. Also, ensure that they are aware of her chances for survival with chemotherapy.

Answering the "ought" question in this case is extremely difficult. The burden of proof belongs to those who advocate overriding the patient's or surrogate's refusal. In order to justify such an override, a real or potential harm to this minor (or a legal constraint) must be shown. Whether the loss of a 20 percent (maximum) chance of survival with chemotherapy counts as a harm is a subjective judgment. Although MT is only 11 years old, how heavily should her capacity as a decision maker and/or her religious convictions weigh? Is she really refusing chemotherapy on religious grounds, or is this an 11 year old's ruse? Maybe she is simply afraid of undergoing such a devastating experience a second time. Perhaps she is in true denial and cannot accept the likelihood of her own death. Perhaps, in light of the 75 to 80 percent chance that chemotherapy will be futile, her treatment refusal is very reasonable. MT's parents ostensibly uphold her refusal because they share her religious beliefs. Are they really acting in her best in-

terest or, by honoring her position, are they simply following the path of least resistance?

The best course of action could be to use the multidisciplinary conference as a fact-finding forum. Most important is knowledge regarding MT's understanding of her prognosis both with and without chemotherapy. How will she and her parents react to the idea of a judicial override? Are they violently opposed or would it offer them a "way out" without the responsibility of personally violating their religious beliefs? Conversely, would they welcome an opportunity to have their religious convictions upheld in a judicial forum? How will MT and her parents react when confronted with the possibility that her refusal might really be grounded in fear or denial, not religious belief?

In keeping with the guidance offered earlier in the chapter, MT's refusal should be upheld if, during the conference, there is consensus regarding her capacity as a decision maker and the capacity of her parents as surrogates. If the family's refusal seems truly grounded in religious conviction, then--given the uncertain benefit of the chemotherapy--the issue can be reduced to whether a 20 percent (maximum) chance of survival justifies an override.

Dr. R requested an ethics consultation, and a multidisciplinary conference was held with MT and her family. MT's refusal appeared to result from her strong denial of the possibility of her death. When gently confronted by Dr. R with the information that she would die soon without chemotherapy, she changed her mind. Stating that she had not understood until then what the true consequence of her refusal would be, she acquiesced to treatment.

With her mother's written permission, MT received a full course of combined chemotherapy. Now 14 years old, she is doing well with no recurrence of cancer. Recently, she wrote a letter of support to another young girl who was having trouble accepting chemotherapy.

XIV. Cases for Further Study

Case 1: *Fresno County Social Services v. Xiong*

During the mid-1980s, Ger Xiong lived with his wife and infant son, Kou, in Ban Vanai, a refugee camp in Thailand. Members of the Hmong people of Laos, the family fled the communist-controlled country after the Vietnam war. While in the camp, American doctors suggested that surgery would help repair Kou's club feet and dislocated hip.

The surgery was performed with incomplete success. At about the same time, Xiong's wife fell ill, prey to what the couple described as cold, fever, and convulsions. Xiong sought Hmong shaman (medicine man) to root out the source of these evils. The shaman traveled into the spirit world to speak with the souls of Xiong's ancestors. He was displeased. He informed the Xiongs that God made the boy with twisted feet in retribution for a wrong committed by an ancestor. The Xiong's should not meddle in God's business. If doctors did not leave the boy alone, bad things would happen to the family.

Further proof was forthcoming. Xiong's next two sons were born in the Thai camp with cleft lips, a signal that God was unhappy with the doctors' efforts to undo His work.

In 1988, the family resettled in Fresno, California, in a Hmong community of about 30,000 persons. Social workers initiated a medical examination of Kou. Physicians again advised surgery. Although Ger Xiong had allowed the boy to be examined, he refused the surgery. The couple wanted more children, and they feared that attempts to fix Kou's problem might provoke an angry God to curse future offspring. God smiled on them. A girl, Joanie, was born in September. No cleft lip. No clubfeet. Perfect.

The Fresno County Department of Social Services sued Kou's parents to force them to allow physicians to perform a series of surgeries that could take as long as two years to complete. Brian A. Shaw, a local orthopedic surgeon, said that Kou's dislocated right hip was retarding growth in his right leg, so that Kou's left leg was already longer than his right. If the dislocation was uncorrected, the difference in the two lengths would become greater, compounding problems elsewhere, such as the spine. "His feet are quite literally upside down," Shaw said. "He walks on the tops of his feet."

Shaw stated that between three and seven surgeries would be required to repair Kou's legs and feet. Surgery and rehabilitation could take two years or longer. Kou would be required to wear a body cast for months. Under the best circumstances, his now-clumsy gait would become normal and he could partake in some athletic events, but as in any major surgery, there is a risk of death. Without the surgery, Kou would suffer increasing pain and would soon be forced into a wheelchair.

In February 1990, Fresno County Superior Court Judge Lawrence J. O'Neill heard Kou's case. The Xiongs appeared in court with two plastic bags. One held a live hen, the other contained incense, strips of paper strung together to represent money, and paper painted silver and gold to signify precious metals. Ger Xiong expected to use these in a ritual ceremony if the judge ruled against him.

He planned to kill the chicken, sprinkle its blood on the papers, and burn them and the incense. He would pray that death or illness resulting from the surgery would fall upon the responsible parties, including physicians, the judge, and the social workers who initiated the lawsuit.

After a two-day trial, Judge O'Neill ruled that Kou's medical interests took precedence over his parents' cultural beliefs. Appellate courts at the state and federal levels, and subsequently the U.S. Supreme Court, refused to overturn O'Neill's decision.

Representatives of all 18 Hmong clans in the United States, frustrated by government attempts to force Kou into the operating room, asked social services officials to reconsider. The National Hmong Council addressed a letter to Ernest Velasquez, director of Fresno County's Social Services Department. In the letter, the council representatives said that the entire Hmong population of the United States (as many as 110,00 people) were concerned about Kou Xiong. "The current case . . . threatens to undermine the foundation of our religion," wrote Cha Yang, President of the Hmong Council. Cases like this, Yang wrote, threaten "the safety and well being of our families." In September 1990, David A. Fox, a Fresno pediatric psychiatrist, was appointed by Judge O'Neill to evaluate Kou. He concluded that "Kou's parents are caring and highly responsible for their family. Kou's future positive psychological development is secure under their care." If forced to undergo surgery, Kou would probably not receive support from his family and would be at "grave psychological risk."

Fox wrote that two tests seemed particularly significant in evaluating the boy's fears about surgery. In one doll-playing sequence, Kou was told about a boy who had successfully had his appendix removed. But in playing, Kou did not allow the boy to return home. The boy had to sleep outside in a car.

In the second game, Kou was told about a man with twisted legs who had become a well-liked school teacher. Kou said he would like to be a teacher, and did not see his clubfeet as an obstacle.

Although the courts had ruled in its favor, the social services department was unable to find a doctor or a hospital that would perform the surgery without the Xiongs' consent. The next step toward a solution would be to remove Kou from his parents custody and place him in a foster home for the duration of his surgical treatment.

Imagine that you are on the ethics committee of the Bay Area Shriner's Hospital. The Fresno County Social Services Department has asked physicians at Shriner's to perform the surgery on Kou. The orthopedic surgeons and hospital administrator have brought the case to the ethics committee for guidance. What should the committee recommend?

[Source: Excerpted from a series of articles by Alex Putaski in the *Fresno* (California) *Bee* which appeared between 4 January and 21 December 1990.]

Case 2: The Case of Angie Carder

Angela C. was a twenty-eight-year old married woman who was approximately twenty-six weeks pregnant. She had suffered from cancer since she was thirteen years old, but had been in remission for approximately two years before she became pregnant. The pregnancy was planned, and she was very much looking forward to the birth. Her health seemed reasonably good until about the twenty-fifth week of pregnancy, when she was admitted to George Washington University Hospital, and a tumor was found in her lung.

Within a few days the physicians determined that her condition was terminal and she would likely die within weeks. At approximately 4:00 p.m. on June 15, 1997, she was told that she might die much sooner. Because her fetus would have a much better chance to be born healthy at twenty-eight weeks or more gestation, she agreed to treatment that might help her survive longer, but insisted that her own care and comfort be primary.

Ms. C's husband, her mother, and her physicians agreed that keeping her comfortable while she died was what she wanted and that her wishes should be honored. The next morning this information was communicated to hospital administration. Legal counsel was consulted, who decided to consult the university's outside counsel. Outside counsel asked a judge to come to the hospital to decide what to do.

Judge Emmett Sullivan of the District of Columbia Superior Court summoned volunteer lawyers, and with police escort rushed to the hospital where he set up "court." Legal counsel was, of course, present for the hospital. In addition, lawyers were appointed to represent Ms. C., and her fetus, and the judge invited the District of Columbia Corporation Counsel to participate as well.

The lawyer for the fetus expressed the view that the fetus was "a probably viable fetus, presumptively viable fetus, age twenty-six weeks," and that the court's task was to "balance" the interests of the fetus "with whatever life is left for the fetus's mother. . . ." Ms. C's lawyer argued simply that she opposed surgical intervention to remove the fetus.

Her attending physician, Louis Hammer, testified that Ms. C agreed to have the child at twenty-eight weeks, but that because the odds of a major handicap were much higher at twenty-six weeks gestation, she did not want the fetus delivered earlier. He said Ms. C was heavily sedated, and would likely die within twenty-four hours.

The patient's mother testified that the previous day, after her daughter had been informed that her condition was terminal, she said, "I only want to die, just give me something to get out of this pain."

Hospital counsel then asked the court to decide "what medical care, if any, should be performed for the benefit of the fetus of Ms. C." The lawyer's arguments not on what Ms. C wanted or even on her best interest, but on the best interests of the fetus and on Ms. C's terminal condition. The lawyer for the fetus, for example, urged that a cesarean be performed because, "sadly, the life of the mother is lost to us no matter what decision is made at this point." Ms. C's lawyer, on the other hand, argued the case on the basis of Ms. C's wishes, noting (correctly) that "we can't order abortions even to protect the post-viable and potentiality of life if a woman objects."

The lawyer for the fetus concluded, "All we are arguing is the state's obligation to rescue a potential life from a dying mother." The judge took a short recess and then issued his opinion orally. The decisive consideration was Ms. C's terminal condition: "The uncontroverted medical testimony is that Angela will probably die within the next twenty-four to forty-eight hours." He did "not clearly know what Angela's present views are" respecting the cesarean section, but found that the fetus had a 50 to 60 percent chance to survive and a less than 20 percent chance for serious handicap. "It is not an easy decision to make, but given the choices, the court is of the view that the fetus should be given an opportunity to live."

Shortly after the court recessed at 4:15 p.m., Hamner informed Ms. C of the decision. Ms. C was on a ventilator, but was able to mouth agreement. The court reconvened upon learning that Ms. was awake and communicating.

The chief of obstetrics, Alan Weingold, reported a more recent discussion with the patient in which she clearly communicated: and after being informed that

Hamner would only do the cesarean section if she consented to it, "very clearly mouthed words several times, I don't want it done. I don't want it done." Hamner confirmed this exchange. Weingold concluded:

I think that she's in contact with reality, clearly understood who Dr. Hamner was. Because of her attachment to him wanted him to perform the surgery. Understood he would not unless she consented and did not consent. This is, in my mind, very clear evidence that she is responding, understanding, and is very capable of making such decisions.

The judge indicated that he was still not sure what her intent was. Counsel for the District of Columbia then suggested that her current refusal did not change anything because the entire proceeding had been premised on the belief that she was refusing to consent. In his words, "I don't think we would be here if she wad said she wants it." The judge concurred and reaffirmed his original order.

Less than an hour later three judges heard by telephone a request for stay of at least fifteen minutes so that arguments could be heard. Ms. C's lawyer told the judges that the cesarean section had been scheduled for 6:30 p.m., which gave them approximately sixteen minutes to hear arguments and make a decision. He argued that the cesarean section would likely end Ms. C's life, and that it was unconstitutional to favor the life of the fetus over that of the mother without the mother's consent. The lawyer for the fetus argued that Ms. C had no important interests in the decision because she was dying; "unintended consequences on the mother" are "insignificant in respect to the mother's very short life expectancy." "The state's interest," she said, "overrides any interest in the mother's continued very short life, which is under heavy medication and very short duration."

A discussion ensued about the possibility of the fetus surviving, which the chief judge cut short by asking: "Let me ask you this, if its relevant at all. Obviously the fetus has a better chance than the mother?" The lawyer for the fetus responded, "Obviously. Right." A few minutes later, the court denied the request for a stay, reserving the right to file an opinion at a later date. The proceeding was concluded at 6:40 p.m.

The cesarean section was performed and the non-viable fetus died approximately two hours later. Ms. C, now confronted with recovery from major surgery and the knowledge of her child's death, died approximately two days later.

[Source: G.J. Annas, "She's Going to Die: The Case of Angela C," *Hastings Center Report* 18, no. 1 (February/March 1988): 23-25.

Case 3: The Case of Robert McFall

In June 1978, Robert McFall, a 39-year-old Pittsburgh asbestos worker, entered Mercy Hospital with an uncontrollable nosebleed. Physicians diagnosed his condition as aplastic anemia, a rare and usually fatal disease in which the bone marrow fails to produce enough red and white blood cells and platelets. McFall's physician recommended a bone-marrow transplant on the grounds that it would increase the patient's chance of surviving for one year from 25 percent to 40 to 60 percent. The search for a compatible transplant donor began with McFall's six brothers and sisters. After they were located in various parts of the country, none turned out to be compatible.

The search continued and McFall's first cousin, David Shimp, aged 43, agreed to undergo some preliminary tests. He was a perfect match for tissue compatibility, but he suddenly refused to be tested for genetic compatibility. He had decided that he would not donate bone marrow to his cousin, even if he was a perfect match. Apparently, some family discussions and disagreements had influenced Shimp's decision. He told his cousin that his wife was angry because he had undergone the first tests without telling her. Shimp's mother also appeared to be bitter about a decades-old disagreement in the family, and she too asked him to stop the testing.

Friends and other McFall relatives believed that disagreements of the past should not affect the present, and they tried to persuade Shimp to change his mind. When McFall called his cousin and told him "You're killing me," Shimp responded that his wife had to come first. Even Shimp's four children tried to persuade him that he would be responsible for his cousin's early death, and they volunteered to be tested themselves; but Shimp would not be moved.

McFall then filed suit to compel his cousin to undergo the bone-marrow transplant. McFall's attorney argued in court that the procedure is essentially harmless to the donor and that the marrow would be replenished, just as blood is replenished after donation. He also cited English common law, dating back to the 13th century, which upheld society's right to force an individual "to help secure the well-being of other members of society." Shimp's attorney argued that his client's right to refuse could not be invaded, and that "no one could be forced to submit to an operation."

Shimp told reporters that he refused to be a donor because he was afraid of becoming paralyzed during the procedure and feared that his marrow might fail to regenerate.

Judge John Flaherty denied McFall's request to force Shimp to undergo the transplant. The judge based his decision on U.S. common-law precedents, which do not recognize a legal duty to take action to save another person's life. "This would defeat the sanctity of the individual," he argued. "Our society is based on the right and sanctity of the individual. It would require forcible submission to the medical procedure. Forcible extraction of bodily tissues causes revulsion to the judicial mind. The rights of the individual must be upheld, even though it appears to be a harsh decision." The judge also declared irrelevant the argument by McFall's attorney that in English law, court-ordered transplants are permitted. Although he thus held that Shimp had no legal obligation to donate his marrow, Judge Flaherty nevertheless called Shimp's refusal "morally indefensible."

After the ruling, McFall told the press, "I feel sorry for my cousin because he and I are friends and he was under a lot of pressure." Shimp made no comment, but his mother said, "He's not a coward the way they are trying to make him out to be. When you get on the table there is no guaranteeing how much bone marrow they will take. It could be my son's death sentence. The doctors don't care about the donors; they care about patients."

On August 10, 1978, Robert McFall died of a cranial hemorrhage. His last request was that his family forgive his cousin, whose actions he found understandable even if not justifiable. A hospital spokesperson said that cranial hemorrhage is a common complication for people with aplastic anemia and that it might have occurred even with the bone-marrow transplant. The day after his cousin died, Shimp said, "I could throw up right now. I feel terrible about Robert dying, but he asked me for something I couldn't give. That's all I can say now. I feel sick."

[Sources for this case include B.J. Culliton, "Court Upholds Refusal to Be Medical Good Samaritan," *Science* 201 (18 August 1978): 596-97; "Bone Marrow Transplant Rejected," *American Medical News* 21 (11 August 1978): 13.]

XV. Study Questions

1. Examine the right to refuse treatment as an American cultural phenomenon. How does this right relate to the intellectual and political assumptions that undergird the U.S. Constitution and Bill of Rights?

2. In light of question 1, is the basic right to refuse treatment universal or culturally relative? Think of this issue relative to the long-standing practice of clitoridectomy and/or radical vulvectomy, performed on young women in Muslim cultures in certain African countries. Think about this issue with regard to both the clinician's and the patient's right to refuse.

3. Review Exhibit 7-1, the "Patient Choice of Care Statement." Should such a document be a standard part of every patient's medical record? What could be added to or deleted from this document?

4. Consider the AC case in relation to the case of Robert McFall. In the McFall case, the judge ruled that U.S. common-law precedents do not recognize a duty to take action to save another person's life, stating: "This would defeat the sanctity of the individual. It would require forcible submission to the medical procedure. Forcible extraction of bodily tissues causes revulsion to the judicial mind. The rights of the individual must be upheld, even though it appears to be a harsh decision."[30] What analogies are there between the two cases? What role, if any, does the patient's gender play?

5. Consider the case of *Fresno County Social Services v. Xiong* from the perspective of refusal to treat. Place yourself in the role of chief of orthopedic surgery at Bay Area Shriner's Hospital. If the ethics committee, in concert with state and federal courts, determined that the surgery should be performed to correct Xou's clubfeet and dislocated hip, would you, as the orthopedic surgeon, perform the surgery over the patient's and his surrogates refusal of treatment?

6. Consider the AC case from the perspective of refusal to treat. Dr. H refuses to perform the cesarian section on AC unless she grants permission for the surgery. AC refuses permission, but the cesarean section is performed anyway, by another physician (let us call her Dr. M). Examine Dr. H's actions in this case relative to Dr. M's. Under what circumstances should clinicians refuse to provide treatment, especially if the patient does not want it? Is civil disobedience a final option in this sort of case?

Notes

1. N. Gibbs, "Love and Let Die," *Time* (19 March 1990): 65.

2. *State v. McAfee*, 259 Ga. 385 S.E. 2d 651 (1989).

3. J.S. Mill, *On Liberty* (New York: Bobbs-Merrill,

1956), 13.

4. G. Dworkin, *Paternalism in Morality and the Law* (Belmont, Calif.: Wadsworth, 1971): 114.

5. H.T. Engelhardt, Jr., *The Foundations of Bioethics* (New York: Oxford University Press, 1986), 264.

6. *Mohr v. Williams*, 95 Minn. 261, 104 N.W. 12 (1905).

7. *Pratt v. Davis*, 118 Ill. App. 161, at 166 (1905), *aff'd*, 224 Ill. 300, 79 N.E. 562 (1906).

8. *Schloendorff v. Society of New York Hospital*, 211 N.Y. 125, at 129, 105 N.E. 92, at 93 (1914).

9. *Natanson v. Kline*, 186 Kan. 393, at 406, 350 P. 2d 1093, at 1104 (1960).

10. R.M. Veatch, *A Theory of Medical Ethics* (New York: Basic Books, 1981), 208.

11. E.H. Loewy, *Textbook of Medical Ethics* (New York: Plenum Medical Book, 1989), 62-63.

12. R. Taylor, "Religion vs. Ethics," *Free Inquiry* 2, no. 3 (1982): 53-57.

13. S.S. Braithwaite and D.C. Thomasma, "Protherapeutic Authoritarianism," in *Medical Ethics: A Guide for Health Professionals* (Rockville, Md.: Aspen, 1988), 327.

14. Ibid.

15. Ibid., p. 1, 333.

16. G.J. Annas, *Judging Medicine* (Clifton, N.J.: Humana Press, 1988), 291.

17. Ibid., p. 298.

18. *Bouvia v. Superior Court*, 179 Cal. App. 3d 1127, 225 Cal. Rptr. 297 (Ct.App. 1986). Adapted from G. Annas, *Judging Medicine* (Clifton, N.J., Humana Press, 1988), 290-301.

19. American Hospital Association, *A Patient's Bill of Rights*, (Chicago: AHA, 1992), 1.

20. President's Commission for the Study of Ethical Problems in Medicine and Biomedical and Behavioral Research, *Making Health Care Decisions* (Washington, D.C.: U.S. Government Printing Office, 1982), 45-46.

21. *United States v. Ballard*, 322 U.S. 78, 86 (1944).

22. *Thomas v. Review Board*, 450 U.S. 707, 714 (1981).

23. G.J. Annas and M.A. Grodin, "The Nuremburg Code," in *The Nazi Doctors and the Nuremburg Code: Human Rights in Human Experimentation* (New York: Oxford University Press, 1992), 2.

24. 45 *Code of Federal Regulations* 46.116 (a)(8).

25. Ibid.

26. Va. Code Ann., sec 54.1-2990 (Michie 1992): "Nothing in this article shall be construed to require a physician to prescribe or render medical treatment to a patient that the physician determines to be medically or ethically inappropriate. However, in such a case, if the physician's determination is contrary to the terms of an advance directive of a qualified patient or the treatment decision of a person designated to make the decision under this article, the physician shall make a reasonable effort to transfer the patient to another physician."

27. Society of Critical Care Medicine Ethics Committee, "Consensus Statement on the Triage of Critically Ill Patients," *Journal of the American Medical Association* 271 (1994): 1200-03.

28. Ibid, 1202.

29. This case was adpated from a report of the Ethics Consultation Service of the University of Virginia.

30. B.J. Culliton, "Court Upholds Refusal to Be Medical Good Samaritan," *Science* 201 (18 August 1978): 596-97.

8

DEATH AND DYING

Charles A. Hite, M.A., and Mary Faith Marshall, Ph.D.

I. Introduction

This chapter discusses a cluster of three problems that face all clinicians who serve patients who are terminally ill: defining death, relieving suffering and pain, and delivering bad news.

The success of modern medicine in preserving life has brought with it a fundamental transformation in our society's attitude toward death. The lifesaving technologies and treatments used to stave off death frequently result in a more agonizing end of life. The power to prolong life too often brings more horror than hope. It is not uncommon for suffering to result, not only from the cause of disease, but also from its treatment. The wisdom of our struggle to gain dominion over death is being questioned. Because the process of fighting death often makes life more unbearable, many choose to embrace death and reject life-sustaining technology.

The place of death has changed. We no longer die among family and friends; more often, we die among strangers. Fifty years ago, 63 percent of Americans died at home. Today, nearly 80 percent take their last breath in a hospital or long-term-care facility. This shift in the venue of death has been accompanied by a change in the relationship between patients and doctors. In the not-too-distant past, most patients were seen by a family doctor--a practitioner who had a limited range of options but who had intimate knowledge of a patient's history and values. Today we live in an age of specialists. In the hospital setting, in particular, these highly trained practitioners have spo-

radic, fragmented relationships with patients. They tend to see not the whole patient but only the particular pathology being treated. Their very specialized and technical knowledge is designed to conquer disease and death and leads patients to demand treatment and expect cure. Stopping treatment and accepting death is tantamount to defeat.

The once-simple act of declaring a person dead is now held hostage by medical technology. "Ours will go down as the era that reinvented death," says ethicist Nancy Dubler. "The motivation," she says, "was the ability to transplant organs."[1] Even in cases of massive brain damage, Dubler notes, organ systems can be maintained for days or weeks. But without an intact brain to regulate them, organs will deteriorate and be unsuitable for transplant. The mere beating of the heart and breathing of the lungs have become an inadequate measure of what constitutes life.

The paradox of modern medicine, that treatment intended to save life often ends up prolonging the agony of dying, is at the heart of two major ethical controversies: euthanasia and physician-assisted suicide. These controversies often explode into public consciousness through dramatic cases that reveal sharp differences over whether or under what circumstances the deliberate taking of life can ever be acceptable.

These cases can involve family members who, frustrated by the medical system's inability to relieve the suffering of loved ones, take the life of someone close to them. In 1985, for example, Roswell Gilbert killed his wife of 51 years by shooting her twice in the head while she sat on the couch. Gilbert, a 76-year-old retired electronics engineer, who lived in Florida, said simply that he could no longer stand to see his wife suffer like an animal. Emily Gilbert had been afflicted by Alzheimer's disease for more than a decade and suffered from a severely collapsed spinal column due to osteoporosis.[2] In 1984, Daniel McKay, a veterinarian in a small Illinois town, was present at the birth of his son, John Francis. The infant was born with a hairlip, cleft palate, webbed hands, and a heart and lung deformity. McKay did not want to see his son suffer and became incensed when the medical team did not involve him in the decision about whether the baby should be treated. McKay took his child from the incubator, walked to a corner of the room, and struck the baby's head to the floor twice.[3]

More recently, attention has focused on participation by physicians in the deaths of their patients. Two examples that follow illustrate why some view physician-assisted suicide with alarm, warning about the dangers of slipping into practices that come close to the involuntary euthanasia of Nazi Germany, while others see it as a logical extension of a physician's duty to relieve suffering.

In June 1990, 54-year-old Janet Adkins died in the back of a Volkswagen van in a Michigan campground. The van belonged to Dr. Jack Kevorkian, a pathologist who publicly promotes the idea of assisted suicide. Kevorkian has invented a "suicide machine" that allows patients to deliver a lethal dose of medication into their bloodstreams by simply throwing a switch. Adkins was newly diagnosed as having Alzheimer's disease, but she was in excellent health at the time of her death. She had known Kevorkian only briefly. Adkins' death outraged many in the medical community. Critics labeled Kevorkian "Dr. Death" and condemned him for failing to explore adequately other alternatives with a patient he barely knew.

A few months later, Dr. Timothy Quill of the University of Rochester wrote about the death of a 45-year-old patient identified as "Diane." Diane had terminal, acute leukemia. She refused treatment that offered her a 25 percent chance of long-term survival, saying she did not want to endure the pain and the loss of dignity and control over her life that would occur with aggressive therapy. Diane told Quill that her desire was to live out her few remaining weeks of life enjoying her family and friends. She asked Quill to provide her with enough medication so that she could take a lethal dose when she felt ready to end her life. Quill, who had treated Diane for more than eight years, was convinced she had thoroughly explored and rejected other options. He provided her the medication. While some questioned Quill's decision, he has been seen, unlike Kevorkian, as a compassionate, caring doctor who struggled to do what was best for a patient for whom he cared deeply.

Although some view the withdrawing and withholding of life-sustaining treatment as "passive euthanasia," we believe a consensus has emerged over the last decade that such a practice is ethical and legal. Ethical problems surrounding the forgoing of life-sustaining treatment are addressed in Chapter 9. In this chapter, we examine proposals that would allow physicians to assist patients with their deaths under certain circumstances, and we examine the system of euthanasia in the Netherlands.

Too frequently, death has become "ghettoized" in the American healthcare system. Terminally ill patients are sent to the enclave of hospice care to spend their final days. Those who do not make it to hospice often receive far less attention and comfort care on acute-care floors than patients who are not terminally ill. This chapter explores how the concepts and techniques of comfort care and pain management developed by hospice can be applied throughout medical practice and why these techniques should become an integral part of medical education.

The final section of this chapter builds on the work of a noted psychiatrist, Robert Buckman, regarding how to talk with patients or family members when disclosing "bad news."

II. Defining Death

Until the last 30 years or so, determining whether a person was dead was a relatively simple matter. Reflecting an earlier era when most people died at home, popular guidance was available to family members to assist them in the determination of a relative's death. In *The Old Person in Your Home*, William Poe described the signs of death as such: "The eyes become fixed, with opened pupils which do not respond to light. The heartbeat and breathing cease. The mouth may be open and motionless. The skin turns pale and cold. The skin in contact with the bed may become bluish or purple--liver mortis. After thirty to sixty minutes the limp extremities may become stiff--rigor mortis."[4]

The cessation of breathing and the absence of an audible heartbeat or a pulse have been death-defining criteria throughout most of history. As with all aspects of medicine, some room for error in the diagnosis of death existed in earlier times, especially prior to the advent of the stethoscope. During the Middle Ages, observers occasionally reported evidence that an individual, assumed to be dead, had been buried alive. The discovery of scratch marks on the inside of coffin lids of exhumed skeletons led to such extraordinary precautions as round-the-clock mortuary attendants who frequently assessed their charges for any signs of life, ropes reaching from buried coffins to an above-ground bell that could be heard by cemetery attendants, and speaking tubes leading from coffins to the ground above so that the cemetery attendant could be summoned should a corpse "awaken."

Modern technology such as the electrocardiogram, which provides an electrical "picture" of heart activity, makes the definition of death via heart/lung criteria essentially infallible. Defining death using the criteria of cessation of heartbeat and breathing, and the absence of a pulse or blood flow is, in essence, a whole-body orientation toward death. This approach to defining death has its roots in Western Judeo-Christian theological traditions. By traditional Jewish standards, death occurred when an individual drew his or her last breath. The Roman Catholic religion, recognizing the soul as encompassed by all of the body, held to the broader heart/lung criteria.[5]

Until recently, American common law also recognized a whole-body definition of death. In 1968, *Black's Law Dictionary* defined death as "the cessation of life; the ceasing to exist; defined by physicians as a total stoppage of the circulation of the blood, and a cessation of the animal and vital functions consequent thereon, such as respiration, pulsation, etc."[6]

The whole-body concept of death, which had historically sufficed as a standard, became inadequate in the 1960s for a number of reasons. The development of intensive care units and their attendant technology allowed for the biological maintenance of persons who previously would have died by heart/lung criteria. Occasional legal cases begged the question

of the timing of death using heart/lung criteria when order of survivorship was at issue.[7]

The capacity of intensive care units to temporarily maintain patients who had lost complete brain function fueled a theoretical debate regarding biological death. The advent of organ transplantation accelerated the debate for pragmatic reasons. Patients who had lost total brain function, including neocortex and brain-stem function, could be biologically maintained on artificial life support for only a period of days before all other organ systems subsequently failed. The opportunities that patients who were brain dead presented as potential organ sources occasioned serious reconsideration of the theoretical and legal definition of death.

In 1968, the Ad Hoc Committee of the Harvard Medical School to Examine the Definition of Brain Death explored this conceptual issue, and subsequently published a report in the *Journal of the American Medical Association* endorsing a whole-brain (versus a whole-body) definition of death.[8] Their criteria for determining brain death included:

1. coma, demonstrated by total unreceptivity and unresponsivity to stimuli;
2. absence of spontaneous breathing given a normal carbon dioxide range;
3. absence of reflexes given the absence of any neurologically depressant medications;
4. a flat or isoelectric electroencephalogram (picture of the electrical activity of the brain).[9]

During the 1970s, some 20 states passed statutes adopting the whole-brain definition of death. In 1975, the American Bar Association even went so far as to propose that whole-brain function be the sole criterion for determining death.[10] Although a few states passed statutes based on this recommendation, its future was foreshortened. In 1981, the President's Commission for the Study of Ethical Problems in Medicine and Biomedical and Behavioral Research proposed a Uniform Determination of Death Act, which endorsed both whole-body (heart/lung) and whole-brain definitions of death. The commission's report stated: "An individual who has sustained either (1) irreversible cessation of circulatory and respiratory functions, or (2) irreversible cessation of all functions of the entire brain, including the brain stem, is dead."[11]

The central thesis behind this conceptual orientation was that the failure of other organ systems (including the heart and lungs) inevitably followed whole-brain death within a relatively short period of time, and that with the loss of either whole-brain or heart/lung function, the breakdown of all other bodily functions would shortly follow.

The current theoretical and conceptual debate regarding the definition of death centers on brain function alone. The controversy is framed by the level of brain function (whole-brain versus partial-brain) necessary to sustain what might be called "life." The conceptual inquiry no longer involves merely biological questions, but includes the philosophical issue of personhood.

The evolution of our concept of death has resulted from the advent of patients who exist in states of permanent unconsciousness (particularly patients who are in a "persistent vegetative state" or PVS). PVS involves the permanent loss of higher cortical brain function. However, the brain stem, which regulates spontaneous vegetative functions such as breathing and sleep/wake cycles and digestion, continues to function. Patients in PVS are capable of involuntary movements (for example eye opening or yawning). They lack any mechanism for sensory input or feeling, lack self-awareness or awareness of their surroundings, and are incontinent. Given adequate maintenance care--including feeding and hydration via nasogastric or gastrostomy tubes, frequent turning to prevent bedsores, physical therapy to prevent contractions, and antibiotics to treat pulmonary infections--such patients can live for years or decades.

Two famous patients, Karen Ann Quinlan and Nancy Beth Cruzan, were in a persistent vegetative state for years. The parents of both young women engaged in protracted court battles for the right to withdraw treatment from their daughters.

The marker on Nancy Cruzan's grave reads:

NANCY BETH CRUZAN
MOST LOVED
DAUGHTER - SISTER - AUNT
Born, July 20, 1957
Departed, Jan 11, 1983
At Peace, Dec 26, 1990

The intrinsic horror that many in the general public feel about continued biological existence in a state of permanent unconsciousness such as PVS has escalated the debate regarding the definition of death. The question arises whether human life is defined simply in biological terms or whether its definition extends to personal qualities such as consciousness and self-awareness. No general consensus exists on this issue among philosophers, clinicians, or laypersons. The issue of whether the definition of death should be extended to cover patients who are in a PVS depends on how one personally views life and death. Some argue that the question is pragmatically moot, because maintenance care can be legally and ethically withdrawn from PVS patients, who will then subsequently "die."

Guidelines for the determination of brain death in newborn infants have evolved more slowly than for adults due to clinical difficulties in making accurate neurological assessments. In infants carried to full term who are less than seven days old, severe neurological injuries may be reversible; the cause of coma is often difficult to establish and may also be reversible; and clinical signs (such as fixed and dilated pupils) may be the result of metabolic imbalances, hypothermia, sedative drugs, and other remedial conditions. The American Academy of Pediatrics Task Force for the Determination of Brain Death in Children published guidelines in 1987 that preclude the diagnosis of brain death in premature infants or in full-term infants less than seven days old.[12] Most of the criteria for determining brain death in full-term infants are similar to those used for adults.

Determining brain death in anencephalic infants has, as yet, proved an impossible task. Anencephaly is a clinical condition in which an infant's membranous skull and the cerebral hemispheres of the brain are absent. The degree of brain-stem development may vary. Anencephalic infants are generally stillborn or die within a few days after birth.[13] The inability to declare brain death in these infants often poses a difficult problem for parents who wish to donate their anencephalic child's organs, seeing this "gift" as one of the only positive aspects of an otherwise tragic situation.

Patients who have been diagnosed as brain dead but who are still being maintained on life supports often pose special problems for family members who may have difficulty conceptualizing the fact that their relative is dead when they see the patient's chest rise and fall from mechanical ventilation and when a cardiac tracing is visible on the electrocardiogram monitor. General clinical wisdom dictates that once the diagnosis of brain death has been made, all artificial life supports should be withdrawn, and the family should be notified that the patient has died.

III. Suffering and Comfort

All too frequently, clinicians who treat terminally ill patients are reluctant to abandon their traditional role of curing the patient and fighting for life. They may be ill-equipped to deal with the complex and idiosyncratic factors that enter into the suffering of patients. They may refuse to recognize that in the care of dying patients, all other goals take a back seat to the relief of suffering. One of the guiding principles of what has come to be called "comfort care" or "palliative care" is that physicians and other clinicians no longer accept suffering as a necessary evil in the patient's treatment.

Eric Cassell, a physician and bioethicist who has written extensively on care for the dying, emphasizes that suffering involves more than pain. "Suffering occurs when an impending destruction of the person is perceived; it continues until the threat of disintegration has passed or until the integrity of the person can be restored in some other manner. It follows, then, that although it often occurs in the presence of acute pain, shortness of breath or other bodily symptoms, suffering extends beyond the physical. Most generally, suffering can be defined as the state of severe distress associated with events that threaten the intactness of the person."[14]

Such events arise from a variety of factors that go into what makes up a person, Cassell notes. This includes relationships with family and friends, cultural background, sexuality, self-esteem, physical traits, skills and abilities, important memories, and even previous experiences with healthcare providers. By way of illustration, Cassell outlines the case of a 35-year-old sculptor with advanced cancer of the breast. The patient was treated with radiation therapy in lieu of a mastectomy, which disfigured one of her breasts. The removal of her ovaries and treatment with a series of medications caused her to become obese, grow facial and body hair, and lose her libido. She lost strength in the hand she relied on for sculpting when cancer invaded nerves near her shoulder. At one point, she became incontinent with watery diarrhea that would occur unexpectedly, often when guests

were present. She sustained a fracture of the thigh, which was caused by cancer and was put in traction. The fracture was repaired, but she was advised not to put weight on the leg because cancer had weakened the bone.

The sculptor certainly suffered physical pain: the nausea and vomiting caused by chemotherapy and the discomfort associated with surgical procedures. But she also suffered from the effect of the disease and its treatment on her personal and social life: "She was housebound and bedbound, her face was changed by steroids, and she was masculinized by her treatment, one breast was twisted and scarred, and she had almost no hair. . . . People can suffer from what they have lost of themselves in relation to the world of objects, events and relationships."[15] Moreover, she suffered from her perception of what the future would bring: "Each tomorrow was seen as worse than today, as heralding increased sickness, pain, or disability--never as the beginning of better times. Despite the distress cause by such thoughts, she could not think otherwise. She felt isolated because she was not like other people and could not do what other people did. She feared that her friends would stop visiting her. She was sure she would die."[16]

In treating the dying and hopelessly ill, clinicians must learn to focus on caring, not curing. They must learn to look beyond simply alleviating physical pain and recognize the complex and highly personal factors that cause suffering. Over the past quarter-century, the modern hospice movement has developed and refined just such an approach in the techniques of comfort care or palliative care. Unfortunately, many of these techniques have not been transferred to the hospital setting, which is where the vast majority of patients die. Ethicists Baruch Brody and H. Tristram Engelhardt, Jr., identify four reasons why hospitals often seem to be unresponsive to the needs of dying patients and their families:

1. The primary concern of physicians and nurses seems to be with those patients who are viewed as having a good chance of surviving. Those who are dying often seem to receive less attention until they suffer an acute crisis.
2. The emphasis in hospitals seems to be on dealing with illnesses and not with painful symptoms. The dying need special attention

to the management of their many painful and degrading symptoms, and this seems to be less central on the hospital agenda.

3. The hospital relegates the patient's family to a secondary place. Visiting hours and the number of visitors are often limited, and little attention is paid to family needs. The special needs of dying patients and their families all seem less central to the agenda of the hospital.

4. Hospitals seem to be organized to fight death until there is nothing left to do. This is, after all, an appropriate attitude for its normal patients. But the terminally ill do not necessarily benefit from such an attitude, so the hospital as normally organized may be inappropriate for them.[17]

The techniques of comfort care and palliative care can be implemented in any clinical setting, but, for the reasons cited above, they are most commonly associated with formal hospice programs.

The modern hospice movement began in 1967 with the founding of St. Christopher's Hospice in England by Cicely Saunders, M.D. The cornerstones of hospice treatment as defined by Saunders are effective control of pain and other symptoms, care of the patient and family as a unit, an interdisciplinary team approach, the use of volunteers, a continuum of care that includes care at home, continuity of care between different settings, and follow-up with family members after the patient's death. By 1993 there were more than 2,000 hospices serving nearly 250,000 people in the United States.[18]

Twenty years ago, Saunders summarized the philosophy of hospice by remembering a young patient who told her as he faced death and leaving his family, "I've fought and I've fought--but now I've accepted."[19] According to Saunders:

We, too, have to learn to accept as well as to fight and to realize that part of our work can have nothing to do with cure but only with the giving of relief and comfort. We will learn by looking at patients, by listening to what they want to say and by meeting their needs as far as we can both practically and philosophically. His readiness finally to say yes to death was in itself an affirma-

tion of life. We need him as much and more than he needs us. Anything which says to the very ill or the very old that there is no longer anything that matters in their life would be a deep impoverishment to the whole of society.[20]

Hospice care has been a major influence on how traditional medical care addresses the relief of pain, one of the major fears of dying patients. Hospice clinicians established the importance of administering medication on a regular schedule so that there would be "constant control" of "constant pain."[21] Hospice clinicians also pioneered and promoted the use of continuous or intermittent parenteral narcotics and patient-controlled analgesia, and they have shown that addiction to pain medications is not a problem for terminally ill patients. The hospice movement has been a leader in responding to the spiritual and social aspects of suffering for the dying. Hospice care providers recognized the importance of patients' fears of loss of control and loneliness and abandonment.[22]

The philosophy and techniques of comfort care can be used in the treatment of patients in any setting, including acute-care hospitals. But many physicians are reluctant to offer comfort care until all possible medical treatments have been used and the patient is near death, according to Timothy Quill, the former medical director of a New York hospice. In *Death and Dignity*, Quill notes that a fundamental characteristic of comfort care is the emphasis on the patient as a person compared to the usual focus on the patient's underlying disease. In comfort care, any treatments or procedures that do not add to the patient's comfort and sense of well-being are stopped. Invasive procedures are used if they help ease pain. Patients are encouraged to share specific fears they may have. The role of family and friends is explored, and patients are aided in repairing broken relationships. The fundamental commitment in comfort care, Quill says, is not to abandon the dying patient in the final stage of life. That begins, he says, by assuring patients that they have power to decide what is best for them.[23] According to Quill:

Comfort care values the uniqueness of each human being, and tries to individualize as much as possible. There are therefore no preset formulas about how to proceed until one has met the patient and begun to understand what is important from his perspective. Comfort care tries to give each individual maximum control, making no assumptions about what choices might be made. . . . One patient may want to die at home no matter what, and another may prefer to stay at home until the end is near, but then return to the hospital to die. Some individuals may easily accept their family's involvement in intimate bodily care as they become weaker, whereas others may find such dependence humiliating and unacceptable. For each decision, the values and expectations of the patient must take precedence over those of the caregivers and the family.[24]

Although proponents of comfort care have made great strides in developing methods to control pain, many patients spend their dying days with their pain inadequately treated. Studies of cancer patients in particular show that millions die each year with uncontrolled pain.[25] One major reason is healthcare professionals' lack of knowledge about appropriate pain management. No formal education programs in pain management exist for medical students and house staff, meaning that the majority of dying cancer patients are cared for by primary-care physicians and nurses who have limited knowledge about pain management and symptom control. Another barrier to pain management is physicians', patients', and families' unsubstantiated fear of addiction. Adding to the problem are barriers in the healthcare system. Control of pain is not considered an adequate reason for admission to a hospital, and there are inadequate community resources and expertise to manage cancer patients' pain at home. Many health insurance programs do not cover the increasingly sophisticated techniques being used for pain control.[26]

Researchers have reported that undertreatment of pain is one reason that some terminally ill patients consider suicide or request their physicians to hasten death.[27] Some maintain that if dying patients were offered adequate pain control and comfort care, the need for physician-assisted suicide or euthanasia would lessen. Quill argues, however, that even in the best hospice programs staffed with highly trained and compassionate caregivers, there are still instances where patients endure intolerable suffering. Like Cassell, Quill believes that the angst of dying involves much more than physical suffering. Suffering is emotional and existential; it involves everything that goes into the concept of an individual's dignity. Loss of dignity robs patients of all meaning and adds to their suffering. Quill asserts: "We have difficulty accepting that for humans, death is sometimes the only escape from intolerable suffering. Allowing someone a peaceful, dignified death under such terrible circumstances can be a very sad, loving gift. Provided that all other options have been thoroughly explored and understood, and we are certain that this is what the patient wants, it may be the best of a very limited number of options one can offer under such dire circumstances."[28]

IV. Euthanasia and Physician-Assisted Suicide

Euthanasia, the intentional taking of another life to promote a "good" or merciful death, can be traced as far back as the ancient Greek and Roman civilizations. Those cultures did not hold the belief that life is precious and should be preserved at all costs. The prevailing attitude was that life, without a chance for a meaningful or happy existence, has little value. The Spartans, for example, required that all deformed infants be put to death. In Athens, the destruction of unhealthy or deformed infants was permitted. For those with an incurable disease who were in great pain, assisting them to end their life was viewed as morally acceptable.[29]

Judaism and Christianity radically changed this view, providing the foundation for the modern Western concept of the sanctity of life. Jewish theologians were uncompromising in their teaching that helping a terminally ill person to die was wrong. In the early Christian church, taking a human life in any form was absolutely forbidden. Suffering was a burden imposed by God that had to be borne until death came naturally. Suffering had meaning. In both Judaism and Christianity, suffering allows the individual to identify with the suffering of others and to share a connection with the larger human community. In this way, the sufferer transcends pain and derives meaning from suffering. Gradually, the Christian church altered its prohibition against taking life to allow killing in a just war or lawfully executing criminals. The guiding principle ultimately became that the intentional killing of innocent humans is wrong. The emphasis on intent allowed the development of the "doctrine of double effect," which means that an act with both good and bad consequences can be carried out so long as certain conditions are met. In the care of a terminally ill patient in terrible pain, for example, the doctrine would permit physicians to administer dosages of pain-relieving drugs so large that they result in killing the patient.[30]

It is against this background that the debate over euthanasia in modern medical history has occurred. During most of the 19th century, physicians generally refused to help incurably ill and dying patients end their lives. Napoleon's physician, for instance, refused the general's request to give a fatal dose of drugs to several mortally ill soldiers who were unable to march and likely to fall into enemy hands. The composer, Hector Berlioz, complained bitterly about the refusal of physicians to end the life of an older sister, who died of breast cancer after six months of excruciating pain.

> My other sister, who went to Grenoble to nurse her, and who did not leave her till the end, all but died from the fatigue and the painful impressions caused by this slow agony. And not a doctor dared to have the humanity to end this martyrdom by making my sister inhale a bottle of chloroform.... The most horrible thing in the world for us, living and sentient beings, is inexorable suffering, pain without any possible compensation when it has reached this degree of intensity; and one must be barbarous, or stupid, or both at once, not to use the sure and easy means now at our disposal to bring it to an end. Savages are more intelligent and more humane.[31]

By the turn of the 20th century, however, physicians and laypersons alike began calling on the medical profession to relax its rigid stance in the treatment of terminally ill patients and patients with incurable disease. Four therapeutic approaches were identified. The first and second applied to patients who were near death. The third and fourth applied to patients who had painful, incurable illness. These approaches continue to shape the euthanasia debate today. They are:

1. The physician could do everything possible to make terminally ill patients as fulfilled and as free

from pain as possible. Nothing could be offered, however, that would hasten death.
2. Physicians could take steps to alleviate suffering, even if they jeopardized the patient's life in the process.
3. The physician could withdraw active therapy that was simply prolonging the patient's suffering. However, the physician was not to abandon the patient.
4. Physicians had the moral right to terminate purposely the life of a patient who suffered from an incurable and agonizing disease and who wanted to die.[32]

This last approach has dominated the debate in recent years over just how far physicians should go in dealing with the requests of incurably ill patients to end their suffering.

This ethical problem received attention in the 1930s. In England, the Voluntary Euthanasia Legalization Society was formed to promote the legalization of painless death. The organization presented a bill to Parliament that proposed allowing euthanasia if the candidate was more than 21 years old and suffering from an incurable disorder involving severe pain. It required a formal written application certified by two witnesses, to be sent to a referee who was to review the request and interview the patient. If permission were granted, someone other than the patient's doctor was to carry out the euthanasia.[33]

In the United States, a group of prominent clergymen that later became known as the Euthanasia Society of America, proposed that it should be legal for "incurable sufferers to choose immediate death rather than await it in agony." In 1938, the founder and chairman of the group, Dr. Charles Potter, a Unitarian minister, said that such a choice was necessary to preserve human dignity. According to Potter: "The problem of euthanasia is one which sooner or later confronts every practicing physician. Perhaps the time has come to forget the Commandment 'Thou Shalt Not Kill,' and listen to Jesus 'Blessed Are the Merciful.' There is no logical argument against euthanasia. Most opposition is based on misunderstanding of the proposed procedure."[34]

In the more than half a century since Potter made that statement, the conflict over euthanasia has continued. In 1988, an article in the *Journal of the Ameri-*

can *Medical Association* (*JAMA*) touched off a new round of debate over when, if ever, to hasten a patient's death.

A. Debbie's Case

In early 1988, an unsigned article in *JAMA* presented a first-person account of a gynecology resident who gave a lethal dose of morphine to a 20-year-old woman who was suffering from ovarian cancer. She had not responded to chemotherapy and was being given supportive care only. The resident described an emaciated, hollow-eyed patient suffering from severe air hunger and unrelenting vomiting. "Debbie" had not eaten or slept in two days. Her only words to the resident, who had never seen her before, were, "Let's get this over with."[35]

Response to the article was overwhelming. Although some sympathized with Debbie's plight, few could defend the resident's handling of the situation. Critics said Debbie's case epitomized many of the worst horrors of physicians' participation in euthanasia: the resident had no established relationship with the patient, had made only a cursory review of the patient's chart, had not talked with the patient's treating physician, and had not talked with the patient's family. The resident relied on a quickly formed, personal reaction to Debbie's plight and a vague request from Debbie herself as the basis for taking a life. To some physician-ethicists, this kind of behavior threatens the soul of medicine. According to Gaylin and colleagues: "This issue touches medicine at its very moral center; if this moral center collapses, if physicians become killers or are even merely licensed to kill, the profession--and, therewith, each physician--will never again be worthy of trust and respect as healer and comforter and protector of life in all its frailty. For if medicine's power over life may be used equally to heal or to kill, the doctor is no more a moral professional but rather a morally neutered technician."[36]

Not all cases, however, are as black-and-white as Debbie's. Less than a year after *JAMA* devoted a special section to the reaction to Debbie's case, the *New England Journal of Medicine* published an update to a five-year-old article that outlined how physicians should care for hopelessly ill patients. This update urged timely discussions with patients about dying, including the use of advance directives. It urged ad-justing the plan of care to suit the needs of each dying patient, including the aggressive use of pain relievers. It acknowledged that it is "certainly not rare" for physicians to assist patients in suicide, either by prescribing medication that could be used in an overdose or discussing required doses and methods of administering drugs that could induce death. All but two of the 11 authors agreed that "It is not immoral for a physician to assist in the rational suicide of a terminally ill person."[37]

B. A Killing Machine or a Compassionate Doctor?

Janet Adkins was not the only person to be assisted in death by Jack Kevorkian. Since June 1990, the self-described "suicide doctor" has acknowledged assisting in 44 suicides. Kevorkian, 68, has been in and out of court on murder charges, stripped of his license to practice medicine, and condemned as "a serial killer on a killing spree" and "a man with a cause, and the cause is immoral, unethical and very dangerous."[38] The governor of Michigan, in signing a law that imposed a temporary ban on assisted suicide while a commission studied the practice, said that Kevorkian "has deliberately flouted the law and taken it upon himself to be his own judge, jury and executioner. . . . No one should have that right."[39]

Reaction has been far less condemning of Dr. Timothy Quill's decision to assist a 45-year-old patient to die by prescribing barbiturates. New York prosecutors declined to seek charges against him, and state medical officials refused to take action against his license to practice. Quill wrote eloquently and movingly about his eight-year relationship with "Diane."[40] He had grown to admire her determination in overcoming personal problems, including the effects of being raised in an alcoholic family and overcoming vaginal cancer as a young woman. In treating her for acute leukemia, he respected the values that went into Diane's decision not to pursue aggressive treatment. He learned about her deep fear that a lingering death would prevent her from enjoying the few months she had left to live. He became convinced that Diane had explored all other options in facing her death and that her decision to choose suicide was well thought out and rational. He found himself advising her on the amount of barbiturates needed for suicide and writing a prescription. He felt uneasy in doing so. "Yet I also felt strongly that I was setting her free to get the most out of the time she had left, and to maintain dignity and control on her own terms until her death."[41]

Despite vast differences in the way Quill and Kevorkian assisted patients with suicide, particularly in the depth of the doctor-patient relationship, they share one thing in common: they are examples of growing public sentiment that it is ethically permissible for physicians to respond to voluntary requests to assist hopelessly ill patients to die. Shortly after Quill's article was published, *Final Exit* surged to the top of the *New York Times* bestseller list. The book, written by the executive director of the Hemlock Society, gives explicit advice on how terminally ill patients can commit suicide.[42] Later in 1991, voters in Washington State defeated a proposal to legalize physician-assisted dying. It lost by fewer than 100,000 votes out of 1.3 million votes cast. In late 1992, a similar initiative was narrowly defeated by California voters. In November 1994, voters in Oregon approved a ballot initiative to legalize physician-assisted suicide. The Oregon Death with Dignity Act was never implemented, however. A court injunction was issued shortly after its passage, and several months later a federal district judge ruled the measure unconstitutional.[43]

Public opinion polls have shown a dramatic turnaround toward euthanasia since the dawn of medicine's technological era. In 1950, 34 percent of Americans said physicians should be allowed to end the lives of patients with incurable disease if the patients and families requested it. By 1991, support for that position had grown to 63 percent of those polled.[44] In late 1993, a national Harris Poll showed 73 percent agreeing that "the law should allow doctors to comply with the wishes of a dying patient in severe distress who asks to have his or her life ended."[45] In a survey of Michigan physicians and the general public in 1994 and 1995, researchers asked whether physician-assisted suicide in the state should be banned or legalized under certain conditions. The researchers found that, given the choice, two-thirds of the public preferred legalization and one-quarter preferred a ban. Most Michigan physicians preferred either the legalization of physician-assisted suicide or no law at all, and fewer than one-fifth preferred a complete ban.[46] Other polls showed strong public support for Kevorkian's crusade to legalize assisted suicide. "The public is scared of the healthcare system, scared of

the intensive care unit, scared of inadequately treated pain," said Steven H. Miles, a geriatrics specialist and chairperson of the ethics committee at Hennepin County Medical Center in Minneapolis. According to Miles, public support for Kevorkian "reflects a kind of keep-your-options-open philosophy rather than an endorsement of assisted suicide."[47]

The Council of Ethical and Judicial Affairs of the American Medical Association defines euthanasia as "bringing about the death of a hopelessly ill and suffering person in a relatively quick and painless way for reasons of mercy," and physician-assisted suicide as when a doctor "facilitates a patient's death by providing the necessary means and/or information to enable the patient to perform the life-ending act."[48] Both practices have been condemned by the American Medical Association, other professional and healthcare organizations[49] as well as by a number of ethicists and theologians.[50] In recent years, however, many physicians and ethicists have proposed or endorsed schemes in which physicians, under certain guidelines, would be allowed to assist patients with suicide.[51] There also are many who would permit physicians to participate in euthanasia.[52]

Arguments favoring euthanasia and physician-assisted suicide focus on two concerns: (1) compassion for the incurably ill who suffer intolerable pain and (2) respect for their human dignity and freedom.[53] These concerns are based on the principle of beneficence, to do what is best for the patient, and the principle of autonomy, the right of the patient to control treatment.[54] Joseph Fletcher, a pioneer in the bioethics field, argued that failure to permit or encourage euthanasia demeans the dignity of persons. People have dignity, he maintained, only if they are able to choose when, how, and why they are to live or to die. "Death control, like birth control, is a matter of human dignity," Fletcher wrote. "Without it persons become puppets. To perceive this is to grasp the error lurking in the notion, widespread in medical circles, that life as such is the highest good."[55]

Opponents of euthanasia and physician-assisted suicide claim that allowing these practices would undermine trust in the patient-physician relationship and lead to the involuntary killing of the handicapped, the poor, or other disenfranchised members of society. They argue that, if physicians were to prescribe adequate pain medication and make sure that patients received necessary comfort care, then there would be no demand for physician-assisted death or euthanasia.[56] Edmund Pellegrino, an ethicist and physician at Georgetown University, makes these points in an article entitled "Doctors Must Not Kill":

- "How can patients trust that the doctor will pursue every effective and beneficent measure when she can relieve herself of a difficult challenge by influencing the patient to choose death? Uncertainty and mistrust are already too much a part of the healing relationship. Euthanasia magnifies these ordinary and natural anxieties. . . . When the proscription against killing is eroded, trust in the doctor cannot survive."[57]

- "It is a short way from the need to contain costs to covertly or overtly planned euthanasia for those members of our society who present the greatest economic burdens. At the beginning, some might suggest rationing needed care to retarded or handicapped infants, very old people, or those with fatal, incurable disease like Alzheimer's. Once euthanasia, in any of its forms, is legalized, the temptation to encourage its use, tacitly or overtly, to alleviate one of our most socially vexing problems--the increasing scarcity of healthcare dollars--will be strong. This could be the first step on the slippery slope, which leads inexorably from voluntary to nonvoluntary and involuntary euthanasia."[58]

- "Hospice programs or palliative care offer comprehensive alternatives to euthanasia that are more respectful of beneficence and autonomy than killing. They relieve pain and anxiety, prepare the patient for the experience of dying, anticipate the need and value of advance directives, and establish understanding between patient and physician about which life-support measures are acceptable to the patient and which are not."[59]

Objections to euthanasia and physician-assisted suicide have also been raised on religious grounds. Speaking from the Christian tradition, for example, William May and Stanley Hauerwas argue that those who favor euthanasia and physician-assisted death place too much emphasis on avoiding the suffering that is a sometimes necessary part of dying. They both see life as a gift from God that puts obligations on the person who is dying and on those who care for the dying person. The Christian prohibition against suicide, Hauerwas maintains, is based on the assumption that our lives are not ours to do with as we please. It is the obligation of caregivers, he adds, to make sure that persons who are dying continue to feel their importance to the larger community. Hauerwas asserts: "The task of medicine is to care when it cannot cure. The refusal to let an attempted suicide die is only our feeble, but real, attempt to remain a community of trust and care through the agency of medicine. Our prohibition and subsequent care of a suicide draws on our profoundest assumptions that each individual's life has purpose beyond simply being autonomous."[60]

May laments that "preoccupation with death has replaced God as the effective center of religious consciousness in the modern world."[61] Those who see death as the absolute evil will view life as sacred, May maintains. Those who see suffering as the enemy will view quality of life as more important than life itself. Like Hauerwas, May believes that society must strike a balance by allowing those near the end of their lives to die and yet not attempting to solve the problem of suffering by eliminating the sufferer.

Modern culture not only denies the right to die by its often mindless prolongation of life, but, just as seriously, it denies with the same heedlessness the right of the person to do his or her own dying. Since modern procedures, moreover, have made dying at the hands of experts and the machines a prolonged and painful business, emotionally and financially as well as physically, they have built up pressure behind the euthanasia movement, which asserts not the right to die, but the right to be killed.

The euthanasia movement encourages engineering death rather than facing dying. Euthanasia would bypass dying to get one dead as quickly as possible. It proposes to relieve suffering by knocking out the interval between the two states of life and death. The moral impulse behind the movement responds understandably to the quandaries of an age that makes of dying such an inhumanly endless business. However, the movement opposes the horrors of a purely technical death by using techniques to eliminate the victim.[62]

In the Netherlands, physician-assisted suicide and euthanasia are illegal but tolerated under certain circumstances. However, prosecution of physicians for these acts has been rare, provided they follow guidelines outlined by a Dutch government commission. In February 1993, national legislation was passed immunizing physicians against prosecution as long as established guidelines were followed. Among the criteria are:

1. The patient must be mentally competent and explicitly and repeatedly request euthanasia;
2. the patient's mental and physical suffering must be severe with no prospect of improvement;
3. the patient must be well-informed about the request;
4. all options of alternative care have been tried or refused by the patient;
5. two physicians must concur with the request.[63]

In 1991, the first nationwide study in The Netherlands on euthanasia and other medical decisions at the end of life was published. The authors of the study concluded that of the approximately 130,000 deaths in the Netherlands in 1990, about 1.8 percent (2,300 persons) were the result of euthanasia by a physician. Another 0.3 percent of total deaths (400 persons) was attributed to physician-assisted suicide. The study also reported that 0.8 percent of deaths (about 1,000 persons) were cases where "drugs were administered with the explicit intention to shorten the patient's life, without the strict criteria for euthanasia being fulfilled." In more than half of these cases, the decision had been discussed with the patient or the patient has previously expressed a wish for euthanasia if suffering became unbearable.[64] Critics say that this last group of deaths in the Netherlands amounts to "involuntary euthanasia" and is evidence that abuse that can occur even in a system with safeguards. They note with alarm that only 200 cases of euthanasia and assisted suicide were reported by physicians to the Dutch government in 1990, despite guidelines to the contrary.[65]

Two additional nationwide studies on euthanasia and assisted suicide in the Netherlands were commissioned in 1995. The first study, which compared the current end-of-life practices with the results of the 1990 study, reported that practices in 1995 were not much different than those in 1990. Researchers estimated that about 2.3 percent of deaths occurred from euthanasia, up slightly from 1990. The number of deaths from physician-assisted suicide remained at about 0.3 percent. Nearly 80 percent of deaths in both these categories involved patients with cancer. In most cases, a general practitioner was involved. The number of deaths where patients' lives were ended without their explicit consent was down slightly, to 0.7 percent. The patients in this category tended to be relatively young and cancer was the predominant diagnosis (60 percent). In about half of all cases where death occurred without explicit consent, the decision to end life was discussed with the patient earlier in the illness or the patient had expressed a wish for euthanasia if suffering became unbearable. In about a third of these cases, life was shortened 24 hours or less; in another 58 percent, life was shortened by one week or less.[66]

The second study evaluated the effectiveness of procedures that had been established in The Netherlands for reporting and reviewing cases of euthanasia and physician-assisted death. The authors found that the rate of notification of cases of euthanasia and physician-assisted suicide rose from an estimated 18 percent in 1990 to about 41 percent in 1995. Cases of physician-assisted death without the patient's explicit request were rarely reported. Two cases were reported in 1990 and three in 1995. The authors of the study expressed cautious optimism about the Dutch system of physician-assisted death.

There seems only to be a small increase in the number of cases of euthanasia, there are indications that decision making has improved, the number of reported cases has greatly increased, and options for further improvement in public oversight have been identified. Nevertheless, there are limits to any system of oversight. Some decisions will continue to be considered by both doctor and patient to be private, and some tension will remain between the public and the private domain, as in other aspects of medicine. Close monitoring of the practice of physician-assisted death is both necessary and possible.[67]

Marcia Angell found the two studies somewhat reassuring. "Are the Dutch on a slippery slope? It appears not," Angell wrote, noting that the rates of euthanasia and physician-assisted suicide were not much different between 1990 and 1995 and that "nearly all cases of euthanasia involved patients who were suffering from a terminal illness and had only a short time to live. The incidence of ending life without an explicit request from the patient, the most disturbing finding of the earlier study, was slightly less in 1995 than in 1990. It would be very hard to construe these findings as a descent into depravity. As far as we can tell, Dutch physicians continue to practice physician-assisted dying only reluctantly and under compelling circumstances."[68] The fact that the majority of cases of physician-assisted deaths in the Netherlands goes unreported might be attributed to the "multiple levels of legal review" and the fact that "euthanasia remains a crime, despite the official status of the guidelines and the legal reporting requirements," Angell wrote. "It is likely that the rate of reporting will remain low unless the notification procedure is made less daunting and the peculiar legal situation is clarified. Ultimately, it is untenable for a medical practice to be simultaneously legal and illegal."[69]

Some proponents of euthanasia and physician-assisted suicide believe that these acts are neither legally nor morally different than withdrawing or withholding life-sustaining treatment. They reject arguments that there is a distinction between actively helping a patient die through administration of drugs and "passively" allowing the patient's death by removing a ventilator.[70] According to Boston College Law School Professor Charles Baron, the potential abuses cited by opponents of euthanasia and assisted suicide --eroding public trust of medicine and exposing the poor and weak to death due to economic considerations--could just as easily occur under the currently accepted "passive" euthanasia of forgoing life-sustaining treatment.

> The competent patient should be the final judge of the level of pain, indignity, discomfort, dependency, meaninglessness and anxiety that he or she should have to put up with before giving up on life. When the patient has competently, knowledgeably, and freely decided that it is time to die, he or she should be able to die. He or she should not have to wait for a life-threatening emergency

and be put through the charade of being "allowed to die" instead of being assisted in suicide or mercifully put to death. He or she should not have to be put through processes of letting nature take its course which are likely to be horrifying to the patient's family, brutalizing to medical personnel, and undignified (if not painful) to the patient. He or she should be able, where practical, to arrange to die surrounded by loved ones in the most meaningful circumstances possible.[71]

Timothy Quill (Diane's doctor) and two colleagues proposed a policy that allows physicians to make the means of suicide available to incurably ill patients.[72] It does not permit active euthanasia. "We believe this position permits the best balance between a humane response to the requests of patients . . . and the need to protect . . . vulnerable people," the authors of the policy say. "In assisted suicide, the final act is solely the patient's, and the risk of subtle coercion from doctors, family members, institutions, or other social forces is greatly reduced. The balance of power between doctor and patient is more nearly equal in physician-assisted suicide than in euthanasia. The physician is counselor and witness and makes the means available, but ultimately the patient must be the one to act or not act."[73] These authors outline seven conditions (similar to those in the Netherlands) that must be met before a physician proceeds in assisting a patient with suicide. They strongly recommend informing family member but leave the ultimate decision about whom to involve to the patient.

In 1994, a more liberal policy that permits voluntary, active euthanasia was endorsed by Quill and other colleagues in an article in the *New England Journal of Medicine*. The authors of this article argue that confining legalized physician-assisted death to assisted suicide "unfairly discriminates against patients with unrelievable suffering who resolve to end their lives but are physically unable to do so. The method chosen is less important than the careful assessment that precedes assisted death."[74] The authors call for the establishment of regional "palliative-care committees" composed of professionals and laypersons. These committees would develop, issue, and revise practice guidelines for physician-assisted death and would educate clinicians and the public about practices of comfort care, ethical standards of informed refusal and discontinuation of life-sustaining treatment, and the option of physician-assisted death. The committees would retrospectively monitor cases of physician-assisted death and prospectively review difficult cases.

Physicians certified as "palliative-care consultants" would report to these committees and provide case-specific oversight of decisions to undertake physician-assisted death. Treating physicians could not undertake physician-assisted death without prior consultation and review by a consultant. These consultants would be physicians with experience in treating dying patients. They would have knowledge about techniques of comfort care and education in the ethics of decision making at the end of life. They would have authority to override agreements by patients and physicians to undertake physician-assisted death. The patient and physician would have a right to appeal to the regional palliative-care committee. No physician would be obligated to help a patient die. Those who do would be required to file reports with the regional committee. The authors of this proposal emphasize that they view physician-assisted death as a "treatment of last resort" that would occur relatively infrequently and "becomes a legitimate option only after standard comfort care measures have been found unsatisfactory by a competent patient in the context of his or her situation and values."[75]

The fact that physicians are willing to address the fears and concerns of their dying patients, including competent requests to help patients relieve suffering by ending their lives, will not undermine trust in medicine, Quill says. Rather, the opposite is true. It is when patients endure the agony of a prolonged death that the real erosion of trust occurs.

The profession appears to turn its back in these horrible moments in order to keep its intentions pure. Doctors cannot intentionally facilitate death, even if death is the only way to relieve a patient's overwhelming suffering. By maintaining this artificial distinction, our profession undermines the true intent of comfort care: to help people maintain dignity, control, and comfort all the way through the final phase of their illness until death. Because so many family members and friends have witnessed such very troubling deaths,

it appears that this experience also undermines the public's trust that doctors will not abandon them if they are unfortunate enough to experience unbearable suffering prior to death.[76]

Helping a patient face death is part of a physician's duty, Quill believes. "Perhaps the most fundamental commitment that physicians make to their dying patients is not to abandon them, no matter how the last stages of their illness may unfold. For many, the fear of dying can be equated with a fear that one will face unspeakable, unknown problems alone at the end. . . . Facing this unknown with dying patients is one of the richest, most rewarding challenges in medicine."[77]

V. Legal Guidance

Forty-four states have laws that make assisted suicide a crime. Oregon voters approved a referendum in 1994 that allows physician-assisted suicide when certain guidelines are met but the Oregon law has been stopped from taking effect pending the outcome of court challenges. A landmark 1997 U.S. Supreme Court ruling declared that there is no constitutional right to assisted suicide. Groups in the states of Washington and New York had challenged laws banning assisted suicide and had been successful in convincing two federal appeals courts that such laws were unconstitutional. Although both appeals courts ruled that terminally ill adults have the right to hasten death with the aid of medications prescribed by their physicians, the courts reached that conclusion by very different routes. Reviewing the arguments of the appeals court decisions lay the groundwork for understanding the reasoning used by justices of the Supreme Court in finding that there is no constitutional right to assisted suicide.

On 6 March 1996, the Ninth Circuit Court of Appeals struck down a law in the state of Washington making physician-assisted suicide a felony. In ruling on the case of *Compassion in Dying v. State of Washington*, the court said the law violated the 14th Amendment's guarantee of personal liberty found in the due-process clause. Judge Stephen Reinhardt, in a lengthy majority opinion, said the right for a terminally ill person to choose assisted suicide had the same basis in law as the right of a pregnant woman to choose to have an abortion or the right of a competent patient to refuse life-sustaining treatment. Both of these rights, Reinhardt said, have been upheld by the U.S. Supreme Court in the 1992 decision *Planned Parenthood v. Casey* and the 1990 decision *Cruzan v. Director, Missouri Dept. of Health*. Quoting language from *Casey* decision, Reinhardt wrote: "Like the decision of whether or not to have an abortion, the decision how and when to die is one of the most intimate and personal choices a person may make in a lifetime, a choice central to personal dignity and autonomy. A competent, terminally ill adult, having lived nearly the full measure of his life, has a strong liberty interest in choosing a dignified and humane death rather than being reduced at the end of his existence to a child-like state of helplessness, diapered, sedated, incontinent."[78]

Reinhardt then turned to the U.S. Supreme Court's *Cruzan* opinion, noting that it makes clear there is a "due process liberty interest in rejecting unwanted medical treatment, including the provision of food and water by artificial means. Moreover, the Court majority clearly recognized that granting the request to remove the tubes through which Cruzan received artificial nutrition and hydration would lead inexorably to her death. . . . Accordingly, we conclude that Cruzan, by recognizing a liberty interest that includes the refusal of artificial provision of life-sustaining food and water, necessarily recognizes a liberty interest in hastening one's own death."[79]

By concluding that assisted suicide is a fundamental right guaranteed by the U.S. Constitution, Reinhardt made it difficult for state governments to justify any interference with this right. He recognized six interests that could be raised by states in regulating assisted suicide:

1. preserving life;
2. preventing suicide;
3. preventing third parties from unduly influencing an individual to end his or her life;
4. safeguarding children, family members, and other loved ones dependent on persons who wish to commit suicide;
5. protecting the integrity of the medical profession; and
6. preventing other adverse consequences that might result if assisted suicide were legal.

After weighing and balancing the individual's constitutional right to assisted suicide against the state's interest to prohibit it, Reinhardt ultimately came down on the side of the individual.

The liberty interest at issue here is an important one and, in the case of the terminally ill, is at its peak. Conversely, the state interests, while equally important in the abstract, are for the most part at a low point here. We recognize that in the case of life and death decisions the state has a particularly strong interest in avoiding undue influence and other forms of abuse. Here, that concern is ameliorated in large measure because of the mandatory involvement in the decision-making process of physicians, who have a strong bias in favor of preserving life, and because the process itself can be carefully regulated and rigorous safeguards adopted.[80]

Less than a month after the Ninth Circuit Appeals Court decision, the U.S. Court of Appeals for the Second Circuit struck down New York laws prohibiting physician-assisted suicide. Judge Robert J. Miner, writing for the majority in the case of *Quill v. Vacco*, refused to declare that the U.S. Constitution gave terminally ill persons a fundamental right to ask for assistance in hastening their deaths by taking medications prescribed by physicians. However, Miner did find that laws prohibiting physician-assisted suicide violated the equal protection clause of the 14th Amendment. He reasoned that, if the state allows citizens to hasten death by refusing life-sustaining treatment, it must also allow similarly situated persons to speed death by taking a prescription for death-producing drugs. Miner wrote: "Withdrawal of life support requires physicians or those acting at their direction physically to remove equipment and, often, to administer palliative drugs which may themselves contribute to death. The ending of life by these means is nothing more nor less than assisted suicide. It simply cannot be said that those mentally competent, terminally ill persons who seek to hasten death but whose treatment does not include life support are treated equally."[81]

The reasoning of both appeals court decisions has been attacked by 46 healthcare groups that have filed a friend-of-the court brief urging the U.S. Supreme

Court not to legalize physician-assisted suicide. The American Medical Association, the American Nurses Association, the American Psychiatric Association, and 43 other groups acknowledge that many patients do not receive proper care at the end of life, but they argue that physician-assisted death is not a compassionate answer to the problem of inadequate palliative care. The brief also maintains that a patient's right to forgo life-sustaining treatment is fundamentally different from assisting in a suicide.[82]

The importance of the distinction between forgoing life-sustaining treatment and requesting physician aid in dying has been pointed out even by those who favor the legalization of physician-assisted suicide. Franklin G. Miller, who favors voluntary active euthanasia, maintains that there is a distinction between assisting a patient in death and allowing the patient to die after withdrawal of life support.

Comparing the significance of the failure to comply with a refusal of life-sustaining treatment and request for assisted suicide manifests that they are not equivalent. When doctors fail to honor a competent patient's refusal of treatment, the patient becomes subjected to unwanted bodily intrusion. If on life support, the patient forced to endure unwanted treatment becomes a prisoner of medical technology. Out of respect for patient autonomy, doctors are duty-bound to honor informed refusals of life-sustaining treatment by competent patients. A terminally-ill patient who requests assisted suicide, by contrast, is asking for a treatment that lies outside standard medical practice, which includes aggressive palliative care that may risk hastening death but not direct intervention with a procedure that induces death. To deny such a request, for example, because the doctor believes that standard palliative care could relieve the patient's suffering, certainly restricts patient self-determination; but it does not amount to bodily invasion or medical imprisonment. And there remain other ways of hastening death than by physician-assisted suicide: the patient can refuse or refrain from food and water to attempt suicide without medical assistance. Unlike a competent refusal of treatment, a competent request for physician-assisted-suicide does not amount to a moral and legal trump that can compel a doctor's compliance. At most, the patient is free to nego-

tiate assisted suicide with a willing physician. But no doctor has a duty to comply.[83]

There is no compelling liberty interest in a fundamental right to physician-assisted suicide, Miller maintains, because the patient who seeks assisted suicide has alternatives to hastening death. On the other hand, the patient who asks for life-support to be withdrawn or the pregnant woman who asks for an abortion has no alternatives. In addition, Miller argues that Miner's equal protection argument is undermined by the real differences between forgoing treatment and assisting in suicide. If prohibiting assisted suicide for the terminally ill violates equal protection of the laws, then it would also stand to reason that it would be a violation to deny voluntary active euthanasia to terminally ill persons who have no physical capacity to self-administer lethal drugs. Miller identifies other problems with the equal protection argument: "The right to refuse life-sustaining treatment, furthermore, is not limited to terminally-ill patients. The equal protection argument would seem to imply that assisted suicide also should not be limited. Moreover, family members frequently decide to forgo life-sustaining treatments that are judged not to be in the best interests of incompetent patients when their prior wishes are unknown. Would equal protection also support active euthanasia by surrogate decision-making in the best interests of similarly situated patients who are not on life support?"[84]

Miller argues that because there is no compelling constitutional protection for the right to assisted suicide, the courts are not the proper vehicles for deciding whether to legalize the practice and how it should be regulated. Rather, state legislatures or statewide referendums should decide the issue, Miller believes. In that way, the practice of physician-assisted suicide can be viewed as a policy experiment that can be tested for its benefits and harms.[85]

In its ruling on the two appeals court cases, the U.S. Supreme Court shifted the focus of debate on assisted suicide to state legislatures. With its dissenting opinions, the Court said the right to assisted suicide is not guaranteed in the U.S. Constitution. The rulings, handed down 26 June 1997, upheld New York and Washington state laws that made it a crime for doctors to give lethal drugs to dying patients who want to end their lives. In both decisions, the Court made it clear that states have a number of reasons for banning the practice of assisted suicide--including protecting the vulnerable groups in society and preserving the ethics and integrity of the medical profession. But the decisions also left the door open for states to pass legislation allowing assisted suicide in circumstances where the rights of a terminally ill patient might be seen as outweighing the interests of the state.[86]

"Throughout the nation, Americans are engaging in an earnest and profound debate about the morality, legality and practicality if physician-assisted suicide," Chief Justice William H. Rehnquist wrote in the decision in the Washington State case. "Our holding permits this debate to continue, as it should in a democratic society."[87]

In its decision on the New York Case, *Vacco v. Quill*, the Court rejected the argument that a ban on assisted suicide violated the 14th amendment's equal protection clause because it treated two groups of people differently. The Court's opinion, written by Rehnquist, said there was a fundamental distinction between terminally ill patients who hasten death by withdrawing life support and terminally ill patients who had to rely on the administration of lethal drugs to hasten death. Rehnquist pointed to a difference in causation and intent.

"(W)hen a patient refuses life-sustaining treatment, he dies from an underlying fatal disease or pathology; but if a patient ingests lethal medication prescribed by a physician, he is killed by that medication," Rehnquist wrote. He added that a physician who withdraws life-support may not intend the death of the patient but rather wants to respect the patient's wishes to refuse what is perceived to be futile or degrading care. A doctor who assists in a suicide, however, clearly wants the patient to die, he said. "By permitting everyone to refuse unwanted medical treatment while prohibiting anyone from assisted suicide, New York law follows a longstanding and rational distinction," Rehnquist concluded.[88]

In the Washington State case, the court rejected the claim that assistance in suicide is a fundamental right protected by the Due Process Clause in the 14th Amendment. Rehnquist, again writing the main opinion, noted that the Supreme Court, in a long line of cases, has used the Due Process Clause to expand the specific freedoms protected in the Bill of Rights to include rights to marry, to marital privacy, to have children, to use contraception, to direct the education of one's children, and to abortion. But a right to assistance in suicide, Rehnquist wrote, "has no place in our Nation's traditions, given the country's consistent, almost universal, and continuing rejection of the right, even for terminally ill, mentally competent adults." To rule in favor of a right to assisted suicide, Rehnquist continued, "the Court would have to reverse centuries of legal doctrine and practice, and strike down the considered policy choice of almost every state."[89]

Rehnquist dismissed the argument that the Court's opinion in the 1990 case of *Cruzan v. Missouri Department of Health*--which recognized a constitutionally protected right to refuse lifesaving hydration and nutrition--could be extended to recognizing a liberty interest for a terminally ill patient to hasten death through assisted suicide. The *Cruzan* opinion was grounded in "the common-law rule that forced medication was a battery, and the long legal tradition protecting the decision to refuse unwanted medical treatment," Rehnquist wrote. "The decision to commit suicide with the assistance of another may be just as personal and profound as the decision to refuse unwanted medical treatment, but it has never enjoyed similar legal protection. Indeed, the two acts are widely and reasonably regarded as quite distinct."[90]

The Court also rejected the notion that it's decision in *Casey v. Planned Parenthood*--upholding a woman's right to an abortion as being "central to personal dignity and autonomy"--could be interpreted to mean that assisted suicide should also be seen as such a right. The fact that many of the personal rights and liberties protected by the due process clause are grounded in personal autonomy "does not warrant the sweeping conclusion that any and all important, intimate, and personal decisions are so protected," Rehnquist wrote.[91]

In those states with specific statutes against assisted suicide, it is defined either as a special offense or a class of murder or manslaughter. Punishment generally consists of a fine ranging from $1,000 to $2,000 and a possible prison term of one or more years. In states without a specific statute, persons aiding in assisted suicide may be charged under common law or general statutory provisions for murder or manslaughter.[92]

Prosecution of physicians or others for assisting someone in suicide appears to depend on the particular circumstances of the case and the publicity and public opinion surrounding it. For example, murder charges against Jack Kevorkian have failed three times. The publicity surrounding Kevorkian's actions prompted passage of a state law that banned assisted suicide. Late in 1996, a Michigan prosecutor made yet another attempt to convict Kevorkian of assisted suicide, charging him with assisting in three suicides earlier that year.[93] On the other hand, a prosecutor in New York initially declined to charge Timothy Quill for his part in the death of Diane, even though the state has a law prohibiting the practice. It was only after Diane's identity was revealed in media reports that the prosecutor brought the case against Quill to a grand jury. The grand jury, however, declined to indict Quill, even though traces of barbiturates were found in Diane's body. A month later, the state's licensing and disciplinary board for healthcare professionals decided Quill was not guilty of any misconduct in his handling of Diane's case. News accounts have described instances where prosecutors and regulatory authorities declined to bring charges against physicians who gave lethal doses of medications to terminally ill patients. In all cases where physicians have been investigated by criminal agencies for compassionately helping a terminally ill person commit suicide, criminal charges have been dismissed or a verdict of not guilty has been returned.[94]

Between 1920 and 1985, 56 "mercy-killing" cases were brought to court in the United States. Of these, 10 defendants were found guilty and imprisoned, 20 were found guilty and given suspended sentences or probation, 15 were acquitted, and six were dismissed.[95]

VI. Professional Guidance

Thomasma and Graber, in an in-depth analysis of duties of healthcare providers to the dying, have suggested a number of "professional axioms" that should be followed. Among the most compelling of their guidelines:

1. The primary guiding principle of therapy ought to be the patient's chosen values, not the latest technology.
2. The patient should be treated as a whole person within the least-threatening technological environment possible. Terminally ill patients may prefer home care over hospital care.

3. The patient's values should be discussed frequently, both before and during treatment, in order to ascertain if the values themselves have changed order of priority in the patient's mind.
4. No assumption should be made that technological intervention is equivalent to compassionate care. The care of any patient involves personal extension of the caregiver to the patient.
5. Quality of life should be assessed so patients and families can make informed judgments about therapies and their side effects.
6. Data about the likelihood of survival from certain treatments can strongly influence a patient's view of quality of life. Patients should be told of longevity and survival data when making decisions about their care.
7. When patients suffer terminal, irreversible illness, the duty to prolong life is overridden by a duty not to prolong dying and/or a duty to relieve suffering.
8. This duty requires attention to the patient's explicit wishes about all interventions, not just the major ones such as cardiopulmonary resuscitation.
9. Comfort care should have pain control as its major objective, although value priorities of the patient should determine how aggressively this is carried out.
10. Controlling pain is a final duty to the dying patient, even if it means the patient's death might be hastened.[96]

VII. Training Clinicians to Deliver Bad News

For healthcare clinicians, delivering bad news (such as a terminal diagnosis or imminent death to patients and family members) is universally an unwelcome responsibility. For the current generation of clinicians, this discomfort stems, in part, from the same inexperience with death that typifies the general population. Most medical and nursing students have never experienced a family member's dying at home. Death, for young clinicians, has been "medicalized" just as it has for others in our society.

Another reason that clinicians fear delivering bad news is that, as students, they are rarely taught the communication skills and practices that ease the messenger's burden. This lack of training is a clear failing on the part of their teachers and those who develop clinical curricula. Student clinicians, if they are lucky, may encounter during their training a mentor who, through long experience or innate sensitivity, models the careful body language and dialogue, the listening and hearing skills, and the empathy and compassion that are required for the successful delivery of bad news. Too often, a different kind of role modeling occurs. Medical students are ordered by harried residents at 3 a.m. to call family members (who may be total strangers) and inform them that a patient has just died. Or they may witness a busy attending physician callously inform a patient that he or she has a terminal diagnosis. They watch while the physician uses medical jargon that the patient does not fully grasp, which ensures a misunderstanding on the patient's part and demonstrates a lack of sincere concern for the patient's reactions, questions, and fears.

Clinicians' qualms about delivering the news of a terminal diagnosis or the death of a family member stem from myriad other factors. These include the fact that most people have never directly examined or confronted their own feelings and attitudes about death. Also, many clinicians harbor rescue fantasies about their patients or too narrowly conceive of their professional roles solely as healers and curers. Such individuals may nurture feelings of defeat and failure when their patients become terminally ill or die, because they failed to "save" their patient. They may sense, and often rightly so, that their patients expected (albeit unrealistically) that the medical armamentarium was complete enough to disallow death or disability.

Also, clinicians nurture legitimate concerns about causing their patients pain and distress. Clinicians may fear the reactions that such news might elicit, such as despair, anger, hopelessness, rage, or even legal recourse. Because most clinicians are, by self-selection, compassionate and caring individuals, they empathize with their patients' plight, and cannot help but share in patients' pain and loss.

Delivering bad news, however onerous a task, remains a professional responsibility of all clinicians. Inherent in this responsibility is the duty to learn and master, to the greatest degree possible, the skills and practices that good messengers possess. Winslade,[97] Buckman,[98] and others maintain that delivering bad news is a skill that can be learned and that should be

an integral part of the clinical curriculum. They emphasize that apart from didactic course work, the most important learning methods involve observing direct interactions between senior clinicians and patients, and that the most instructive element in the entire learning process is the patient.

At the University of Toronto, Robert Buckman and Yvonne Kason have developed a course, "Breaking Bad News," which has generated a book by the same title.[99] Buckman maintains that certain communication skills are basic prerequisites to productive encounters during which bad news is delivered to patients. He cites studies that have repeatedly shown that patients' dissatisfaction with clinicians' communication skills outweigh any concerns that they might have about clinical competence.[100] Such sources of dissatisfaction include the appearance that the clinician is not listening to the patient, the use of technical medical jargon, or the appearance of patronizing or "talking down to" the patient.[101] Buckman sites one study that found that patients usually present with between 1.2 and 3.9 major complaints. Unfortunately, physicians generally allow their patients a scant 18 seconds to begin relating their histories before they interrupt them. A mere 23 percent of patients are allowed to complete their initial statements.[102]

As an aid to effective communication between patients and clinicians, Buckman and his colleagues endorse the following listening skills. First, clinicians must prepare for listening by staging the appropriate setting. This includes:

- Maintaining auditory and visual privacy: taking the patient to a private waiting room, closing the office door, or pulling the curtain around the patient's bed (which offers visual if not auditory privacy).

- Making complete introductions: the clinician should always address the patient first, irrespective of who or how many persons are involved in a meeting; this practice emphasizes the primacy of the patient's importance in the proceedings and is a subtle message from clinician to patient.

- Addressing the patient by the appellation that he or she prefers ("Mrs. Jones" rather than "Mary," or vice versa).

- Sitting down at face-to-face level with the patient: if the patient is bedridden, the clinician should find a place to sit so that he or she is not standing above the bed; sitting on chairs, stools, the patient's bed, even a bedside commode (if that is the only seat available) is preferable to literally talking down to the patient from a standing position.

- Asking open-ended, not closed, questions so that the patient is encouraged to voice feelings, fears, and the need for information or support.
- Not interrupting the patient unless necessary.
- Being comfortable with silences: silences often signal that the patient is gearing up to address a painful and/or very important issue.[103]

Once the clinician has set the stage for effective listening, the next step to a successful interaction is to ensure that a complete dialogue occurs between the clinician and the patient. This is facilitated by hearing (not just listening to) what the patient says (or, more important, what the patient doesn't say); by paying attention to how the patient phrases comments and questions; and by paying close attention to body language, since the patient's physical behavior may send a different message than his or her words. For example, the display of denial, indifference, or complete acceptance by the patient may be belied by physical acts such as failure to make eye contact, hand wringing, foot tapping, or other signs of anxiety or distress. Responses such as reiterating the patient's comments, making nonjudgmental observations of behavior, or trying to assess the patient's feelings are important and effective mechanisms in establishing human connections and assuring the patient that his or her message is being understood. If the patient or family member responds with anger, hostility, or even rage, the clinician must not personalize this reaction. When the patient or family directs blame or invective against the clinician, this response may manifest frustration with the overall situation. The clinician (or messenger) is merely a convenient target.

Delivering the news to family members that a relative has just died can be just as stressful as delivering bad news to a patient. If the death is sudden and unexpected, it may even be more difficult. In general, the same precepts that apply to delivering bad news to a patient apply when dealing with family members. It is important to assess the family members' most recent understanding of the patient's con-

dition. This may provide a general opening to explain that the patient's condition worsened, that attempts to revive the patient (if they were attempted) failed, and that the patient has died. Any euphemisms for death such as "expired" or "passed on" should be avoided. All opportunities to provide support for family members should be made in advance, if possible, including involving a chaplain or counseling services. Providing a chance to spend time alone with the dead patient and responding to family members' requests for information about the circumstances of the patient's death or about the patient's medical condition may be important factors in alleviating the family members' acute pain and in allowing for a healthy grieving process.

Ideally, the news that a family member has died should be given in person. Circumstances do not always allow for this, and sometimes tragic news must be imparted over the phone. Buckman has identified some ground rules for this situation that include:

- Always make sure that you know to whom you are speaking.
- Introduce yourself and say what you do, indicating whether you have met the family member.
- Speak slowly and give the relative time to adjust (this is particularly important for phone calls in the middle of the night).
- Let the relative know that you would rather be speaking to him or her in person.
- Precede the news with a warning statement such as, "I am afraid that I have some bad news about your wife."
- If the relative then interrupts to ask whether the patient has died, tell the truth, using a narrative statement such as "I'm sorry to say that she has died."
- Find out who is with the relative, or who is available to provide support, and suggest that the relative contact this person, and not be alone.
- Offer further contact, such as being available when and if the relative visits the hospital.[104]

VII. Buckman's Six-Step Method for Delivering Bad News

In their course for medical students, Buckman and his colleagues have developed a six-step protocol to prepare students for effective clinical encounters during which they must be the messengers of bad news:

1. Get off to a good start by:
   - Optimizing the physical context (ensure privacy and a quiet environment if at all possible, make eye-to-eye contact with the patient, sit at the patient's level).
   - Ensuring that all participants who should be at the meeting are there (who does the patient want present for support), and that those whom the patient doesn't want present aren't there; this is another means of providing for the patient's privacy and psychological support.
   - Making introductions, shaking hands with or touching the patient if he or she is receptive to physical contact; ensure that the patient is always addressed first, both with verbal and physical contact regardless of the presence of others, to reinforce the message that the patient is of primary concern.
2. Find out how much the patient knows about his or her medical condition by using open-ended questions such as "Can you tell me why Dr. Jones suggested that you see me today?" or "What can you tell me of your understanding of your medical problem?"
3. Find out how much the patient wants to know about his or her clinical situation, by asking such questions as:
   - "If this condition turns out to be serious, are you the kind of person who likes to know exactly what is going on?"
   - "Would you like me to tell you the full details of your condition--or is there somebody else that you would like me to talk to?"

Remember that cultural traditions may affect not only the patients reception of bad news but future interactions with the patient and family members. In some Asian cultures, for example, it is considered unkind to deliver the news of a terminal diagnosis directly to the patient. Often when an Asian person is terminally ill, all aspects of treatment are directed by close relatives. The diagnosis of terminal illness is never disclosed to the patient. While such traditions may run counter to the Western cultural ethic of informed consent and respect for autonomy, honoring the conventions and traditions of other cultures should be practiced by clinicians when possible (within the standards of good clinical, ethical, and legal practice) in light of the culturally diverse society in which we practice.

4. Share information according to the patient's needs and desires; make a mutually-agreed upon plan for the future:
   - Decide on a mutual agenda (diagnosis/treatment plan/prognosis/support).
   - Start from the patient's starting point; patients may be in varying degrees of denial, may have misunderstood or forgotten previous information, or may simply need to have details reconfirmed to allay fears of misdiagnosis. Also, remember that what is of primary importance to the patient (loss of hair, for example) may not coincide with clinical priorities.
   - Give information in small chunks; it is difficult for persons under stress to retain information. Patients often relate in subsequent interviews that "Once I heard the word cancer I blocked out everything else that you said."
   - Use English, not Medspeak or jargon.
   - Check the patient's understanding frequently by asking such questions as "Does what I am saying make sense to you?" and by asking the patient to reiterate in his or her own words what you have just said.
   - Reinforce and clarify information frequently.
   - Check your communication level. Speak to an adult patient on adult terms; do not patronize, offer false reassurance, or speak to an adult as if he or she was a child.
   - Listen for the patient's agenda. What are his or her desires in terms of therapy; life goals; important accomplishments prior to death; or fears regarding disability, pain, or loss of dignity?
5. Responding to the patient's feelings
   - Identify and acknowledge the patient's reaction to bad news. Feelings such as anger, despair, and hostility are common and should not be ignored by the clinician.
6. Planning and follow-through
   - Make a contract with the patient on a plan of care and follow-through. Establish the patient's priorities about medical treatment as well as plans for the future. When appro-

priate, discuss advance directives regarding aggressive therapy, an acceptable quality of life, preferences about the circumstances of dying (where, for example), and preferences regarding surrogate decision makers in the event of future incapacity.

- Remember that the competent adult patient has the right to accept or reject any suggestions.[105]

XI. Cases for Further Study

Case 1: A Request for a "Humanized" Death

EF is a 75-year-old male suffering from herpes zoster, the medical term for shingles. Herpes zoster is an infection of the nerves that supply certain areas of the skin. It causes a painful rash of crusting blisters that can cover extensive portions of the torso and face. In cases where the face is affected, it can cause blindness. The physician who initially diagnosed him (in 1985) and the several specialists who treated EF told him that it was the most severe case they had ever seen. The rash covered his body from the lower part of his ribs up beyond his neck and onto his face. Although he is not yet blind, his physicians expect that he will lose his sight in the near future. After being diagnosed in 1985, he was given complete sedation and painkilling drugs. Later, as the effectiveness of these medications waned, he was put on prednisone, Darvon, Bentyl, Talwin, Mepergan, Prolixin, Elavil, and Trilafon. In addition, he has had nerve blocks, special electrical nerve stimulation, and spinal surgery. His condition is not terminal, but combined with his treatments, it is extremely painful and debilitating. Normally a man who weighs 150 pounds, he is down to 94 pounds and has begun to have "more pain in my spine, sides and body than I can handle each day and night." There is no cure for his illness, and his quality of life will only deteriorate as he gets older.

By the end of 1990, after months of careful thought, EF decided that he could not take the pain any longer and that he wanted to end his life. Because of his own discomfort with violence and his fear that he might be unsuccessful as well as his genuine concern for any family members who might find his body, he decided it was important to take his life with a lethal dose of medication. He consulted his physicians for advice on how best to take his life and to get a prescription for the medication to do it.

His physicians, while empathizing deeply with his situation, felt they could not in good conscience pro-

vide him with the assistance he needed. They believed doing so was inappropriate because he was not terminally ill and because it would violate their professional duty to act as healers, rather than as agents of death. In addition, they noted that EF was a Roman Catholic from a very religious family, and that his wife and the rest of his family (who had been extremely supportive and actively involved in his care) would be strongly opposed to EF's plans to commit suicide. EF's physicians believed that these factors made it totally inappropriate for them to comply with EF's request. To improve his efforts at persuasion, EF did some research in the bioethics literature and came across a defense of assisted suicide and "active" euthanasia by Joseph Fletcher: "It is harder morally to justify letting somebody die a slow and ugly death, dehumanized, than it is to justify helping him escape from such misery. . . . The case for euthanasia depends upon how we understand benefit of the sick and harm and wrong. If we regard dehumanized and merely biological life as sometimes real harm and the opposite of benefit, to refuse to welcome or even introduce death would be quite wrong morally."[106]

Despite the power of Fletcher's arguments and EF's persistent pleas for help, EF was unable to convince his physicians to help him. He opted instead to search on his own for a physician who might be willing to help him. He called up several physicians in a nearby town and explained his difficult situation and begged for them to help him end his suffering. One physician, Dr. G, was intrigued by the story. Being himself an advocate of assisted suicide and even active euthanasia (in certain carefully monitored circumstances) he decided to help EF. After a lengthy conversation with EF about his history and reasons for wanting to die, in addition to confirmation of his condition through EF's regular physicians, Dr. G said he would honor EF's request. He stipulated that, although he had every intention of complying, he needed a few days to discuss the situation with some of his colleagues. He promised that in his discussions he would not do anything that would expose EF's identity.

As a conscientious physician interested in reforming the practice of medicine, Dr. G notified the local state university hospital of the case and his intentions (although he did not reveal the patient's name or other medical facts that would compromise EF's identity).

As a member of the ethics consultation service of the ethics committee, you are asked to identify the ethical issues in the case, and provide a recommendation for the ethics committee to consider.

[Source: Ethics Consultation Service, University of Virginia.]

Case 2: Suffering and the Sanctity of Life

Mr. P is a 76-year-old man who resides at the Home for the Jewish Aged. He had been well until age 70, when he began to exhibit signs and symptoms of senile dementia of the Alzheimer's type. This resulted in placement at the home five years ago. Since that time, he has followed a slowly progressive downhill course; for the past year he has been mute and bedbound. A complete demential evaluation within the past year revealed only cortical atrophy with no other anatomic or biochemical abnormalities. Attempts at rehabilitation have met with limited success.

Ten days prior to this ethics committee meeting, Mr. P was found to be febrile to 104 degrees F and was transferred here to Academia Hospital. Work-up revealed probably postobstructive pneumonia with an 8-cm mass in the left upper lobe. Mr. P was placed on antibiotics and IV [intravenous] fluids for his pneumonia. On the second hospital day, Mr. P was noted to be moaning and resisting movement. On exam, the right leg was found to be foreshortened and externally rotated. X-rays revealed a pathologic fracture of the femur. The diagnosis of metastatic carcinoma with an unknown primary, probably lung, was made. The attending physician and house staff agreed that the most appropriate therapy was to keep the patient comfortable with fluids and, if needed, narcotics and to withhold all further diagnostic and therapeutic measures.

In view of the patient's poor overall prognosis, the physicians felt it advisable to inquire as to the family's wishes regarding resuscitation and to discuss the overall treatment plan. The attending physician contacted the only known relative, a daughter, Mrs. R, a 50-year-old woman who came in the following day with her husband and their son, Stanley R, a pulmonary physician. Upon hearing the physician's proposed management plan, the family became very upset. Not only did they not wish to take the small but (to the physicians) reasonably undertaken risk of respiratory depression and even pulmonary arrest associated with the use of narcotic analgesics, they also refused to agree to a DNR [do-not-resuscitate] order and demanded a thorough workup and aggressive treatment for the cancer, including a bone scan and bronchoscopy, and, if necessary, chemotherapy or radiation therapy. It seems that all of the R's belong to an orthodox Jewish community which holds that all life is infinitely valuable and every means must be taken to prolong each life to the greatest extent. The attending physician then suggested that the family members might wish to think the matter over carefully and discuss it with their rabbi.

Mrs. R agreed to this and called back to say that she, her husband, her son, and the rabbi had discussed the situation and had concluded that her father should be resuscitated and that no narcotics should be used, and that the aggressive medical workup as proposed by the grandson be done promptly. To the physician's inquiry as to whether these views corresponded with what the patient might have wanted, had he been competent to decide, the daughter responded that she felt sure that he would agree. The physicians have been unable to find any other source of information about the patient's own religious values and preferences. Meanwhile, the patient cries out in pain constantly, yanks out his IVs, and resists all examinations and procedures. On seeing the patient's discomfort, the family has agreed to small doses of narcotics after the physicians have promised to watch carefully for respiratory depression. It has been explained to the family that Mr. P will need restraints for any procedures and that these procedures may cause discomfort without necessarily prolonging his life or improving his quality of life, but they feel very strongly that he doesn't understand what is happening, and that they know what is best for him.

The attending physician requests the advice of the ethics committee as how to proceed at this point.

[Source: R. Macklin and R. Kupfer, *Hospital Ethics Committees: Manual for a Training Program* (New York: Albert Einstein College of Medicine, March 1988.]

Case 3: She Doesn't Need to Know

Mrs. N is a 60-year old, Korean-American woman who immigrated to the United States when she was in her early 30s. She possesses basic skills in the English language and has worked as a member of the cafeteria staff at Memorial Community Hospital for 13 years. A vivacious and pleasant woman, Mrs. N is known by all of the staff in this small hospital and is universally liked, often referred to as "Grandma."

In November 1992, Mrs. N was admitted as a patient to Memorial Community Hospital with an undiagnosed pulmonary illness. At first, clinicians suspected that Mrs. N might be afflicted with tuberculosis. Further workup revealed that Mrs. N had lung cancer.

Upon learning of the diagnosis, Mrs. N's husband and children insisted that she not be informed of her terminal diagnosis. In keeping with their cultural traditions, Mrs. N's family felt that it would be cruel to reveal her condition to her, that "she doesn't need to know," and demanded that all decision making be made by family members. Mrs. N underwent a left lower lobe lobectomy, after her physicians explained to her that it would make her "breathing easier," but without revealing her diagnosis of pulmonary cancer.

Mrs. N's son served as a translator during discussions of her medical condition with physicians.

Although Mrs. N has never directly asked her physicians about her condition, she has often made allusions to the patient in the next bed, referring to the patient's cancer and to its ultimate outcome. Also, in a thank-you note written to hospital staff, Mrs. N stated that she had come to feel that the staff were like members of her family, and that she never thought that she would be saying "goodbye" to all of them.

Many clinicians, most especially the nurses providing care for Mrs. N, are uncomfortable with the secrecy surrounding her diagnosis. They are not convinced that Mrs. N wished to remain uninformed about her condition; they are also afraid that, because she is so well known to the entire hospital staff, someone might inadvertently disclose diagnostic information to her out of ignorance of the family's position.

A request for assistance with this dilemma is made to the ethics committee.

[Source: This case is adapted from a presentation made at "Developing Hospital Ethics Programs," a conference held in March 1992 at the Center for Biomedical Ethics at the University of Virginia.]

X. Study Questions

1. What are the criteria for determining brain death? What is the difference between brain death and death as defined by heart/lung criteria? Why can't a premature infant be declared brain dead?
2. What is PVS? Are PVS patients "persons"? What rights, if any, do patients in PVS hold; what duties, if any, are they owed?
3. Should the definition of death center on biological criteria or the issue of personhood?
4. What do Eric Cassell and Timothy Quill mean when they state that the suffering of the dying is not only physical, but emotional and existential?
5. Is there such a thing as rational suicide?
6. What is your position on physician-assisted suicide? On active euthanasia?
7. Consider Case 1, "A Request for a 'Humanized' Death." EF's physicians denied his request for assisted suicide for a number of reasons listed below. Evaluate each reason individually:

   a. EF was not terminally ill.
   b. Assisting EF would violate the physicians' professional duty to act as healers.

c. Because EF came from a Roman Catholic family, his wife and others would be strongly opposed to EF's plans to commit suicide.

Notes

1. N.N. Dubler and D. Nimmons, *Ethics on Call* (New York: Harmony, 1992), 156.
2. D.C. Thomasma and G.C. Graber, *Euthanasia: Toward An Ethical Social Policy* (New York: Continuum, 1990), 183.
3. Ibid., 159.
4. W.D. Poe, *The Old Person in Your Home* (New York: Scribners, 1969), 68.
5. B.A. Brody and H.T. Engelhardt, Jr., *Bioethics: Readings and Cases* (Englewood Cliffs, N.J.: Prentice-Hall, 1987), 377.
6. *Black's Law Dictionary*, 4th ed. rev., (St. Paul, Minn.: West Publishing, 1968): 488-89.
7. *Gray v. Sawyer*, 247 S.W.2d 496 (Ky. Ct.App. 1952).
8. Ad Hoc Committee of the Harvard Medical School to Examine the Definition of Brain Death, *Journal of the American Medical Association* 205 (1968): 337-40.
9. Ibid., p. 337-38.
10. See note 5 above, p. 378.
11. President's Commission for the Study of Ethical Problems in Medicine and Biomedical and Behavioral Research, *Defining Death* (Washington, D.C.: U.S. Government Printing Office, 1981), 2.
12. American Academy of Pediatrics, Task Force on Brain Death in Children, "Guidelines for the Determination of Brain Death in Children," *Pediatrics* 80 (1987): 298-300.
13. R.E. Behrman and V.C. Vaughan III, *Nelson Textbook of Pediatrics*, 13th ed. (Philadelphia: W.B. Saunders, 1987), 1299.
14. E.J. Cassell, *Nature of Suffering* (New York: Oxford University Press, 1991), 33.
15. Ibid., 39.
16. Ibid., 31.
17. See note 5 above, p. 369.
18. Harvard Medical School Health Publications Group, "A Guide to Hospice Care," *Harvard Health Letter*, (September 1994), Special Reprint, First Printing.
19. C.M.S. Saunders, "The Care of the Dying Patient and His Family," in S.J. Reiser, A.J. Dyck, and W.J. Curran, ed., *Ethics in Medicine: Historical Perspectives and Contemporary Concerns* (Cambridge,

Mass: Massachusetts Institute of Technology Press, 1977), 513.

20. Ibid., 513.

21. Ibid., 512.

22. See note 18 above, p. 127; see note 19 above, p. 512.

23. T.E. Quill, *Death and Dignity: Making Choices and Taking Charge* (New York: W.W. Norton, 1993).

24. Ibid., 80.

25. K.M. Foley, "The Relationship of Pain and Symptom Management to Patient Requests for Physician-Assisted Suicide," *Journal of Pain and Symptom Management* 6 (1991): 289.

26. Ibid., 289-97.

27. Ibid., 289.

28. See note 23 above, p. 113.

29. See note 2 above, pp. 1-2; J. Rachels, *The End of Life: Euthanasia and Morality* (New York: Oxford University Press, 1986), 7-19.

30. Rachels, see note 29 above; see note 14 above, p. 45.

31. S.J. Reiser, "The Dilemma of Euthanasia in Modern Medical History: The English and American Experience," in S.J. Reiser, A.J. Dyck, and W.J. Curran, eds., *Ethics in Medicine: Historical Perspectives and Contemporary Concerns* (Cambridge, Mass.: Massachusetts Institute of Technology Press, 1977), 488.

32. Ibid., 488-90.

33. Ibid., 491.

34. See note 2 above, p. 186.

35. "It's Over Debbie," *Journal of the American Medical Association* 259, no. 2 (1988): 272. (Unsigned article in "A Piece of My Mind" column, edited by R.K.Young).

36. W. Gaylin et al., "Doctors Must Not Kill," *Journal of the American Medical Association* 259 (1988): 2140.

37. S.H. Wanzer et al., "The Physician's Responsibility toward Hopelessly Ill Patients: A Second Look," *New England Journal of Medicine* 320 (1989): 848.

38. M.A. Nevins, "From the Beside . . .," *Trends in Health Care, Law & Ethics* 7, no. 2 (Winter 1992): 23.

39. Associated Press, "Kevorkian Helps Pair Kill Selves Before Ban," *Roanoke Times & World-News*, 16 December 1992, p. A6.

40. T.E. Quill, "Death and Dignity: A Case of Individualized Decision Making," *New England Journal of Medicine* 324 (1991): 691-94.

41. Ibid., 693.

42. D. Humphry, *Final Exit* (Secaucus, N.J.: Hemlock Society, 1991).

43. M.A. Lee et al., "Legalizing Assisted Suicide --Views of Physicians in Oregon," *New England Journal of Medicine* 334, no. 5 (1996): 310-15.

44. R.J. Blendon, U.S. Szalay, and R.A. Knox, "Should Physicians Aid Their Patients in Dying?" *Journal of the American Medical Association* 267 (1992): 2658-62; Council on Ethical and Judicial Affairs, American Medical Association, "Decisions Near the End of Life," *Journal of the American Medical Association* 267 (1992): 2229-33.

45. B. Knickerbocker, "Assisted-Suicide Issue More Active as Citizens Appear to Change Mood," *Wall Street Journal*, 2 May 1994, p. 6.

46. J.G. Bachman et al., "Attitudes of Michigan Physicians and the Public toward Legalizing Physician-Assisted Suicide and Voluntary Euthanasia," *New England Journal of Medicine* 334, no. 5 (1996): 303-09.

47. D. Colburn, "Debate on Assisted Suicide Gains Steam: Court Decisions and Public Polls Suggest Distrust of the Present System of End-of-Life Care," *Washington Post*, 10 May 1994, p. Z8.

48. Council on Ethical and Judicial Affairs, see note 44 above.

49. President's Commission for the Study of Ethical Problems in Medicine and Biomedical and Behavioral Research, *Deciding to Forego Life-Sustaining Treatment* (Washington, D.C.: U.S. Government Printing Office, 1983), 72; American Geriatrics Society Public Policy Committee, "Voluntary Active Euthanasia," *Journal of the American Geriatrics Society* 39 (1991): 826.

50. D. Callahan, "To Kill and to Ration: Preserving the Difference," in *What Kind of Life: The Limits of Medical Progress* (New York: Simon and Schuster, 1990), 221-49; A.J. Dyck, "An Alternative to the Ethic of Euthanasia," in S.J. Reiser, A.J. Dyck, and W.J. Curran, ed., *Ethics in Medicine: Historical Perspectives and Contemporary Concerns* (Cambridge, Mass.: Massachusetts Institute of Technology Press, 1977), 529-35; Gaylin, see note 36 above; B. Jennings, "Active Euthanasia and Forgoing Life-Sustaining Treatment: Can We Hold the Line?" *Journal of Pain and Symptom Management* 6 (1991): 312-16; H. Arkes et al., "Always to Care, Never to Kill," *Wall Street Journal*, 27 November 1991, 8; T.D. Sullivan, "Active and Passive Euthanasia: An Impertinent Distinction?" in T.A. Mappes and J.S. Zembaty, ed., *Biomedical Ethics* (New York: McGraw-Hill, 1991), 371-74; R.I. Misbin, "Physicians Aid In Dying," *New England Journal of Medicine* 325 (1991): 1307-11; G.R. Scofield, "Physician-Assisted Suicide: Part of the Problem or Part of the So-

lution?" *Trends in Health Care, Law & Ethics* 7, no. 2 (Winter 1992); 15-18; A.J. Dyck, "Physician-Assisted Suicide: Is It Ethical?" *Trends In Health Care, Law & Ethics* 7, no. 2 (Winter 1992): 19-22; S.M. Wolf, "Holding the Line on Euthanasia," *Hastings Center Report* 19 (January-February 1989): 13-15; R.A. McCormick, "Physician-Assisted Suicide: Flight from Compassion," *Christian Century* 108, no. 35 (4 December 1991): 1132-34.

51. T.E. Quill, C.K. Cassel, and D.E. Meier, "Care of the Hopelessly Ill: Proposed Clinical Criteria for Physician-Assisted Suicide," *New England Journal of Medicine* 327 (1992): 1380-84; N.S. Jecker, "Giving Death a Hand: When the Dying and the Doctor Stand in a Special Relationship," *Journal of the American Geriatrics Society* 39 (1991): 831-35; H. Brody, "Assisted Death --A Compassionate Response to a Medical Failure," *New England Journal of Medicine* 327 (1992): 1384-88; M. Angell, "Doctors and Assisted Suicide," *Annals of the Royal College of Physicians and Surgeons of Canada* 24, no. 7 (1991): 94-95; C. Cassel and D. Meier, "Morals and Moralism in the Debate over Euthanasia and Assisted Suicide," *New England Journal of Medicine* 323 (1990): 750-52; R.F. Weir, "The Morality of Physician-Assisted Suicide," *Law, Medicine & Health Care* 20 (1992): 116-26.

52. G.I. Benrubi, "Euthanasia--The Need for Procedural Safeguards," *New England Journal of Medicine* 326 (1992): 197-99; J. Rachels, "Active and Passive Euthanasia," in T.A. Mappes and J.S. Zembaty, ed., *Biomedical Ethics* (New York: McGraw-Hill, 1991), 367-70; "Physician-Assisted Suicide and the Right to Die with Assistance," *Harvard Law Review* 105 (1992): 2021-40; E.H. Loewy, "Healing and Killing, Harming and Not Harming: Physician Participation in Euthanasia and Capital Punishment," *The Journal of Clinical Ethics* 3 (1992): 29-34; C.H. Baron, "The Fictional Distinction between Active and Passive Euthanasia and the Danger It Poses to the Civil Liberties of Patients," paper presented at American Civil Liberties Union Biennial Conference, University of Vermont, 26-30 June 1991; P. Singer, "A Consequentialist Argument for Active Euthanasia," in B.A. Brody and H.T. Engelhardt, Jr., *Bioethics: Readings and Cases* (Englewood Cliffs, N.J.: Prentice-Hall, 1987), 165-69.

53. Dyck, "An Alternative to the Ethic of Euthanasia," see note 50 above, p. 530.

54. E.D. Pellegrino, "Doctors Must Not Kill," *The Journal of Clinical Ethics* 3 (1992): 96-97.

55. J.C. Fletcher, "The Patient's Right to Die," in *Euthanasia and the Right to Death*, A.B. Downing, ed.

(New York: Humanities Press, 1971).

56. Gaylin et al., see note 36 above; Dyck, "An Alternative to the Ethic of Euthanasia," see note 50 above; Callahan, see note 50 above; Council on Ethical and Judicial Affairs, see note 44 above; Wolf, see note 50 above; McCormick, see note 50 above; Arkes et al., see note 50 above.

57. See note 54 above, pp. 98-99.

58. Ibid., p. 100.

59. Ibid., pp. 97-98.

60. S. Hauerwas, *Suffering Presence* (Notre Dame, Ind.: University of Notre Dame Press, 1986), 107.

61. W.F. May, *Physician's Covenant* (Philadelphia: Westminister Press, 1983), 67.

62. Ibid., pp. 83-84.

63. Council on Judicial and Ethical Affairs, see note 44 above; Wanzer et al., see note 37 above.

64. P.J. Van Der Maas et al., "Euthanasia and Other Medical Decisions Concerning the End of Life," *Lancet* 338 (1991): 669-74; M. Battin, "Voluntary Euthanasia and the Risks of Abuse: Can We Learn Anything from the Netherlands?" *Law, Medicine & Health Care* 20 (1992): 133-43.

65. Dyck, see note 50 above; Pellegrino, see note 54 above; National Conference of Catholic Bishops Secretariat for Pro-Life Activities, "Dutch Euthanasia Program Called a Disaster," *Life at Risk* 3 (1991): 1.

66. P.J. Van Der Maas et al., "Euthanasia, Physician-Assisted Suicide and Other Medical Practices Involving the End of Life in the Netherlands, 1990-1995," *New England Journal of Medicine* 335, no. 22 (1996): 1699-1705.

67. G. Van Der Wal et al., "Evaluation of the Notification Procedure for Physician-Assisted Death in the Netherlands," *New England Journal of Medicine* 335, no. 22 (1996): 1706-11.

68. M. Angell, "Euthanasia in the Netherlands--Good News or Bad?" *New England Journal of Medicine* 335, no. 22 (1996): 1676-78.

69. Ibid., 1677.

70. See note 52 above.

71. Baron, see note 52 above; 12-13.

72. Quill, Cassel, and Meier, see note 51 above.

73. Ibid., pp. 1380-81.

74. F.G. Miller et al., "Regulating Physician-Assisted Death," *New England Journal of Medicine* 331 (1994): 119-23.

75. Ibid., p. 119.

76. See note 23 above, 108.

77. Ibid., p. 83-84.

78. *Compassion in Dying v. State of Washington,*

79 F.3d 790 (9th Cir. 1996).

79. Ibid, p. 816.

80. Ibid, p. 836.

81. *Quill v. Vacco*, 80 F.3d 716, p. 729 (2d Cir. 1996).

82. D.M. Gianelli, "AMA to Court: No Suicide Aid," *American Medical News*, 25 November 1996.

83. F.G. Miller, "Legalizing Physician-Assisted Suicide by Judicial Decision: A Critical Appraisal," *Bioethics Matters* 5, no. 3 (July 1996): insert 1-4.

84. Ibid., p. 3.

85. Ibid.

86. J. Biskupic, "High Court Allows Ban on Assisted Suicide, Strikes Down Law Restricting Online Speech," *Washington Post*, 27 June 1997, p. A1.

87. *Washington v. Glucksberg*, 117 S. Ct. 2258, p. 2275.

88. *Vacco v. Quill*, 117 S. Ct. 2293, p. 2301.

89. See note 87 above, p. 2260.

90. Ibid., p. 2270.

91. Ibid. p. 2271.

92. *Harvard Law Review*, see note 52 above, pp. 2024, 2031; Weir, see note 51 above, p. 119.

93. "Departing Prosecutor Charges Dr. Kevorkian in 10 Deaths," *American Medical News*, 18 November 1996, 31.

94. Weir, see note 51 above, pp. 118-19; A. Meisel, *The Right to Die* (New York: John Wiley & Sons, 1992), 45; Quill, Cassel, and Meier, see note 51 above, p. 1381.

95. D. Cundiff, *Euthanasia Is Not The Answer: A Hospice Physician's View* (Totowa, N.J.: Humana Press, 1992), 56. [The breakout of cases given by Cundiff does not total 56--Ed.]

96. See note 2 above, 129-40.

97. W. Winslade, "Teaching about Dying," *Choice in Dying News* 1, no. 4 (Winter 1992): 1-6.

98. R. Buckman, *How to Break Bad News: A Guide for Health Professionals* (Baltimore: Johns Hopkins University Press, 1992).

99. Ibid.

100. Z. Ben-Sira, "The Function of the Professional's Affective Behavior in Client Satisfaction," *Journal of Health and Social Behavior* 17 (1976): 3-11.

101. R.J. Baron, "An Introduction to Medical Phenomenology: I Can't Hear You When I'm Listening," *Annals of Internal Medicine* 101 (1985): 606-11.

102. H.B. Beckman and R.M. Frankel, "The Effect of Physician Behavior on the Collection of Data," *Annals of Internal Medicine* 101 (1984): 692-96.

103. See note 98 above, pp. 44-50

104. Ibid., 187-88.

105. See note 98 above, pp. 96-97.

106. J.F. Fletcher, *Humanhood: Essays in Bioemedical Ethics* (Buffalo, N.Y.: Prometheus Books, 1979): 149.

9

THE DECISION TO FORGO LIFE-SUSTAINING TREATMENT WHEN THE PATIENT IS INCAPACITATED

John C. Fletcher, Ph.D.

I. Introduction

This chapter is about ethical problems in decisions to forgo (not start or stop) treatments that sustain life when the patient (1) is seriously or irreversibly incapacitated; or (2) never was a capable decision maker. Cases B and C below illustrate these two situations. Chapter 7 deals with ethical problems in capable patients' refusals of life-sustaining treatment.

The hardest cases of forgoing treatment have a mixture of technical uncertainty, pain, suffering, poor quality of life due in some degree to treatment, costly technologies, and a probability of death without treatment.[1] Ethical problems related to such cases are among the most frequent faced by clinicians, family members, and guardians in critical-care settings and nursing homes.[2] The Study to Understand Prognosis and Preferences for Outcomes and Risks of Treatment (SUPPORT), which is the largest controlled trial ever done to study medical and ethical issues in critically ill patients with one or more of nine illnesses, focused in large part on quality of decision making to forgo life-sustaining treatment.[3] The results of SUPPORT are discussed more fully below.

This chapter traces briefly the history of the problem and its causes. It then sketches the evolution of ethical and legal norms and describes the types of cases that most frequently arise. Finally, the chapter provides guidelines for clinicians and surrogates to consider and a discussion of the ethical reasons for seeking the goals that shape the guidelines.

II. History of the Problem

A. Early History of Medical Technology and Its Uses

Reiser surveyed the history of medical care for the most hopelessly ill persons,[4] beginning in ancient Greek medicine with Hippocrates and his students. He noted that the main theme in Hippocrates' essay on "Epidemics"[5] is balancing treatment aimed to benefit patients with the possibility of inflicting harm on them. The Hippocratic medical ethic, widely misunderstood as a simple maxim of "do no harm," is much more complex and integral to the main theme of this chapter. Hippocrates said: "As to diseases, make a habit of two things--to help, or at least to do no harm."[6] Hippocrates also advised students "to refuse to treat those who are overmastered by their diseases, realizing that in such cases medicine is powerless."[7] These ethical concerns are similar to the issues discussed in this chapter, and there is evidence of ancient predecessors of intensive care.

Researchers have found there are records of intensive monitoring of extremely sick persons in ancient Egypt and other civilizations,[8] and Bloom and Lundberg have identified the roots of modern intensive care in many ancient settings.[9] "Rescue" technologies may have begun with Vesalius's (1543) experiment with an animal to maintain breathing with a bellows and tube. Rescue workers in England used this method in the 19th century to resuscitate drowned persons. The first tank respirator was invented in 1832. Use of the Drinker/Shaw "iron lung" (1929) in the polio epidemic resulted in the earliest ethical dilemmas of selection and weaning.[10] Technologies to support heart and kidney function came next. Reiser notes that Albert Hyman, in the 1930s, placed a needle electrode into the chest of 43 patients in cardiac arrest and saved 14, but the press condemned his work.[11] Willem Kolff invented the dialysis machine in the 1940s in Holland during the Nazi occupation; selection of patients for dialysis dramatized ethical conflicts and was one of the causes for the "birth of bioethics" (see Chapter 12).

The intensive care unit (ICU) had its origins in England in the mid-19th century with small rooms next to surgical amphitheaters for extra care in patient recovery, as noted by Florence Nightingale.[12] ICUs for premature infants began in France and spread to many nations. The number of general ICUs to treat acute trauma in adults grew in the years of World War II, especially after the 1942 Coconut Grove fire in Boston. The specialized ICU of today took several decades to evolve.[13] ICU care blossomed in the 1960s from a place of brief interventions for trauma to a setting for long-term treatment that, debatably, was extended to everyone. With this change came the agenda of ethical and legal concerns that are the main subject of this chapter.

B. Recent History of the Problem

Today, at least three major factors contribute to the high incidence of cases involving the decision to forgo life-sustaining treatment when the patient is incapacitated:

1. the rapid growth of technologies for critical-care medicine and the changing role of physicians, including the expectation that physicians control these technologies;
2. increasing numbers of incapacitated patients in hospitals and nursing homes; and
3. a cultural demand to use technology to prolong the lives of dying patients.

1. Technology and the Physician's Role

Lewis Thomas, the late medical essayist, told a story of being invited to a county medical association in the 1950s to inaugurate the president-elect. At dinner, the physician-honoree received a phone call. He left, and returned just as the evening was ending. Having missed his own inauguration, he explained to Thomas that his patient, near death for days, had just died. He left the meeting, in his words, because "the family was in distress and needed him." Thomas ended the story, "This was in the early 1950s when medicine was turning into a science, but the old art was still in place."[14]

Thomas's story is in a book by Winslade and Ross that traces the change in the role of the physician in the 20th century.[15] In the "old art" of medicine, doctors treated the patient in the context of the family. With the "new science," the physician's goal was to diagnose and treat disease processes. The person with the disease was not the center of attention. The physician's task today, the book argues, is to combine the old art and the new science. The authors argue that only the "prepared" patient and family will benefit from the new science and avoid the harms that can result from inappropriate use of technologies found mainly in large teaching or community hospitals (kidney dialysis, respirators, organ transplantation, chemotherapies, coronary bypass operations, artificial feeding and hydration, and so forth). One of the tasks of an ethics program in a healthcare organization is to prepare members of the community by educating them to be patients and surrogate decision makers in the context of high-technology treatment.

2. Increasing Numbers of Incapacitated Patients

Today, there are many more incapacitated adult patients in the clinical setting than there were a generation ago. One major cause is the aging of the population. A second cause is that more patients survive after head trauma, stroke, and alcohol and other substance abuse.

Americans in very large numbers are aging. Those over the age of 65 will soon be the majority of patients routinely seen by internists.[16] The fastest-growing age group is the population above the age of 85. With this phenomenon comes a percentage of patients with diminished capacity due to dementia and Alzheimer's disease. The number of people with severe dementia is expected to increase by 60 percent between 1987 the year 2000.[17] Chapter 5 discusses patients' capacity to participate in routine healthcare decisions, a major issue in each clinician-patient encounter.

Concern about incapacity is well justified when the focus is on decision making for patients in the ICU setting. Critically ill patients are more often incapable of communicating. Investigators found that only 45 percent of the 4,301 seriously ill patients in Phase I of SUPPORT (a two-year prospective observational study) were able to communicate.[18] Decisions to forgo treatment are decisions about death, and that is why these decisions ought to be and are so difficult. In the medical-surgical ICUs of two large hospitals in San Francisco, researchers reported that only five of 115 patients were capable.[19] In a general medical ICU in a Rochester, New York community hospital, researchers found that only five of 28 patients could participate in decision making.[20] In the latter two studies, however, family members were available to be surrogates in 90 percent of cases. In SUPPORT, 87 percent of incapable patients' surrogates were willing to be interviewed.[21] Thus, family members can almost always be found to serve as surrogate decision makers.

3. Prolonging Life: What Kind of Life?

Anthropologist Lynn Payer asserts that American medicine is much more aggressive with technology at the end of life than is true in other cultures.[22] Lewis Thomas coined the term "halfway technologies," because the patient eventually dies.[23] Where Americans die is strong evidence of a cultural shift, despite the "halfway" measures. In 1949, half of those who died in the United States died at home or at the scene of accidents. Only 49 percent died in hospitals or nursing homes. By 1983, the President's Commission for the Study of Ethical Problems in Medicine and Biomedical and Behavioral Research found that about 80 percent of Americans died in hospitals or nursing homes.[24] Nearly a decade later, the National Center for Health Statistics reported deaths in hospitals (61 percent) and in nursing homes (17 percent).[25] There are large variations in specific states.[26]

The findings reported by the SUPPORT investigators provide empirical confirmation of Payer's observation. In Phase I, observers documented shortcomings in communication and frequency of aggressive treatment. They also recorded that dying in the hospital was often sad and painful. For example, only

47 percent of physicians knew when their patients desired to avoid cardiopulmonary resuscitation (CPR); 46 percent of do-not-resuscitate (DNR) orders were written within two days of death; 38 percent of patients who died spent at least 10 days in an ICU; and for 50 percent of patients who died in the hospital, family members reported moderate to severe pain at least half of the time.[27]

Phase II of SUPPORT was a controlled trial, with 4,804 patients and their physicians assigned randomly by specialty group to an intervention group ($n = 2,652$) or a control group ($n = 2,152$). For the intervention group, specially trained nurses had multiple contacts with patient, family, physician, and hospital staff to elicit preferences, improve understanding of outcomes, encourage attention to pain control, and facilitate advance-care planning and communication. Investigators reported that, as a result of this intervention, there was no improvement on any of the following outcomes:

1. physician-patient communication (37 percent of control patients and 40 percent of intervention patients discussed CPR preferences);
2. incidence or timing of DNR orders;
3. physicians' knowledge of patients' preferences about CPR;
4. days spent in an ICU;
5. use of mechanical ventilation;
6. days comatose before death;
7. level of reported pain; and
8. use of hospital resources.[28]

SUPPORT also confirms that the term *life-sustaining technology* may be misleading. Aggressive measures can rescue some gravely ill patients from certain death. However, these interventions may only prolong the process of dying, cause needless suffering, or maintain a vegetative or profoundly impaired existence that is of no benefit to the patient. In referring to any life-sustaining technology, the question posed in the title of Daniel Callahan's book, *What Kind of Life?* is always relevant.[29]

III. What Are the Sources of the Norms? Evolution of Ethical Guidelines for Clinicians

What norms should guide clinicians in forgoing treatment? And what are the sources of these norms?

Ethical guidance for choices to forgo life-sustaining treatment began in ancient Greece and continues to evolve. An older guideline, widely regarded as outworn, is based on a distinction between ordinary and extraordinary or "heroic" treatment. The guideline was that "ordinary treatments" which carried hope of benefit to the patient, were obligatory but "extraordinary treatments" were optional.

A. Ordinary and Extraordinary Treatment

Ordinary treatments were seen as:

1. of potential benefit to the patient;
2. of a type described as "usual" (every hospital had them);
3. not unusually complex;
4. not excessively invasive;
5. not burdensomely expensive; and
6. available to virtually everyone who needed them.

Extraordinary treatments could carry both benefits and burdens but were described in opposite terms from ordinary treatments: unusual, complex, invasive, very painful, expensive, and available to few.

The distinction broke down. Continual advances in technology and the demand to use all available means to sustain life meant that treatments initially seen as extraordinary were seen quickly as routine. A good example is artificial feeding and hydration. What was once given by mouth became a very powerful medical technology when given parenterally (intravenously or subcutaneously) or enterally (via any route to the alimentary canal or gastrointestinal system).

The original meaning of ordinary versus extraordinary care was uncovered in the President's Commission's historical studies of the origins of the benefits/burdens guideline (see below).[30] Catholic moral theologians, like Banez in 1595, used the distinction to explain how the ethical principle of proportionality worked in actual cases. While holding it to be reasonable that a person must try to maintain his or her life, Banez taught that it was not obligatory to use extraordinary means to live. It was obligatory to preserve life by nourishment, medicine, clothing, with a level of pain and anguish "common to all." He argued that any extraordinary deeds (*sumptos*) sharply disproportionate to one's state in life were not re-

quired. However, this older tradition was overwhelmed by biomedical technology's growth and the conventional wisdom that grew up alongside it.

B. Withholding Versus Withdrawing: Is It a Distinction with a Difference?

The conventional wisdom was that it was morally harder to withdraw treatment than to withhold it in the first place. For example, in the mid-1970s, a physician wrote: "By not starting a 'routine IV' I am not committed to that modality of therapy. It is easier not to start daily intravenous parenteral fluids than to stop them, once begun--just as it is easier not to turn on the respiratory assistance machine than to turn the switch off, once started."[31]

By the early 1980s, this way of thinking probably was widely shared by clinicians in emergency and critical-care settings. One can question, however, what the physician meant by "easier." If he meant "morally easier," then the claim is open to serious challenge, which the President's Commission did with real effect. In perspective, easier likely meant that when resources were virtually unlimited, clinicians felt that more conflict was avoided if they used more technology for the sickest patients. However, what may feel easier emotionally does not add up to a sound moral judgment.

A preference for withholding treatment was also based on an argument that an important distinction lay between an "act" (leading to death) and an "omission" (leading to death). Withdrawing, in contrast to withholding, was seen as killing the patient. On its face, to act to withdraw appeared to have more moral responsibility attached than to omit to act and let the disease take its course.

There are other reasons why it is hard to stop treatments that become marginally beneficial or even futile (for example, loyalty to the patient, gestures aimed toward the family to show that one is doing "everything possible," denial of death, and so forth). A further reason is a misconception, by clinicians or hospital administrators, that the law always requires maintaining life-sustaining treatment.[32] This is untrue in any state, although there are many important variations among states in their laws on forgoing treatment.[33]

Is there a real moral difference--with a sharp bite and a bright line--between withholding and withdrawing treatment? The President's Commission strongly challenged but did not silence the conventional wisdom.[34] The commission argued that it ought to be morally harder to withhold any treatment, especially if it has not yet been tried, than to withdraw any treatment that has been tried and has failed to benefit the patient or is physiologically futile. When in doubt if one or more treatments will benefit a patient, clinicians should examine whether they should conduct a brief therapeutic trial. However, if they know that a treatment is not effective or beneficial, there is no moral obligation to continue it.

This point can be reinforced by clarifying the goals of treatment when patients are dying or hopelessly ill. The goals for such patients should shift from prolonging life to providing comfort and relief of suffering. Continuing aggressive treatment, such as mechanical ventilation, may cause discomfort without producing any compensating benefit for the patient. In caring for dying patients, withdrawing burdensome treatment is just as important as withholding aggressive treatment such as CPR.[35]

IV. Landmark Legal Cases: Forum for Ethical Debate

From the 1960s through the 1980s, the legal forum was the major arena for the evolution of "right-to-die" cases. In a secular society, court cases are an important forum for debating ethical issues and clarifying legal principles and guidelines for decision making. The ethical issues have mainly concerned questions about the basis for decisions to forgo treatment and questions about who has the moral (and legal) standing to make such decisions for incapacitated patients. Decisions to withdraw treatment (and cause death) are decisions to withdraw life-sustaining technologies. In recent years, such cases have often been debated in the context of "medical futility."

A. *Quinlan*: Withdrawing the Ventilator

Karen Ann Quinlan was the patient in a landmark legal case involving withdrawal of a ventilator (*In Re Quinlan*).[36] In 1975, Quinlan, a 21-year-old New Jersey woman, suffered severe brain damage from anoxia after an alcohol/drug overdose. Brought to an emergency room, she eventually needed a respirator to breathe and a nasogastric feeding tube. She was

not "brain dead," but she was eventually diagnosed as being in a persistent vegetative state (PVS).

Several months later, her father asked the court to appoint him guardian to authorize removal of the respirator. He was opposed by her physicians, who argued that maintaining the respirator was "standard treatment" and removing it would be an act of euthanasia because it would cause her death.

A lower court, the local prosecutor, and the state's attorney-general agreed with the physicians. The New Jersey Supreme Court, however, granted the request. Her doctors weaned her slowly from the ventilator over a two-month period. She continued in a PVS for 10 more years until her death. About withdrawing the ventilator, the New Jersey Supreme Court's reasoning was: "the State's interest (i.e., in the preservation of life) weakens and the individual's right of privacy grows as the degree of bodily invasion increases and the prognosis dims. Ultimately, there comes a point at which the individual's rights overcome the State's interest."[37]

Quinlan's parents wanted the ventilator stopped, but they never asked that artificial feeding and hydration be withdrawn. Other important legal cases became forums for moral debate about withdrawing artificial feeding and hydration.

B. Herbert: Withdrawing Artificial Feeding and Hydration

In the 1980s, controversy shifted to feeding and hydration by intravenous lines, nasogastric tubes (tubes leading into the stomach by way of the nasal passages), or tubes placed surgically into the gastrointestinal tract. The Clarence Herbert case (*Barber v. Superior Court*)[38] was a legal landmark, because the California court was the first to use the President's Commission's benefits/burdens approach in its decision.

In California in 1982, Dr. Neil Barber and Dr. Robert Nejdl were charged with homicide after they stopped life-sustaining treatment at the request of the spouse and family. On 26 August 1981, a patient with cancer, Mr. Herbert, had surgery to close an ileostomy. In the recovery room, he stopped breathing and his heart stopped (he had a history of heart problems). He was placed on a respirator. On August 27, the hospital neurologist diagnosed the patient as severely brain damaged and with a poor prognosis. Dr. Barber recommended to Mrs. Herbert that the respirator be stopped, and she consented. The respirator was stopped on August 29. However, the patient did not die, and he began to breathe on his own. The next day, the family signed a consent form and wrote that "all machines [be] taken off that are sustaining life." The nasogastric tube and fluids were stopped on August 31, and Mr. Herbert died on September 6 from dehydration and pneumonia.

A nursing supervisor, Sandra Bardenilla, was concerned about Dr. Nejdl's decision to stop the air mist after removing the respirator. She believed that without it, the patient would develop a mucous plug and die. Unable to locate either doctor, she received permission from another doctor to restart the air mist. She was angrily reprimanded by Dr. Nejdl, who told her that "patients are taken off respirators so that they will die." Angered, she reported the incident to the district attorney, who brought criminal charges, alleging that forgoing both treatments was part of a conspiracy to kill Mr. Herbert to hide malpractice. A hearing and two trials resulted. Finally, the court of appeals found the criminal charges baseless. The court cited the reasoning of the President's Commission that the main approach to such cases was the proportionality of benefits and burdens of each treatment that sustains life.

Some opponents of removing feeding tubes from hopelessly ill patients claim that it "starves them to death." Richard A. McCormick questioned this reasoning.[39] He compared the impact of the disease on the patient to the smashing of a tree by a hurricane, and feeding and hydration to "propping up" the tree in the aftermath. McCormick doubted that a moral fault can be found in removing props from a smashed tree that will die shortly but is putting forth a few leaves as a result of the props. The damage is irreversible. Further, Lynn and Childress[40] asserted that continuing to feed hopelessly ill patients can actually cause harm to them. Such patients typically have little interest in food, and problems from a lack of nutrition can be alleviated by medication. The experience of starving in healthy persons is very different than in patients with an incurable disease.[41]

C. *Cruzan*: The Persistent Vegetative State

Many important cases of forgoing life-sustaining treatment have involved patients in the vegetative state. The vegetative state is defined as follows:

a clinical condition of complete unawareness of the self and the environment, accompanied by sleep-wake cycles with either complete or partial preservation of hypothalamic and brain-stem autonomic functions. The condition may be transient, marking a stage in the recovery from severe acute or chronic brain damage, or permanent, as a consequence of the failure to recover from such injuries. "Persistent" vegetative state is a diagnosis of a wakeful unconscious state that lasts longer than one month. "Permanent" vegetative state exists when irreversibility can be established with a high degree of clinical certainty.[42]

Most persons would want treatment withdrawn if they were to be devastated by a neurological disorder that progressed to a permanent vegetative state (which could be viewed as a condition worse than death itself). However, many state laws on living wills require that death be "imminent" before the directive to limit treatment to comfort care be respected. Patients in a vegetative state can survive for years with food and fluids given by surgical placement of a tube into the stomach.

The most recent landmark case involving vegetative state was the case of Nancy Cruzan, a case originating in Missouri that was acted on by the U.S. Supreme Court (*Cruzan v. Director, Missouri Department of Health*) (see Case B below). Legislation since the Supreme Court decision, such as the Virginia Health Care Decisions Act of 1992, broadens the law to include PVS as a condition in which forgoing life-sustaining treatment is permitted.

D. *Wanglie* and *Baby K*: Medical Futility

After the *Cruzan* case, the debate about withholding and withdrawing treatment took a new turn. Rather than focusing on particular technologies, the debate turned to "medical futility" and how accurately this concept could guide decision making. The 1991 case of Helga Wanglie in Minnesota became the first case in which a hospital went to court to ask permission for treatment to be withdrawn (*In Re the Conservatorship of Helga M. Wanglie*).[43]

Helga Wanglie was an 86-year-old woman diagnosed as in a PVS. Her husband and adult children, motivated by religious beliefs, insisted that she be kept alive at all costs. Physicians in the case looked upon mechanical ventilation, artificial feeding and hydration, and intensive care as futile. They were unable to transfer Mrs. Wanglie to another hospital or another physician from Hennepin County Hospital in Minneapolis. The physicians believed that Mr. Wanglie was not weighing and considering the medical facts of the case in an appropriate way and did not have his wife's best interest at heart. Unable to resolve the dispute, and after a four-to-three vote of the county board that controlled the hospital, the institution asked a court to appoint an independent conservator. The court denied the request, affirming that Mr. Wanglie was the proper decision maker and surrogate. Mrs. Wanglie died several months after the hearing, still supported by the ventilator.

In moral debate, *medical futility* can be understood in two senses:

1. in a narrow sense as physiological futility (that is, when a treatment is ineffective in producing a desired effect, such as using laetrile to treat cancer or administering CPR in the presence of cardiac rupture or severe outflow obstruction); or
2. in a broad sense as the lack of benefit (that is, even if a treatment might be physiologically effective in a given case, it is futile because it fails to restore consciousness, to prevent total dependence on intensive care, to alleviate suffering, to restore the patient to an acceptable quality of life, or to prevent the patient's dying).

One can immediately see that, if it is used in this second sense, the concept of medical futility is a large tent under which many other disputes can be gathered (such as, quality-of-life issues, questions about rationing expensive end-of-life care, and the issue of who has the authority to make decisions about forgoing treatment).

The literature in clinical ethics on "futility" or "futile care" is large and controversial. After the *Wanglie* decision, there was sharp debate as to how to resolve cases that were seen to involve medical futility. Famous cases included Baby L,[44] *Baby K* (see case 2 at end of chapter),[45] and other cases involving expensive technology.[46] No consensus about futility emerged, especially as defined in the broad (second) sense. Physicians' unilateral decisions, especially to withdraw treatments regarded as qualitatively futile, are arguably unethical without a broad consensus in the nation about allocation of expensive resources for

critical care. However, the United States had neither a political nor an ethical consensus about health policy. We have no consensus about allocation of expensive resources at the end of life, except for organ transplantation.

The literature on futility focuses heavily on resuscitation.[47] Proposals have been made to save money at the end of life by avoiding "futile care,"[48] especially by reducing the incidence of resuscitation for patients with terminal cancer and other poor prognoses.[49] These proposals lack empirical support for the prospect of cost savings. Data from the SUPPORT investigators,[50] expert analysis of Medicare hospital expenditures in the last year of life, and discussion of relatively small economic savings from universal palliative care[51] cast doubt on the prospects of such proposals. Nonetheless, debate about cost savings in critical-care medicine is important, because ICU care is estimated to consume about 1 percent of the U.S. Gross National Product (GNP) or 20 percent of all hospital expenditures.[52]

Some discussions of futility are also open to criticism because they convey more medical certainty than can be proved and argue that physicians ought to make unilateral decisions to withhold or withdraw treatment in such a context. Several articles challenge the usefulness of the concept of futility for clinical ethics when it is understood in the broad sense, because it masks so many value judgments.[53] The debate about medical futility can also be a vehicle to "smuggle in" concerns about rationing expensive treatment to the national debate on healthcare reform. Even in the face of disputes about the meaning of futility, some institutions have implemented policies to support and encourage physicians' authority in decisions to withhold treatment in this context.[54]

Stell lucidly explores the historical beginnings and continuing debate about futile treatment.[55] He is critical of defining futility with the concept of lack of benefit.[56] He defines a futile effort in terms of its desired end, due to an "intrinsic defect" (that is, the effort cannot achieve its desired end). He argues that futile efforts, when "undertaken voluntarily and expressing the agent's will, can ennoble the doer and inspire others."[57] In short, futile efforts can have important symbolic meanings for persons, although such expressions clearly have their limits. This issue was clearly part of the dynamics in the *Baby K* case (*In Re Baby K*) (see Case 2 at end of chapter). One cannot "do" clinical ethics or develop hospital or nursing home policies today without a concept of futility and a strategy for futility disputes.

V. Ethical and Legal Standards When the Patient Lacks Capacity

In addition to the benefits/burdens standard, which is discussed in the next section, legal cases have clarified two standards for the decision making process when the patient is incapacitated: (1) substituted-judgment standard and (2) the best-interest standard. The first standard should be used where there is evidence that the patient communicated her or his preferences and values before becoming incapacitated. The second standard should be used by clinicians and surrogates when the patient's views are unknown or unknowable.

A. The Substituted-Judgment Standard

A substituted judgment attempts to approximate the moral choices that the patient would have made if he or she could express these choices. If the patient has been capable of making decisions but is presently incapacitated, clinicians and family should ask, "What would be the patient's preferences, if she or he could speak?" This standard was first clarified in the Clare Conroy case in New Jersey, (*In Re Conroy*),[58] and it was described as a "subjective standard." Justice Schreiber wrote:

> We hold that life-sustaining treatment may be withheld or withdrawn from an incompetent patient when it is clear that the particular patient would have refused the treatment under the circumstances involved. The standard we are enunciating is a subjective one, consistent with the notion that the right that we are seeking to effectuate is a very personal right to control one's own life. The question is not what a reasonable or average person would have chosen to do under the circumstances, but what the particular patient would have done if able to choose for himself.[59]

The best evidence decision makers can have is from the patient's own statements, verbal or written. Substituted judgment based on verbal statements

played a role in the *Cruzan* case (see Case B below), because Nancy Ann Cruzan did not have a written advance directive. The U.S. Supreme Court ruled that Missouri could require "clear and convincing" evidence of a person's prior wishes, such as a written document.

B. The Best-Interest Standard

If the patient's preferences for or against life-sustaining treatment are unknown or unknowable, or if the patient has never been capable, then the clinicians, in consultation with the family or guardian, are morally obliged to shape a plan of care regarded as in the "best interest" of the patient. *Best interest* in this context means "best medical interest" as evaluated in the framework of the benefits and burdens guideline, discussed in Guideline 2 below, and illustrated by the Saikewicz case, which is Case C below.

VI. Guidelines for Clinicians with Case Discussions

The guidelines recommended below are from the American Medical Association,[60] a task force of the Society of Critical Care Medicine,[61] and interdisciplinary groups for the study of ethical problems in medicine. These groups include the President's Commission,[62] the Office of Technology Assessment of the U.S. Congress,[63] a Hastings Center task force,[64] and an international consensus conference of 33 delegates from 10 nations who worked for two years on this subject.[65]

Four guidelines for clinicians can be adapted from these sources. There appears to be an ethical consensus about guideline 2, which answers the question, "On what basis ought decisions to forgo life-sustaining treatments be made when the patient is incapacitated?" The benefit/burden standard prevails in clinical ethics today, in continuity with older ethical traditions. McCormick explains this standard as follows: "If a proposed treatment will offer no benefit, or the benefit will be outweighed by the burdens, the treatment is morally optional."[66]

Cases posing difficult choices about forgoing life-sustaining treatment can vary factually and in how clinicians interpret them. Other duties of disclosure and communication can become more difficult in these situations. The cases in this section and those at the end of the chapter illustrate this variety and the potential for misunderstanding. Throughout this section, the guideline is given first, accompanied by a case with discussion to illustrate how the guideline is used.

A. *Guideline 1*: Respect Advance Directives

When an incapacitated patient who is terminally ill or in a state of PVS has a living will and/or has appointed a surrogate with a durable medical power of attorney, clinicians and family have moral and legal duties to honor such directives and to share authority with the patient's proxy in decisions to forgo life-sustaining treatment. However, statements that persons make in living wills about their preferences in the event that they are in a terminal stage of illness are not helpful when they are not yet in that stage. Case A presents a situation in which a patient who is now incapacitated wrote personal instructions on a living will, which are not ethically or legally binding unless the patient is terminally ill. The instructions do not anticipate the facts of the medical situation in which the patient's physicians must now make decisions about diagnosis and treatment.

Case A: Do Advance Directives Trump Everything Else?

Ms. B, a 70-year-old, single woman with severe hypertension, suffers her first stroke at home resulting in right-sided hemiplegia (paralysis of one-half of the body). Mrs. N, a widowed sister who lives with Ms. B, calls the rescue squad. They respond and keep the patient's airway open. Ms. B is unable to communicate. On admission to the emergency room, she is intubated and has cardiac arrhythmias. Later that day, in an ICU, she remains intubated and a nasogastric tube is placed to remove gastric secretions and to prevent aspiration pneumonia.

Mrs. N, her only living, close relative, brings to the hospital a properly witnessed living will, dated and signed one year earlier by the patient. Ms. B had specifically refused CPR and artificial feeding and hydration if "in the opinion of my physicians I cannot be restored to a state of health with the capacity to be in meaningful communication with my loved ones and companions. This

communication might be nonverbal, but unless I can meaningfully understand and appreciate it, I prefer to die rather than exist in such a condition. I fear death less than the indignity of dependence and deterioration."

Her physicians tended to view advance directives in terms of the law of the state--that directives are effective when the patient is "terminally ill." In the ICU, Mrs. N objects to intubation and the placement of the nasogastric tube, saying, "That is just what she was talking about. I live with her and know what she meant. You are ignoring me." Ms. B had also appointed Mrs. N to hold a durable power of attorney for healthcare decisions.

Physicians persuaded Mrs. N to consent to another computed tomography (CT) scan. Afterwards, a neurologist wrote a note that the patient had experienced a large stroke of the dominant hemisphere. Her speech will definitely be affected. It is unclear how much recovery, if any, she will have.

Does the living will and durable power of attorney trump everything else? Some state laws say that the patient's instructions to forgo life-sustaining treatment may only be implemented when the patient is [in the view of two physicians] "terminally ill" and when "death is imminent." How should her personal instructions be understood?[67]

Advance directives do not trump a benefits/burdens assessment. Ms. B's living will ought to be interpreted in the context of her diagnosis and prognosis. It will take time to evaluate the effects of a stroke and develop a plan of care, but treatment cannot proceed unilaterally over Mrs. N's objections. The ethical issues are complex given Ms. B's known wishes, her refusal of specific technologies, and Mrs. N's power of attorney. Ms. B's views of quality of life and death are known, and Mrs. N has authority to consent or refuse treatment. Meanwhile, physicians need time to answer the questions: How dependent and impaired will she be? Will she deteriorate? It is not unusual for physicians to decline a family's request to stop treatment. An informative recent survey on physician's practices found that 34 percent of a sample of 879 critical-care physicians had declined requests by family members to withdraw ventilation, because they believed the patient had a reasonable chance to recover.[68]

If the patient worsens and becomes terminally ill, the nasogastric tube--even if it were begun to permit feeding, hydration, and administration of other medications during the evaluation period--can ethically be withdrawn; this is true for intubation as well. Mrs. N's agreement is necessary to begin feeding and hydration by the nasogastric tube and for each major step of the case. If she does not agree, the attending physician is obligated to try to resolve the dispute while continuing to evaluate Ms. B's condition and prognosis. There are two acceptable moral options in this case:

1. Continue to treat while establishing a prognosis, assuming that physicians can persuade Ms. B's sister that this is the best course.
2. Stop treatment if Ms. B's sister can persuade the physicians that this would be her sister's decision if she could make it and regardless of an ambiguous prognosis.

Recognition of Mrs. N's role as surrogate decision maker in this case is a major factor in moral problem solving. Mrs. N felt ignored by the ICU physicians. Clinicians frequently fail to recognize surrogates' authority. Dubler discusses the fragility of the surrogate/proxy-physician relationship.[69] There are similar cases in the literature, but in these published cases the patients were more grievously ill than Ms. N.[70] Elizabeth Hansot, a faculty member of Stanford University, wrote to a medical journal about physicians' dismissing her role as surrogate in spite of her having a durable power of attorney for healthcare.[71] Dr. Hansot's mother, 87 years old, was a stroke patient like Ms. B, but she was in a terminal condition. Hansot reported that despite the fact that her mother had developed an advance directive with her physician, her lawyer, and her offspring, the document was "invisible" when most needed because her mother's physician failed to notify the medical team of its existence. Recalling her harsh interaction with the attending pulmonologist, she said that he challenged her defense of her mother's prior instructions, asking her if she "was an ageist, or an ideologue interested only in abstract principles." After several days, a tech-

nician was delegated to extubate her mother, and no physician was present. Gilligan and Raffin presume that Hansot's gender lessened her power in the eyes of male physicians, and they prescribe education.[72]

Another important issue is Ms. B's "broad" or nonconforming advance directives. This case occurred in a state with a living will statute that restricts clinicians from honoring the declarant's instructions unless the declarant is diagnosed with a terminal illness or persistent vegetative state. Ms. B's instructions in her advance directive were broader than the statute permits in that she directed that treatments be withheld or withdrawn if she suffered irreversible brain damage but was not terminally ill. Her advance directive, as discussed by Meisel, was a "nonconforming" type.[73] Should it have been respected? Her physicians believed that the moral limits of their relationship with her were bound only by the legal limits imposed by the state and that their aggressive plan of care was permitted. However, their interpretation is subject to serious ethical and legal challenge, especially since Mrs. N was on the scene within a few hours of the patient's admission.

A broad advance directive exceeds the narrow scope of most state laws. Is it any the less morally weighty or *prima facie* invalid for that reason? Meisel counsels that nonconforming directives should be "presumed to be valid even in a jurisdiction that has enacted advance directive legislation."[74] He states that "the better view, and the one likely to prevail," is that state legislatures do not create a right to make decisions about treatment in a future situation when they pass living-will or durable-power-of-attorney statutes. Indeed, this right already exists and the legislation affirms it and provides immunity from legal liability if physicians honor this right, as it did in this particular state. Meisel depicts statutes regarding advance directives as cumulative--intended to "preserve and supplement existing common law and constitutional rights and not to supersede or limit them."[75] Susan Wolf also reasons that "a directive broader than the state statute is not out of bounds."[76] She, like Meisel, argues that common-law rights recognized by judges and constitutional protections, as acknowledged by the U.S. Supreme Court majority in the *Cruzan* decision, also support physicians honoring broader directives.

B. *Guideline 2*: Use the Benefit/Burden Standard as the Major Guideline

Benefits and burdens can be defined as follows:

1. Treatment *benefits* of two types can increase the well-being of the patient: (a) health benefits--positive and empirically measurable effects in curing, arresting, or relieving the patient's disease, condition, symptoms, and pain; or (b) quality-of-life benefits--improvements in mental status or added days or months of life that are mutually rewarding to the patient and others.
2. Treatment *burdens* of two types can diminish the well-being of patients: (a) when treatment provides no measurable health benefits with increased pain, suffering, or debilitation; or (b) when treatment reduces the patient's quality of life.

An ethically sound basis on which to evaluate choices to forgo life-sustaining treatments in incapacitated patients is to assess the benefits and burdens for the patient of each treatment. The following guidelines are suggested:

1. Physicians have a duty to make recommendations to other decision makers based on benefit/burden assessments.
2. Benefits and burdens should be assessed within the framework of the patient's prior expressed wishes or known values, beliefs, and previous decisions about treatment, and a substituted judgment made if possible; if it is not possible, the best-medical interest standard should be followed.
3. Family members are usually the best source of information about a patient's preferences, supplemented by information from other members of the clinical team.
4. When the benefits of treatment are proportionate to or exceed the burdens, it is obligatory to give treatment (unless refused by the patient in an advance directive).
5. It is obligatory for clinicians to withhold and strive to withdraw treatment(s) that clearly will harm or are harming the patient.

Cases B and C present complications in using the benefit/burden standard with incapacitated patients.

If the patient has no written advance directives and resides in a state with a very high legal standard of evidence for patient preferences, serious problems can arise. Also, if the patient never had capacity to make decisions, the best-interests standard is the preferred approach.

Case B: The Patient's Preferences Are Known but Legally Contested (*Cruzan v. Harmon*)[77]

On 11 January 1983, Nancy Beth Cruzan, then 25 years old, was injured in a single-car accident and found lying face down in a ditch. She had been thrown approximately 35 feet from her overturned vehicle. A state trooper who first arrived at the accident examined her and found "no detectable respiratory or cardiac function." Paramedics were able to revive her breathing and heartbeat but she suffered permanent brain damage. In the hospital, a gastrostomy tube was implanted on 5 February 1983 to permit nutrition and hydration, and rehabilitation efforts were begun, but without success. In October 1983, she was transferred to the Missouri Rehabilitation Center in Mount Vernon.

After four years, her parents (as coguardians) asked the hospital administration to end the gastrostomy feedings. Her parents reported that their daughter had made statements to friends that she would never want to be kept alive if she was seriously brain-injured. The administration refused the request and, on 23 October 1987, the Cruzans filed a declaratory judgment action seeking judicial sanction of their instructions. As presented to the Missouri Supreme Court, the medical facts were:

Ms. Cruzan's respiration and circulation were not artificially supported and are within normal limits. She was oblivious to her environment except for reflexive responses to sound and painful stimuli. She had cerebral cortical atrophy, which is irreversible, permanent, progressive, and ongoing. A spastic quadriplegic, her arms and legs were contracted with irreversible muscular and tendon damage. She had lost all cognitive ability. She could not swallow food or water and will never recover this function. Medical experts testified that she could live for another 30 years in a persistent vegetative state, which was her condition at that time.[78]

In March 1988, a three day hearing began, at the family's request. Her parents argued that Nancy had a common-law right to be free from unwanted medical treatment as well as state and federal constitutional rights to privacy that protected her right to refuse unwanted medical treatment. Her parents also testified that Nancy had told her housemates that she would not want to continue to live if she could not be "at least halfway normal." Knowing her stated preferences made a substituted judgment possible.

On 27 July 1988, Probate Judge Charles Teel approved the request. On 3 August 1988, Missouri Attorney General William Webster filed a notice that the state would appeal to the Missouri Supreme Court. On 16 November 1988, by a vote of four to three, the Missouri Supreme Court overturned Judge Teel's decision. While recognizing a right to refuse treatment embodied in the common-law doctrine of informed consent, the court questioned whether it applied in this case. The court also declined to read into the state constitution a broad right of privacy that would support an unrestricted right to refuse treatment and expressed doubt that the Federal Constitution embodied such a right. The court then decided that Missouri's living-will statute embodied a state policy strongly favoring the preservation of life, and that Nancy's statements to her housemates were unreliable for the purpose of determining her intent. The court rejected the argument that her parents were entitled to order the termination of her medical treatment, concluding that no person can assume the choice for an incapacitated person in the absence of the formalities required by the living-will statute or clear and convincing evidence of the patient's wishes. Further, the majority opinion (written by Judge Edward D. Robertson, Jr.) based its decision in part on a refusal to engage in "quality-of-life" considerations. Robertson stated, "Were quality of life at issue, persons with all manner of handicaps might find the state seeking to terminate their lives. Instead, the state's interest is in life; that issue is unquali-

fied."[79] The court declared that the state's "interest in life" required that the feeding tube not be removed, even though Nancy Beth Cruzan was in a persistent vegetative state. This decision was appealed by the family to the U.S. Supreme Court (*Cruzan v. Director, Missouri Department of Health*).[80]

On 25 June 1990, the U.S. Supreme Court, by a vote of five to four, rendered a decision (written by Chief Justice William H. Rehnquist) with two main parts: (1) the court "assumed that the United States Constitution would grant a competent person a constitutionally protected right to refuse lifesaving hydration and nutrition"; (2) the U.S. Constitution did not prohibit the state of Missouri from "requiring clear and convincing evidence of a person's expressed decision while competent to have hydration and nutrition withdrawn in such a way as to cause death." The Court held that even though her parents were "loving and caring," Missouri could "choose to defer" only to Nancy Cruzan's wishes (which were not written but reportedly oral), and ignore both the parents' own wishes and their views about what their daughter would want.[81]

On 30 August 1990, the Cruzans asked Judge Teel for a second hearing, saying that they had new evidence that their daughter once indicated to three other people that she would rather die than live in a vegetative state. On 17 September 1990, Attorney General Webster said that the state no longer had a "recognizable legal interest" in the case, and asked Judge Teel to drop the state health department and the director of the rehabilitation center from future litigation. Judge Teel dropped the state as a defendant. On November 1, three former coworkers told Judge Teel that they recalled conversations with Ms. Cruzan in which she said she never would want to "live as a vegetable" on medical machines. Her physician, who had opposed removing the feeding tube, termed her life "a living hell" and testified that she should be allowed to die.

On 5 December 1990, Ms. Cruzan's court-appointed guardian recommended that the feeding tube be removed so she could die. Judge Teel approved on December 14. Between December 18 and December 24, anti-euthanasia groups attempted to stay the court's order and asked state and federal courts for injunctions, which were denied. At one point, some members of the group stormed the clinic in an attempt to reattach the tube. Ms. Cruzan died on December 26, 13 days after the feeding tube was removed.

The U.S. Supreme Court's decision, in effect, affirmed the competent person's right to refuse any life-sustaining treatment, including artificial feeding and hydration. Regarding the incapacitated person, the court left to the states the choice of whether the legal standard for a substituted judgment would be satisfied if the patient had made only verbal statements. The Virginia Health Care Decisions Act encourages written advance directives and also accepts the validity of prior verbal statements, as do many other states. Weir and Gostin reviewed 50 legal cases about forgoing treatment with incapacitated patients in U.S. state courts. Only four (three in New York and the *Cruzan* case in Missouri) were decided on grounds with such a high standard of evidence of the patient's preferences that the thrust of the benefit/burden standard and prior verbal statements would not be sufficient to resolve the problem.[82] For these reasons, clinicians should be familiar with the law of the state in which they practice.

Case C: The Patient Never Had Capacity

Joseph Saikewicz, at the age of 67, was diagnosed with acute nonlymphoblastic leukemia, at that time (1967) an invariable fatal illness. He has resided at the Belchertown State School, a Massachusetts facility for the mentally retarded, for 40 years. In this era, chemotherapy for this form of leukemia had limited results (that is, short term remission from two to 13 months in 30 to 50 percent of cases), but much poorer results in patients over 60 years of age. Side effects were serious: nausea, anemia, and infections. Mr. Saikewicz had never been a capable decision maker. He was severely retarded from birth with an IQ of 10. He communicated with others by gestures and could not speak except in grunts. He did not understand common dangers and became disoriented when away from his most familiar surroundings.

Officials at the school approached the probate court with the question of whether Mr. Saikewicz should be treated. The court appointed a guardian *ad litem* to consider the relevant issues and to make decisions about his care and treatment. The guardian recommended that "not treating Mr. Saikewicz would be in his best interests" for these reasons: his disease is incurable, treatment would have very serious and painful side effects that he would neither understand not be able to put into perspective, and that the patient had never been a capable decision maker. This review was upheld by the Supreme Judicial Court of Massachusetts, but the court used a substituted-judgment standard, rather then the argument of the guardian based upon best interests. [83]

The Saikewicz case is important, because the court erroneously proposed that a substituted-judgment standard should be used to make the decision. Saikewicz had never been capable of making any decisions and had no knowable preferences regarding treatment or any other matter. This particular court wanted to avoid even the appearance of quality-of-life reasoning in using the best-interest standard, which was the argument made by the guardian. The court had been deeply divided on the ethical and legal principles relevant to such cases. To use the substituted-judgment standard was fictional in this case and should not be done with patients who have never been capable. The only meaningful standard in such cases is the best-interest standard.

There are also famous cases (*Linares* and *Baby K*) in which an ethically defensible decision to forgo life-sustaining treatment is blocked by legal arguments that state law (*Linares*) or federal law (*Baby K*) does not permit the decision explicitly. These cases are presented at the end of the chapter (Cases 1 and 2).

C. *Guideline 3*: Disclose Poor Prognosis or Futility

If the patient's prognosis is poor or if one or more treatments are futile, physicians have a duty to disclose this assessment and the reasoning that underlies it and to recommend to other decision makers that futile treatment be withheld or withdrawn. The duty to inform falls within the larger scope of duties of disclosing poor prognosis and of limiting medical care when no overall improvement results (see Chapter 6).[84]

Case D is about informing families about poor prognosis or futility (for example before writing DNR orders) or not offering other treatments deemed *futile* for an incapacitated patient.

Case D: Informing about Poor Prognosis or Futility

On morning rounds outside the room of Mrs. A, a 62-year-old unconscious woman who is dying from ovarian cancer, the healthcare team reaches consensus that CPR would be "worse than useless, it would harm her." Her family, large and contentious, has been keeping a bedside vigil and fighting among themselves and with the healthcare team about "doing everything" for the patient. The patient's nurse asks the attending physician, "Are you going to speak with the family about DNR?" The attending physician responds, "Do I have a clear duty to speak with them? I ought to be able to write a DNR order because CPR is not medically indicated. If I do speak with them, they will think I am asking them to 'pull the plug' on their mother. They will want to fight about it. They are burdened enough already without having to hear about this medical decision. Why leave them feeling guilty? It is our job to manage the medical matters." The nurse says, "The hospital policy and state law says that the surrogate decision maker needs to be consulted before the DNR order can be written." The physician says, "That may be, but we differ about whether informing them will do more harm than good." What should be done?[85]

In the case of Mrs. A, there is a disagreement between a physician and a nurse about disclosure to family members of the reason for a DNR order. The nurse's position is in keeping with the guideline to disclose futility. This guideline reflects respect for the norms of family life and also for shared decision making. But before such disclosure can occur, the family needs help with their inner turmoil and their reasons for fighting with the staff. The physician wants to avoid turmoil by not discussing the DNR order with the family. However, his proposal involves violating the principle underlying the guideline, unless he can defend it on ethical grounds. Is such a defense possible? The only valid argument is that family members were incapacitated as decision makers by their

emotional problems, which begs a question about what kind of help is appropriate. Psychiatric or pastoral help and assessment of the situation is indicated. The higher priority is for the physician to inform the family, in the context of supportive help for them, without unreasonable delay.

CPR and DNR decisions are frequently very difficult choices in critical-care units. After reviewing the recent literature on withholding CPR on medical grounds, Brunetti and Stell advise that the attending physician should decide to forgo CPR only when there is enough information to make an adequately informed judgment that the results will be unfavorable to the patient.[86] Discussions with patients and surrogates regarding CPR should be recorded in the chart. It is also crucial to record the reasons for writing DNR orders in the progress notes of the patient's medical record.

Six steps for writing DNR orders follow:

1. The physician makes a benefit/burden assessment of CPR in the context of the patient's overall prognosis.
2. If the assessment is negative, the physician consults with other members of the healthcare team about the issue and discusses the need for a DNR order.
3. If there is no remaining substantive objection to a DNR order among the team, the physician approaches the patient (if capable) or the designated decision makers (if the patient is incapacitated) and explains a DNR order and why healthcare team recommends writing such an order.
4. If no substantive objection is made, the physician writes the order in the patient's chart, with the reasons for the DNR order in the progress notes.
5. The DNR order is reviewed regularly, at least every seven days.
6. The DNR order can be revoked if the benefit/burden assessment changes.

D. *Guideline 4*: In Mediating Disputes with Surrogate Decision Makers, Treat the Patient until the Dispute is Resolved, Except When Treatment is Harmful

The fourth and final guideline concerns disputes between clinicians and surrogate decision makers about decisions to forgo life sustaining treatment.

Points A, B, and C below are well settled in clinical ethics. Point D is the least established and is open to further exploration.

If the surrogate of an incapacitated patient demands:

a. *Withholding beneficial treatment that the patient may have wanted*: Clinicians should not acquiesce to the demand. They should strive to resolve the dispute by ethics consultation and other help. Clinicians should put the best medical interest of the patient above all other considerations. The burden of seeking legal action to stop treatment falls on the family in this situation.

b. *Starting clearly harmful treatment*: After good-faith efforts to resolve the disputes by ethics consultation and other help as indicated, with prior institutional approval, physicians should withhold the treatment, even over the objections of guardians or family members.

c. *Continuing clearly harmful treatment*: After using ethics consultation and other help as indicated (see Chapter 14) to resolve the dispute, physicians should, with institutional approval, strive to withdraw the treatment, even over the objections of guardians or family members. In these cases, the institution should seek a court's approval for withdrawal of life-sustaining but harmful treatment(s).

d. *Withholding or withdrawing "medically futile" (defined in the broad sense above in Section IV.D) treatments that are not harmful* How to resolve these disputes continues to be debated in clinical ethics and law (see *Baby K* case below).

Case E describes a dispute between surrogates and clinicians about forgoing physiologically futile treatment when an incapable patient's prior wishes were unknowable. This case was one of several that led to an amendment in Virginia state law to permit physicians to refuse to provide treatment under such circumstances. Federal court decisions in the *Baby K* case (see case 2 at end of chapter) have preempted Virginia law in such cases.

Case E: "Code Him Until He's Brain Dead!"[87]

In 1988, a 61-year-old widowed patient with a 30-year history of alcohol abuse and a history of previous strokes, was brought to the Emergency Department by the rescue squad from a nursing home. He was unconscious, with a high fever, and cyanotic. He could not breathe on his own and a breathing tube was placed. He had twice been a patient in the hospital for treatment of strokes. He had not spoken or communicated with anyone since his strokes two years earlier. He had no advance directive. He was transferred to the intensive care unit and treated with several antibiotics, as well as intubated. Physicians were unable to discover the true source of infection.

His three daughters came quickly to the hospital from a neighboring community. One daughter, Pam, was the spokesperson. Physicians in the ICU recommended that a DNR order was appropriate. She objected vehemently and began every discussion about her father's condition with: "Code him until he's brain dead!" She had learned the term "Code him" in a previous admission (one year prior) of her father to the hospital for treatment of a stroke. On that occasion, a resident had approached her to discuss a DNR order and made the statement, according to Pam, that her father's condition was "hopeless." She refused the DNR order. At the time, the state law was that no life-sustaining treatment could be withheld or withdrawn without concurrence of surrogate decision makers. Her father survived. She stated, "The doctors were wrong before and they can be wrong now; code him until he's brain dead!"

The daughters said that their father had never made his wishes clear about what he wanted done in this kind of situation, and that they had never talked about this issue with him before his strokes. They did discuss his history of alcohol abuse and said that he had been abusive to them as children. They had never had a good relationship with him. They described a process of "coming together" around his care in the nursing home, and that they believed that he responded to them and heard them, although there were no data to support this impression. ICU physicians requested an ethics consultation, which began on the night of the patient's admission.

The sisters were staunchly opposed to any suggestion of withholding or withdrawing treatment. They made a religious argument, saying, "Where there is life there is hope." They also said that "When God decides to take him, we will accept it, but we will not accept any human decisions to end his life." They insisted that "everything be done." Physicians recommended continuing to search for the cause of his infection, treatment with antibiotics, but no cardiac resuscitation if an arrest occurred.

During a week of "stand-off" between the family and health care team, the ethics consultation continued. The consultant arranged several meetings between physicians, nurses, social workers, and family. The patient had not responded to treatment and became steadily worse. His physicians and nurses stated further treatment was "futile." Also, other patients who could benefit more from intensive care were being denied the bed. The clinicians recommended to the daughters that the breathing machine be removed and, if his heart stopped, that he be allowed to die without massaging his chest or restarting his heart by electroshock. They needed to write a DNR order. Pam objected, saying again, "You are asking us to murder our father. This is our belief. We want him coded (resuscitated) until he is brain dead!" In desperation, a physician turned to a nurse and said, "Do we have to take this? What can physicians and nurses do when the law gives the family the upper hand in a dispute like this? What can we do about our own ethical position of not inflicting torture on this hopelessly ill patient? And what about the injustice to other patients?"

The resources of clinical ethics program (see Chapter 14) clearly are needed but may be ineffective in disputes about medical futility in incapacitated patients. In such disputes, the surrogates tend to mistrust anyone connected with the healthcare organization (HCO).

Following "Code Him" and similar cases, the Virginia General Assembly was persuaded to amend the Virginia Health Care Decisions Act in 1992. The amendment stipulates that physicians are not required to prescribe or render treatment that the physician determines to be "medically or ethically inappropriate."[88] The law requires that a good-faith effort be made to transfer the patient to the care of another physician. In Maryland, as well, the state legislature amended its Health Care Decisions Act to support the authority of physicians not to render "medically ineffective treatment," which the legislature defined as

that which, "to a reasonable degree of medical certainty, will neither prevent nor reduce the deterioration of the health of a patient, nor prevent the impending death of a patient."[89]

Bridging between state law and hospital policy, the University of Virginia Health Sciences Center amended its DNR policy in 1992 to permit physicians to write a DNR order over a surrogate's objection when CPR clearly would be harmful or physiologically futile. This step is a last resort. All efforts to resolve the dispute must have failed, including an offer of ethics consultation as well as unsuccessful efforts to transfer the patient to the care of another physician. At the time the DNR policy was amended, the hospital required consultation by the attending physician with the chair of the ethics committee, who could assemble an *ad hoc* group to consider the situation. That requirement has now been made an option in a current and revised policy.

The policy was first used in 1993 in a case of a 53-year-old woman with multiorgan system failure, whose husband and family opposed a DNR order. The chair of the ethics committee convened an *ad hoc* group to meet with the attending physician and others. They developed a plan; and a DNR order was written. The patient died eight days later.

Later a dispute arose between the hospital's billing department and the family. Risk Management at UVA believes that aggravation over billing was the primary causation for an ensuing suit. The patient's total bill was approximately $105,000, and her insurance paid for all but about $2,000. The family, already bitter over the outcome of the case, received repeated bills with a final notice that the unpaid bill would be turned over to a collection agency. They turned the letter over to their attorneys, who sought and received the medical record. Within the record was a report from the Ethics Committee chairperson about the consultation and recommendations supporting writing a DNR order.

In a context of this unresolved grievance and the wake of court decisions in the *Baby K* case, the family's attorneys filed two lawsuits: one against the hospital in federal court alleging a violation of the federal "anti-dumping" law, the Emergency Medical Treatment and Active Labor Act (EMTALA); and the other in state court alleging a violation of the Health Care Decisions Act. This second case (*Cindy Bryan v. Rector and Visitors of the University of Virginia*), is discussed in Chapter 14, because it named members of the ethics committee and others. The suit in a state court was dismissed. The federal appeals court upheld a lower court's dismissal of the EMTALA charge, stating that "emergency treatment" presumed by EMTALA was not in question, as the patient had received stabilizing treatment for almost two weeks.[90]

In some cases, the use of the benefit/burden guideline has been blocked by arguments that no law exists to permit withdrawing treatment (see *Linares*, Case 1 see below) or that federal law does not permit forgoing treatment under emergency conditions (see *Baby K*, Case 2 below). In both situations, and where it is unclear that treatment would be harmful to the patients, it is advisable for the HCO to seek legal guidance for its actions. The hospital's attorney in the *Linares* case acted irresponsibly in arguing that it was the family's duty to seek a legal resolution of the case, rather than placing the burden on the hospital itself.

Recommendations for action to implement Guideline 4 are outlined in Exhibit 9-1.[91]

VII. Ethical Reasons for Clinicians to Support Guidelines

The ethical problems in these cases are caused by clinicians' conflicting moral obligations to patients. On the one hand are obligations to sustain life and benefit patients. On the other hand are obligations not to harm or unduly burden patients for unsound reasons.

Different ethical views about forgoing life-sustaining treatment compete and contend in this society. The prevailing view strives to combine clinical objectivity with respect for the patient's values and preferences. Decisions ought to be made by weighing the best clinical information about the benefits and burdens to the patient of each treatment that sustains life in the light of what is known about the patient's preferences and values. An influential report of the President's Commission for the Study of Ethical Problems in Medicine and Biomedical and Behavioral Research took this position.[92] Competing views depend more on other subjective and cultural factors. One view is that the struggle for life should be continued at all costs, out of respect for the sanctity of human life. This view is often expressed in the context of strong religious commitments. A third view, which is rarely found, places the highest value on quality of life as defined by a society's needs for contributing members. This view would support unilateral, socially approved decisions to withhold or stop all treatment if such qualities were no longer present in the patient.

Guideline 1 (respect advance directives) reflects duties consistent with the principle of respect for persons and the self-determination exercised before persons become incapacitated. These duties also reflect care for the relationships of patients, families, and the larger community. The care shown in planning advance directives strengthens bonds in families and inspires courage to face death with realism. Although children are legally incompetent and their parents are the legally authorized proxy decision makers, several states now have laws permitting proxy decision makers to initiate advance directives on behalf of terminally ill children.[93]

Guideline 2 (use the benefit/burden standard) grows out of claims of the ethical principles of beneficence and nonmaleficence. When clinicians are faced with situations in which harm cannot be avoided, they are still obliged in their actions to attempt to produce a positive ratio of benefits over burdens. The benefit/burden approach to decision making responds to this obligation. This guideline would lead clinicians to avoid harm to a patient and discontinue futile treatments and to be fair and just in their allocation of expensive treatments. The guideline also places the burden of proof on those who hold that some medical treatments (such as feeding and hydration) have a higher moral status than other treatments.

Guideline 3 (disclose poor prognosis or futility) is consistent with other guidelines on truthtelling and informed consent. It is supported by studies that report that the more family members understand the course of a patient's illness and the cause of death, the better they can acknowledge their grief and have fewer physical and psychological problems.[94] Full disclosure of clinically relevant information for family members of patients who die tends to promote their mental and physical health in the aftermath of loss and bereavement. Keeping the family abreast of clinicians' decision making is medically and ethically sound, but some clinicians clearly violate this norm by their own admission.

Asch and colleagues surveyed 879 critical-care physicians. They found that of 713 who withdrew life-sustaining treatment for reasons of futility, 105 (15

Exhibit 9-1
Recommendations for Action in Disputes with Surrogates about Incapacitated Patients

Medical Opinion	Surrogate Evaluation		
	"Worth a Try"	"Don't Know"	"Not Worth It"
Standard treatment; benefits patient	Treat	Treat	Treat; possible legal action by family?
Uncertain	Trial of treatment	Trial of treatment	No treatment
Highly unlikely to work	Trial or transfer	Permissive no treatment and review	No treatment
No medical benefit; possible harm to patient	Treat and review	No treatment	No treatment
"Won't work"; physiological futility and certain harm to patient	No treatment and review; notice of public policy about withholding; possible legal action by hospital to withdraw	No treatment	No treatment

Source: Adapted with permission from material presented by Christine Mitchell at the "Bioethics Summer Retreat," 29 June 1994.

percent) did so without the knowledge of the patient or family. Of interest in the context of futility disputes is their finding that 23 (3 percent) withdrew life supports despite the objections of the patient or family.[95] A rule of thumb about what should be disclosed is that if forgoing specific treatments is supported by a consensus in rounds by the clinical team, this fact should be communicated to the surrogate by the physician in charge of the case.

Guideline 4 (In mediating disputes with surrogate decision makers, treat the patient until the dispute is resolved, except when treatment is harmful) is the newest and least established guideline for clinicians. This guideline rests on a premise that favors sustaining life while vigorously seeking to resolve the dispute with attention to the goals of treatment and respect for all parties. The one exception appears when treatment is physiologically futile, and emotional appeals from families to "do everything possible" are demands that clinicians know would harm the patient. Clinicians ought not to consider these demands without real evidence that such would be the clear wish of the patient and, even then, caution should prevail. The policy of hospitals and nursing homes should state that clinicians are not required to render or prescribe therapy that they know to be physiologically futile or harmful.

Ethics case consultation (see Chapter 14) may not be an ideal process to mediate bitter futility disputes, since the surrogates tend to mistrust anyone related to the HCO. A better strategy may be to recruit a few well-respected persons from the community as mediators in futility disputes. If attempts fail to resolve such disputes and demands persist, there must be a good-faith attempt to transfer the patient to another facility. Failing transfer, the recommendation is that the HCO should ask a court for approval to withdraw futile treatment. The guideline assumes that an institutional policy permitting the withholding of treatment (especially CPR) under these circumstances is ethically acceptable. The outcome of the *Baby K* case is unusual in that the court order applied to emergency hospital treatment for apnea in the case of an anencephalic infant residing in a nursing home. The outcome of *Cindy Bryan v. Rector and Visitors of the University of Virginia* clarified EMTALA's scope with respect to patients hospitalized for a period of days. Seeking legal relief for ethical problems is a last but sometimes necessary resort.

In cases where the dispute is mainly about the patient's quality of life, respect for family wishes should prevail, since families are better situated to evaluate issues related to quality of life. To act unilaterally to withdraw treatment (for example to turn off a ventilator or to remove feeding tubes) over family objections runs contrary to a moral perspective allowing families to be the final interpreters of what quality of life means for their members. Views on quality of life differ greatly among individuals and from family to family. However, if the case clearly involves *harm* to patients by continuing treatment, clinicians' first loyalty is to the patient and to prevent harm.

Guideline 4, section D on withholding futile or harmful treatments even over family objections, has been shown in one study to be an effective practice.[96] In this study, Massachusetts General Hospital, one of the first institutions to have a patient care ethics committee for intensive care, reported on 20 cases in which clinicians wrote DNR orders, after prolonged attempts to mediate disagreements, over the objections of family members. Brennan described one of these cases in detail.[97] In this same hospital in 1994, physicians decided to write a DNR order and then to wean a patient from a ventilator over her daughter's objection. The patient died and her daughter brought a lawsuit that named, among others, the chairperson of the committee.[98] The jury of a trial court decided in favor of physicians defending their decisions on the basis of "medical futility." Capron argues that the trial court did not settle the question of whether society would truly favor health professionals' unilateral decisions to withhold or withdraw life-sustaining treatments over the objections of surrogates, based on the professionals' evaluation of the "worth of the outcome."[99] The decision is being appealed to a higher court. This case, *Gilgunn v. Massachusetts General Hospital*, is also discussed in Chapter 14.

Guideline 4, section C and the recommendations in Exhibit 9-1 run counter to the President's Commission's morally inflexible, "failsafe" policy to continue treatment in the context of all types of disputes.[100] This unguarded policy can lead to harm to patients and the demoralization of clinicians. Section C assumes that the approach of the President's Commission is too lenient by permitting families to dictate treatment choices. The responsibility of physicians to protect patients from harm--even the harm that results from desperate attempts by families to avoid death--is a well-established norm in clinical ethics.

Can futility disputes be prevented? How can the culture that spawns them be changed? Some of the

same problems that were identified in the SUPPORT study are at work here. Just as there are many physicians who are uninhibited therapeutic activists in critical care, there are patients and families who, under any circumstances, refuse to "give up" even when massive resources are involved. They may not feel part of a community that expects treatment to be limited. Lo and Brody each note in reflections on the SUPPORT study that change in the culture of critical care requires fundamental shifts in U.S. healthcare policy, physicians' values, and medical education.[101] These three areas of reform also influence the context of futility disputes. Reform in healthcare policy must precede economic and medical rationing of treatments and to discourage treatment in cases where it would be futile. The values of family practitioners rather than therapeutic activists need to be more in evidence in ICUs and critical care. Medical education must emphasize the quality of a "relationship-centered model"[102] and the need to learn the patient's whole story.

VIII. Cases for Further Study

Case 1: The Linares Case

When he was eight months old in September 1988, Samuel Linares swallowed a balloon. His father was with him and responded to the child quickly. He smelled rubber on his breath and tried to revive him, unsuccessfully. He ran with the child to a firehouse where emergency CPR was performed. The child showed no vital signs for at least 20 minutes. He was intubated at the hospital and admitted to the pediatric intensive care unit of Rush Presbyterian Hospital in Chicago and placed on a ventilator. Severe brain damage was diagnosed.

The child did not improve and was diagnosed as being in a persistent vegetative state. As months passed, his father and mother, Rudy and Tammy Linares, became despondent and requested that physicians stop the ventilator. Neighbors described the parents as devoted to the child. The Linares's financial problems were heavy. Medical bills in the case were estimated to exceed $200,000. Mr. Linares, a 23-year-old laborer, earned about $300 a week. Mrs. Linares was notified in February that she must repay nearly $20,000 that she collected in welfare payments by claiming that she was a single parent.

At this time, the hospital had no ethics committee and offered no ethics consultation. Max Brown, the hospital's attorney, was the most involved person in the case, other than Samuel's physicians and nurses. Mr. Brown took the position that while Illinois law did clearly permit hospitals to withdraw life supports from patients who are "brain dead" (the Illinois Definition of Death Act), there was no precedent for withdrawing a ventilator in a patient with "minimal brain function." Illinois accepts funds for child protection from the federal government. In such cases, the federal "Baby Doe" law applies. This law permits withholding or withdrawing treatment from infants under one year of age who are in "irreversible coma." Mr. Brown, however, did not interpret federal law to permit withdrawal in this case.

After the child was in the ICU for eight months, hospital officials advised the parents to seek a court order authorizing the removal of the respirator. They made an appointment with a lawyer on 28 April 1989 to discuss the matter. On April 26, they returned to their apartment to find a message on the answering machine from hospital officials that Samuel was about to be transferred to a long-term care facility about 70 miles away. They had been aware of the hospital's plans but were shocked that the move was to be made so soon.

Later that day, Mr. Linares entered the ICU with a .357 Magnum pistol. "I'm not here to hurt anyone," he said, as he unplugged his child's respirator, "I just want to let my son die." Within moments, the 16-month-old child's heart stopped. Mr. Linares continued to rock Samuel in his arms for 20 minutes. Then, he slid the gun across the floor to the police and collapsed in wrenching sobs. Linares was charged with first-degree murder. Freed on bond, he appeared in Cook County Criminal Court on May 18.

The child's physician, Gilbert Goldman, said, "There was no ethical difference of opinion here. The physicians agreed that the child was in an irreversible coma and would not recover. There was no medical opposition to removing the ventilator. What we faced was a legal obstacle."

Brown said that he advised the medical staff not to remove the life support. "There is an absence in the law," he said. "I told the medical staff there was a possibility they would face criminal charges. I can't speculate with the careers of doctors and nurses."

The murder charge against Linares was later dismissed by the judge in criminal court, who held that the child's condition was hopeless before the father's action.

[Sources: Adapted from S.H. Miles, "Taking Hostages: The Linares Case," *Hastings Center Report* 19, no. 4 (1989): 4; D. Johnson, "Father Speeds Baby's

Death as Question of Law Lingers," *New York Times*, 7 May 1989, A26; D.C Thomasma, "Clinical Care Ethics and Public Policy: Reflections on the Linares Case," *Law, Medicine & Health Care*, 17. no. 4 (1989): 335-38.]

Case 2: The Case of Baby K

Baby K was born with anencephaly at Fairfax Hospital (hereinafter "the Hospital") in Virginia on 13 October 1992. Anencephaly is a congenital malformation resulting in lack of cerebral hemispheres and with only a brain stem. The infant is permanently unconscious and presumably cannot experience pain. The condition had been diagnosed prenatally. Ms. H, the baby's mother, and Mr. K, the baby's father, are unmarried. One year prior to Baby K's birth, Ms. H's nine year old daughter died in the same hospital of injuries suffered in a motor vehicle accident in which Ms. H was driving.

Anencephaly was diagnosed at Ms. H's first prenatal and ultrasound examination at six months gestation. Ms. H's obstetrician and neonatologist had discussed the option of abortion. They explained that most anencephalic infants die soon after birth, and if death did not occur, the infant would be permanently unconscious and without feeling. Ms. H refused abortion. She requested that the child be treated maximally at birth, because she believes that all human life has value, including her anencephalic daughter. She believed that God would work a miracle if it was God's will. Mr. K, the baby's father, disagreed with Ms. H about her wishes for treatment.

A cesarean section was needed. Ms. H had a general anesthetic and was incapacitated during and after delivery. Physicians intubated Baby K at birth for three reasons: (1) in response to the earlier request of Ms. H, (2) to confirm the diagnosis, and (3) to give Ms. H a full opportunity to understand the diagnosis and prognosis of anencephaly. The physicians hoped that she would change her mind about treatment upon viewing the infant's condition. She did not change her mind. Physicians discussed a DNR order with Ms. H, and she refused. The physicians made many attempts to communicate about the prognosis, and they attempted unsuccessfully to transfer the infant to other neonatal care units and children's hospitals (the clinicians' and hospital administrators interpreted that the Virginia Health Care Decisions Act required them to do so).

Physicians asked the ethics committee to meet with Ms. H, and a three-person team (family practitioner, psychiatrist, and minister) was unsuccessful in resolving the dispute on 22 October 1992. According to the district court, her "treating physicians requested the assistance of the Hospital's 'Ethics Committee' in overriding the mother's wishes." The ethics committee noted that the care was "futile" and advised that the Hospital "attempt to resolve this through our legal system" if, after a waiting period, no change occurred in Ms. H's position.[103]

During this period, Ms. H contacted the staff of a state agency for protection of the rights of the disabled, which advised the Hospital of its concerns about state and federal nondiscrimination and medical neglect statutes. The Hospital filed a proceeding in federal court in January, 1993 to determine the level of care it is obligated to render and requested appointing a guardian *ad litem*. Having weaned Baby K from the ventilator, physicians transferred her to a nursing home with an agreement that she could return to the Hospital if breathing problems occurred. After her third admission (3 March 1993), a tracheostomy was performed for placement of a breathing tube, and she was transferred back to the nursing home on 13 April 1993.

Federal Judge Claude Hilton ruled on 1 July 1993 that the Hospital has a duty to provide full medical care (including ventilator support) to Baby K under the Federal Rehabilitation Act of 1973, the Americans with Disabilities Act of 1990, and the Emergency Medical Treatment and Active Labor Act (EMTALA). No weight was given to the guardian *ad litem*'s recommendation that further prolongation of Baby K's dying process was futile and inhumane. The judge made no finding regarding a standard of care for anencephaly or pertaining to the issue of the best interest of the infant.

A key section of the court's ruling was: "The use of a mechanical ventilator to assist breathing is not 'futile' or 'inhumane' in relieving the acute symptoms of respiratory difficulty which is the emergency medical condition that must be treated under EMTALA. To hold otherwise would allow hospitals to deny emergency treatment to numerous classes of patients, such as accident victims who have terminal cancer or AIDS, on the grounds that they eventually will die anyway from these diseases and that emergency care for them would therefore be 'futile.'"[104]

The U.S. Fourth Circuit Court of Appeals heard arguments on 26 October 1993 in the Hospital's appeal of Judge Hilton's decision. Their two to one opinion on 10 February 1994 affirmed the earlier judgment of the trial court. The appeals court examined only one question: Did Congress in passing EMTALA provide an exception for anencephalic infants (or anyone else) in respiratory distress? The court found EMTALA's language clear--that is, hospitals are re-

quired to stabilize the medical condition creating the emergency. The decision, in effect, informed Congress that it could clarify EMTALA, if it wanted. The dissenting justice argued that EMTALA was passed to prevent "dumping" for economic reasons, and because no treatment for anencephaly existed, there was no legal duty to ventilate the infant on an emergency basis. A key section of the dissent was: "I simply do not believe, however, that Congress, in enacting EMTALA, meant for the judiciary to superintend the sensitive decision-making process between family and physicians at the bedside of a helpless and terminally ill patient under the circumstances of this case. Tragic end-of-life hospital dramas such as this one do not represent phenomena susceptible to uniform legal control."[105]

The Hospital requested an *en banc* hearing with all sitting judges on the Fourth Circuit. The court denied this request. The Hospital, Baby K's father, and the guardian *ad litem* appealed to the U.S. Supreme Court. On 3 October 1994, the Supreme Court declined to review the case without comment as to its reasons. Congress has made some effort to draft language for federal legislation to clarify congressional intent that EMTALA's requirement for stabilization be "consistent with reasonable medical standards."

Baby K continued to be cared for in a nursing home until she died at the Hospital of cardiac arrest on Wednesday, 5 April 1995, after being vigorously resuscitated.[106] This was her sixth and final admission to the Hospital. She had medical bills of nearly $500,000, which were covered by her mother's insurance and Medicaid. Her hospital bill before her death, nearly $250,000, had been paid in full by Kaiser Permanente, a health maintenance organization in which Ms. H was enrolled in her job as a cafeteria worker before Baby K's birth.

[Sources: Adapted from *In Re Baby K*, 832 F.Supp. 1022 (E.D. Va 1993); *In Re Baby K*, 16 F.3d 590 (4th Cir. 1994); M. Tousignant and B. Miller, "Death of Baby K Leaves a Legacy of Legal Precedents," *Washington Post*, 6 April 1995, A1.]

IX. Study Questions

1. Why is the distinction between ordinary and extraordinary treatment considered outworn?
2. Examine the guidance that there is no ethical difference between withholding and withdrawing medical treatment from the perspective of "act" versus "omission."
3. You think that CPR is medically inappropriate for your comatose patient, Mr. R. How do you initiate this discussion with his family/surrogate decision

makers? What are the strengths and weakness of the following approaches. What is your recommended approach?

   a. Ask the family whether they want "everything done" for Mr. R.
   b. Ask the family's permission to write a DNR order.
   c. Discuss the medical inappropriateness of CPR for Mr. R. Tell the family that this is not an option for treatment, and discuss other treatment plans such as comfort care.
   d. Tell the family that you have written a DNR order in Mr. R's chart, as this is your medical prerogative.

4. Consider Case B, "*Cruzan v. Harmon.*" What are the ethical and legal issues in this case? What are the two major components of the U.S. Supreme Court's decision? Did Nancy Cruzan die on 11 January 1983 (the date of her accident) or on 26 December 1990 (after feeding and hydration had been forgone)?
5. Consider Case 1, "The *Linares* Case." Discuss the clinicians' responsibilities to their patient and his family regarding their approval of removing the ventilator versus the hospital attorney's opposition? Should the clinicians have acted differently?
6. Discuss Case E, "Code Him until He's Brain Dead!" in light of Virginia's new Health Care Decisions Act. What course of action should clinicians take if this were a current case?
7. Discuss Case 2, "The Case of *Baby K*," and its effects on the guidelines for clinicians in this chapter.

Notes

1. The terms *treatment* and *technology* are used interchangeably in this chapter. However, there is a point in some cases at which the term *treatment* loses its moral content, because it assumes an intent to benefit patients.

2. Local, state, and national experience lies behind this estimate of frequency. Two-thirds (66 percent) of the requests for ethics consultation at the University of Virginia Hospitals concern decisions to forgo life-sustaining treatment. J.C. Fletcher and H. Boverman, "Ethics Consultation at the Medical Center of the University of Virginia," see *Newsletter of the Society for Bioethics Consultation* 1, no. 1 (15 July 1988): 3-6; J.C. Fletcher, "Decisions to Forgo Life-Sustaining Treatment," *Virginia Medical Journal* 116 (1989): 462-65.

A survey of healthcare professionals in 10 Virginia hospitals was conducted in 1990 to rank the needs that ethics programs in hospitals can meet. The survey also asked respondents to identify the most frequent ethical problems they saw in the hospital. Decisions to forgo life-sustaining treatment was by far the most frequent ethical problem named by 1,541 respondents. Of 22 types of ethical problems identified by respondents as frequent and difficult, 35 percent of all answers referred to forgoing life-sustaining treatment. See E.M. Spencer et al., "Ethics Programs at Community Hospitals in Virginia," *Virginia Medical Quarterly* 119 (1992): 178-79. A study of ethics committees in nursing homes reported that decisions to forgo treatment are the most frequent ethical problem for which such groups are used. See G. Glasser, N.R. Zweibel, and C.K. Cassel, "Ethics Committees in the Nursing Home: Results of a National Survey," *Journal of the American Geriatrics Society* 36 (1988): 150-56. Also, for an excellent "ethical assessment" of the environment of intensive care units, see C. Marsden, "An Ethical Assessment of Intensive Care," *International Journal of Technology Assessment* 8, no. 3 (1992): 408-18.

3. SUPPORT Investigators, "A Controlled Trial to Improve Care in Seriously Ill Hospitalized Patients," *Journal of the American Medical Association* 274 (1995): 1591-98.

4. S.J. Reiser, "The Intensive Care Unit: The Unfolding and Ambiguities of Survival Therapy," *International Journal of Technology Assessment in Health Care* 8, no. 3 (1992): 382-94.

5. Hippocrates, "Epidemics II," in, *Hippocrates_I*, trans. W.H.S. Jones (Cambridge, Mass.: Harvard University Press, 1923).

6. G.E.R. Lloyed, ed., *Hippocratic Writings* (New York: Penguin Books, 1978), 94.

7. Ibid., p. 103.

8. G. Majno, *The Healing Hand: Man and Wound in the Ancient World* (Cambridge, Mass.: Harvard University Press, 1975).

9. B.S. Bloom and D. Lundberg, "Intensive Care: Where Are We?" *International Journal of Technology Assessment in Health Care* 8, no. 3 (1992): 379-81.

10. P. Drinker and C.F. McKhann, "The Use of a New Apparatus for the Prolonged Administration of Artificial Respiration," *Journal of the American Medical Association* 92 (1929): 1658-60.

11. See note 4 above, p. 386.

12. F. Nightingale, *Notes on Hospitals*, 3rd ed., (London: Longman, 1863).

13. J.S. Hassett, "Technology's Front Line: The

Intensive Care Unit," in *The Machine at the Bedside*, ed. S.J. Reiser and M. Anbar (Cambridge, England: Cambridge University Press, 1984), 95-104.

14. W.J. Winslade and J.W. Ross, *Choosing Life and Death* (New York: Free Press, 1986), 5.

15. Ibid.

16. H.R. Moody, *Ethics in an Aging Society* (Baltimore, Md.: Johns Hopkins University Press, 1992), 20.

17. U.S. Congress, Office of Technology Assessment, *Losing a Million Minds: Confronting the Tragedy of Alzheimer's Disease and Other Dementias*, OTA-BA-323 (Washington, D.C.: U.S. Government Printing Office, 1987), 15-22.

18. See note 3 above, p. 1592.

19. N.G. Smedira, et al., "Withholding and Withdrawal of Life Support from the Critically Ill," *New England Journal of Medicine* 322 (1990): 309-15.

20. D.K.P. Lee et al., "Withdrawing Care: Experience in a Medical Intensive Care Unit," *Journal of the American Medical Association* 271 (1994): 1358-61.

21. See note 3 above, p. 1592.

22. L. Payer, *Medicine and Culture* (New York: Penguin Books, 1988).

23. L. Thomas, *The Youngest Science: Notes of a Medicine-Watcher* (New York: Viking, 1983).

24. President's Commission for the Study of Ethical Problems in Medicine and Biomedical and Behavioral Research, *Deciding to Forego Life-Sustaining Treatment* (Washington, D.C.: U.S. Government Printing Office, 1983), 17-18.

25. National Center for Health Statistics, "Mortality. Part A. Section 1," in *Vital Statistic of the United States, 1991*, (Washington, D.C.: U.S. Government Printing Office, 1996--DHHS Publication no. (PHS) 96-1101), 380-81.

26. In a personal conversation with the author dated 7 December 1996, S. Tolle reported: "Figures from the Oregon Health Division Vital Statistics for 1995 are almost evenly divided between three locations: acute care hospitals (32%), nursing homes (32%), and home (31%)."

27. See note 3 above, p. 1594.

28. Ibid., 1596.

29. D. Callahan, *What Kind of Life?* (New York: Simon & Schuster, 1990).

30. See note 24 above, pp. 82-83.

31. L.S. Baer, "Nontreatment of Some Severe Strokes," *Annals of Neurology* 4 (1978): 381-82.

32. R. Zussman, *Intensive Care* (Chicago: University of Chicago Press, 1992): 136-38.

33. A. Meisel, *The Right to Die* (New York: John Wiley & Sons, 1993) and cumulative supplements.

34. See note 30 above, pp. 60-90.

35. P. Ramsey, *The Patient as Person* (New Haven, Conn.: Yale University Press, 1971), 113-57.

36. *In re Quinlan*, 70 N.J. 10, 355 A.2d 647 (1976).

37. Ibid.

38. *Barber v. Superior Court*, 147 Cal. App. 3d 1006, 195 Cal. Rptr. 484 (1983). This account of the case is adapted from B. Steinbock, "The Removal of Mr. Herbert's Feeding Tube," *Hastings Center Report* 13, no. 5 (October 1983): 13.

39. R.A. McCormick, "The *Cruzan* Decision," *Midwest Medical Ethics* (Winter-Spring 1989): 3-9.

40. J. Lynn and J.F. Childress, "Must Patients Always Be Given Food and Water?" *Hastings Center Report* 13 (October 1983): 17-21.

41. P. Schmitz and M. O'Brien, "Observations on Nutrition and Hydration in Dying Cancer Patients," in *By No Extraordinary Means*, ed. J. Lynn (Bloomington, Ind.: University of Indiana Press, 1986), 29-38.

42. The Multi-Society Task Force on PVS, "Medical Aspects of the Persistent Vegetative State," *New England Journal of Medicine* 330 (1994): 1499.

43. M. Angell, "The Case of Helga Wanglie. A New Kind of Right to Die Case," *New England Journal of Medicine* 325 (1991): 511-12.

44. J.J. Paris, R.K. Crone, and F.E. Reardon, "Physicians' Refusal of Requested Treatment: The Case of Baby L," *New England Journal of Medicine* 329 (1990): 1012-15.

45. G.J. Annas, "Asking the Courts to Set the Standard of Emergency Care--The Case of Baby K," *New England Journal of Medicine* 330 (1994): 1542-45.

46. J.J. Paris et al., "Beyond Autonomy: Physicians' Refusal to Use Life-Prolonging Extracorporeal Membrane Oxygenation," *New England Journal of Medicine* 329 (1993): 354-57.

47. L.J. Blackhall, "Must We Always Use CPR," *New England Journal of Medicine* 317 (1987): 1281-83; J.D. Lantos et al., "The Illusion of Futility in Clinical Practice," *American Journal of Medicine* 87 (1989): 81-84; L.J. Schneiderman, N.S. Jecker, and A.R. Jonsen, "Medical Futility: Its Meaning and Ethical Implications," *Annals of Internal Medicine* 112 (1990): 949-54; T. Tomlinson and H. Brody, "Futility and the Ethics of Resuscitation," *Journal of the American Medical Association* 264 (1990): 1276-80; N.S. Jecker and L.J. Schneiderman, "An Ethical Analysis of 'Futility' in the 1992 American Heart Association Guidelines for Cardiopulmonary Resuscitation and Emergency Cardiac Care," *Archives of Internal Medicine* 153, no. 19 (1993):

2195-98; J.R. Curtis et al., "Use of the Medical Futility Rationale in Do-Not-Attempt-Resuscitation Orders," *Journal of the American Medical Association* 273 no. 2 (1995): 124-28.

48. J.F. Fries et al., "Reducing Health Care Costs by Reducing the Need and Demand for Medical Services," *New England Journal of Medicine* 329 (1993): 321-25; G.D. Lundberg, "American Health Care System Management Objectives: The Aura of Inevitability Becomes Incarnate," *Journal of the American Medical Association* 269 (1993): 2554-55.

49. D.J. Murphy and T.E. Finucane, "Do Not Resuscitate Policies: A First Step in Cost Control," *Archives of Internal Medicine* 153 (1993): 1641-48.

50. J.M. Teno et al., "Prognosis-Based Futility Guidelines: Does Anyone Win?" *Journal of the American Geriatrics Society* 42 (1994): 1202-07.

51. J. Lubitz, J. Beebe, and C. Baker, "Longevity and Medicare Expenditures," *New England Journal of Medicine* 332 (1995): 999-1003; E.J. Emanuel and L.L. Emanuel, "The Economics of Dying: The Illusion of Cost Savings at the End of Life," *New England Journal of Medicine* 330 (1994): 540-44.

52. This figure has been constant since the early 1980s. See W.A. Knaus, E.A. Draper, and D.P. Wagner, "The Use of Intensive Care," *Milbank Quarterly* 61, no. 4 (1983): 562; L. Jaroff , "Health: Knowing When to Stop," *Time*, 4 December 1995, 76.

53. S.J. Youngner, "Who Defines Futility?" *Journal of the American Medical Association* 260 (1988): 2094-95; R.D. Truog, "Beyond Futility," *The Journal of Clinical Ethics* 3 (1992): 143-45; R.D. Truog, A.S. Brett, and J. Frader, "The Problem with Futility," *New England Journal of Medicine* 326 (1992): 1560-64; B.A. Brody and A. Halevy, "Is Futility a Futile Concept?" *Journal of Medicine and Philosophy* 20, no. 2 (1995): 122-44.

54. K.A. Koch, B.W. Meyers, and S. Sandroni, "Analysis of Power in Medical Decisionmaking: An Argument for Physician Autonomy," *Law, Medicine & Health Care* 20 (1992): 320-26.

55. L.K. Stell, "Real Futility," *North Carolina Medical Journal* 56, no. 9 (1995): 432-38.

56. L. Schneiderman, "The Futility Debate: Effective versus Beneficial Intervention," *Journal of the American Geriatrics Society* 42 (1994): 883-86.

57. See note 55 above, p. 435.

58. *In re Conroy*, 98 N.J. 321, 486 A.2d 1209 (1985).

59. Ibid., 98 N.J. 321 at 360.

60. American Medical Association, Council on Ethical and Judicial Affairs, "Withholding or Withdrawing Life-Sustaining Medical Treatments," in *Code of Medical Ethics* (Chicago: AMA, 1994), 36-50.

61. Task Force on Ethics of the Society of Critical Care Medicine, "Consensus Report on the Ethics of Foregoing Life-Sustaining Treatments in the Critically Ill," *Critical Care Medicine* 18, no. 12 (1990): 1435-39.

62. See note 30 above, p. 3.

63. U.S. Congress, Office of Technology Assessment, *Life-Sustaining Technologies and the Elderly*, OTA-BA-306 (Washington, D.C.: U.S. Government Printing Office, July 1987).

64. Hastings Center, *Guidelines on the Termination of Life-Sustaining Treatment and the Care of the Dying* (Briarcliff Manor, N.Y.: Hastings Center, 1987).

65. J.M. Stanley et al., "The Appleton Consensus: Suggested International Guidelines for Decisions to Forgo Medical Treatment," *Journal of Medical Ethics* 15 (1989): 129-36.

66. See note 39 above, p. 8.

67. This case was conposed for teaching by the faculty at the University of Virginia.

68. D.A. Asch, J. Hansen-Flaschen, and P.L. Lanken, "Decisions to Limit or Continue Life-Sustaining Treatment by Critical Care Physicians in the United States: Conflicts between Physicians' Practices and Patients' Wishes," *American Journal of Respiratory and Critical Care Medicine* 151 (1995): 288-92.

69. N.N. Dubler, "The Doctor-Proxy Relationship: The Neglected Connection," *Kennedy Institute of Ethics Journal* 5, no. 4 (1995): 289-306.

70. S.S. Hall, "The Medical Machine: The Rapps," *Health* (October 1991): 91-102; M.S.D. Bosek, "Ethics from the Other Side of the Bed: A Daughter's Perspective," *Medical Surgical Nursing* 3, no. 4 (1994): 316-18, 334.

71. E. Hansot, "A Letter from a Patient's Daughter," *Annals of Internal Medicine* 125 (1996): 149-51.

72. T. Gilligan and T.A. Raffin, "Whose Death Is It, Anyway?" *Annals of Internal Medicine* 125 (1996): 137-41.

73. A. Meisel, *The Right to Die*, 2nd ed. (New York: John Wiley & Sons, 1995), 2: 25-30. Also see Meisel's discussion of the varied terminology for the surrogate decision maker's role in forgoing life-sustaining treatment (pp. 11-13). Meisel also reports that all states, except Alabama, now have statutes that permit appointment of healthcare proxies (p. 133, 211-13).

74. Ibid., 26-27.

75. Ibid., 27.

76. S.M. Wolf, "Honoring Broader Directives," *Hastings Center Report* 21, no. 5 (1991): S8-S9.

77. Sources for *Cruzan* case: *Info Trends: Medicine, Law, and Ethics*, Spring, 1989, p. 1; *Cruzan v. Harmon*, 760 S.W. 2d 408 (Mo. 1988) (*en banc*); *Cruzan v. Director, Missouri Dept. of Health*, 497 U.S. 261 (1990); E.D. Robertson, Jr., *Personal Autonomy and Substituted Judgment* (Corpus Christi, Tex.: Diocesan Press, 1991); G.J. Annas, "Nancy Cruzan and the Right to Die," *New England Journal of Medicine* 323 (1990): 670-72; M. Gladwell, "Woman in Right-to-Die Case Succumbs," *Washington Post*, 27 December 1990, A3.

78. *Cruzan v. Harmon*, 760 S.W.2d 408, at 411 (Mo. 1988) (*en banc*).

79. Ibid., 420.

80. *Cruzan v. Director, Missouri Department of Health*, 497 U.S. 261 (1990).

81. Ibid.

82. R.F. Weir and L. Gostin, "Decisions to Abate Life-Sustaining Treatment for Nonautonomous Patients," *Journal of the American Medical Association* 264 (1990): 1846-53.

83. *Superintendent of Belchertown v. Saikewicz*, Mass. 370 N.E. 2d 417 (1977); the Saikewicz case is also included in T.L. Beauchamp and J.F. Childress, *Principles of Biomedical Ethics*, 4th ed. (New York: Oxford University Press, 1994), 522.

84. Also, for a complete review of studies of CPR as a source of information from which to discuss CPR with colleagues and patients, see an important article by A.H. Moss, "Informing the Patient about Cardiopulmonary Resuscitation: When the Risks Outweigh the Benefits," *Journal of General Internal Medicine* 4 (1989): 349-55. For a review of the subject of in-hospital CPR, see: A.P. Schneider, D.J. Nelson, and D.D. Brown, "In-Hospital Cardiopulmonary Resuscitation: A 30-Year Review," *Journal of the American Board of Family Practice* 6, no. 2 (1993): 91-101.

85. This case was composed for teaching by the faculty at the University of Virginia.

86. L.L. Brunetti and L.K. Stell, *A Physician's Guide to the Legal and Ethical Aspects of Patient Care* (Charlotte, N.C.: Charlotte Area Health Education Center, 1994), 148.

87. Ethics Consultation Service, University of Virginia, 1988; J.C. Fletcher and P.J. Eulie, "Code Him Until He's Brain Dead!" In *Ethics at the Bedside*, ed. C.M. Culver (Dartmouth, N.H.: University of New England Press, 1990), 8-28.

88. According to the Virginia Health Care Decisions Act of 1992, Va. Code Ann., sec. 54.1-2990 (Michie 1994): "Nothing in this article shall be construed to require a physician to prescribe or render medical treatment to a patient that the physician determines to be medically or ethically inappropriate. However, in such a case, if the physician's determination is contrary to the terms of an advance directive of a qualified patient or the treatment decision of a person designated to make the decision under this article, the physician shall make a reasonable effort to transfer the patient to another physician."

89. Maryland Health Care Decisions Act of 1993, Md. Code Ann., Health-Gen sec. 5-601-618 (1993); "Maryland Addresses Right-to-Die Issue with New Surrogate Law," *Medical Ethics Advisor* 9, no. 5 (May 1993): 57-9.

90. *Cindy Bryan v. Rector and Visitors of the University of Virginia*, 95 F.3d 349, (4th Cir. 1996).

91. This table was adapted from material presented by Christine Mitchell, R.N., M.A., at the "Bioethics Summer Retreat," 29 June 1994. Used with permission.

92. See note 30 above, p. 3.

93. L.S. Jefferson et al., "Use of the Natural Death Act in Pediatric Patients," *Critical Care Medicine* 19 (1991): 901-05.

94. J.J. Lynch, *The Broken Heart* (New York: Basic Books, 1977).

95. See note 68, above, p. 291.

96. T.A. Brennan, "Incompetent Patients with Limited Care in the Absence of Family Consent," *Annals of Internal Medicine* 109 (1988): 819-25.

97. T.A. Brennan, "Do-Not-Resuscitate Orders for the Incompetent Patient in the Absence of Family Consent," *Law, Medicine & Health Care* 14 (1986): 13-19.

98. *Gilgunn v. Massachusetts General Hospital*, a jury trial verdict recorded at Super. Ct. Civ. Action No. 92-4820, Suffolk Co., Mass., April 21, 1995.

99. A.M. Capron, "Abandoning a Waning Life," *Hastings Center Report* 25, no. 4 (1995): 24-26.

100. See note 30 above, p. 247.

101. B. Lo, "End-of-Life Care after Termination of SUPPORT," *Hastings Center Report* 25, no. 6 (1995): S6-S8; H. Brody, "The Best System in the World," *Hastings Center Report* 25, no. 6 (1995): S18-S21.

102. Brody, see note 101 above, p. 520.

103. *In re Baby K*, 832 F.Supp. 1022 (E.D. Va. 1993).

104. Ibid.

105. *In re Baby K*, 16 F.3d 590 (4th Cir. 1994).

106. M. Tousignant and B. Miller, "Death of Baby K Leaves a Legacy of Legal Precedents," *Washington Post*, 6 April 1995, A1.

10

DECISIONS ABOUT TREATMENT FOR NEWBORNS, INFANTS, AND CHILDREN

Robert J. Boyle, M.D.

Cases

Baby B was the 1800-gram product of an uncomplicated, full-term pregnancy. At birth he was noted to have multiple congenital anomalies including a small omphalocele (protrusion of abdominal contents through an opening at the umbilicus), overlapping fingers, scalp defects, cleft lip and palate. He was transferred by air to the University Medical Center five hours by car from the family's hometown. Evaluation revealed that the infant had a congenital heart defect, which was causing respiratory distress. The cardiologist reported that the infant had severe pulmonary valve stenosis, which could be easily palliated with a shunt procedure. Physicians also suspected that he had trisomy 13. Infants with trisomy 13 rarely live beyond infancy, and those who do survive have severe developmental delay. Chromosome analysis using bone marrow cells required 24 hours. In the interim, the infant was supported on the respirator. The family was informed by phone about the potential diagnosis. The local pediatrician was also notified so that she could help inform the family and answer their questions. The following day, the diagnosis was confirmed as trisomy 13. The neonatal intensive care unit (NICU) team (attending physician, residents, nurses, social workers) agreed that the most reasonable option was to recommend to the family to discontinue the respirator and to provide only comfort care to the infant. The social worker was to arrange transportation for the family so they could visit the infant and participate in the decision face-to-face.

Baby Doe was the full-term product of an uncomplicated pregnancy. At birth, the infant was noted to have the typical features of Down syndrome, (trisomy 21). Shortly thereafter, the infant was also diagnosed as having tracheoesophageal fistula/esophageal atresia, a lesion that would be relatively easily repaired in a newborn. Without repair, the infant would not be able to be fed. The family's obstetrician informed the family that infants with Down syndrome had very delayed development and should be institutionalized. He suggested that the family allow the infant to die. The infant's physician approached the family for permission to transfer the infant to the regional children's hospital for surgery, but the family denied permission for surgery and for transfer. The infant died several days later after unsuccessful appeals through the state courts.

Baby CD was born at 25 weeks' gestation (15 weeks early) following premature labor. The infant has moderate respiratory-distress syndrome and requires a respirator. She is at risk for chronic lung disease; bleeding into the ventricles of the brain; retinopathy of prematurity which may cause blindness; and infection of the bloodstream. A hospital stay of three months is anticipated if there are no severe complications. The family does not want anything done for the infant because she may be "slow" when she grows up; they do not feel that they would be able to handle the burden and educational expense of a child who is mentally retarded. They also are concerned that this will have a negative effect on their other child.

EF, an 18-month-old male was admitted to the local hospital with the diagnosis of croup. During his hospitalization he was found to have failure to thrive, rickets, iron-deficiency anemia, and probable kwashiorkor (severe malnutrition). When taking the child's medical history, the treatment team learned that his parents were members of a religious sect that required a strict vegetarian diet to which they had adhered. When clinicians confronted the parents with an explanation of the child's problems, which were caused by the diet, the parents refused to allow further testing and demanded to take the child home immediately.

I. Introduction

This chapter examines the particular ethical issues associated with clinical decision making for infants and children. The decision-making processes and guidelines are basically the same as those recommended for decision making in clinical situations involving adults. However, there are uncontested differences between pediatrics and other medical specialties that require special attention.

Children represent the future of their families, their communities, the nation, and the world. They require special protection because of their immature status. The infant and young child have remarkable reparative and adaptive potential. Their propensity for dramatic and rapid change demands specific and continuing attention. For these reasons, particular ethical questions asked about pediatric patients may be answered differently from the same questions asked about people nearing the normal end of their lives.

The areas of ethical concern particularly related to pediatric patients have to do with standards for parents and others as surrogate decision makers, the difficulty in establishing specific guidelines for newborn and pediatric issues, the increase in capacity for decision making with normal intellectual develop-

ment, the dual responsibility of healthcare professionals who care for infants and children to their patients and to their patients' parents and families, the question of moral standing of very young infants, and the use of children in research and as sources of tissue and organs for their family members and others.

This chapter has a particular focus on the issues associated with newborn infants, because these issues have led to difficult ethical dilemmas associated with high-technology medical care, quality of life, the authority of parents and others to make decisions for children, and what guidelines should be followed when making these decisions. Any moral precepts or ethical guidelines that can be applied to issues associated with the care of newborns can also be applied to the care of older infants and children, up to the age at which they are considered capable decision makers in their own right.

The issues and guidelines presented in the previous chapters certainly apply to newborns and pediatric patients as well as adults. Specifically, the chapters on capacity, disclosure, informed consent, refusal, death and dying, and forgoing life-sustaining treatment contain material related directly to the pediatric patient.

Micro-allocation and macro-allocation of healthcare resources, covered in later chapters, are also critical to pediatric medicine. The intensity and expense of care for the extremely low birthweight infant was a controversial item in the state of Oregon's healthcare allocation plan that prioritizes several hundred types of medical treatment. Healthcare spending for months of neonatal intensive care must be evaluated in relation to underfunded prenatal care, which has been shown to prevent many premature births. Many nurseries have faced the problem of too many babies for their space and nursing personnel, raising critical issues in triage. Care of older critically ill children in intensive care units often presents similar allocation problems. In addition, clinicians are often faced with decisions concerning the proper balance between medical and economic considerations in the everyday office practice of pediatrics in a managed-care environment.

Much of this chapter focuses on the issues of forgoing life-sustaining therapy in critically ill, malformed, or handicapped neonates and in critically ill older children. Should these decisions ever be made? How are the decisions made? Since these patients are not capable and never have been capable, the issue of surrogate decision making is central. Who should make the decision? In addition, the chapter addresses the proper role of the parents and others in decision making for children in all clinical situations, relating this general role to decision-making authority in critical-care situations.

II. Background and Historical Issues

The history of providing special consideration to children is a brief one. Infanticide and abandonment were relatively common until the early 1800s. Children in the Middle Ages were considered "chattel" and were put to work as early as age three. Although infanticide was forbidden by church law, it was recognized as only a minor offense. Child labor laws were unknown until the 20th century, and there were laws against using children in any manner in the workplace. Removal of a child from the parents' custody because of flagrant battering was first authorized by a court in 1881 based on a statute protecting animals from cruelty.[1] Death in childhood was common until the advent of antibiotics and universal immunizations after World War II, and before that time children were considered to be an easily replaceable resource.

During the early part of this century and particularly since World War II, our culture has paid increasing attention to children's needs. There have been numerous legislative attempts to afford children a safer and better life, and the courts are paying more attention to children and children's issues. Laws requiring universal immunizations, access to public health clinics, strictly enforced child labor laws, attempts to ensure children's economic security in divorce, recently promulgated guidelines for state court judges that address decision making of children, and many other activities all point to society's continuing emphasis on the interests of children. On the other hand, political decisions concerning allocation of money have often seemed to favor other more vocal and politically astute constituencies than children. Be that as it may, children are now considered of significant, if not overriding, value to our society. Our culture funding this position by supporting educational and healthcare amenities for children and by paying particular heed to certain conditions of infancy and childhood, including the care of sick newborns.

III. Ethical Issues in the Care of Newborns

Attention to issues of ethical concern related to the care of newborns began in the 1970s with a dramatic growth in technology and understanding related to the care of critically ill newborn infants. The "premature nurseries" of the 1960s--in which primitive incubators, oxygen, and tube feedings were the extent of the technology available--rapidly evolved into high-tech intensive care units with multisystem monitoring, mechanical ventilators, micro-intravenous (IV) lines, routine brain ultrasound, and so forth. Infants who were five weeks premature, had respiratory distress, and weighed three pounds often died in the 1960s, but by the 1970s had become straightforward cases with extremely low mortality and morbidity rates.

In the 1990s, NICUs began using extracorporeal membrane oxygenation (ECMO) heart-lung machines for up to four weeks to support newborns with respiratory failure; for the majority of such patients, the results have been impressively positive. Infants born 15 to 16 weeks early, weighing approximately one pound, now reside for months in the NICU. The dramatic technological advances in adult medical care have been applied to younger and younger patients; these advances include kidney, heart, liver, and bone marrow transplants; cardiac pacemakers; and cardiac surgery techniques. Neonatal heart transplants are now limited only by the short supply of donor hearts.

As has been the case in other areas of medical care, these technological advances have been accomplished without (or with a moderate lag in) philosophical or policy reflection on the use of these technologies--either at the level of the individual patient or at the regional or national level.

IV. Selective Nontreatment of Newborns

The ethical and medical debate over selective nontreatment of newborns did not become public until the early 1970s. In England, Lorber defined clinical criteria to determine which children with spina bifida were to be treated in his clinic. He believed that his criteria were based on factors that predicted better prognosis.[2] Others in the United States began to question his approach, because many of the children who were untreated did not die, and their outcomes were worse than they would have been with appropriate treatment.

In 1971, bioethicists directed a great deal of attention to a landmark case at the Johns Hopkins Hospital involving an infant with Down syndrome (trisomy 21) who was born with duodenal atresia. The parents decided that they did not want to parent a child with Down syndrome and requested that he be allowed to die. Believing that the parents had the right to make decisions for this child, the hospital agreed to their request. Without a surgical repair, the child could not be fed and was allowed to die of dehydration and starvation.[3]

In a series of articles and commentaries beginning in 1973, pediatricians Duff and Campbell reported on a practice of selective nontreatment at Yale-New Haven Hospital that resulted in the deaths of 43 infants over a period of 30 months. They stated that infants with anencephaly have a "right to die," that some defective infants need to escape a "wrongful life" characterized by cruel treatment in institutions, and that families need to be spared the chronic sorrow of caring for infants with little or no possibility for meaningful lives. The decisions about nontreatment were made jointly by the physicians and parents, with the physicians sometimes yielding to parental wishes.[4]

Also in 1973, Shaw--a pediatric surgeon--wrote that the presence of mental retardation and/or severe physical malformations is an important consideration in deciding whether to treat neonates.[5]

Surveys at that time indicated that many pediatricians and pediatric surgeons agreed with a policy of selective nontreatment of seriously impaired newborns. Researchers who conducted a 1977 survey of Massachusetts pediatricians reported that 54 percent did not recommend surgery for an infant with Down syndrome and duodenal atresia, and 66 percent would not recommend surgery for an infant with a severe case of spina bifida.[6] Researchers who conducted another survey of pediatricians in the San Francisco area reported that 22 percent favored nontreatment for infants who had Down syndrome with no complications, and over half of the respondents recommended nontreatment in cases of Down syndrome with duodenal atresia.[7]

Outside of the United States, physicians held similar views. A physician in England was accused of "murdering" a patient born with Down syndrome and bowel obstruction by feeding him only water and prescribing large doses of painkiller; the physician was acquitted, having been supported by ranking members of the Royal College of Physicians. In addition, observers in England reported that cardiac surgery routinely performed on nonhandicapped children was withheld from infants with Down syndrome.[8]

These and other reports opened a debate in the ethics and pediatrics literature on the issues of selective nontreatment and "forgoing life-sustaining treatment" in infants in various clinical situations with varying degrees of long- and short-term morbidity.

V. Baby Doe Regulations

In April 1982, the Reagan administration intervened in response to outcry from right-to-life advocates and advocacy groups for people with disabilities over the "Baby Doe" case, which involved forgoing the life-sustaining treatment of an infant. The exact details of the original case are not known, because the case was sealed by the court. President Reagan directed the U.S. Department of Health and Human Services (HHS) to propose regulations to prevent hospitals from withholding care from imperiled newborns. The regulations that followed were based on Section 504 of the 1973 Rehabilitation Act that prohibited discrimination against individuals with handicaps. The purpose of these regulations was to ensure that handicapped infants received all potentially efficacious lifesaving treatment without consideration of quality of life. The regulations appeared to require maximal treatment in all cases except those in which treatment was futile because the infant was irreversibly and imminently dying. A "hotline" was set up for individuals to anonymously report instances of nontreatment. "Baby Doe squads" were organized and dispatched to medical institutions where violations had been reported. Signs were to be posted in all nurseries and intensive care units defining the regulations and indicating the hotline number. Hospitals that were found in violation risked of loosing their federal funding and federal reimbursements.[9] These regulations were challenged in the courts and eventually overturned on procedural grounds.

In March 1983, the President's Commission for the Study of Ethical Problems in Medicine and Biomedical and Behavioral Research advocated full treatment for infants with Down syndrome, but the committee also suggested that families and medical teams needed latitude for judgment in complex cases.[10]

HHS proposed modified rules, which were finalized in January 1984:

1. All such disabled infants must under all circumstances receive appropriate nutrition, hydration and medication.
2. All such disabled infants must be given medically indicated treatment.
3. There are three exceptions to the requirement that all disabled infants must receive treatment, or stated in other terms, three circumstances in which treatment is not considered "medically indicated." These circumstances are:

   a. If the infant is chronically and irreversibly comatose.
   b. If the provision of such treatment would merely prolong dying, not be effective in ameliorating or correcting all of the infant's life-threatening conditions, or otherwise be futile in terms of the survival of the infant.
   c. If the provision of such treatment would be virtually futile in terms of the survival of the infant and the treatment itself under such circumstances would be inhumane.

4. The physician's "reasonable medical judgement" concerning the medically indicated treatment must be one that would be made by a reasonably prudent physician, knowledgeable about the case and the treatment possibilities with respect to the medical conditions involved. It is not to be based on subjective "quality of life" or other abstract concepts.[11]

The Baby Doe rules did identify a role for parents: "Given these requirements and the crucial role of the physician in carrying out these requirements, it must be emphasized that the parents of the disabled infant also play a crucial role in this process, particularly with regard to choices among alternative medical treatments. They too must have assistance and supportive services available during this difficult time and access to current and comprehensive information on the treatment, rehabilitation, and supportive services available for the infant."[12]

The courts heard another case at approximately the same time, involving Baby Jane Doe, who was born with spina bifida and hydrocephalus and whose parents had refused surgery. A "right-to-life" attorney had become aware of the case and filed a petition with the courts. The court refused HHS access to the hospital records. The U.S. Supreme Court eventually ruled that the government had no authority "to give unsolicited advice either to parents, to hospitals or to State officials who are faced with difficult treatment decisions concerning handicapped children."[13]

The federal government continued to pursue the issue. Eventually, after negotiations among hospital associations, physicians' groups, advocates for people with disabilities, and right-to-life groups, Congress passed amendments to the Child Abuse Protection Act.[14] Enforcement was placed in the hands of each state's child protection program. In addition, the rules for implementation of the law suggested, but did not require, the establishment of "infant care review committees" in healthcare institutions.[15] These committees were the seed for the development of hospital ethics committees in many institutions.

Although the original Baby Doe rules were deemphasized and the government's enforcement power was significantly deflated, these regulations continued to have a significant effect on clinical practice. A 1986 survey of pediatricians found that 60 percent believed that the regulations did not allow for adequate consideration of the infant's suffering. Of the respondents, 33 percent reported that the regulations had altered the care that they provided to infants; 56 percent believed that infants with extremely poor prognoses were being overtreated because of these recommendations. In response to several hypothetical cases, 32 percent of the neonatologists thought that heroic treatment was not in the infants' best interest but was required by the regulations.[16]

The Baby Doe episode and the unique administrative, judicial, and legislative events that transpired, while extremely unpleasant to many, certainly stimulated discussion and highlighted problems with decision making in some circumstances. Today, the overall effect of the regulations in most nurseries has been tempered, and the process by which such decisions are made has evolved and become more routine; researchers estimate that 65 to 90 percent of deaths in NICUs follow withdrawal of life support.[17] However, some court rulings still adhere strictly to the regulations, (such as the *Linares* case presented in Chapter 9). Likewise, several book-length studies, accounts from parents, and essays by neonatologists have suggested that overtreatment may be a significant problem in some areas of newborn care.[18] However, the authors of a recent study reported that significant numbers of neonatologists would not recommend lifesaving surgery for an infant born to an HIV (human immunodeficiency virus)-positive mother. The authors concluded that neonatologists may be guilty of discrimination against these infants based on their estimate of medical condition as well as quality of life.[19]

VI. Approaches to Decision Making

Although neonatologists' approach to treatment of critically ill, malformed, or handicapped newborns has evolved during the past 20 years, the imperiled newborn still presents a special dilemma for the healthcare team. Robert Weir summarizes the problem in stark detail:

> The moral decision making process in the NICU is complex. This complexity precludes the selection of any particular persons or groups of persons as automatically the best qualified to make all such decisions. . . . The complicating factors are these: the high stakes involved in decisions, the uncertainty of making proxy decisions for incompetent patients who have never been competent, serious time constraints, maximum emotional stress on parents, occasional disagreements between parents about the morally correct course of action, conflicts of interest (between parents and child, physician and child, parents and physicians), the difficulty of predicting neurologic impairment and future handicaps, inadequate communication of information between parties in cases and the logistical problems in using hospital committees or courts of law.[20]

Weir has identified five basic options for approaching the problem:

1. *Treat all nondying neonates.* Ramsey suggests that clinicians have no moral right to choose that some live and some die when the medical indications for treatment are the same.[21] He and others see no role for judgments about quality of life.
2. *Terminate the lives of selected nonpersons.* How one defines personhood becomes critical. This option has no application to critically ill older children, because they are by definition "persons."

3. *Withhold treatment according to parental discretion.* The traditional role of parents is emphasized. Parental rights are strongly supported. Consideration is given to the emotional, financial, and other effects of the infant's condition on the parents and family.
4. *Withhold treatment according to projections about quality of life.* Considerations about quality of life were specifically prohibited in the Baby Doe regulations, and others have criticized the approach as subjective.
5. *Withhold treatment judged not in the child's best interest.* Defining the child's best interest often overlaps with consideration about quality of life.

Although Weir's discussion specifically addresses newborns, his concepts can be easily adapted to decisions affecting older children. Should nontreatment decisions be made? If so, who should be involved in the decision making? What criteria should be used to make the decision?

VII. Moral Status of the Infant

Some have argued that the newborn, especially the handicapped or extremely premature newborn, may not have the same moral and legal protection as the older child or the adult. They find it problematic to define birth as the point at which to draw a major moral distinction between a fetus with very limited rights and the newborn infant. Is the newborn morally closer to the unborn fetus than to an adult? Tooley concludes that the infant cannot be considered a person because it lacks advanced brain function until at least three months of age. The infant has no self-consciousness, ability to suffer, or sense of the future.[22] Engelhardt softens this view by concluding that newborns are not persons in the strict sense, but are persons in a deeply held social and cultural sense.[23] Others believe that infants have value, based on a relational view that results from interpersonal bonding, affection, and care by parents and other adults.[24]

What role does our society acceptance of abortion, especially for fetuses with handicapping conditions, play on our judgments about newborns when they are born extremely prematurely or with handicapping conditions? Mahowald describes the "premium baby" mentality, a result of reduced family size, contraception, abortion, and antenatal diagnosis.[25]

Why does the older child have a deeper value both to parents and to society? Parental refusal of treatment for a five-year-old hit by a car who has severe head trauma and risk of neurological impairment would be quickly challenged. Why do many individuals tolerate requests for nontreatment of at-risk, extremely preterm infants. Some people believe that, with time, the parent and family have formed a more personal relationship with the older child, have invested emotionally and psychologically in the child, and have had rewarding two-way interactions with the child.

In an interesting anthropological review of maternal-infant attachment in the context of infanticide over the centuries, Daly and Wilson note that maternal (and probably paternal) bonding entails at least three distinct processes proceeding over widely variable time courses. First, in the immediate postpartum period, the mother assesses the quality of the child and the quality of the present circumstances. Many mothers experience an initial indifference to the infant. In the second stage, which usually begins during the following week, the mother feels that the baby is wonderful; this feeling grows over the next several weeks as the baby begins to smile and respond, and an individualized love is established. The third phase continues over several years with a gradual deepening of love. In earlier times, mothers demonstrated a growing disinclination to abandon or damage older children (such as in times of famine).[26] When a child is not attractive at birth or is removed from the parents' presence for days to weeks, this process is affected to some degree.

Blustein describes the neonate as "not born into the family circle so much as outside it, awaiting inclusion or exclusion. The moral problem the family must confront is whether the child should become part of the family unit."[27] It is not unusual for parents to delay naming a child who may die or refer to the infant as "it."

It seems unreasonable in our culture to argue that newborns do not have moral worth. In fact, most of the arguments both for and against nontreatment are couched in terms that respect the moral worth (of whatever degree) of these infants.

VIII. Decision Makers

Weir proposes that proxy decision makers must meet the following criteria, which are also generalizable to critically ill older children:

1. relevant knowledge and information about medical facts, prognosis, family setting;
2. impartiality;
3. emotional stability;
4. consistency--process should end with same result in similar cases.[28]

Our legal system has traditionally recognized parental autonomy as parents' authority to make decisions about treatment for their children. During the Baby Doe period when parental decision making was challenged, many authoritative groups, ethicists, and the courts strengthened and validated the parental role. Parents' authority to make decisions about treatment is considered part of the power that society grants parents in other important matters regarding their children, (such as housing, clothing, nutrition, schooling, and religious upbringing). Parents are recognized as having a moral responsibility for the care of their children, and they should be in a position to judge what is best for their infant in most cases. Buchanan and Brock have defined several reasons for this stance: parents are generally most knowledgeable and interested in their children and most likely to do the best job for them; the family usually bears the consequences of the choices that are made; and children learn values and standards within their families, and different values and standards may lead to different healthcare choices.[29]

Parents need unbiased, full disclosure of information pertaining to their infant's diagnosis, prognosis, and options for treatment. Unfortunately, a variety of factors complicate this process. Many infants in neonatal units have been transported there from their hospital of birth. This may be a distance of a few city blocks to several hundred miles. In some cases, the parents may only briefly or never see the infant before her or she is transported. The infant's mother may be ill herself or may be recovering from anesthesia. It is extremely important for the family to see their infant and communicate face-to-face with the healthcare team whenever possible.

Families who are faced with the birth of an infant with unexpected life-threatening problems face major emotional issues. The perinatal period has been recognized as extremely sensitive for both parents. They have expected the birth of a full-term, healthy infant; instead they are faced with tragedy. They may be emotionally devastated, and they grieve the loss of the normal infant that they expected. Denial, anger, depression, fear, and even disgust often overwhelm them. Parent-infant attachment suffers in this setting.

Some clinicians feel strongly enough about the right of the parents to make decisions that they would not override the parents' decisions, even when clinicians disagree. They believe that parents are the best possible proxies, because the parents face the prospect of long-term, emotionally and financially draining treatment of a seriously handicapped child. The validity of this viewpoint is discussed below. Shaw and colleagues reported in 1977 that most pediatricians and pediatric surgeons believe that selective nontreatment is appropriately a matter of parental discretion.[30]

However, most clinicians believe that the parents' role is not unlimited. The parents' decision must benefit the well-being of the child. Most of the time this occurs. However, the parents' decision should be questioned when a decision is made that reflects not the child's best interest but other interests (for example, in the cases of Baby Doe and Baby CD presented at the beginning of this chapter). It is not unusual for the court to intervene, if necessary, overriding the parents' authority by proving them unable to protect the child's health or welfare. Parents are not legally at liberty to refuse consent for life-sustaining treatment. Courts usually overturn Jehovah's Witness parents' refusal of blood for their children. Likewise, Christian Science parents have been prosecuted for refusing or denying care for their children. The courts have seen the need to protect the best interest of such children.

According to Fost, "The history of childhood is one that does not support idyllic notions of parents as decision makers for their children."[31] Whitelaw and Thoresen state that "The statistics on non-accidental injury and sexual abuse indicate that parents' wishes for their children are not necessarily always in the child's best interest."[32]

Families may be unwilling to accept emotionally the "less-than-perfect child." They may be overwhelmed with the prospects of chronic medical care, financial burdens, educational challenges, potential harm to other children in the family, and so forth. Dellinger and Kuszler assert: "It is naive to posit an identity of interest between infant and parent [in all situations]. Parents guard their own interests, those of the family as a unit, and those of current and future siblings--all of which may be gravely threatened by the newborn."[33] According to Weir: "In promoting their own psychological and financial interests, protecting their chosen life-style and other children at home, some parents cannot make impartial judgements."[34]

The current emphasis on autonomy in informed consent means that there has been some attempt to apply these concepts to parental decision making. The distinction between informed consent and proxy or substitute consent is often overlooked. Parents provide the latter. Legal and moral grounds for requiring informed consent are stronger than those for substitute consent. Mahowald observes that "The parents' right to decide about their infant's treatment is legally less binding than their right to decide about their own treatments."[35]

Bartholome suggests that the language of "consent" should be replaced by the language of "permission" with regard to parental decision making, in order to distinguish what persons may do for themselves from what they do on behalf of another. He sees the parents' role as a *duty* rather than a *right*. The parent has a duty to ensure the provision of necessary medical care: "Parental permission for interventions into children's lives must not be seen as the unconditional right to demand or refuse a particular intervention because it is a proper exercise of parental authority over the lives of children. That children are largely dependent, at least for a time, on their parents is to be affirmed, but that dependency does not warrant the second-class social standing implied by a parental right of 'consent' in decisions affecting the health care of their children."[36]

Weir also raises the problem of consistency when parents are the sole decision makers: "If birth-defective neonates sometimes live or die merely on the basis of parental discretion, the decisions in these cases may adhere to no ethical principles or criteria generally acceptable by other persons . . . there exists virtually no possibility for consistency from case to case."[37]

IX. The Clinician's Role as Advocate

Physicians, nurses, and other professionals who care for children have traditionally seen themselves as advocates for their patients. They have a responsibility to promote the child's best interest and to seek intervention if the dilemma cannot be resolved. Beauchamp and Childress reflect this point of view: "Our view is that physicians have a primary responsibility to the patient. . . . The physician ought to act in the patient's best interests, even if it is necessary to seek a court order to authorize surgery, blood transfusion or the like. Other familial interests, such as avoiding the depletion of family resources, should not be considered until a certain threshold is reached, viz., when significant patient interests would not be served by continued treatment or by particular treatment."[38] Bartholome defines clinicians' social roles and relationships with their child-patients that impose "legal and ethical duties and obligations which exist independently of any parental wishes, desires and/or 'consentings.' "[39] A recent conference sponsored by the New York Academy of Medicine concluded that "professionals must maintain an independent obligation to protect the child's interests."[40] Others have suggested that clinicians have some insight into a community standard of best interest for the individual patient.[41]

Some have taken this argument to the point of suggesting that physicians should be the decision makers in these cases, because they have the medical knowledge and insight and are seen as advocates for their patients. However, physicians are not completely objective either. They may have their own biases about treatment or nontreatment of handicapped children. They may have a conflict of interest relating to nursery census, outcome statistics, and so forth.

Ramsey is convinced that neither parents nor physicians are the best proxies. Instead, he suggests that any decision about the possible termination of an individual's life should be made by a disinterested party.[42] Using this approach, the Baby Doe deliberations and the President's Commission suggested that hospital or unit-based committees address these treatment decisions. Many hospitals set up such committees, not as decision-making bodies, but with advisory or review responsibility. As decision-making bodies, committees have a tendency to be formalistic, slow-moving, and cumbersome. However, they certainly can be useful when there is conflict among the decision makers or when the parties request outside assistance.

X. Process of Decision Making

The most realistic and functional approach to decision making about treatment of imperiled newborns is similar to the approach discussed in earlier chapters--a shared process that involves the surrogates (the parents) and the clinicians involved in the infant's care. The clinician's role is to diagnose the infant's condition--seeking consultation as needed--and present the diagnosis; prognosis; options for treatment; and recommendations, where appropriate, to the family. This process of communication and disclosure should provide the family insight into all of the issues involved in the child's care. The family then brings their values, goals, and preferences to the discussion, and ideally all can reach a decision. Involvement of all of the members of the caregiving team (rather than parents and physicians alone) ensures a more open process. This model, although occasionally difficult to achieve, can be considered the basic model for decision making in all pediatric medical care, and more broadly, for all medical care for individual patients. King adapts Brody's "transparency" model described in Chapter 4 to the neonatal intensive care setting.[43]

XI. Basis for Decision Making

What criteria should be used as a basis for decision making for imperiled newborns? Should any consideration be given to the quality of life, long-term outcome, degree of handicap, or family burden?

A. Medical Indications

Ramsey uses an approach that emphasizes medical indications. He contends that there is an obligation to use a treatment that is medically indicated as long as the patient is not dying. He argues that decision makers should avoid making judgments about the quality of life because such judgments violate the principle of equality of life.[44]

The Baby Doe rules took a similar stance. Clinicians were required to provide treatment for infants in all cases except where the infant was permanently comatose, or where treatment would not correct other life-threatening conditions or was virtually futile and inhumane. The commentary that accompanied the regulations said that it is a discriminatory act under the law to withhold surgery to correct an intestinal obstruction in an infant with Down syndrome, when the decision to withhold is based upon the future mental retardation of the infant and there are no medical contraindications to the surgery. However, withholding of treatment from an infant with anencephaly would not constitute a discriminatory act, because the treatment would be futile and would only prolong the act of dying. Furthermore, withholding of certain treatments from a severely premature and low-birthweight infant on the grounds of reasonable medical judgment concerning the improbability of success or risks of potential harm to the infant would not be in violation. Even the Baby Doe rules involved some consideration beyond life as an absolute, taking into account the issues of futility and burdens and benefits of treatment.

B. Quality of Life

"Quality-of-life" terminology carries negative connotations from the Baby Doe era. Quality of life can be defined subjectively; what one clinician sees as a good quality of life may be unacceptable to another professional or a parent. A family may see the life of a child who is profoundly visually handicapped but with normal intelligence as qualitatively poor. Although many families do not feel burdened with a moderately mentally retarded child, others consider learning disability with normal intelligence unacceptable. Clinicians who work with developmentally impaired children often have a very different appraisal than laypersons of quality of life in this patient population.

However, it may be possible to use quality of life as a basis for decision making when considering more fundamental issues. Richard McCormick proposes a minimal condition for defining "quality": the capacity for experience or social interrelating. If the condi-

tion is not met, as with anencephaly, treatment is not required.[45]

Coulter et al. have also defined interests that would constitute a "minimal quality of life":

1. Freedom from intractable pain and suffering. Mental retardation, paralysis, cerebral palsy would not be considered physical suffering; dyspnea or intractable physical pain would.
2. Capacity to experience and enjoy life--the ability to enjoy food, warmth or the caring touch of another; the ability to give or receive love.
3. Expectation of continued life--heroic treatment, when death will likely occur in a few weeks or months, may be cruel.[46]

C. Technical Medical Criteria

Using a technical medical approach (such as Lorber's criteria for treatment of spina bifida), while based on data from populations of patients, still presupposes value judgments about probable results.

D. Nonmaleficence/Best Interest

Jonsen and Garland argue that neonatal intensive care may violate the obligation of nonmaleficence if one or more of three conditions (the converse of Coulter's quality-of-life criteria) are present: inability to survive infancy, inability to live without severe pain, and inability to participate at least minimally in human experience.[47]

Some conclude that using a best-interest standard --weighing benefits and burdens for the particular patient and, in some cases, for the family--represents the mainstream ethical position in the United States.[48] Weir and Bale[49] suggest eight variables for evaluating "best interest":

1. the severity of the patient's medical condition;
2. the achievability of curative or corrective treatment;
3. the important medical goals in the case, (such as prolongation of life, relief of pain, or amelioration of disabling conditions);
4. the presence of serious neurologic impairments;
5. the extent of the infant's suffering;
6. the multiplicity of other serious medical problems;

7. the life expectancy of the infant; and
8. the proportionality of treatment-related benefits and burdens.

However, quality of life is still involved in the considerations, and the various approaches overlap and complement one another. Brock's discussion reflects this approach:

> A narrowly constrained role for quality of life considerations is inevitable if competent patients, or incompetent patients' surrogates, are to be free to decide whether a life-sustaining treatment and the life that it makes possible are on balance a benefit or excessively burdensome. Using this standard, the infant's prospects in relatively few cases will be so poor that it is reasonable to hold that continued life is clearly not in its interests. The clearest cases are probably when its life will be filled with substantial and unrelievable suffering and when the infant has suffered such severe brain damage as to preclude any significant social or environmental interaction. Other cases of very severe disabilities are more controversial and problematic, in part because of the wide variation in the weight adult patients give to such considerations and the fact that infants do not yet have preferences or values of their own.[50]

Clinicians who care for critically ill infants and children have always had both a short-term and a long-term focus to outcome and care. A child's day-to-day survival and survival to discharge have always been interpreted in light of long-term issues of development and the child's ability to perform in school and function in society. The child's interests likewise have this short-term and long-term focus. Buchanan and Brock describe these as "current interests" and "future-oriented or forward-looking interests." The current interests of infants are expressively experiential and functional: they are interests in achieving pleasure and in avoiding pain and discomfort. Developmental interests are especially prominent among the forward-looking interests: interests in the development of agency (having the capacity necessary for being an agent), opportunity, and human relationships.[51]

Another difficult issue in this benefit-burden analysis has to do with benefits and burdens to parties other than the infant, especially the family and, in some circumstances, society. Some individuals argue that the burdens of caring for and raising a severely impaired child (often over a lifetime), the difficulties of providing education, the financial burden of chronic medical care, and the effects on normal siblings should all be considered in benefit-burden analysis. According to Silverman, "Parents of a badly damaged baby often resent the implied demand that their family is required to pass a 'sacrifice test' to satisfy the moral expectations of those who do not have to live, day by day, with the consequences of diffuse idealism. It is easy . . . to demand prolongation of each and every new life that requires none of one's own . . . resources to maintain that life later."[52] Others focus on the burden on society, the expense of caring for the handicapped, the burden of additional numbers of children who require special education, and so forth.

Rarely are these issues considered in proxy decisions for adult patients. Why should we accept this stance for infants and children? According to Beauchamp and Childress: "Proxies should not refuse treatment against the incompetent patient's interests in order to avoid burdens to the family or to society. The incompetent patient's best medical interests generally should be the decisive criterion for a proxy, even if these interests conflict with familial interests."[53]

The recent New York Academy of Medicine conference reached the following conclusion:

> Although parents may have legitimate concerns about the effect of treatment decisions on themselves and their other children, the desire to avoid emotional, financial or other hardships cannot justify the denial of clearly beneficial medical care to an ill or injured child. . . . If parents are unable or unwilling to provide essential medical treatment, healthcare professionals should first assure that social counseling and supports are made available to the family to assist them. If the parents remain unwilling to consent to the needed medical treatment, then we must utilize legal mechanisms to ensure social support or supervision to provide those treatments which are clearly in the best interests of the child."[54]

If decisions are soundly based on what is truly in the best interest of the child, treatment should rarely if ever be forgone because of the burdens the infant's continuing existence would place on others. On the other hand, it is insensitive to deny the effects of these burdens. The caregivers have an obligation to assist the family, by all possible means, to prevent such burdens (assistance with funding, insurance, educational opportunities, parent support groups, diagnosis-specific information, and so forth). In fact, one of the major criticisms of the Baby Doe regulations was that the administration required care, but little was being done to develop and fund adequate programs for the survivors.

In addition, caregivers themselves may be influenced by other factors in considering withholding or withdrawing care. Chiswick warns against being overly influenced by:

1. the frustration of caring for an infant on a long-term basis;
2. the appearance of the infant, who may be relatively wasted, with skin lesions, and the narrow head of prematurity;
3. the lack of family involvement;
4. a biased impression of prognosis.[55]

XII. Economic Factors in Decision Making

The increasingly prominent economic issues associated with healthcare may add a difficult dimension to decision making about treatment for imperiled newborns. If certain types of available but very expensive treatment are precluded under a healthcare plan, issues of justice for those who cannot afford such care for their children will continue to haunt the country.

XIII. Certainty/Uncertainty

Pediatricians--especially neonatologists, geneticists, and developmentalists--have developed a large and constantly updated literature on prognosis, both for survival and morbidity, for most of the common neonatal conditions that might lead to questions about nontreatment. This body of information allows better-informed disclosure to family and better-informed decision making by all of those involved in the care of the infant. For example, 60 to 70 percent of premature infants who develop hemorrhage in the ventricles

of the brain but do not require a shunt to treat hydrocephalus do quite well neurodevelopmentally. Even infants whose bleeding involves the cortex of the brain do not necessarily have mental retardation although they usually have some element of cerebral palsy. For extremely premature infants who survive beyond four days of age, the overall mortality is equivalent to much more mature preterm infants. Premature infants born 12 to 14 weeks early usually have a long-term (two to four month) oxygen requirement, possibly on the respirator; but, of those who survive beyond the first one to two weeks, the vast majority have clinically normal pulmonary function by 6 to 12 months of age. On the other hand, infants born with severe perinatal asphyxia--who in the first 24 hours of life have seizures that are difficult to control, transient renal and myocardial failure, and flaccidity--have a high rate of mortality in the immediate newborn period; those who survive have at least a 90 percent chance of severe neurodevelopmental impairment, approaching McCormick's criterion for lack of potential for human relationships.

Valid disclosure and careful decision making require that clinicians have current and accurate data available regarding the infant's condition. However, data do not solve all of the problems of prognostication. Interpretation of the data may differ from clinician to clinician, and parent to parent. A 60 percent survival rate may sound hopeful to some, and dismally poor to others. Some may insist that this patient will be one of the 5 percent to survive or one of the 10 percent who will not be severely neurologically impaired. Some may demand to continue treatment until the prognosis is certain. Decision makers must still make judgments about how much of a burden the infant will be required to bear to possibly be the 1 survivor out of 20; they must weigh the relatively low burden of tube feedings against the higher burden of surgeries and ventilators.

Rhoden describes several strategies for approaching decisions in the absence of sufficient information to make the prognosis immediately:[56]

- *Wait until certain*: Continue until the patient is actually dying or comatose. Letting one patient die who would have had a tolerable life would be worse than saving one whose life would be devastated. Err on the side of life. Rhoden believes that this approach pays insufficient attention to suffering; that it is governed by technology rather than using technology as a tool; and that it sees parents only as onlookers.

- *Statistical prognosis*: Use statistical cutoffs and aggressively treat all those selected. Few will live with handicaps. But the few who die may die slowly. This approach sacrifices some potentially normal infants. Decision making is psychologically easier, because it is a "go-by-the-book" approach. Withdrawing therapy is not an issue. Several European countries have taken this approach with premature infants of a specific birthweight.

- *Individualized prognosis*: Decide for each infant using the available data, the present condition, and a benefit-burden analysis. This approach allows a role for the family in decision making. It also can be a source of confusion, uncertainty, error, and agony. However, Rhoden believes that this is justified, given the tragic nature of the situations. Fischer and Stevenson have applied this strategy in their NICU at Stanford and make suggestions for its application in other settings.[57] The American Academy of Pediatrics has endorsed this approach, as well.[58]

There are few, if any, absolute certainties in medical prognostication. Therefore, it is unreasonable to expect or await situations where issues are completely defined. Beauchamp and Childress summarize the issue:

> In cases of incompetent patients, including seriously ill newborns, we should begin with the normal presumption in favor of the prolongation of life. Decision makers should then work diligently to determine the patient's actual interests. Judgements about the best interests of seriously ill newborns must be made by considering the prospective benefits and burdens as objectively as possible, in light of the patient's condition.... Although the possibility of error is substantial, it is no greater than in many other judgements in medicine. Because of potential error in diagnosis, prognosis, and judgements about the patient's interests, the normal obligation to preserve life dictates erring on the side of sustaining life, at

least in cases of serious doubt about the available evidence.[59]

XIV. Specific Clinical Issues

A. Extremely Premature Infants

Infants who are born at a gestational age of 26 or more weeks or weighing greater than 800 grams have mortality rates of 10 to 25 percent with serious morbidity rates of 15 to 20 percent in the survivors. Based on this information, most neonatal physicians believe that aggressive treatment of this population is the standard of care. Infants of lower birthweight or gestational age pose real problems related to the uncertainty of their prognosis for survival and morbidity; necessity for prolonged, very expensive care; questions about quality of life; and effect on the family during the hospitalization and in the future. (See, for example, the case of Baby CD presented at the beginning of this chapter.) Mortality, at 23 weeks, based on compiled national data, varies from 70 to 90 percent (mean 85 percent); at 24 weeks mortality is 20 to 70 percent (mean 66 percent; at 25 weeks mortality is 25 to 53 percent (mean 40 percent). The ethical problems begin even before delivery when attempts to plan care are frustrated by inability to predict exact gestational age accurately. Obstetrical estimates may be two to three weeks less than actual age. These differences may have major implications for mortality and morbidity. Risks change following delivery, depending on initial condition, response to therapy, and postnatal age. For infants who survive the first 96 hours, overall mortality rates fall to 10 to 20 percent. Parents should be properly informed before about potential mortality and risks and also about the uncertainties that exist until the infant is born and evaluated. After birth, parents should be allowed to participate in decisions about their infant's care, with clinicians giving parental choices more weight as the uncertainty of survival and outcome increases.

There is a growing consensus on guidelines for approaching decisions about this population. For infants less than 23 weeks or 500 grams at birth, the presumption should be against resuscitation unless the parents request full support and the infant is potentially viable. For older or larger infants, the presumption should be in favor of resuscitation unless the parents request no aggressive care and the infant is in poor clinical condition. Ideally, experts with sufficient experience to assess the infant should be present at delivery. These infants usually require immediate tracheal intubation and ventilation. Treatment should be wholehearted or not at all. Parents should be informed that the infant will be constantly evaluated, and that any decision to resuscitate does not mean that aggressive care cannot be withdrawn if a negative prognosis seems likely.[60] The Canadian Pediatric Society recommends against treatment for infants under 23 weeks, recommends that parents be given the option of treatment for babies at 23 to 24 weeks, and strongly recommends continued treatment for babies born at 25 or more weeks of gestational age.[61]

A recent Michigan case, *State v. Messenger*, highlights the difficulties of decision making about treatment for extremely premature infants. Dr. Messenger, a dermatologist, and his wife, who was in preterm labor at 25 weeks, had discussed their wishes that no resuscitation be performed at birth. The neonatologist believed that the infant should be assessed and, if vigorous, supported. Unfortunately, the neonatologist was not present at the birth, and a physician's assistant resuscitated the baby who was described as lifeless and cyanotic at birth. Following resuscitation, the infant was taken to the NICU in poor condition. The father denied permission to treat the infant with surfactant (a natural material that coats the alveoli and prevents collapse of the lungs) or to place central arterial and IV lines. The neonatologist believed that the infant had improved somewhat after adjusting the respirator, and she asked the family for permission to treat the baby with surfactant. When the family asked about the infant's gestational age, they were told it was 25 weeks. They then asked to be left alone with the infant. The parents then removed the baby from the ventilator and held him. He was pronounced dead approximately 75 minutes later. The father was charged with manslaughter. The treating neonatologist testified that, given the patient's situation, she would have backed the parents' decision if she had been consulted. A jury later found the father innocent. They believed that the parental choice was in the child's best interest. The case has generated heated discussion, and it highlights the need for communication, the presence of experts at delivery, and careful evaluation.[62]

B. Infants with Life-Threatening Congenital Anomalies

Life-threatening congenital anomalies represent a wide spectrum--from a single defect with an extremely poor prognosis such as anencephaly (absence of the cerebral cortex); to a lesion with long-term developmental implications such as meningomyelocele (spina bifida); to cardiac lesions that are life-threatening but relatively easily repaired with excellent long-term prognosis, such as transposition of the great vessels of the heart; to multiple congenital anomalies that require multiple surgical repairs but present little or no risk of developmental delay or mental retardation, such as the VATER complex (vertebral defects, anal atresia, tracheoesophageal fistula with esophageal atresia, and radial and renal anomalies). Therefore, accurate diagnosis and prognostic data are critical for valid decision making. In addition, one or both parents may feel guilty about the defect, the likelihood of the child having an abnormal appearance, or the prognosis of some degree of continuing disability.

C. Infants with Chromosomal Defects

The short-term prognosis for survival of infants with trisomy 13 or trisomy 18 is extremely poor, even when those infants do not have major anomalies. Those who survive beyond the first year of life are extremely mentally retarded. Infants with trisomy 21 (Down syndrome) on the other hand, very often can function in the family setting, attend school, and work in a protected environment. Decisions about treatment for infants with chromosomal defects raise concerns about futile therapy for dying infants and quality of life for those who survive with chronic medical problems and/or mental retardation. See the cases of Baby B and Baby Doe presented at the beginning of this chapter.

D. Infants with Severe Birth Asphyxia

Infants with severe birth asphyxia are usually full-term infants who suffer multisystem damage due to lack of adequate oxygen and blood flow before, during, or immediately after birth. Some of these infants survive their multisystem failure; they may have severe central nervous system dysfunction and often require long-term tube feeding, physical therapy, and seizure medication. These patients are later diagnosed as having "cerebral palsy," but early prognostication is difficult for many of them.

E. Infants with Brain Death or Persistent Vegetative State

Most experts agree that the adult parameters for the determination of death by neurologic criteria validly apply to full-term infants older than seven days of age. The immature nervous system makes the determination in younger infants problematic.[63] Ashwal and colleagues have recently defined guidelines for the determination of persistent vegetative state in children, which allow the same considerations for care as for adults.[64]

F. Infants with Hypoplastic Left Heart Syndrome

Until recently, infants with hypoplastic left heart syndrome, born without a functional left side of the heart, died within several days after birth. First, prostaglandin E became available to maintain patency of the ductus arteriosus and allow blood flow to the body. Second, a series of surgical procedures was developed that palliates the lesion, but the infant still has a significant cardiac defect. The results of such procedures are guarded, at best. Finally, infant heart transplantation became available; this allows for reasonably good outcomes. However, the child requires lifelong immunosuppression, and the supply of donor hearts is extremely limited. Of the candidates, 30 to 50 percent die before receiving their transplants. Whereas families were informed in the past that no therapy was available, now they are routinely offered options of no therapy, surgical palliation, or heart transplant.

G. Drug Screening and HIV Testing of Newborns

Screening of a newborn infant's stool or urine for drugs has important implications for the baby's mother, because the test also screens the mother for recent drug use. This potentially violates the mother's privacy. If the information is important for the infant's medical treatment, there may be valid reasons to risk the violation. If the test is being done solely to identify drug-using parents, the mother's informed consent should be sought.

Likewise, HIV testing of the neonate tests for antibodies acquired across the placenta from the mother and therefore screens the mother for antibodies. Until recently, there were valid reasons for respecting the mother's privacy. However, early identification of this infection has recently shown to benefit the infant's subsequent health and mortality. This issue has raised heated debate in the arenas of public health, ethics, and legislation.[65]

H. Healthy Children as a Source for Tissue and Organs

Clinicians have encountered an increasing number of requests for using a child as a source for organ or tissue harvesting (particularly for kidney or bone marrow) for a family member. The risks attending such procedures are relatively well known, but the possible benefits for the family member who needs the organ donation, for the family, and for the donor child are much more difficult to evaluate. Is there a conflict of interest in the consent process when one of the parents is the recipient of the tissue/organ? Should another party be appointed to attend to the child's interests? Most bone marrow transplant programs accept parental consent as the only permission necessary for sibling donation. In a survey of transplant programs, Chan and colleagues reported that 64 percent think that, when a parent is the recipient, the other parent or both parents together can consent. The remainder of the respondents believe that an independent entity should be involved either as sole decision maker or working with the parents.[66] Most believe that the benefits to the donor are related to continued emotional bonds to the recipient, increased self-esteem, and prevention of the grief from death of a sibling or parent. For procedures with higher risk to the donor, outside evaluation or even court oversight (including appointment of a guardian *ad litem*) may be warranted.[67]

I. Children Needing Therapy Disallowed by Their Parents' Religious Beliefs

Should parents be able to refuse needed treatment for their child because of the parents' religious convictions? (See, for example, the Case of EF, presented at the beginning of this chapter.) Presently, different states have different laws concerning this issue. Most states allow overriding the parents' refusal of treatment for their child in a life-threatening situation, but this is not universal. For example, Jehovah's Witness parents' refusal of blood transfusion for their child is usually overridden. However, some states provide an exemption to neglect statutes for faith healing or spiritual treatment. Even in those situations, when the child's health is in danger, courts have ordered medical treatment. When death has occurred, convictions have been overturned if the parents could be characterized as "well-intentioned."[68]

XV. Statements by Authoritative Bodies

A. American Academy of Pediatrics, Committee on Bioethics, "Treatment of Critically Ill Newborns" (1983)

[The] ambiguities and differences of opinion . . . should not preclude consensus on some ethical principles. The most basic of these principles is that the pediatrician's primary obligation is to the child. While the needs and interests of parents, as well as of the larger society, are proper concerns of the pediatrician, his or her primary moral and legal obligation is to the child-patient. Withholding or withdrawing life-sustaining treatment is justified only if such a course serves the interests of the patient. When the infant's prospects are for a life dominated by suffering, the concerns of the family may play a larger role. Treatment should not be withheld for the primary purpose of improving the psychological or social well-being of others, no matter how poignant those needs may be.

The complexity and importance of these decisions require that they be made with the utmost care. The traditional method of a single physician making such judgements, without exposure to other persons having additional facts, experience, and points of view, may lead to decisions that, in retrospect, cannot be justified.[69]

B. President's Commission for the Study of Ethical Problems in Medicine and Biomedical and Behavioral Research, *Deciding to Forego Life-sustaining Treatment* (1983)

Many therapies undertaken to save the lives of seriously ill newborns will leave the survivors with permanent handicaps, either from the underlying defect (such as heart surgery not affecting the retardation of a Down Syndrome infant) or from the therapy itself (as when mechanical ventilation for a premature baby results in blindness or a scarred trachea). One of the most troubling and persistent issues in this entire area is whether, or to what extent, the expectation of such handicaps should be considered in deciding to treat or not to treat a seriously ill newborn. The Commission has concluded that a very restrictive standard is appropriate: such permanent handicaps justify a decision not to provide life-sustaining treatment only when they are so severe that continued existence would not be a net benefit to the infant. Though inevitably somewhat subjective and imprecise in actual application, the concept of "benefit" excludes honoring idiosyncratic views that might be allowed if a person were deciding about his or her own treatment. Rather, net benefit is absent only if the burdens imposed on the patient by the disability or its treatment would lead a competent decision maker to choose to forego the treatment. As in all surrogate decision making, the surrogate is obligated to try to evaluate benefits and burdens from the infant's own perspective. The Commission believes that the handicaps of Down Syndrome, for example, are not in themselves of this magnitude and do not justify failing to provide medically proven treatment, such as surgical correction of a blocked intestinal tract.[70]

C. American Academy of Pediatrics, "Principles of Treatment of Disabled Infants" (1984)

Discrimination of any type against any individual with a disability/disabilities, regardless of the nature or severity of the disability, is morally and legally indefensible.

These rights for all disabled persons must be recognized at birth.

When medical care is clearly beneficial, it should always be provided. When appropriate medical care is not available, arrangements should be made to transfer the infant to an appropriate medical facility. Consideration such as anticipated or actual limited potential of an individual and present or future lack of available community resources are irrelevant and must not determine the decisions concerning medical care. The individual's medical condition should be the sole focus of the decision.

It is ethically and legally justified to withhold medical or surgical procedures which are clearly futile and will only prolong the act of dying.

In cases where it is uncertain whether medical treatment will be beneficial, a person's disability must not be the basis for a decision to withhold treatment.[71]

D. American Academy of Pediatrics, Committee on Bioethics, "Guidelines on Forgoing Life-Sustaining Medical Treatment" (1994)

The burdens of [life-sustaining medical treatment] may include intractable pain; irremediable disability or helplessness; emotional suffering; invasive and/or inhumane interventions designed to sustain life; or other activities that severely detract from the patient's quality of life. The phrase "quality of life" refers to the experience of life as viewed by the patient, i.e., how the patient, not the parents or health care providers, perceives or evaluates his or her existence. The American Academy of Pediatrics specifically rejects attempts to equate quality of life with "social worth" as judged by others.

Our social system generally grants patients and families wide discretion in making their own decisions about health care and in continuing, limiting, declining, or discontinuing treatment, whether life-sustaining or otherwise. Medical professionals should seek to override family wishes only when those views clearly conflict with the interests of the child.[72]

E. American Medical Association, Council on Ethical and Judicial Affairs, "The Use of Minors as Organ and Tissue Donors" (1994)

In general minors should not be permitted to serve as a source when there is a very serious risk of complications (e.g., partial liver or lung donation, which involve a substantial risk of serious immediate or long-term morbidity). . . . Minors may be permitted to serve as a source when the risks are low (e.g., blood or skin donation, in which the donated tissue can regenerate and . . . anesthesia is not required), moderate (e.g., bone marrow donation, in which the donated tissue can regenerate but brief general or spinal anesthesia is required) or serious (e.g., kidney donation, which involves more extensive anaesthesia and major invasive surgery).

If a child is capable of making his or her own medical treatment decisions, he or she should be considered capable of deciding whether to be an organ or tissue donor. However, physicians should not perform organ retrievals of serious risk without first obtaining court authorization. Courts should confirm that the mature minor is acting voluntarily and without coercion.

If a child is not capable of making his or her own medical decisions, all transplantations should have parental approval, and those which pose a serious risk should receive court authorization. In the court authorization process the evaluation of a child psychiatrist or psychologist must be sought and a guardian ad litem should be assigned to the potential minor donor in order to fully represent the minor's interests.

When deciding on behalf of immature children, parents and courts should ensure that a transplantation presents a "clear benefit" to the minor source, which entails meeting the following requirements:

a. ideally, the minor should be the only possible source;
b. for transplantations of moderate or serious risk, the transplantations must be necessary with some degree of medical certainty to provide a substantial benefit . . .;

c. the organ or tissue transplant must have a reasonable probability of success . . .;

d. generally, minors should be allowed to serve as a source only to close family members;

e. psychological or emotional benefits to the potential source may be considered, though evidence of future benefit to the minor source should be clear and convincing. Possible benefits to a child include the following: continued emotional bonds between the minor and the recipient; increased self-esteem; and prevention of adverse reaction to death of a sibling.[73]

F. American Academy of Pediatrics, "Perinatal Care at the Threshold of Viability" (1995)

Ethical decisions regarding the extent of resuscitation efforts and subsequent support of the neonate are complex. Parents should understand that decisions about neonatal management made before delivery may be altered depending on the condition of the neonate at birth, the postnatal gestational age assessment, and the infant's response to resuscitative and stabilization measures. Recommendations regarding the extent of continuing support depend on frequent reevaluations of the infant's condition and prognosis.[74]

G. American Academy of Pediatrics, Committee on Fetus and Newborn, "The Initiation or Withdrawal of Treatment for High-Risk Newborns" (1995)

The following dilemma . . . exists: intensive treatment of all severely ill infants sometimes results in prolongation of dying or occasionally iatrogenic illness; nonintensive treatment results in increased mortality and unnecessary morbidity. The overall outcomes of either approach are disappointing.

A reasonably acceptable approach to this dilemma is an individualized prognostic strategy. In this setting, care is provided for the individual infant at the appropriate level based on the expected outcome at the time care is initiated. In this strategy, the infant is constantly reevaluated, and the prognosis is reassessed based on the best

available information in conjunction with the physician's best medical judgment. This approach places significant responsibility on the physician and healthcare team to evaluate the infant accurately and continuously. The family of the infant must be kept informed of the infant's current status and prognosis. They must be involved in major decisions that ultimately could alter the infant's outcome.

The rights of parents in decision making must be respected. However, physicians should not be forced to undertreat or overtreat an infant if, in their best medical judgment, the treatment is not in compliance with the standard of care for that infant.[75]

H. American Academy of Pediatrics, Committee on Bioethics, "Informed Consent, Parental Permission, and Assent in Pediatric Practice" (1995)

In attempting to adapt the concept of informed consent to pediatrics, many believe that the child's parents or guardians have the authority or "right" to give consent by proxy. Most parents seek to safeguard the welfare and best interests of their children with regard to healthcare, and as a result proxy consent has seemed to work reasonably well.

However, the concept encompasses many ambiguities. Consent embodies judgments about proposed interventions and, more importantly, consent expresses something for one's self: a person who consents responds based on unique personal beliefs, values and goals.

Thus "proxy consent" poses serious problems for pediatric healthcare providers. Such providers have legal and ethical duties to their child patients to render competent medical care based on what the patient needs, not what someone else expresses. . . . The pediatrician's responsibilities to his or her patient exist independent of parental desires or proxy consent.[76]

I. American Academy of Pediatrics, Committee on Bioethics, "Ethics and the Care of Critically Ill Infants and Children" (1996)

The American Academy of Pediatrics supports individualized decision making about life-sustaining medical treatment for all children, regardless of age. These decisions should be jointly made by physicians and parents, unless good reasons require invoking established child protection services to contravene parental authority. At this time, resource allocation (rationing) decisions about which children should receive intensive care resources should be made clear and explicit in public policy, rather than made at the bedside.[77]

XVI. Plan of Care

In the clinical setting, most pediatric cases would benefit significantly from the development of a prospective plan of care. At the beginning of the clinical relationship, whether focused on a specific life-threatening diagnosis or on a less dramatic aspect of care, the clinical team (all of those involved with the care of the child, including--but not limited to--attending physicians, residents, consultants, nurses, and social workers) and the family should begin to consider the important issues related to that child's care. For critically ill infants and children, this approach requires considering the meaning of the diagnosis, seeking appropriate information before and after diagnosis, requesting appropriate consultation and support, identifying possible options, and so forth.

An overall plan of care for infants and children is a goal of the primary-care clinicians from whom these patients receive their everyday medical interventions and advice. To achieve this goal, it is necessary for clinicians to maintain an ongoing relationship with the child and his or her family. Primary-care clinicians can be the source of invaluable knowledge and advice when it is necessary to make critical decisions in a tertiary-care center.

XVII. Conclusion

Decision making for imperiled newborn infants and more recently for critically ill older children has evolved dramatically over the past 20 years under some unusual pressures. Our society has attempted to dictate rigid standards of care, while at the same time criticizing caregivers for their poor outcomes and lack of respect for parents' wishes. There is no doubt that at times specific decisions have erred with regard to under treatment or overtreatment, but the re-

flection and evaluation of past mistakes, while often unpleasant, has benefited individual decision makers and society. Our society has reached a consensus that it is justifiable in some circumstances to withhold or withdraw life-sustaining treatment from severely impaired newborns and children.

Because of the relative frequency and complexity of these issues, clinicians should develop a prospective plan of care that addresses current and potential ethical concerns.

Decisions regarding withdrawing or withholding treatment should be based primarily on the best interest of the child as determined by his or her caregivers and family. The process should be open; it should involve full disclosure of accurate and complete information, with the provision of consultation as necessary. One or more avenues for review of the decisions and the decision-making process can be invaluable for the family and clinicians.

XVIII. Cases for Further Study

Case 1: "When the Bough Breaks"

Baby John Davis was born 12 weeks prematurely, the product of a gestation complicated by recurrent episodes of premature labor. His mother was hospitalized for six weeks prior to delivery. She and her husband have been married for six years. they had lost four previous pregnancies, all at approximately 10-22 weeks gestation. On her doctor's advice, she quit work early in the pregnancy. Her husband has been out of work for several months. The family lives approximately three hours from the medical center.

Baby John weighed 1,000 grams (2.2 pounds) at birth. He immediately developed respiratory distress syndrome and required mechanical ventilation. He developed a patent ductus arteriosus that did not respond to medical therapy and required a thoracotomy for closure. He developed a pneumothorax (leak of air into the chest cavity) that required a chest tube for drainage.

He is now six months old. He has been mechanically ventilated since birth. His chest X-ray shows extremely severe bronchopulmonary dysplasia, with scarring and emphysema. He has been receiving maximal medical therapy with bronchodilators, antibiotics, and several courses of steroids. However, he has shown no improvement over the past month.

John is very developmentally delayed. His physicians believe that this delay is caused primarily by his debilitation from his severe lung disease. However, he has had so many episodes of severe hypoxemia and bradycardia (low heart rate) that he may also have a neurologic injury. Recently, he has required chronic sedation. Otherwise, he is agitated most of the time due to hypoxia. When he becomes agitated, he becomes even more hypoxic and air hungry.

The attending physicians and house staff all agree that it is very unlikely that John will ever go home. They are also concerned that, because he requires sedation most of the time, he is unable to interact with his environment; thus, his development is falling farther behind. They believe that the time has come to approach John's parents about withdrawing the ventilator. The case is discussed at the weekly "family rounds." Most of the nursing staff is in agreement. However, two of the primary-care nurses who have taken care of him since birth feel that this would be euthanasia.

John's parents initially visited each weekend. However, over the past two to three months, they have visited less frequently. The nurses believe John's parents cannot make an informed decision about their son's care, because they seem to have lost interest in him.

The attending physician has requested an ethics consultation about how to proceed. She has asked for help with two questions: Is it ethically justifiable to withdraw the ventilator from this child? Who should participate in the decision?

[Source: This case was modified from the author's clinical experience at the University of Virginia.]

Case 2: "Should They Have a Choice?"

Baby Sarah is the eight-pound, full-term product of an uncomplicated gestation born to a 30-year-old mother. Sarah's parents have been married eight years. They have two other children, ages three and six. Both parents are college-educated and employed.

Approximately 12 hours after birth, the infant was noted to be pale and in respiratory distress. Chest X-ray showed pulmonary congestion. Arterial blood gas revealed a severe acidosis. The infant was intubated and placed on a respirator. Echocardiogram demonstrated hypoplastic left heart syndrome with atresia of the mitral valve, small left ventricle, and aortic atresia. The ascending aorta was extremely small and fed in a manner opposite to the usual direction through the ductus arteriosus. The infant was begun on prostaglandin to maintain a patent ductus, and her condition improved. However, she was not able to be weaned from the ventilator.

The attending neonatologist and the cardiology consultant met with the parents and explained the diagnosis and the uniformly fatal prognosis without surgery. They presented three options:

1. *Norwood procedure.* This procedure is actually a three-stage surgical procedure that palliates the lesion. Even when it is successful, it leaves the child with a significant cardiac lesion. The procedure has not been successful in the institution where Baby Sarah is being treated. The family is presented the option of transferring to another institution in the Northeast where the results have been better.
2. *Cardiac transplant.* Improving immunosuppression and surgical technique have improved the transplantation statistics, and the chances of long-term survival are excellent. However, the children require lifetime immunosuppression and frequent medical checks. Unfortunately, there is a shortage of donor hearts. The average wait for a donor heart is 27 days, but may it reach 3 to 4 months. Of the candidates for heart transplant, 50 percent die while waiting for a donor heart. Many transplant candidates become progressively sicker, ventilator dependent, and moderately hypoxic. On the other hand, it is possible that a heart could become available within the next few days.
3. *No surgery.* The third option is to withdraw the ventilator and prostaglandins, provide comfort care, and allow the infant to die. Until several years ago, this was the only approach possible.

The family was offered the option of taking their infant home or remaining in the hospital. The team suggested that the family think about the options. They were given no recommendations, because the team had adopted the philosophy that all three options were equally valid.

The parents spoke with the infant's grandparents and their minister. The following day, they again met with the medical team and presented their decision that aggressive care be withdrawn and comfort care be provided.

Some members of the nursing and resident staff were uncomfortable with the decision. The believed that it did not give the infant a chance to live and that this family should be able to cope easily with the issues of long-term care. An ethics consultation has been requested to deal with this question and with the policy of presenting the three options.

[Source: This case was modified from the author's clinical experience at the University of Virginia.]

Case 3: "It Will Ruin My Life"

Baby Adam was born after 27-weeks of gestation (13 weeks premature), weighing 1,140 grams (2.5 pounds). The gestation had been uncomplicated until the sudden onset of vaginal bleeding which required an emergency cesarean section. The infant was resuscitated in the delivery room, intubated, and placed on the ventilator. Arrangements were made to transfer the infant to the regional NICU.

The mother is Hispanic; she speaks limited English but seems to understand fairly well. The father is a professional with a prosperous practice in the area. The couple has been married for five years, and they have a four-year-old daughter.

When the transport team from the regional center arrived at the referring hospital and was preparing the infant for transport, the father entered the nursery and informed the team that he did not want this infant to live if there was any chance that the child could be retarded. He did not want any [censored] ruining his life. The team reassured him that infants this size usually do very well, and the majority are normal children.

The infant was transported and did well over the next several days. On the third day of the baby's life, a routine head ultrasound revealed a mild, grade-2 intraventricular hemorrhage. When the father visited that afternoon, he was informed of the result of the ultrasound and that infants with grade-2 hemorrhage have approximately the same prognosis as children without hemorrhage. He again told the resident and nurse that he did not want the infant to live if there was a possibility of retardation, and he said that he was opposed to the current treatment. However, he did not pursue the issue that day.

Attempts to reach the infant's mother at the referring hospital were only partly successful. At times, the father answered the phone and would not permit the mother to speak. At other times, the mother answered but told the staff that they should talk to her husband.

Intravenous access became difficult, and a central line was required to continue hydration. The attending physician called the father who again expressed his view about the current treatment and refused permission for the central line. When told that the infant would die without fluid therapy, he confirmed that this was what he intended.

The attending physician discussed the case with the staff and with another attending physician. He called the hospital administrator, who filed a petition with the juvenile court to conduct permission for the procedure. A hearing was held by conference call. On questioning by the judge, the father stated that he was opposed to the procedure because of the risk of infection and pneumothorax. The judge gave permission for the procedure.

How should the staff now proceed? How vigorously should the mother's input be sought? What should be the approach toward the father?

[Source: This case was modified from the author's clinical experience at the University of Virginia.]

XIX. Study Questions

1. Richard McCormick has proposed a minimal condition for defining quality of life: the capacity for experience or social interrelating. How would you define "quality of life"? Would you apply a different standard to a neonate than to a child or an adult? If so, why?

2. The Joint Policy Statement of the American Academy of Pediatrics, "Principles of Treatment of Disabled Infants," says: "Discrimination of any type against any individual with a disability/disabilities, regardless of the nature or severity of the disability, is morally and legally indefensible . . . Consideration such as anticipated or actual limited potential of an individual and present or future lack of available community resources are irrelevant and must not determine the decisions concerning medical care." Do you agree with this statement? How does benefit/burden assessment apply under this guideline?

3. The author of this chapter states: "The prospect of mature adolescents implementing advance directives against the wishes of their parents or physicians has not been examined." Take the opportunity to do so now, and discuss this general issue.

Notes

1. S.X. Radbill, "Children in a World of Violence: A History of Child Abuse," in *The Battered Child*, ed. H. Kempe and R.E. Helfer (Chicago: University of Chicago Press, 1980).

2. J. Lorber, "Results of Treatment of Meningomyelocele," *Developmental Medicine and Child Neurology* 13 (1971): 279.

3. W.G. Bartholome, "The Child-Patient: Do Parents Have the "Right to Decide," in *The Law-Medicine Relation: A Philosophical Exploration*, ed. S.F. Spicker,

J.M. Healey, and H.T. Engelhardt, Jr. (Boston: D. Reidel, 1981), 271-77.

4. R.S. Duff and A.G.M. Campbell, "Moral and Ethical Dilemmas in the Special Care Nursery," *New England Journal of Medicine* 289 (1973): 890.

5. A. Shaw, "Dilemmas of 'Informed Consent' in Children," *New England Journal of Medicine* 289 (1973): 885-90.

6. D. Todres et al., "Pediatricians' Attitude Affecting Decisionmaking in Defective Newborns," *Pediatrics* 60 (1977): 197-201.

7. "Treating the Defective Newborn: A Survey of Physicians' Attitudes," *Hastings Center Report* 6, no. 2 (1976): 2.

8. A. Davis, "All Babies Should Be Kept Alive as Far as Possible," in *Principles of Health Care Ethics*, ed. R. Gillon (London: John Wiley, 1994), 629-41.

9. U.S. Department of Health and Human Services, "Interim Final Rule 45 CFR Part 84, Nondiscrimination on the Basis of a Handicap," *Federal Register* 48 (7 March 1983): 9630-32.

10. U.S. President's Commission for the Study of Ethical Problems in Medicine and Biomedical and Behavioral Research, "Seriously Ill Newborns," in *Deciding to Forego Life-Sustaining Treatment: A Report on the Ethical, Medical, and Legal Issues in Treatment Decisions* (Washington, D.C.: U.S. Government Printing Office, 1983), 197-229.

11. U.S. Department of Health and Human Services, "Nondiscrimination on the Basis of Handicaps: Procedures and Guidelines Relating to Health Care for Handicapped Infants," *Federal Register* 49 (12 January 1984): 622-54.

12. Ibid.

13. *Bowen v. American Hospital Association*, 476 U.S. 610, at 611 (1986) discussed in K. Kerr, "Reporting the Case of Baby Jane Doe," *Hastings Center Report* 14, no. 4 (1984): 7-9.

14. 42 U.S.C. sec. 5103 (1982).

15. 50 Federal Register 14893 (1985).

16. L.M. Kopelman et al., "Neonatologists Judge the 'Baby Doe' Regulations," *New England Journal of Medicine* 318 (1988): 677-83.

17. E.B. Pearson, C.L. Bose, and E.N. Kraybill, "Decisions about Futile Treatment in an Intensive Care Nursery," *North Carolina Medical Journal* 56 (1995): 462-66; and S.N. Wall and J.C. Partridge, "Withdrawal of Life Support in the Intensive Care Nursery: Decisions and Practice by Neonatologists," *Pediatric Research* 33 (1993): 30A.

18. Committee on Bioethics, American Academy of Pediatrics, "Ethics and The Care of Critically Ill Infants and Children," *Pediatrics* 98 (1996): 149-52.

19. B.W. Levin et al., "The Treatment of Non-HIV Related Conditions in Newborns at Risk for HIV: A Survey of Neonatologists," *American Journal of Public Health* 85 (1996): 1507-13.

20. R. Weir, *Selective Treatment of Handicapped Newborns: Moral Dilemmas in Neonatal Medicine* (New York: Oxford University Press, 1984).

21. P. Ramsey, *Ethics at the Edges of Life* (New Haven, Conn.: Yale University Press, 1978), 155.

22. M. Tooley, "Abortion and Infanticide," *Philosophy and Public Affairs* 2 (1972): 37-65.

23. H.T. Engelhardt, Jr. *The Foundations of Bioethics* (New York: Oxford University Press, 1988) 116-19, 145, 217.

24. W.F. May, "Parenting, Bonding and Valuing the Retarded," in *Ethics and Mental Retardation*, ed. L.M. Kopelman and J.C. Moskop (Dordrecht, The Netherlands: D. Reidel, 1984), 141-60.

25. M.B. Mahowald, *Women and Children in Health Care* (New York: Oxford University Press, 1993), 170.

26. M. Daly and M. Wilson, *Homicide* (New York: Aldine De Gruyer, 1988), 71-72.

27. J. Blustein, "The Rights Approach and the Intimacy Approach: Family Suffering and Care of Defective Newborns," *Mount Sinai Journal of Medicine* 56 (1989): 164-67.

28. See note 20 above.

29. A.E. Buchanan and D.W. Brock, *Deciding for Others: The Ethics of Surrogate Decisionmaking* (New York: Cambridge University Press, 1989).

30. A. Shaw, J.G. Randolph, and B. Manard, "Ethical Issues in Pediatric Surgery: A National Survey of Pediatricians and Pediatric Surgeons," *Pediatrics* 60 (1977): 588.

31. N. Fost, "Parents as Decision Makers for Children," *Primary Care Clinics of North America* 13 (1986): 285-93.

32. A. Whitelaw and M. Thoresen, "Ethical Dilemmas Around the Time of Birth," in *Principles of Health Care Ethics*, ed. R. Gillon (London: John Wiley & Sons, 1994), 617-27.

33. A.M. Dellinger and P.C. Kuszler, "Infants: Public-Policy and Legal Issues," in *Encyclopedia of Bioethics*, ed. W.T. Reich (New York: Simon & Schuster MacMillan, 1995), 1214-20.

34. See note 20 above, p. 259.

35. See note 25 above, p. 169-72.

36. See note 3 above, p. 271-72.

37. See note 20 above, p. 260.

38. T.L. Beauchamp and J.F. Childress, *Principles of Biomedical Ethics* (New York : Oxford University Press, 1983), 241.

39. W.G. Bartholome, "Withholding/Withdrawing Life-Sustaining Treatment," in *Contemporary Issues in Pediatric Ethics*, ed. M.M. Burgess and B.E. Woodrow (Lewiston, N.Y.: Edwin Mellen Press), 17.

40. A.R. Fleischman et al., "Caring for Gravely Ill Children," *Pediatrics* 94 (1992): 422-39.

41. C.H. Rushton and J.J. Glover, "Involving Parents in Decisions to Forego Life-Sustaining Treatment for Critically Ill Infants and Children," *Pediatric Annals* 18 (1989): 206-14.

42. See note 21 above.

43. N.M.P. King, "Transparency in Neonatal Intensive Care," *Hastings Center Report* 22 (May-June 1992): 18-25.

44. See note 21 above.

45. R.A. McCormick, "To Save or Let Die: The Dilemma of Modern Medicine," *Journal of the American Medical Association* 229 (1974): 172.

46. D.L. Coulter, T.H. Murray, and M.C. Cerreto, "Practical Ethics in Pediatrics," *Current Problems in Pediatrics* 18 (1988): 168-69.

47. A.R. Jonsen and M.J. Garland, "A Moral Policy for Life/Death Decisions in the Intensive Care Nursery," in *Ethics of Newborn Intensive Care*, ed. A.R. Jonsen and M.J. Garland (Berkeley: University of California, Institute of Governmental Studies, 1976), 176.

48. R.F. Weir, "Infants: Ethical Issues," in *Encyclopedia of Bioethics*, ed. W.T. Reich (New York: Simon and Schuster MacMillan, 1995), 1206-14.

49. R.F. Weir and J.D. Bale, "Selective Nontreatment of Neurologically Impaired Neonates," *Neurologic Clinics of North America* 7 (1989): 807-22.

50. D.W. Brock, "Death and Dying," in *Medical Ethics*, ed. R.M. Veatch (Boston: Jones and Bartlett, 1989), 352.

51. See note 29 above.

52. W. Silverman, "Overtreatment of Neonates? A Personal Retrospective," *Pediatrics* 90 (1992): 971-76.

53. See note 38 above, p. 158.

54. See note 40 above, pp. 433-39.

55. M.L. Chiswick, "Withdrawal of Life Support in Babies: Deceptive Signals," *Archives of Disease in Childhood* 65 (1990): 1096-97.

56. N.K. Rhoden, "Treating Baby Doe: The Ethics of Uncertainty," *Hastings Center Report* 16 (August 1986): 34-42

57. A.F. Fischer and D.K. Stevenson, "The Consequences of Uncertainty: An Empirical Approach to Medical Decisionmaking in Neonatal Intensive Care," *Journal of the American Medical Association* 258 (1987): 1929-31.

58. Committee on Fetus and Newborn, American Academy of Pediatrics, "The Initiation or Withdrawal of Treatment for High-Risk Newborns," *Pediatrics* 96 (1995): 362-63.

59. See note 38 above, p. 162.

60. J. Tyson, "Evidence-Based Ethics and the Care of Premature Infants," *The Future of Children* 5 (1995): 197-213; J.R. Botkin, "Delivery Room Decisions for Tiny Infants: An Ethical Analysis," *The Journal of Clinical Ethics* 1, no. 4 (1990): 306-11; A. Whitelaw and M. Thoresen, "Ethical Dilemmas around the Time of Birth," in *Principles of Health Care Ethics*, ed. R. Gillon (London: John Wiley & Sons, 1994), 617-27; D.L. Coulter, T.H. Murray, and M.C. Cerreto, "Practical Ethics in Pediatrics," *Current Problems in Pediatrics* 18, no. 3 (1988): 143-95.

61. Fetus and Newborn Committee, Canadian Pediatric Society; Maternal Fetal Medicine Committee, Society of Obstetricians and Gynecologists of Canada, "Management of the Woman with Threshold Birth of an Infant of Extremely Low Gestational Age," *Canadian Medical Association Journal* 151 (1994): 547-53.

62. J.J. Paris and M.D. Schreiber, "Parental Discretion in Refusal of Treatment for Newborns: A Real but Limited Right," *Clinics in Perinatology* 23, no. 3 (1996): 573-95; F.I. Clark, "Making Sense of *State v. Messenger*," *Pediatrics* 97, no. 4 (1996): 579-83.

63. M.M. Farrell and D.I. Levin, "Brain Death in the Pediatric Patient: Historical, Sociological, Medical, Religious, Cultural, Legal and Ethical Considerations," *Critical Care Medicine* 21, no. 12 (1993): 1951-65; M.A. Fishman, "Validity of Brain Death Criteria in Infants," *Pediatrics* 96 (1995): 513-15; Task Force on Brain Death in Children, "Guidelines for the Determination of Brain Death in Children," *Annals of Neurology* 21 (1987): 616-17.

64. S. Ashwal et al., "The Persistent Vegetative State in Children," *Annals of Neurology* 32 (1992): 570-76.

65. J.T. Berger, F. Rosner, and P. Farnsworth, "The Ethics of Mandatory Testing in Newborns," *The Journal of Clinical Ethics* 7, no. 1 (1996): 77-84; D.S. Davis, "Mandatory HIV Testing in Newborns: Not Yet, Maybe Never," *The Journal of Clinical Ethics* 7, no. 2 (1996): 191-92.

66. K.W. Chan et al., "Use of Minors as Bone Marrow Donors: Current Attitude and Management," *Jour-

nal of Pediatrics 128 (1996): 644-48.

67. W.J. Curran, "Beyond the Best Interests of the Child--Bone Marrow Transplant among Half-Siblings," New England Journal of Medicine 324 (1991): 1818-19; T.E. Williams, "Legal Issues and Ethical Dilemmas Surrounding Bone Marrow Transplantation in Children," American Journal of Pediatrics Hematology Oncology 6 (1984): 83-88; G.R. Bungio et al., "Bone Marrow Transplantation in Children: Between Therapeutic and Medico-Legal Problems," Bone Marrow Transplantation 4, suppl. 4 (1989): 34-37; A.R. Holder, "Adolescents," in Encyclopedia of Bioethics, ed. W.T. Reich (New York: Simon & Schuster Macmillan, 1995), 69-70; Council on Ethical and Judicial Affairs, American Medical Association, "The Use of Minors as Organ and Tissue Donors," Code of Medical Ethics Reports 5, no. 1 (1994): 229-43.

68. R. Swan, "Faith Healing, Christian Science and the Medical Care of Children," New England Journal of Medicine 309, no. 26 (1983): 1639-41; K.H. Rothenberg, "Medical Decision Making for Children," in Biolaw 8: 149-73.

69. Committee on Bioethics, American Academy of Pediatrics, "Treatment of Critically Ill Newborns," Pediatrics 72 (1983): 565-66.

70. President's Commission for the Study of Ethical Problems in Medicine and Biomedical and Behavioral Research, Deciding to Forego Life-Sustaining Treatment (Washington, D.C.: U.S. Government Printing Office, 1983), 6-8, 218-219.

71. American Academy of Pediatrics, "Principles of Treatment of Disabled Infants," Pediatrics 73 (1984): 559-60.

72. Committee on Bioethics, American Academy of Pediatrics, "Guidelines on Forgoing Life-Sustaining Medical Treatment," Pediatrics 93 (1994): 532-36.

73. Council on Ethical and Judicial Affairs, American Medical Association, "Report 56: The Use of Minors as Organ and Tissue Donors," Code of Medical Ethics Reports 5, no. 1 (January 1994): 229-43.

74. American Academy of Pediatrics, "Perinatal Care at the Threshold of Viability," Pediatrics 96 (1995): 974-76.

75. Committee on Fetus and Newborn, American Academy of Pediatrics, "The Initiation or Withdrawal of Treatment for High-Risk Newborns," Pediatrics 96 (1995): 362-63.

76. Committee on Bioethics, American Academy of Pediatrics, "Informed Consent, Parental Permission, and Assent in Pediatric Practice," Pediatrics 95 (1995): 314-17.

77. Committee on Bioethics, American Academy of Pediatrics, "Ethics and the Care of Critically Ill Infants and Children," Pediatrics 98 (1996): 149-52.

11

REPRODUCTIVE ISSUES

Mary V. Rorty, Ph.D., Joanne D. Pinkerton, M.D.,
and John C. Fletcher, Ph.D.

I. Introduction

Issues involving reproduction generate conflict, misunderstanding, and differences of attitude. A multitude of values are at stake in reproductive decisions --at the personal, professional, group, and societal level.

In the United States, a pluralistic culture creates large paradoxes and wide extremes in reproductive choices. For example, as a people Americans are extremely reluctant to coerce choices about reproduction; respect for autonomy and privacy is very strong in this realm. Ironically, hardly any other aspect of human behavior is subjected to such strong regulation. Some laws are designed to protect the vulnerable and others to restrict reproductive options.

Reproduction is clearly a woman's issue but not in any isolated or private sense. Women, their partners, healthcare providers, and the state face a wide range of choices about the conduct and regulation of reproduction. Many of these choices are highly controversial and will remain so. There are good reasons why thoughtful persons continue to disagree on many of the topics considered in this chapter.

This chapter has three goals:

1. to identify important types of cases with ethical significance involving reproductive choices;
2. to provide starting points for discussion among those who are professionally and personally involved in moral questions about reproduction; and
3. to encourage clinicians to plan for the ethical conflicts that are most likely to arise in the clinical setting.

The plan-of-care approach to clinical ethics recommended in Chapters 1 and 2 is especially pertinent to the third goal.

The discussion is divided into six major topics:

1. sterilization, castration, and genital surgery;
2. contraception, contragestion, and abortion;
3. reproductive technologies;
4. maternal-fetal relations;
5. prenatal diagnosis; and
6. pregnancy and terminal or life-threatening illness.

The goal of this chapter is not to persuade the reader that one position or another is morally right. We do not argue for a consensus view where none exists. In the rare instance where a moral consensus exists regarding a particular reproductive issue, it is described along with the relevant ethical considerations. For most of these topics, however, the best one can do in a spirit of "clinical pragmatism" (see Chapter 2) is to raise good questions, appreciate the complexity of the problems, and find the best literature on the subject. Today, many important legal cases and state and federal laws regulate certain reproductive choices. Clinicians should know enough about these laws and current controversies to recognize when they need legal help.

In two areas--"old" reproductive choices (sterilization) and "new" technologies (abortion in the context of embryo reduction)--cases are presented in which an ethics consultation was requested, along with a brief summary of research that may shed light on these cases.

II. Sterilization, Castration, and Genital Surgery

Although they differ in intent and context, these three types of surgical intervention share an important characteristic: they permanently alter the function of the reproductive organs.

Tubal ligation surgically sterilizes women. Castration, a more radical operation in men, removes the testes entirely, thus preventing both sexual pleasure and reproduction. The closest parallel for women is ovary removal, or oophorectomy. Various forms of genital surgery, including clitoridectomy or infibulation, are practiced in some African cultures. Male circumcision is widely practiced in Western societies. Female genital surgery has recently become an issue for healthcare providers in the United States due to immigration from cultures in which it is practiced.

A. Sterilization

Voluntary surgical sterilization is one of the most widely used means of contraception, especially for married women. The percentage of married couples using sterilization as a method of contraception more than doubled from 1972 to 1988, a trend associated with higher costs of other contraceptive methods and a shrinking range of options.[1]

Voluntary sterilization raises different issues than compulsory sterilization. Questions of capacity and consent complicate decisions about sterilization procedures for some populations, including people with mental retardation, the institutionalized, and minor children. Surgical sterilization (vasectomy or tubal ligation) was debated in the 1960s and 1970s because of widespread eugenic sterilization of individuals with mental retardation, and grossly high sterilization rates of some social groups.[2] There are alarming statistics about the number of Native American women who have been sterilized. Criminals convicted of repeated crimes were also sterilized in some states. In both kinds of coerced sterilization, eugenic and punitive,

the intent of advocates has been to solve a social problem through legalization of medical means.

1. The Case of AB

A grandmother whose 11-year-old granddaughter was her ward asked a pediatrician if the granddaughter could be sterilized. The girl was mildly mentally retarded. The grandmother's motives seemed to be fear of future sexual promiscuity and pregnancy out of wedlock, which would complicate taking care of her. The pediatrician called a pediatric surgeon, who requested an ethics consultation.

The consultation service believed that the reports of the girl's functional capacity indicated that this was not a decision that the grandmother should be making for the child. It was possible that, in the future, the granddaughter could operate functionally on her own in society, marry, and decide to bear children. Whether to have children was a decision she would have to make at the time. Further, there were other alternatives to preventing conception, such as an intrauterine device (IUD) or an implant. The consensus was that sterilization would be wrong, although other means of birth control might be appropriate.

The ethics consultants prepared a letter for the surgeon with ethical consideration of the proposal, as well as reference to the existing legal process that made sterilization in this case very unlikely if not impossible. Also, advice on contraception for a girl of this age was secured for the pediatrician from an obstetrician-gynecologist.[3]

2. Ethical Considerations

There is now a societal consensus that nonconsensual sterilization in cases like AB, even in the context of family life, violates so many values and ethical principles that it is not a morally acceptable option. In children with mild to moderate retardation, the options are how best to protect the child short of sterilization and how to aid her development as a person. Societal views about respect and help for persons with mental retardation have changed. In cases where children and adults are profoundly retarded and sexually vulnerable, genuine ethical concerns about reproduction do arise. How much weight should be given to a family's wishes to sterilize a profoundly retarded family member?[4] To the interests of the state? To the wishes of a retarded girl or woman, boy or man? Curran provides an excellent overview of the ethical issues in sterilization and other forms of fertility control.[5]

Moral repulsion about the ideology and consequences of an earlier eugenics movement was a main impetus behind this societal consensus. Earlier in this century, tens of thousands of persons were involuntarily sterilized across the United States. From the 1920s through the 1950s, more than 7,000 mentally ill or retarded individuals were sterilized involuntarily in Virginia institutions alone. More than 300 mandatory sterilizations occurred in Virginia between 1960 and 1979.[6] By the mid-1930s, 32 states had passed sterilization laws that assumed the heritability of maladies such as mental illness, alcoholism, and epilepsy--as well as associated social conditions such poverty. Sterilization laws extended to many whose medical diagnoses made them potential parents of "socially inadequate" offspring.[7]

Eugenic aims, along with racial prejudice and bias against the mentally retarded, formed the basis for these actions. Undoubtedly, some degree of popular sentiment remains about restraining fertility individuals who are dependent on welfare or people who are mentally ill.[8]

3. Professional Statements

The Committee on Ethics of the American College of Obstetricians and Gynecologists (ACOG) published guidelines, *Sterilization of Women Who Are Mentally Handicapped* (1988) and *Ethical Considerations in Sterilization* (1989).[9] Among the committee's recommendations are:

The initial premise should be that nonvoluntary sterilization is generally not ethically acceptable in our society.... [But] four categories of concern should be considered in any decision to sterilize a person who is mentally incapacitated or incompetent:

1. identification of an appropriate decision maker;
2. alternatives to sterilization;
3. best interests of the person who is mentally incapacitated or incompetent; and

4. current understanding of applicable laws."[10]

The ACOG committee also urged that "because a patient's ability to procreate may significantly affect the lives of others, the physician should encourage the patient to include other appropriate persons in the counseling process."[11] Writing primarily about institutionalized persons, the committee urged physicians to seek legal and/or ethical consultation when they find themselves in a dilemma in which it is necessary to protect the choices of vulnerable women.

4. Legal Landscape

Those involved in cases where involuntary sterilization is an issue should obtain legal advice, because this procedure is heavily regulated. It is important to review state law to determine what the age, informed consent, and waiting requirements are.[12] Nonpublic hospitals may choose which (if any) sterilizations they want to offer patients.

The U.S. Supreme Court decided in 1927 in *Buck v. Bell*[13] that Virginia's statute permitting compulsory sterilization for "feeble-mindedness" and other conditions was constitutional. This decision has never been overturned, but it is not a reliable legal precedent today. *Skinner v. Oklahoma*,[14] which overturned an Oklahoma law permitting compulsory sterilization of three-time felons ("three strikes and you're out"), is a sounder source of authority from the U.S. Supreme Court; it has been echoed approvingly in later cases involving reproductive rights. Some state statutes, such as California's, make involuntary sterilization almost impossible.[15]

In the early 1970s, the case of the Relf sisters came to light and to court (*Relf v. Weinberger*).[16] In Montgomery, Alabama, two teenage girls were surgically sterilized in federally funded health programs without the valid consent of their parents. Congress then acted to restrict the conditions for sterilizations in such programs. Federal regulations ruled out use of federal funds to sterilize any person under 21 years of age. Further, a federally mandated consent form must be signed and dated at least 30 days but no more than 180 days prior to the sterilization procedure.[17]

Today, almost all states have statutes or case law that tightly control sterilization of persons who have not given voluntary, informed consent--especially minors and mentally disabled individuals. In 1979, California and the District of Columbia banned the sterilization of any person under the government's care.[18] However, as recently as 1985, at least 19 states had laws that permitted the sterilization of mentally retarded persons.[19] Dubler and White describe the current legal and regulatory situation in sterilization and other forms of fertility control.[20]

B. Castration and Genital Surgery

Orchiectomy (surgical castration) involves removal of the male sex organs, a much more radical operation than is required for sterilization. Castration was used as a punishment for sex crimes and repeated rapes in a number of states for more than 100 years. A nonsurgical procedure labeled "chemical castration" uses hormone-inhibiting drugs to create so-called erotic apathy. It has been used for about 25 years in the same context. In the United States, 50 sex offender clinics use this therapy.[21] In Denmark, where chemical castration is allowed, recidivism rates are reported to be less than 3 percent, compared to 30 to 50 percent for noncastrated offenders.[22]

Recently, there has been renewed debate about castration. Some sex offenders have requested castration. For example, Larry McQuay recently asked to be castrated before leaving prison in California; he argued that unless he is castrated, he will be unable to resist repeating his offenses.[23] A bill has been introduced in the California legislature to legalize chemical castration for sex offenders.

Female genital surgery has become an issue in the U.S. literature and in U.S. courts because of immigration cases. Virtually unknown in Western countries until recently, a variety of operations are performed on the genitals of pubescent girls in some Middle Eastern and African societies, as initiation rites. The operations range in severity from ritual incisions to full clitoridectomy (excision of the clitoris) and in some cultures are accompanied with infibulation (stitching the labia together).[24] Western and non-Western feminists have been involved in international discussion of female genital surgery, but it has been difficult to reach a consensus because of debate about the importance of respecting cultural differences. The literature on this topic is growing. Kopelman and others helpfully discuss whether ethical or cultural relativism ought to be given a strong voice in this issue.[25]

1. The case of LO

In 1994 a Nigerian woman succeeded in halting deportation proceedings against herself and her five- and six-year-old daughters, of whom she had custody, by appealing for "cultural asylum." She claimed that her country's practice of female genital mutilation was a threat to her daughters. The immigration judge found that the threat of genital mutilation to the daughters established the "extreme hardship" required to establish residency status, and described the practice as "cruel" and serving "no known medical purpose."[26]

2. Professional Statements

The American Medical Association's Council on Scientific Affairs has released guidelines on female genital mutilation,[27] and the U.S. Congress has considered a bill making female genital surgery illegal in the United States.[28] International health groups such as the World Health Organization (WHO) and the United Nations Educational, Scientific, and Cultural Organization (UNESCO) have protested such practices and have provided guidelines that can be consulted by Western healthcare providers. The 1994 United Nations Population Conference in Cairo included this sentence: "Governments are urged to prohibit female genital mutilation wherever it exists and to give vigorous support to efforts among non-governmental and community organizations to eliminate such practices."[29]

III. Contraception, Contragestion, and Abortion

Contraception, contragestion (which is a contraction of contragestation), and abortion are methods of preventing an unintended or undesired pregnancy. These interventions form a continuum of preventive methods from conception to birth. Different beliefs about the moral status of a fertilized ovum or a previable or viable fetus lead to a wide range of attitudes in our society about these alternatives.

Policar and Joffee provide current reviews of the medical, technical, and social issues in the field of contraception.[30] Because of liability risks for pharmaceutical firms and reduced economic investment in contraceptive development, U.S. women have fewer birth control choices than women in other industrialized nations, and contraception is more expensive than elsewhere.[31] Abstinence from sexual activity is the only noncontroversial form of contraception; debate continues about the appropriateness, availability, ease of use, and safety of all other forms of preventing birth.

A. Contraception and Contragestion

In 1990, a California judge ordered a heroin addict not to get pregnant as a condition of probation. "I want to make it clear that one of the reasons I am making this order is you've got five children. . . . You're 30 years old. None of your children are in your custody or control. Two of them are on Aid for Dependent Children. And I'm afraid that if you get pregnant, we're going to get a cocaine or heroin-addicted baby." The order was overturned on appeal.[32]

Legislation has been introduced in California, Hawaii, and Tennessee providing financial incentives for voluntary insertion of Norplant in mothers on welfare. In each of two recent legislative sessions, bills have been introduced in Washington State to require involuntary insertion of Norplant into mothers whose children are born with fetal alcohol syndrome.[33]

1. Ethical Questions for Debate

Use of medical measures for social purposes is highly problematic as a moral matter, especially when these measures are compelled, rather than used with consent. How should healthcare professionals respond if asked to participate in "creative sentencing" of women offenders, such as mandating the use of Norplant as a condition for probation? What should professionals do if asked by a woman to remove an implant that was inserted pursuant to a legal order?

Seeing morally relevant differences between contraception, contragestion, and abortion depends on one's moral views. Are there moral differences between using postcoital methods of birth control such as using oral contraceptives as a "morning after" pill

or emergency contraceptive and using RU-486?[34] RU-486 is a glucocorticoid agent that induces menstruation; if the drug taken by a woman who desires to avoid pregnancy and has missed a period, it results in dislodging the newly implanted embryo from the wall of the uterus. The drug should be administered under the care of a physician because of the risk in some women of heavy bleeding and incomplete miscarriage. RU-486 is also therapeutically useful for cancer, hypertension, and diabetes.

Regelson's account of RU-486 is a rich case study in how ethics and politics interact in the United States.[35] Under political pressure in the early 1990s, the U.S. Food and Drug Administration (FDA) imposed an "import alert" on testing RU-486 for contragestion, although the drug could be imported for research for other medical purposes.[36] President Clinton revoked the prohibition in 1993. The nonprofit Population Council is the principal U.S. sponsor of the drug as a contragestive. Cahill carefully explores the morally relevant similarities and differences between abortion and the use of RU-486.[37]

2. Professional Statements

The San Francisco Medical Society and the California Medical Association supported testing of RU-486.[38] The American Medical Association (AMA) later supported testing the drug and, if found safe and effective, its clinical use in the United States.[39]

3. Legal Landscape

In the contemporary legal environment, decisions about contraception and contragestion fall under the protection of the privacy rights and the protection under the First and Fourteenth Amendments. *Skinner v. Oklahoma* recognized marriage and procreation as fundamental rights that required equal protection under the U.S. Constitution.[40] Rights to state noninterference with contraception were secured in *Griswold v. Connecticut* and *Eisenstadt v. Baird*.[41] These cases struck down state statutes forbidding the prescription of contraceptives to adults, whether married or unmarried. The court found a constitutional right of privacy inherent in such decisions. The abortion rights protected in *Roe v. Wade* were based upon an extension of the right to privacy established in the contraception cases.[42]

B. Abortion

Of all interventions to prevent birth, abortion remains the most controversial. Despite various court cases that have made elective abortion, with some restrictions, legal in the United States, abortion remains a socially divisive issue. The focus on elective abortion tends to overshadow discussion of other justifications for terminating pregnancies, including selective abortions done to prevent the birth of physically or genetically impaired children and "reductions" of multiple pregnancies to enhance the chances of live birth for some.[43] Genetic or eugenic abortions intended to prevent the birth of severely impaired children, have more social and medical sanction and are less controversial among some social groups than elective abortions.

1. Ethical Considerations and Questions

Elective abortion is a legally protected but morally controversial option. A woman's right to abortion is protected against unwarranted interference by the state or third parties. But what may be legal can be morally controversial. There are strongly clashing moral views about abortion that reflect differences among religious and philosophical traditions.[44] A prevailing moral approach to abortion can be described, although defending it is not a subject of this chapter.

U.S. public opinion studies over a long period report that the prevailing moral view in this society is to permit abortion within limits and for serious reasons.[45] On the one hand, the limits are designed to protect the health, safety, and well-being of women; and on the other hand, they protect the interests of viable fetuses. Many people hold that there are morally relevant differences between cases and reasons for abortions. Abortion to protect the health and safety of a woman is the clearest and most justifiable case. At the other extreme are abortions for highly suspect reasons (such as for sex selection apart from a diagnosed genetic disorder). Although abortion for sex selection is legal, many people believe that it is extremely difficult to justify on moral grounds because it violates the principle of equality and is a precedent for eugenics.[46]

Out of respect for reproductive autonomy, most people would leave evaluation of what counts as "serious" reasons for abortion to the consciences of women as informed by their physicians and their spiritual or moral advisers. An older and discredited practice is to require women to justify their reasons for abortion publicly, (that is to have their reasons and life situations reviewed by a special committee). Also, a well-established social practice is that healthcare professionals as individuals are free to decide whether to participate in abortions, depending upon the circumstances and their personal moral commitments.

Ethical questions have been raised about what information should be provided to pregnant women about the option of abortion. Many healthcare professionals in family planning clinics supported by federal funds had significant ethical concerns when government regulations prohibited speaking about abortion when counseling clients.[47] President Clinton rescinded these regulations. Another often-debated ethical and legal questions is whether healthcare professionals should notify parents of adolescents who request abortions.

Pregnancy reduction is a form of abortion. If a patient requests it for reasons that do not involve serious risk to the woman's health, as in the case below, what are the limits of a physician's duty to perform the procedure?[48] Are hospital ethics committees appropriate forums to debate whether elective abortions or pregnancy reductions should be permitted?[49]

2. Case: "Why Not Two to One?"

Mr. and Mrs. D, busy professionals in their early 30s, had a two-year-old son. Mrs. D was 12 weeks pregnant with naturally conceived, healthy-appearing twins. Mr. and Mrs. D felt that carrying, delivering, and raising twins would create excessive strain on them. They were concerned about the medical risks and the physical and emotional demands that twins would place on Mrs. D. They were concerned that they would not have adequate time to give proper attention to raising three young children. They were also concerned that twins would make it necessary for Mrs. D to take substantially more time off work, which would stunt her professional growth.

A perinatology consultant informed the couple of the option of selective termination of the most anterior (lowest in the uterus) twin. Other options included abortion of the whole pregnancy, giving up one twin for adoption, keeping both, or going out of state to have the selective termination done at a university center that specializes in this procedure. The couple requested that a selective termination be done locally, finding all of the other options unacceptable. The perinatologist, who had only performed selective terminations for genetic indications in a twin, requested an ethics consultation. The hospital where the perinatologist performed procedures did not have a policy on the issue of whether physicians should cooperate with requests to reduce normal pregnancy of twins from two to one.

The perinatologist asked the hospital ethics committee for consultation. After considerable discussion, the committee recommended that he not cooperate with the request. The group reasoned that fetal reduction in this case carried some risk to the other twin without the same benefits as in a multifetal pregnancy (more than three) or in selective termination of an affected twin.[50] They viewed the risk-benefit ratio as not proportionate. The physician declined their advice and performed the procedure without mishap to the other twin. The physician reasoned that if his and society's views permitted first-trimester abortion in the first place (reducing one fetus to none), then there was no morally relevant difference between that action and reducing two fetuses to one. "Why not two to one?" he asked, "since society permits abortion for any reason."[51]

3. Professional Statements

In *Further Ethical Considerations in Induced Abortion*, ACOG issued the following statement:

> The College recognizes that situations of conflict may arise between a pregnant woman's health interest and the welfare of her fetus. Both legally and ethically this conflict can lead to a justification for inducing abortion. The College affirms that the resolution of such conflict by inducing abortion in no way implies that the physician has an adversary relationship toward the fetus and therefore, the physician does not view the destruction of the fetus as the primary purpose of abortion. The College consequently recognizes a continuing obligation on the part of the physician towards the survival of a possibly viable fetus

where this can be discharged without additional hazard to the life of the mother.[52]

In *Multifetal Pregnancy Reduction and Selective Fetal Termination*, ACOG stated: "Even for some who do not believe that abortion is acceptable, multiple pregnancy reduction can be justified ethically when the risks of carrying the pregnancy are considerable and could be reduced if the number of fetuses were fewer. Varying degrees of risk will be interpreted differently by individual patients."[53]

4. Legal Landscape

Abortion decisions are regulated by both federal and state law. The fundamental right of abortion protected in *Roe v. Wade*[54] (1973) has not been overturned by later legal challenges, but U.S. abortion law has been somewhat modified. *Planned Parenthood Association of Southeastern Pennsylvania v. Casey* (1992) affirmed a woman's right to terminate pregnancy until viability, and thereafter if necessary to protect her life or health.[55] The court held that state laws regulating abortion will be found valid if they do not impose an "undue burden" or "substantial obstacle" on access to abortion. The Pennsylvania statute's requirements of information disclosure, 24-hour waiting period, and parental consent were upheld under this standard, but its requirement for spousal notification was found unconstitutional. Federal laws prohibit federal funding under Medicaid for elective abortions (and for research involving abortion or risks to the fetus) that are not therapeutic in intent.[56] President Bush's executive order that blocked federal funds for research or transplanting fetal tissue was rescinded by President Clinton in 1993. Fetal tissue for such research is obtained with the woman's consent from a dead fetus following elective abortion.

Allen's review of abortion law in the United States and other nations is informative.[57] Clinicians are strongly advised to be familiar with their own state laws on abortion.

IV. Reproductive Technologies

Since ancient times, third parties have played a role in pregnancy to overcome infertility, sterility, or incapacity to carry to term. Today's reproductive technologies have increased in complexity and are used more frequently. The traditional definition of "parents" as the gestational partners cannot encompass all of today's genetic, gestational, nurturant and emotional possibilities. Although forms of surrogacy are described in some of our oldest cultural records, technological advances of the 20th century have greatly increased the variety of ways in which individuals or couples can achieve parenthood, and have increased disputes and ethical perplexity about who is the "real" parent and who "owns" the raw materials and the results of conception. Individuals and couples, who during an earlier era would have been childless, are assisted to bear children and raise families; at the same time, ethical and legal questions have been raised that earlier generations would have found incredible.

A. Case

Sally Morgan is 46 years old and has been divorced for 10 years. She has one child, a 25-year-old daughter. Recently, she married Frank Charlton, a 49-year-old childless widower. They would like to start a family of their own, but she is now infertile.

Mrs. Charlton consults a university in vitro fertilization (IVF) program, where she is told that she is not a suitable candidate for the procedure. However, her husband's sperm could be used to fertilize an ovum (egg) from an anonymous donor. The embryo could then be implanted in a surrogate mother and carried to term.

Since Mrs. Charlton would like her child to be genetically related, her daughter offers to donate ova for the IVF process. Each of the daughter's eggs contains 50 per cent of her mother's genetic material; therefore, the baby would have one-half of that amount, or 25 per cent. In this manner, the child would be genetically related to Mrs. Charlton. Mrs. Charlton would be in the unusual position of being both mother and grandmother to the child; her daughter would be the child's biologic mother and sister.[58]

B. Ethical Questions

Assisted reproductive technologies are fraught with unsettled ethical questions. Lauritzen asks whether more reproductive choices are necessarily better?[59] To what extent does the expansion of choices result in more freedom of choice? Rothman emphasizes that the capacity to reproduce, potentially a source of power for women, may also subject them to more control.[60] Like Annas,[61] Rothman is persuaded that--because so much manipulation and money, and so many different parties are involved--reproductive technologies result in "commodification" of women's bodies and of children. The moral judgment of these authors points to the dehumanization that occurs by viewing persons and reproduction only as economic tools or as means to an end.

To what extent do these technologies contribute to the alienation of women from procreation, robbing them of a significant source of power?[62] Should the use of reproductive technologies (such as artificial insemination and IVF) be discouraged for single women, lesbian couples, or postmenopausal women --even if they can pay for them?[63] Should medical technology be used to help postmenopausal women have children? How old is "too old" to be a mother? In cases of "surrogate" or host mothers, who should be considered the mother--the woman who nurtures the fetus in her womb and gives birth, or the women whose egg is fertilized and then implanted as an embryo?[64] Can commercial or even noncommercial surrogacy be truly voluntary?[65] How should extracorporeal embryos be treated?[66] Can they be frozen? Sold? Given away? Used for research? Owned? If so, by whom? Can they be given into custody? Can they inherit? Do the resulting children, if any, have a right to know their genetic inheritance? What limits should be placed on the number of years embryos are frozen?[67] What should be done with frozen embryos if the couple divorces?

2. Professional Statements

In 1986, ACOG described current IVF practices and briefly discussed the ethical issues in *Ethical Issues in Human In Vitro Fertilization and Embryo Placement*.[68] ACOG took positions favoring several practices: (1) freezing and storage of eggs and embryos, (2) a nonprofit system of collecting sperm and eggs for IVF, and (3) the conduct of research with embryos. ACOG avoided comment on whether embryos to be used for research were to be those not transferred at IVF to treat infertility or those fertilized solely for the purpose of research. ACOG recommended that research was not to be done on embryos past the 14th developmental day, after which the embryos were to be destroyed. ACOG also developed guidelines for the practice of surrogacy in *Ethical Issues in Surrogate Motherhood*,[69] based on the model of a preconception adoption agreement. ACOG recommended that the surrogate be regarded as the mother for all medical and other purposes, and that she could decide at birth whether to place the child for adoption.

3. Legal Landscape

In the strict sense, the only federal actions affecting reproductive technologies have been executive orders and bans on funding research with the human embryo in relation to IVF.[70] In 1993, Congress removed obstacles to research. The action was intended to improve the safety and efficacy of IVF as a procedure to treat infertility.[71] Nevertheless, Congress also banned federal funding for any investigative research with human embryos, even "spare" embryos not transferred after IVF.[72]

In the private sector, professional guidelines prepared by ACOG and the American Fertility Society are presumed to operate. These guidelines permit research with spare human embryos up to 14 days. Presumably, no U.S. researchers are creating embryos for the sake of research only, although a National Institutes of Health (NIH) panel recommended that this would be sound policy to permit important research that could not be done otherwise. President Clinton rejected this part of the NIH report; to date, the NIH has not invited any proposals involving research with human embryos.[73]

In the area of state laws, there are several cases involving parental rights of children conceived by artificial insemination. Many states prohibit, do not enforce, or tightly regulate contracts for surrogacy. Cases of particular interest to medical ethicists include *In re Baby M* and *Davis v. Davis*.[74] Baby M was the first reported legal case involving surrogacy and was widely discussed in the bioethics literature (see Case 1 at end of this chapter). In *Davis v. Davis*, the Tennessee Supreme Court decided that a divorced man's constitutionally protected right to avoid procreation outweighed his former wife's interest in donating their pre-embryos produced by IVF. Other

state and federal courts have not addressed contracts involving IVF.

V. Maternal-Fetal Relations

Although the law has not invested the fetus with legal personhood, there is a tendency in medicine, when treating a late-term pregnancy, to consider the fetus a "second patient." Occasions may thus arise when a third party becomes an advocate for the "rights" of the fetus, calling into question the usual presumption that the woman bearing a wanted child is the best and most appropriate advocate for fetal interests. Such conflicts have come to be called "maternal-fetal conflicts." It is well known that fetal development can be harmed by a variety of causes that operate before or after conception--including exposure to environmental toxins; maternal infections and diseases; and maternal behavior such as smoking, alcohol abuse, or other substance abuse. The mother's refusal to follow medical recommendations, can directly involve physicians.[75]

Medical personnel can combine with law enforcement officials to coerce pregnant women into treatment or confinement to protect the fetus. One of the most important examples of such partnerships in the United States is a program begun in 1989 by the Medical University of South Carolina, which required pregnant women who tested positive for cocaine to seek drug counseling and prenatal care under the threat of criminal sanctions.[76] In five years, 42 pregnant women, who were predominantly African Americans, were arrested. The university discontinued the policy in a settlement with the civil rights division of the U.S. Department of Health and Human Services. A jury trial is now underway, in which the university and the city of Charleston face a multimillion dollar class-action lawsuit brought on behalf of several women jailed under the policy.[77] A jury trial found that the plaintiffs deserved no damages, but the decision is on appeal. Other issues in the case remain under judicial review.

See case 2 at the end of this chapter for an example of maternal-fetal conflict.

A. Ethical Considerations

What limits, if any, should constrain a woman's medical decision that seems to conflict with the welfare of the fetus?[78] Positive incentives to align maternal interests more closely with those of the fetus are seldom considered, although there is considerable discussion of how much pressure, coercion, or punishment is appropriate to shape the behavior of pregnant women.[79] Is it ever ethical for physicians to resort to the use of force to impose treatment on an unwilling pregnant woman? Pinkerton and Finnerty reviewed the ethical and legal aspects of this question in a recent article.[80] How should physicians decide whether to seek a court order in the absence of a statute that requires or authorizes them to do it? Should punishment also apply to men if risk to children from sperm damaged by substance abuse is demonstrated?[81]

Ethical and legal views vary widely on these questions. Rhoden argued that parents have a duty to rescue their children (in effect, to be "good Samaritans"), but that they have no duty to be "splendid Samaritans" by embarking on rescues that risk their life or health.[82] Robertson, softening his earlier position justifying forced treatment to prevent harm, argued that "no physician should be required to seek a mandatory Cesarean section."[83] However, he argued that women affected by phenylketonuria (PKU) who were noncompliant with dietary restrictions during pregnancy and risked harm to the fetus could be restrained and forced to comply.

B. Professional Statements

In *Patient Choice: Maternal-Fetal Conflict*, ACOG concludes: "Every reasonable effort should be made to protect the fetus, but the pregnant woman's autonomy should be respected. . . . Obstetricians should refrain from performing procedures that are unwanted by a pregnant woman."[84]

Most obstetricians concur with the ACOG statement that court-ordered intervention should "almost never" be considered.[85] The American Medical Association (AMA) advises physicians not to seek court-ordered interventions in pregnancy, despite the frustration of witnessing preventable harm to a fetus.[86] The AMA statement recommends that physicians remain in the role of "medical counselor and advisor," rather than policing the decisions of women regarding their pregnancies. The statement points out that legal measures might be justified under exceptional circumstances (such as where interventions involve minimal risks to the mother and promise large benefits to the fetus).

C. Legal Landscape

No federal law directly bears on maternal-fetal conflicts. At the state level, in *Jefferson v. Griffin Spalding County Hospital Authority*,[87] the Georgia Supreme Court upheld a lower court order for a cesarean section to be performed on a woman with placenta previa at term who had refused the procedure. This decision has been heavily criticized. Other lower-court decisions involving forced obstetrical interventions have been reported and discussed in the literature.[88]

A pivotal "paradigm case" of a judicially imposed cesarean section involved Angela Carder, a pregnant woman who was dying of cancer in the 26th week of pregnancy at George Washington University Hospital in Washington, D.C. (see Chapter 7). She clearly refused surgery in her last hours of life, although she had earlier said "yes." The trial judge's reasoning balanced the rights of the mother against the interests of the state in the life of the fetus. The fetus died shortly after delivery, as did the patient. Her family successfully sued the hospital and her physicians for violation of her rights, and an appeals court overturned the judge's decision.[89] The appeals court argued strongly that a process of substituted judgment should have occurred when making decisions about the care of Ms. Carder. The court questioned whether there would ever be circumstances to justify such a massive intervention over a woman's or a surrogate's objections.

Since *Carder*, there has been no instance of a court-ordered cesarean section. One subsequent Illinois case of placental insufficiency at 36 weeks was brought to court by the Cook County State's Attorney who asked that a cesarean section be ordered. The appeals court resoundingly rejected his plea and referred to the *Carder* court's opinion.[90]

VI. Prenatal Diagnosis

Prenatal diagnosis can now be done in virtually any pregnancy to detect disorders in cases of known higher genetic risk or to detect chromosomal abnormalities. There is a strong trend toward earlier and safer methods of prenatal diagnosis for pregnant women.[91] In addition to the diagnostic techniques of ultrasonography, first-trimester chorionic villus sampling, amniocentesis, and cordocentesis, it is now possible to perform DNA diagnosis of a single cell of an early embryo after IVF to test for genetic disease.[92] Combining this technique with improved methods of gene therapy would make treatment possible in the embryo and fetus.[93] Fetal therapy is now possible in some cases. Currently, treatment through drugs, blood products, and vitamins is more effective than fetal surgery, which is still under study in a few centers for some congenital malformations.[94]

Prenatal diagnosis raises an array of difficult ethical and psychological issues for patients and clinicians. The most acute moral and emotional issues concern choices about selective abortion. Researchers who have conducted empirical studies have found that genetic abortion choices are more stressful and morally complex than choices to end an unwanted pregnancy.[95] This is because, in most cases, the pregnancy is wanted and parents have already bonded with the fetus by viewing ultrasound images. Abortion of a wanted pregnancy, especially for individual eugenic reasons, is morally and emotionally problematic. The standard of care is to provide emotional support and counseling before and after the procedure.

Another factor that contributes to a stressful and morally complex choice is uncertainty about the degree of severity in some disorders. Some disorders are more treatable and less burdensome than others. If the family has a living child with the disorder, they may be concerned that abortion would be harmful to the child's mental health. Wertz and colleagues reported this concern presented itself in a study of parents who were receiving prenatal diagnosis for cystic fibrosis.[96] In addition, parents may share the concern of persons with disabilities that selective abortion sets a precedent for neglect of genetically affected persons who survive. Critics of prenatal diagnosis are also concerned that environmental contributions to some genetic orders will be underestimated and obscured. Parents listen to these concerns, and many take them to heart.

Some reasons to seek prenatal diagnosis are far more ethically controversial than a family history of a hereditary disorder or advanced maternal age. A woman in her 20s or early 30s who appreciates the general risks of chromosomal disorders can be very anxious about her pregnancy and want reassurance. Some couples want to know the gender of the fetus in advance for cultural reasons or to select their child's gender. Some couples have moral reasons to oppose abortion but seek prenatal diagnosis strictly for information. In rare cases, the diagnosis is sought only to benefit a third party, (such as compatibility for bone marrow donation or for paternity testing).

Using DNA technology, scientists are now currently working to locate and sequence all genes that cause disease. Once these genes have been identified and located, physicians can correctly diagnose the disorder, even in the fetus, and develop drugs and other therapies. Therapy is usually many years behind progress in diagnosis. In the interim, scores of dilemmas abound. The following case raises difficult ethical questions in the context of prenatal diagnosis in a society that deeply respects diversity and toleration of cultural differences.

A. Case: A Deaf Couple Wants a Child

Mr. and Mrs. Harris are deaf. Mrs. Harris has inherited two copies of a recessive gene that is the cause of her deafness. She, one brother, and one sister are deaf. Her parents were first cousins, and consanguinity increases the risks of genetic disease, including genes that cause deafness. Mr. Harris has a form of deafness known as Waardenburg syndrome, caused by a dominant gene transmitted from his grandfather, to Mr. Harris's mother, to him. His mother and one of her brothers were deaf. Mr. Harris has one sister who is deaf and one sister who can hear. The dominant gene for Mr. Harris's deafness has been mapped to chromosome number 2.

If Mr. and Mrs. Harris have a child, there is a 50 percent chance that the child will be deaf. They visit a geneticist to ask for help having a deaf child. They say that deafness is not a handicapping condition but mainly a language problem. (This view is widely held by hearing-impaired persons today. "Deaf pride" is a cultural movement that insists that deafness is not a disease and that deaf persons are as qualified as others for any profession or occupation.) Mr. and Mrs. Harris believe that they can more successfully raise a deaf child rather than a hearing child, and they are willing to use selective abortion after prenatal diagnosis to achieve their goal.[97]

B. Ethical Considerations

Although prenatal diagnosis constantly improving in safety, variety, and possible range of discovery, it is not without its risks. To what extent it should be offered to various populations and for what indications remain subject to discussion.

What options does the geneticist have in the case of Mr. and Mrs. Harris? To what extent should the geneticist cooperate? Should an obstetrician-gynecologist who is skilled in prenatal diagnosis perform the procedure? Does parental autonomy prevail? Should a healthcare provider participate in the selective abortion of a presumably healthy fetus in order to produce a deaf child as the parents desire? Is there an ethical difference between selecting a deaf child by prenatal diagnosis and abortion and surgically rendering a hearing child deaf after birth?

The options are to cooperate, to refuse, or to refuse and refer the Harrises to a physician who will serve them. One argument for cooperation is respect for the parents' autonomy and for fairness. If one helps other parents who reason, "We do not want this particular child," one ought to respect the Harris's desire for a deaf child. Another consideration is the desire to nurture human diversity. Rather than judge the parents' motives, one could concentrate on helping the couple to have a deaf child. Deafness is not an overwhelming handicap; indeed, the Harrises arguably do not see it as a handicap at all.

Arguments for refusal begin with the argument that it violates responsible parenthood to choose deliberately that one's child be born handicapped. Further, it is wrong to abort a normal fetus to select a hearing-impaired child. A final argument is that the Harrises' choice appears to be a precedent for eugenics--selecting traits that are culturally desirable for genetic tampering. In this respect the couple's wish is analogous to permissive sex selection, because they are selecting for a desirable (to them) trait. If one ought to oppose sex selection because of the consequences for women around the world and violation of equality, (an estimated 60 to 100 million women are missing from the world's population, mostly in China and

India), then one ought not to take steps that lead in that direction.[98]

C. Professional Statements

There are no statements of professional guidance for geneticists on the particular ethical problem represented by the case of Mr. and Mrs. Harris. A close parallel to this situation is the use of prenatal diagnosis to further parents' desire to have a child of the preferred sex. In this setting, abortion prevents have a child of the "wrong" gender. In 1983, the President's Commission for the Study of Ethical Problems in Medicine and Biomedical and Behavioral Research recommended against using prenatal diagnosis for sex choice, because it violated equality between the sexes.[99] Earlier, a Hastings Center task force on prenatal diagnosis took essentially the same position, but it stated that laws prohibiting sex selection were unwise because these laws could be a wedge further to limit abortions.[100] Organizations of human geneticists in other nations and international conferences have also discouraged sex selection in this form.[101] Most recently, the Institute of Medicine's Committee on Assessing Genetic Risk criticized the use of prenatal diagnosis for sex selection as a "misuse of genetic services that is inappropriate" and that "should be discouraged by health professionals."[102]

These statements assume that prenatal diagnosis ought to be done only to give parents and physicians information about the health of the fetus. Because gender is not a disease, diagnosis of gender is not needed.

D. Legal Landscape

Most states have statutes that address some aspects of prenatal diagnosis, but prenatal diagnosis is not legally proscribed in any state. Courts in many jurisdictions have decided cases involving the tort of "wrongful birth." These cases involve charges by parents that negligence deprived them of their right to information in order to make decisions about pregnancy. Such a case might arise if an infant with trisomy was to born to a woman over the age of 35, and the physician failed to inform the pregnant woman that a prenatal diagnosis test was indicated for chromosomal disorders linked to advanced maternal age.

Only a few courts have decided "wrongful-life" cases. Such cases involve charges brought on behalf of the child that it would have been better not to be born. At least one commentator believes the issue is dead in the courts.[103] One widely discussed wrongful-life case is *Curlender v. Bio-Science Laboratories*.[104] (see Case 3 at the end of this chapter.)

VII. Pregnancy and Terminal or Life-Threatening Illness

Our usual social expectations about the role of pregnancy in the life of the parents are disrupted when the mother faces a terminal illness of either short or longer duration. Questions arise about the effect of pregnancy on the course of the mother's illness; in addition, questions arise about the effect of the illness, or treatments for it, upon the normal development of the fetus. What are the obligations of care providers in such a situation?

The Angela Carder case briefly discussed above (see Chapter 7) poses the ethical and legal issues of surgical intervention in pregnancy when the woman is terminally ill. In this case, a pregnant woman who was dying of cancer had never been asked, "If it comes down to it, should we perform an emergency cesarean section or should we let the baby die with you?" As she worsened, her capacity to consent or refuse treatment was at issue, the fetus was marginally "viable," and hospital authorities were very concerned about their legal position. Even as a judicial hearing began at the hospital, the hospital's ethics committee had convened for its regular meeting. The committee was neither informed nor consulted about the ethics emergency.[105]

A. Ethical Considerations

Experience with court-ordered obstetrical interventions has led to a consensus that coerced surgery to save the fetus (as in the Angela Carder case) is ethically and legally indefensible, because of the degree of violation of bodily integrity and respect for the autonomy of a competent decision maker. This consensus extends to the situation of a competent, dying, pregnant woman who refuses surgery. Clini-

cians who are in such a situation should regard her as the only decision maker with moral standing to consent to or refuse surgery.[106] If the patient is incapable of decision making and has left no prior instructions regarding her preferences in these circumstances, then the criterion of substituted judgment should prevail (see Chapters 5 and 9). McCullough and Chervenak argue that well-documented and complete placenta previa is the one clinical situation in which court-ordered cesarean section would be ethically justified.[107] Placental previa is a truly life-threatening situation for the woman, and the chance that the fetus would survive vaginal delivery is very small.

Pregnant patients with human immunodeficiency virus (HIV) infection have an incurable disease that is transmissible to the fetus, which can be effectively prevented in a majority of cases by early treatment with AZT (zidovudine).[108] The benefits of AZT to the fetus and the need to know whether the pregnant patient has antibodies to HIV have created advocates for mandatory testing in pregnancy, which would put great pressure on women to accept AZT therapy.[109] Bayer argues against mandatory testing because it violates the rights to privacy and self-determination, and because he believes that it will lead to mandatory treatment.[110] Although controversy still exists because of duties to infants and children, an important theme in the ethics literature is to respect the self-determination of pregnant patients who have HIV equally with any other patient--pregnant or not.[111] Pregnancy is not a pretext for forgoing one's rights or self-respect. In our view, if the woman is pregnant, at high risk for HIV infection, and untested, directive advice to be tested is justified by the woman's interests and most certainly by the future child's interests.

B. Professional Statements

The ACOG recommends the following regarding treatment and counseling of HIV-infected women: "An individual woman's reproductive choices should be respected regardless of her HIV status. In discussing options for contraception and childbearing, the physician should make the woman aware of the implications of her infection for a child and of the potential effects of pregnancy on her own health. If the woman is pregnant, she should be provided with the information needed to decide whether to continue her pregnancy."[112]

C. Legal Landscape

Many state "living-will" statutes include pregnancy exceptions that prevent women from directing, in advance, that life-sustaining treatment be stopped while they are pregnant or while they are carrying a viable fetus. However, some commentators have forcefully argued that such exceptions are unconstitutional.[113] To date, procreative choices by HIV-infected women are not regulated by statute; however, some states are developing "springing guardianships" that would permit HIV-infected mothers to give up child custody temporarily while they are ill, and regain custody when they are physically able.

VIII. Conclusion

A. Preventive Planning

Several of the issues discussed above are amenable to "preventive ethics" or a "plan-of-care" approach. Some examples illustrate this point.

- *Develop a plan of care.* In the case of AB, the pediatric surgeon was advised to work with the pediatrician to help the grandmother develop a plan to prevent pregnancy within an overall plan of care for the granddaughter.
- *Prepare institutional policy statements.* Prenatal diagnosis centers can prepare policy statements outlining any conditions for which services will not be provided, such as requests for sex selection or reasons that do not concern the health of the fetus. Such reasons include paternity testing and HLA testing for compatibility as a bone marrow or organ donor. Such policy positions are needed now and in the future, as envisioned in the hypothetical case of the deaf couple. The choices available should be discussed in advance, and caregivers and patients with individual moral compunctions about abortions should be realistic about what alternatives are available for various conditions revealed by prenatal diagnostic tests.
- *Encourage patients to complete advance directives.* Women like Angela Carder who have life-

threatening illnesses can be encouraged to complete advance directives before their capacity is questioned; planning can reduce ethical uncertainty about decisions at the end of life. Testing for preexisting conditions allows even more time than prenatal testing for women with chronic or terminal illnesses to make reproductive decisions.

- *Use informed consent, negotiation, and respectful persuasion.* Chervenak and McCullough proposed three strategies for preventive ethics in cases of drug abuse during pregnancy: the use of informed consent as an ongoing dialogue with the pregnant woman, negotiation, and respectful persuasion.[114]
- *Follow professional guidelines.* The Tennessee Supreme Court, which decided *Davis v. Davis*, laid out guidelines to obtain advanced informed consent for preventing irresolvable disputes about disposition of unused and frozen preembryos. The options include donating the embryos to other infertile couples, donating them for research, or destroying them. The American Fertility Society had developed similar guidelines long before the Davis conflict gave rise to a legal dispute.[115] If the physician who served the couple had followed these existing professional guidelines, a legal case would probably have been prevented and the consent document respected (even though there was conflict between the spouses). It is likely that the Tennessee court's suggestions will encourage couples and fertility centers to plan ahead when practicing IVF and freezing embryos.

B. A Multitude of Values

Clinicians are well advised to approach moral problems in reproductive choices with respect for a multitude of values that are unlikely ever to fit into a coherent and consistent whole. Daniel Callahan identified many of these values: respect for an individual's right to life; protection of the weak and powerless; the legitimacy of writing moral convictions and principles into law; the legitimacy of accepting accidents and mischance as a part of life; the obligation on the part of the community to provide support for women who suffer unwanted pregnancies; the value of upholding moral ideals even at the cost of individual difficulties and travail; freedom of choice; the principle that those who must personally bear the burden of their moral choices ought to have the right to make those choices; the enfranchisement of women in controlling their own destinies; freedom to procreate without control from the state; the value of adapting to a world that no longer needs, nor can afford, unlimited childbearing; and the injustice of *de facto* discrimination in favor of the affluent and powerful when reproductive decisions prove costly.[116]

IX. Cases for Further Study

Case 1: The Case of Baby M

William and Elizabeth Stern were a childless couple who desired to have a child. Mary Beth Whitehead responded to an advertisement by the Infertility Center of New York, was quickly approved, and became pregnant by artificial insemination with William Stern's semen. She was to earn $10,000 on the day she delivered a baby to the Sterns. If she miscarried, she would have earned a nominal fee.

Immediately after the birth of the baby girl, Mrs. Whitehead became distraught at the thought of giving her up. She convinced the Sterns to let her have the baby for a few days, and then fled to Florida, where she remained despite a court order directing her to deliver the baby into the custody of Mr. Stern. The baby lived with Mrs. Whitehead for four months until Mr. Stern regained temporary custody of the child. Baby M then lived with the Sterns for 8 months while a trial went on in Hackensack [New Jersey] to determine whether the surrogacy contract signed by the Whiteheads and the Sterns was enforceable.

On March 31, 1987, the judge issued a 120-page ruling in which he awarded permanent custody to Mr Stern. Further, he permanently canceled Mrs. Whitehead's visitation privileges, terminated her parental rights, and processed Mrs. Stern's petition for adoption. The court based its ruling both on the enforceability of the underlying surrogacy contract, and upon a finding that it was in the best interests of the child to live with the Sterns.

On February 3, 1988, the New Jersey Supreme court reversed the trial court, finding that the surrogacy contract violated New Jersey law concerning babyselling, adoption, and termination of parental rights. The court voided Mrs. Stern's adoption proceeding, reinstated Mrs. Whitehead's status as legal mother of the child, but upheld the trial court's order (based on the best interests of the child) to award custody to the Sterns, with visitation privileges to be worked out by the families and the trial courts.

[Source: U.S. Congress, Office of Technology Assessment, *Infertility: Medical and Social Choices*, OTA-BA-358 (Washington, DC: U.S. Government Printing Office, May 1988), 268.]

Case 2: Case of Ms. W

Ms. W is a 19-year-old, unmarried woman who is pregnant for the third time. She had an abortion when she was 15; and she has a 10-month-old daughter. She was admitted to the hospital in the 26th or 27th week of gestation and placed on intravenous medications (magnesium sulfate) to stop her preterm labor. Two days later, Ms. W asked her physician, Dr. C, to discontinue the medications because she was "tired of being in the hospital and the medications and the fetus were too painful and uncomfortable." Dr. C explained that the potential risks of premature delivery included respiratory immaturity, intraventricular hemorrhage, neurologic handicaps, and even fetal death. He advised her to continue the medications for two or three more weeks to give the fetus more time to mature. These critical weeks would enhance the fetus's chances of survival (from 50 percent at 26 weeks of gestation to 90 percent at 30 weeks of gestation) and decrease morbidity, reducing the risk of chronic lung disease (from 50 percent at 26 weeks' to 20 percent at 30 weeks' gestation) and neurologic handicaps later on in life.

Ms. W continued to refuse treatment, and a psychiatric consultation was obtained. The consultant found Ms. W to be extremely immature, emotionally labile, and unrealistic, with a very poor social situation. She had been battered by family members. She sometimes had suicidal ideas. She had used illegal drugs in the past, but not recently. She was diagnosed with a long-standing personality disorder. Meanwhile, she continued to refuse the medication to stop labor and threatened to leave the hospital.

Dr. C contemplates three options: (1) to respect Ms. W's wishes and risk delivering a very premature fetus who might expire or might survive with handicaps secondary to prematurity and its complications; (2) to refuse to abide by her wishes, but transfer care to a physician who is willing to do so; (3) to refuse to abide by her wishes and try to obtain a court order to force Ms. W to undergo treatment.

[Source: Ethics Consultation Service, University of Virginia.]

Case 3: *Curlender v. Bio-Science Laboratories*

The plaintiff, Sauna Tamar Curlender, was born with Tay-Sachs disease. Her parents had previously retained the laboratory named as defendant to administer tests to determine whether they were carriers for Tay-Sachs disease. The tests were reported to have been negative. The parents relied on these tests. Because of the alleged negligence in the laboratory's performance, they had a child with Tay-Sachs disease, subject to severe suffering and a life expectancy of approximately four years.

The child's lawsuit for "wrongful life" brought damages for emotional distress and the deprivation of 72.6 years of life. She sought an additional $3 million in punitive damages on the grounds that the defendants knew their testing procedures were likely to produce a substantial number of false-negatives and yet proceeded to use them "in conscious disregard of the health, safety, and well-being of the plaintiff. . . ." The court could not determine whether the parents relied upon the test to conceive a child or to forego amniocentesis, nor did the court seem to care.

The court first distinguished between this case and others that had been brought by illegitimate children for "wrongful life" against their fathers. The latter suits had been denied, and the court pointed to the injury of a severe genetic disease as contrasted with the injury of illegitimacy. Second, the court noted a trend in the law to recognize that there should be recovery when an infant is born defective and "its painful existence is a direct and proximate result of negligence by others." Third, the court observed that children have continued to sue for wrongful life because of the seriousness of the wrong, the increasing understanding of its causes, and "the understanding that the law reflects, perhaps later than sooner, basic changes in the way society views such matters."

The case reportedly was settled for $1.6 million, but the court denied recovery based on a 70-year life expectancy.

[Source: S. Elias and G.J. Annas, *Reproductive Genetics and the Law* (Chicago: Year Book Medical Publishers, 1987), 115-16; used with permission]

X. Study Questions

1. Many ethical issues in human reproduction turn on the question of the moral status of the embryo and developing fetus in relation to the scope of a competent woman's or parents' autonomous choices. Under what circumstances can a woman's or parents' choices be limited? Taking a clear position on this question is one important "baseline" from which to examine various conflicts that occur between men and women, fetus and pregnant woman, and clinicians and pregnant women. What position do you hold and why?

2. If a criminal offender agrees to sterilization as a term of sentencing, should healthcare professionals participate in the sterilization? If chemical "castration" by administering hormones can reduce sex crimes, should child molesters have the option of choosing this procedure as punishment instead of serving time?

3. What is your opinion of the bill introduced into the Washington State legislature in 1992, permitting involuntary insertion of Norplant in mothers who have given birth to a child with fetal alcohol syndrome?

4. Consider the case, "Why Not Two to One?" in the abortion section. What do you think of the ethics consultants' advice? What is your opinion of the physician's reasoning that there is no morally relevant difference between first-trimester abortion and selected termination of a twin fetus?

5. Discuss the New Jersey Supreme Court's decision in Case 1, "The Case of Baby M." Do you agree or disagree with it? What do you think would be the best legal opinion?

6. What is your response to the case, "A Deaf Couple Wants a Child"? What ethical position would you take and why?

Notes

1. L. Speroff and P. Darney, *A Clinical Guide for Contraception* (Baltimore, Md.: Williams & Wilkins, 1992), 8.

2. P.R. Reilly, *The Surgical Solution: A History of Involuntary Sterilization in the United States* (Baltimore: Johns Hopkins University Press, 1991), 158.

3. Ethics Consultation Service, University of Virginia

4. R. Macklin and W. Gaylin, eds., *Mental Retardation and Sterilization: A Problem of Competency and Paternalism* (Hastings-on-Hudson, N.Y.: Hastings Center, 1981).

5. C.E. Curran, "II. Fertility Control: Ethical Issues," in W.T. Reich, ed., *Encyclopedia of Bioethics*, 2nd ed. (New York: Simon & Schuster Macmillan, 1995), 832-39.

6. See note 2 above, p. 158.

7. M. Haller, *Hereditarian Attitudes in American*

Thought (New Brunswick, N.J.: Rutgers University Press, 1963).

8. In 1981, a Texas legislator asked his constituency whether women on welfare who had at least three children should be sterilized. The majority voted in favor of making welfare benefits conditional upon sterilization, *Texas Observer*, 20 March 1981. About 20 percent of respondents to a telephone poll conducted by the *Boston Globe* in 1982 were in favor of involuntary sterilization of mentally ill individuals, *Boston Globe*, 31 March 1982.

9. American College of Obstetricians and Gynecologists, Committee on Ethics, #63 *Sterilization of Women Who are Mentally Handicapped*, (Washington, D.C.: ACOG, 1988); American College of Obstetricians and Gynecologists, Committee on Ethics, #73 *Ethical Issues in Sterilization* (Washington, D.C.: ACOG, 1989).

10. See note 9 above, *Sterilization of Women*, p. 2.

11. See note 9 above, *Ethical Issues in Sterilization*, p. 1

12. For a good discussion of the legal and ethical issues in medical decisions related to sexual activity in minors see, A. Holder, *Legal Issues in Pediatrics and Adolescent Medicine*, 2nd ed. (New Haven, Conn.: Yale University Press, 1985), 267-93.

13. *Buck v. Bell*, 274 U.S. 200 (1927).

14. *Skinner v. Oklahoma*, 316 U.S. 535 (1942).

15. See note 2 above, p. 148.

16. "Alabama: A Well-Meaning Act," *Newsweek*, 16 July 1973, 30-31; *Relf v. Weinberger*, 372 F. Supp 1196 (D.C. Dist. 1974), 565 F.2d 722 (D.C. Cir. 1977).

17. 42 *Code of Federal Regulations* 50.202.

18. See note 2 above, p. 148.

19. Ibid. (These states are Arkansas, Colorado, Connecticut, Delaware, Georgia, Idaho, Kentucky, Maine, Minnesota, Mississippi, Montana, North Carolina, Oklahoma, Oregon, South Carolina, Utah, Vermont, Virginia, and West Virginia).

20. N.N. Dubler and A. White, "IV. Fertility Control: Legal and Regulatory Issues," in W.T. Reich, ed. *Encyclopedia of Bioethics*, 2nd ed. (New York: Simon & Schuster Macmillan, 1995), 839-47.

21. "At Issue: Castration for Sex Offenders?" *American Bar Association Journal* 78 (July 1992): 42.

22. C.M. Coyle, "Sterilization: A 'Remedy for the Malady' of Child Abuse?" *Journal of Contemporary Health Law & Policy* 5 (1990): 245.

23. L.D. McQuay, "The Case for Castration, Part I," *Washington Monthly* 26, no. 5 (1996): 26-28; F.S. Berlin, "The Case for Castration, Part II," *Washington Monthly* 26, no. 5 (1996): 28-30.

24. C.L. Annas, "Irreversible Error: The Power and Prejudice of Female Genital Mutilation," *Journal of Contemporary Health Law & Policy* 12, no. 2 (1996): 325-53; N. Toubia, "Female Genital Mutilation and the Responsibility of Reproductive Health Professionals," *International Journal of Obstetrics and Gynecology* 46, no. 2 (1994): 127-35.

25. R.L. Schwartz, "Multiculturalism, Medicine and the Limits of Autonomy," *Cambridge Quarterly of Health Care Ethics* 3, no. 3 (1994): 431-39; E. Winkel, "A Muslim Perspective on Female Circumcision," *Women & Health* 23, no. 1 (1995): 1-7. An interesting aspect of the discussion is the analogy with male circumcision, which is not practiced by 80 percent of the world's population, but is well accepted in some industrialized nations. For a criticism of this practice, see E. Wallerstein, *Circumcision: An American Health Fallacy* (New York: Springer Publishing, 1980). For discussion of cultural differences and ethical arguments, see L.M. Kopelman, "Female Circumcision/Genital Mutilation and Ethical Relativism," *Second Opinion* 20, no. 2 (1994): 55-71; O.A. Koso-Thomas, "I. Female Circumcision," in W.T. Reich, ed., *Encyclopedia of Bioethics*, 2nd ed. (New York: Simon & Schuster Macmillan, 1995), 382-87.

26. *In re Oluloro*, Portland, Oregon, Immigration Court, No. A72 147 491 (March 23, 1994) (oral discussion). The case is described in Annas, see note 24 above. For discussion of female circumcision in the context of public health, see N. Toubia, "Female Circumcision as a Public Health Issue," *New England Journal of Medicine* 331, no. 11 (1994): 712-16.

27. Council on Scientific Affairs, American Medical Association, "Female Genital Mutilation," *Journal of the American Medical Association* 274, no. 21 (1995): 1714-16.

28. Female Genital Mutilation Act of 1993, H.R. 3247. See also P. Schroeder, "Female Genital Mutilation: A Form of Child Abuse," *New England Journal of Medicine* 331, no. 11 (1994): 739-40.

29. A.M. Rosenthal, "A Victory in Cairo," *New York Times*, 6 September 1994, A19.

30. M. Policar, "I. Fertility Control: Medical Aspects," in W.T. Reich, ed., *Encyclopedia of Bioethics*, 2nd ed. (New York: Simon & Schuster Macmillan, 1995), 818-27; C. Joffe, "II. Fertility Control: Social Issues," in W.T. Reich, ed. *Encyclopedia of Bioethics*, 2nd ed., (New York: Simon & Schuster Macmillan, 1995), 828-31.

31. M. Potts, "Birth Control Methods in the United States," *Family Planning Perspectives* 20 (1988): 288,

cited in Speroff and Darney (see note 1 above, p. 12). Potts argues that the limited choices of contraceptives cause both the high rates of unintended pregnancies in the United States (estimated at 50 percent of all pregnancies) and the high rates of abortion (estimated at 50 percent of all unintended pregnancies). Also see C.F. Westoff, "Unintended Pregnancy in America and Abroad," *Family Planning Perspectives* 20 (1988): 254.

32. *People v. Zaring*, 8 Cal. App. 4th 362, 10 Cal. Rptr. 2d 263 (1992).

33. H.B. 2909, 52nd Leg., Washington (1992); S. 5249, 53rd Leg., Washington (1993).

34. A. Glasier et al., "Mifepristone (RU-486) Compared with High-Dose Estrogen and Progestogen for Emergency Postcoital Contraception," *New England Journal of Medicine* 327, no. 15 (1992): 1041-44.

35. W. Regelson, "RU-486: How Abortion Politics Has Impacted on a Potentially Useful Drug of Broad Medical Application," *Perspectives in Biology and Medicine* 35, no. 3 (1992): 330-39.

36. J. Palca, "The Pill of Choice," *Science* 245 (1989): 1319-23.

37. L.S. Cahill, "Abortion Pill RU-486: Ethics, Rhetoric, and Social Practice," *Hastings Center Report* 17, no. 5 (1987): 5-8.

38. K. Gervais and S. Miles, *RU-486: New Issues in the American Abortion Debate* (Minneapolis, Minn.: Center for Biomedical Ethics, 1990), 25-39; C. Holden, "Update: RU-486," *Science* 248 (20 April 1990): 306.

39. See note 38 above, Gervais and Miles, pp. 25-26.

40. See note 14 above.

41. *Griswold v. Connecticut*, 381 U.S. 479 (1965); *Eisenstadt v. Baird*, 405 U.S. 438 (1972).

42. *Roe v. Wade*, 410 U.S. 113 (1973).

43. M.V. Rorty and J. Pinkerton, "Fetal Reduction: The Ultimate Elective Surgery," *Journal of Contemporary Health Law & Policy* 13, no. 1 (1997): 53-77.

44. The range of views are presented fairly in W.T. Reich, ed., *Encyclopedia of Bioethics*, 2nd ed. (New York: Simon & Schuster Macmillan, 1995) by R. Macklin, "Contemporary Ethical Perspectives," 6-16; D.M. Feldman, "Jewish Perspectives," 26-30; L.S. Cahill, "Roman Catholic Perspectives," 30-34; B.W. Harrison, "Protestant Perspectives," 34-38; O. Bakar, "Islamic Perspectives," 38-42.

45. University of Chicago, National Opinion Research Center, *General Social Surveys 1972-1995: Cumulative Codebook* (Chicago: National Opinion Research Center, 1995).

46. D.C. Wertz and J.C. Fletcher, "Fatal Knowl-

edge? Prenatal Diagnosis and Sex Selection," *Hastings Center Report* 19, no. 3 (1989): 21-27.

47. B. Spielman, "*Rust v. Sullivan*: Legal Issues and Ethical Concerns," *Women's Health Issues* 1, no. 4 (1991): 172-79.

48. A.R. Holder and M.S. Henifin, "Case Studies--Selective Termination of Pregnancy," *Hastings Center Report* 18, no. 1 (February/March 1988): 21.

49. J. LaPuma et al., "A Perinatal Ethics Committee on Abortion: Process and Outcome in Thirty-One Cases," *The Journal of Clinical Ethics* 3, no. 3 (1992): 196-203; H. Rodman, "The Microethics and Macroethics of Hospital Abortion Committees," *The Journal of Clinical Ethics* 3, no. 3 (1992): 234-38; J.F. Drane, "Abortion: Doomed Only to an Immoderate Response?" *The Journal of Clinical Ethics* 3, no. 3 (1992): 238-40; J. Edelwich, "Commentary on 'A Perinatal Ethics Committee on Abortion,' " *The Journal of Clinical Ethics* 3, no. 3 (1992): 240-41.

50. M.I. Evans et al., "International, Collaborative Experience of 1789 Patients Having Multifetal Pregnancy Reduction: A Plateauing of Risks and Outcomes," *Journal of the Society for Gynecologic Investigation* 3, no. 1 (1996): 23-26. This up-to-date report states that the overall loss rate was 11.7 percent; the rates varied from a low of 7.6 percent for triplets to twins and increased with each additional starting number of fetuses to 22.9 percent for sextuplets or higher. Loss rates by finishing numbers of remaining fetuses were lowest for twins. This study did not report on reduction of twins to one.

51. This case was contributed by Kenneth N. Scissors, M.D., chairman of the Bioethics Program, Emanual Hospital, Portland, Oreg. This case was considered by the ethics committee of this program.

52. American College of Obstetrics and Gynecology, *Statement of Policy: Further Ethical Consideration in Induced Abortion* (Washington, D.C.: ACOG, 1977).

53. American College of Obstetrics and Gynecology, Committee on Ethics, *Multifetal Pregnancy Reduction and Selective Fetal Termination* (Washington, D.C.: ACOG, 1991).

54. See note 42 above.

55. *Planned Parenthood Association of Southeastern Pennsylvania v. Casey*, 112 S.Ct. 2791 (1992).

56. The Hyde Amendment, named for its sponsor Henry Hyde (R.-Ill.), limits federal funding only to cases where two physicians attest that continuation of the pregnancy will result in severe and long-lasting damage to the woman's physical health, and in cases of reported rape and incest. The language of the original amend-

ment is found in *Congressional Record* 122 (24 June 1976): 20410. The Family Planning Services and Population Research Act of 1970 (Public Law No. 91-572, 84 Stat. 1504 [19070]) prohibited research on abortion as a method of birth control. In the Health Extension Act of 1985 (Public Law No. 99-158, 99 Stat. 820 [1985]), Congress prohibited fetal research in the context of abortion that added any risk to the fetus.

57. A. Allen, "II. Abortion, Contemporary Ethical and Legal Aspects: B. Legal and Regulatory Issues," in W.T. Reich, ed., *Encyclopedia of Bioethics*, 2nd ed., (New York: Simon & Schuster Macmillan, 1995), 16-26.

58. Case appears as "When Baby's Mother Is also Grandma--and Sister," *Hastings Center Report* 15, no. 5 (October 1985): 29.

59. P. Lauritzen. "What Price Parenthood?" *Hastings Center Report* 20, no. 2 (March/April 1990): 38-45.

60. B.K. Rothman, *Recreating Motherhood* (New York: W.W. Norton, 1989).

61. G.J. Annas, "The Baby Broker Boom," *Hastings Center Report* 16, no. 3 (1986): 30-34.

62. J.G. Raymond, "Reproductive Gifts and Gift Giving: The Altruistic Woman," *Hastings Center Report* 20, no. 6 (1990): 7-10.

63. D. Wikler and N.J. Wikler. "Turkey-Baster Babies: The Demedicalization of Artificial Insemination," *Milbank Quarterly* 69, no. 1 (1991): 5-35.

64. G.J. Annas, "Using Genes to Define Motherhood--The California Solution," *New England Journal of Medicine* 326, no. 6 (1992): 417-20.

65. See note 59 above.

66. G.J. Annas, "Redefining Parenthood and Protecting Embryos: Why We Need New Laws," *Hastings Center Report* 14, no. 5 (1984): 50-54.

67. A.L. Bonnicksen, "Embryo Freezing: Ethical Issues in the Clinical Setting," *Hastings Center Report* 18, no. 6 (1988): 26-29; in Great Britain on 1 August 1996, more than 10,000 frozen embryos had to be destroyed because the legal limit of five years in storage imposed by a 1991 law had passed. See P.R. Brinsden et al., "Frozen Embryos: Decision Time in the U.K.," *Human Reproduction* 10, no. 12 (1995): 3083-84.

68. American College of Obstetrics and Gynecology, Committee on Ethics, *Ethical Issues in Human In Vitro Fertilization and Embryo Placement* (Washington, D.C.: ACOG, 1986).

69. American College of Obstetrics and Gynecology, *Ethical Issues in Surrogate Motherhood* (Washington, D.C.: ACOG, 1990).

70. J.C. Fletcher, "Human Fetal and Embryo Research: Lysenkoism in Reverse--How and Why?" in R.H. Blank and A.L. Bonnicksen, eds., *Emerging Issues in Biomedical Policy: An Annual Review*, vol. 2 (New York: Columbia University Press, 1993), 200-31.

71. NIH Revitalization Act of 1993, Public Law 103-43. This law nullified the requirement that all IVF research had to be reviewed by an ethics advisory board and opened the way for the NIH to receive proposals.

72. G.J. Annas, A. Caplan, and S. Elias, "The Politics of Human-Embryo Research--Avoiding Ethical Gridlock," *New England Journal of Medicine* 334, no. 20 (1996): 1329-32.

73. J.C. Fletcher, "U.S. Public Policy on Embryo Research: Two Steps Forward, One Large Step Back," *Human Reproduction* 10, no. 7 (1995): 1875-78.

74. *In re Baby M*, 109 N.J. 396, 537 A.2d 1227 (1988); *Davis v. Davis*, 842 S.W.2d 588 (Tenn. 1992).

75. M. Schwartz, "Pregnant Woman versus Fetus: A Dilemma for Hospital Ethics Committees," *Cambridge Quarterly of Health Care Ethics* 1, no. 1 (1987): 51-62. See also C.R. Daniels, *At Women's Expense: State Power and the Politics of Fetal Rights* (Cambridge, Mass.: Harvard University Press, 1993).

76. P.H. Jos, M.F. Marshall, and M. Perlmutter, "The Charleston Policy on Cocaine Use During Pregnancy: A Cautionary Tale," *Journal of Law, Medicine & Ethics* 23 (1995): 120-28.

77. *Ferguson and Roe et al. v. City of Charleston et al.*, No. 2-93-26242-2 (D.S.C. filed 5 October 1993).

78. L.J. Nelson and N. Milliken, "Compelled Medical Treatment of Pregnant Women," *Journal of the American Medical Association* 259, no. 7 (1988): 1060-66; D. Brown, H.F. Andersen, and T.E. Elkins, "An Analysis of the ACOG and AAP Ethics Statements on Conflict in Maternal-Fetal Care," *The Journal of Clinical Ethics* 2, no. 1 (1991): 19-22; F.A. Chervenak and L.B. McCullough, "Inadequacies with the ACOG and AAP Statements on Managing Ethical Conflict During the Intrapartum Period," *The Journal of Clinical Ethics* 2, no. 1 (1991): 23-24; S.S. Mattingly, "The Maternal-Fetal Dyad: Exploring the Two-Patient Obstetric Model," *Hastings Center Report* 22, no. 1 (January-February 1992): 13-17.

79. V.E. Kolder, J. Gallagher, and M.T. Parsons, "Court-Ordered Obstetrical Interventions," *New England Journal of Medicine* 316, no. 19 (1987): 1192-96; J.A. Robertson and J.D. Schulman, "Pregnancy and Prenatal Harm to Offspring: The Case of Mothers with PKU," *Hastings Center Report* 17, no. 4 (1987): 23-26; D. Johnsen, "A New Threat to Pregnant Women's Au-

tonomy," *Hastings Center Report* 17, no. 4 (1987): 33-37.

80. J.D. Pinkerton and J. Finnerty, "Resolving the Clinical and Ethical Dilemmas Involved in Fetal-Maternal Conflicts," *American Journal of Obstetrics and Gynecology* 175, no. 2 (1996): 289-95.

81. H.L. Nelson, "Paternal-Fetal Conflict," *Hastings Center Report* 22, no. 2 (March-April 1992): 3.

82. N.K. Rhoden, "Cesareans and Samaritans," *Law, Medicine & Health Care* 15 (1987): 118-25.

83. See note 79 above, Robertson, p. 30.

84. American College of Obstetrics and Gynecology, *Patient Choice: Maternal-Fetal Conflict* (Washington, D.C., ACOG, 1987).

85. T.E. Elkins et al., "Maternal-Fetal Conflict: A Study of Court-Ordered Cesarean Sections," *The Journal of Clinical Ethics* 1, no. 4 (1990): 316.

86. American Medical Association, Board of Trustees, "Legal Interventions During Pregnancy," *Journal of the American Medical Association* 264 (1990): 2663-64.

87. *Jefferson v. Griffin Spalding County Hospital Authority*, 247 Ga. 86, 274 S.E.2d 457 (Sup. Ct. 1981).

88. See notes 78 and 79 above. Also a District of Columbia court (*In re Madyun*) ordered cesarean delivery over the religious objections of a Muslim woman, when her labor failed to progress 60 hours after her membranes ruptured. The case is described in C. Gorney, "Whose Baby Is It, Anyway?" *Washington Post*, 13 December 1988, D-1.

89. The Angela Carder case is reported in G.J. Annas, "She's Going to Die: The Case of Angela C.," *Hastings Center Report* 18, no. 1 (1988): 23-25. For discussion of the appeals court reversal, see G.J. Annas, "At Law-Foreclosing the Use of Force: A.C. Reversed," *Hastings Center Report* 20, no. 4 (July-August 1990): 27-29, also see L. Greenhouse, "Appeals Court Vacates Forced-Caesarean Ruling," *New York Times*, 22 March 1988, A4.

90. In re *Baby Boy Doe v. Mother Doe*, 632 N.E.2d 326 (Ill. App, 1st Dist. 1994).

91. M.I. Evans, ed., *Reproductive Risks and Prenatal Diagnosis* (Norwalk, Conn.: Appleton & Lange, 1992).

92. A.H. Handyside et al., "Birth of a Normal Girl after in Vitro Fertilization and Preimplantation Diagnostic Testing for Cystic Fibrosis," *New England Journal of Medicine* 327, no. 13 (1992): 905-09.

93. J.C. Fletcher and G. Richter, "Human Fetal Gene Therapy: Moral and Ethical Questions," *Human Gene Therapy* 7, no. 13 (1996): 1605-14.

94. J. Yankowitz and C. Weiner, "Medical Fetal Therapy," *Ballieres Clinical Obstetrics and Gynaecology* 9, no. 3 (1995): 553-70; F. Luks, "Fetal Surgery," *Ballieres Clinical Obstetrics and Gynaecology* 9, no. 3 (1995): 571-77.

95. N.E. Adler, S. Keyes, and P. Robertson, "Psychological Issues in New Reproductive Technologies: Pregnancy-Inducing Technology and Diagnostic Screening," in J. Rodin and A. Collins, eds., *Women and New Reproductive Technologies: Medical, Psychosocial, Legal, and Ethical Dilemmas* (Hillsdale, N.J.: Lawrence Erlbaum, 1991), 111-31.

96. D.C. Wertz et al., "Attitudes toward Abortion among Parents of Children with Cystic Fibrosis," *American Journal of Public Health* 81, no. 8 (1991): 992-98.

97. This case, contributed by Dr. Walter Nance, chair of the Department of Genetics at the Medical College of Virginia, is hypothetical. However, Nance says, "Based on my genetic counseling with several hearing-impaired couples, the ethical questions are already being asked." Namely, should geneticists help deaf couples to have a deaf rather than a hearing child?

98. See note 46 above.

99. President's Commission for the Study of Ethical Problems in Medicine and Biomedical and Behavioral Research, *Screening and Counseling for Genetic Conditions* (Washington, D.C.: U.S. Government Printing Office, 1983), 44.

100. T.M. Powledge and J.C. Fletcher, "Guidelines for the Ethical, Social, and Legal Issues in Prenatal Diagnosis," *New England Journal of Medicine* 300 (1979): 168-73.

101. J.C. Fletcher et. al, "Ethical, Legal, and Societal Considerations of Prenatal Diagnosis," in J.L. Hamerton and N.E. Simpson, ed., "Prenatal Diagnosis: Past, Present and Future," *Prenatal Diagnosis* (special issue) (1980): 43; "Empfehlung der Ethikkommission der Gellschaft fur Anthropologie und Humangenetik" ("Against the Disclosure of Fetal Sex before the 14th Week of Gestation"), in J. Murken, *Pranatale Diagnostik und Therapie* (Stuttgart, Germany: Ferdinand Enke Verlag, 1987), 321; Danish Council of Ethics, *Fetal Diagnosis and Ethics: A Report* (Copenhagen, Denmark: Clausen Offset, 1991), 58; Z. Bankowski and A.M. Capron, ed., *Genetics, Ethics, and Human Values*, Reports of the Working Groups, 24th Council of International Organizations of Medical Sciences, Roundtable Conference (Geneva, Switzerland: World Health Organization, CIOMS, 1991), 178.

102. L.B. Andrews et al., ed., *Assessing Genetic Risks* (Washington, D.C.: National Academy Press,

1994), 8.

103. G.J. Annas, *Judging Medicine* (Clifton, N.J.: Humana Press, 1988).

104. *Curlender v. Bio-Science Laboratories*, 106 Cal. App.3d 811, 165 Cal. Rptr. 477 (1980).

105. Gail Povar, M.D., chair of the committee, stated that the ethics committee had not yet been authorized to do consultations and was not in a legitimate position to be consulted (personal communication, 14 April 1994).

106. See note 89 above.

107. L.B. McCullough and F.A. Chervenak, *Ethics in Obstetrics and Gynecology* (New York: Oxford University Press, 1994), 248-53.

108. E.M. Connor et. al, "Reduction of Maternal-Infant Transmission of HIV-1 with Zidovudine Treatment," *New England Journal of Medicine* 331, no. 18 (1994): 1173-80.

109. C.A. Hoffman and R. Munson, "Ethical Issues in the Use of Zidovudine to Reduce Vertical Transmission," *New England Journal of Medicine* 332, no. 13 (1995): 891-92.

110. R. Bayer, "Ethical Challenges Posed by Zidovudine Treatment to Reduce Vertical Transmission of HIV," *New England Journal of Medicine* 331, no. 18 (1994): 1223-25; R. Bayer, "Ethical Issues in the Use of Zidovudine to Reduce Vertical Transmission," *New England Journal of Medicine* 332, no. 13 (1995): 892.

111. L. Walters, "Ethical Issues in HIV Testing in Pregnancy," in R. Faden, G. Geller, and M. Powers, ed., *AIDS, Women and the Next Generation* (New York: Oxford University Press, 1991), 274-87; J.D. Arras, "HIV and Childbearing: AIDS and Reproductive Decisions: Having Children in Fear and Trembling," *Milbank Quarterly* 68 (1990): 353-82.

112. American College of Obstetrics and Gynecology, Committee on Ethics, *Human Immunodeficiency Virus Infection: Physicians' Responsibilities* (Washington, D.C.: ACOG, 1990).

113. T.J. Burch, "Incubator or Individual? The Legal and Policy Deficiencies of Pregnancy Clauses in Living Will and Advance Health Care Directive Statutes," *Maryland Law Review* 54, no. 2 (1995): 528-70; K.H. Rothenberg, "Feminism, Law, and Bioethics," *Kennedy Institute of Ethics Journal* 6, no. 1 (1996): 69-84.

114. F.A. Chervenak and L.B. McCullough, "Preventive Ethics Strategies for Drug Abuse During Pregnancy," *The Journal of Clinical Ethics* 1, no. 2 (1990): 157-62.

115. American Fertility Society, "Ethical Statement on *In Vitro* Fertilization," *Fertility and Sterility* 41 (1984): 12-17; American Fertility Society, "Minimal Standards for Programs of *In Vitro* Fertilization," *Fertility and Sterility* 41 (1984): 13-18.

116. D. Callahan, "The Abortion Debate: Is Progress Possible?" in S. Callahan and D. Callahan, *Abortion: Understanding Differences* (New York: Plenum Press, 1984), 309-24.

12

PATIENT SELECTION: TRAGIC CHOICES

Mary Faith Marshall, Ph.D.

She and the children were undergoing at this very moment the ordeal she had heard about--rumored in Warsaw a score of times in whispers--but which had seemed at once so unbearable and unlikely to happen to her that she had thrust it out of her mind. But here she was, and here was the doctor. While over there--just beyond the roofs of the boxcars recently vacated by death-bound Malkinia Jews--was Birkenau, and the doctor could select for its abyssal doors anyone whom he desired. . . .

"You may keep one of your children."

"Bitte?" said Sophie.

"You may keep one of your children," he repeated. "The other one will have to go. Which one will you keep?. . ."

Her thought processes dwindled, ceased. Then she felt her legs crumple. "I can't choose! I can't choose! She began to scream." Oh, how she recalled her own screams! Tormented angels never screeched so loudly above hell's pandemonium. *"Ich kann nicht wahlen!"* she screamed.

The doctor was aware of unwanted attention. "Shut up!" he ordered. "Hurry now and choose. Choose, goddamnit, or I'll send them both over there. Quick!"

"Don't make me choose," she heard herself plead in a whisper, "I can't choose."

"Send them both over there, then," the doctor said to the aide, *"nach links."*

"Mama!" she heard Eva's thin but soaring cry at the instant that she thrust the child away from her and rose from the concrete with a clumsy stumbling motion. "Take the baby!" she called out. "Take my little girl!"

At this point the aide--with a careful gentleness that Sophie would try without success to forget--tugged at Eva's hand and led her away into the waiting legion of the damned. She would forever retain a dim impression that the child had continued to look back, beseeching. But because she was now almost completely blinded by salty, thick, copious tears she was spared whatever expression Eva wore, and she was always grateful for that. For in the bleak honesty of her heart she knew that she would never have been able to tolerate it, driven nearly mad as she was by her last glimpse of that vanishing small form.[1]

I. Description of the Problem

According to Joseph Fletcher:

Hegel, in his short essay on logic, reasoned that the headachy business of choosing between one good and another, or obversely between one evil and another, is true tragedy, whereas the simplistic collision of good and evil--black and white--is only melodrama, Sunday School ethics. It is hard for Shakespeare's Othello to decide between his love of Desdemona and Iago's testimony, or for Sophocle's Antigone to choose between her loyalty to her brother and her loyalty to King Creon. So it is with all competing value problems. All serious ethics, as in a socially just healthcare system, deal with tragedy, not with melodrama--with choices between competing values, not with obvious matters of good and evil, right or wrong."[2]

Choosing between persons who are competing for basic healthcare services seems a grossly unfair, if not impossible task. The choice assumes tragic dimensions when life itself hangs in the balance. What moral calculus exists to tip the scale in favor of one person over another? How do we weigh competing claims to life or health? The dilemma faced by William Styron's tragic heroine, Sophie, generates pathos and horror in the reader. There is no right answer, no golden rule, no yardstick or measure to calibrate the tragic elements of the situation.

Although this headachy business of choosing between competing goods or competing evils involves heartache as well, there must be criteria for making a choice when a choice, however unfortunate, has to be made. Whether unconscious or well-reasoned--or motivated by malice, greed, efficacy, or compassion --selection criteria are a necessary preliminary for choosing.

II. Options

There are two fundamental approaches to choosing when the choice is between persons: consequentialism and egalitarianism. Consequentialist principles focus priority on the results or consequences of choices. Consequentialism is outcome-based decision making. One important example of a consequentialist approach often used in emergency medicine is utilitarianism. Utilitarian principles allow for methods of maximizing the greatest good (however interpreted) for the greatest number of persons or of minimizing potential or actual harm for the greatest number. Conversely, egalitarian principles minimize the differences among persons; they frustrate the consideration of individual traits or characteristics in decision making. All persons in need are treated as equals.

The following organizational summary of the major consequentialist and egalitarian principles was formulated by bioethicist Gerald Winslow:[3]

A. Consequentialist Principles

- *The principle of medical success.* Priority is given to those patients for whom treatment has the highest probability of medical success.
- *The principle of immediate usefulness.* Priority is given to the most useful option under the immediate circumstances.
- *The principle of conservation.* Priority is given to those who require proportionately smaller amounts of the resources.
- *The principle of parental role.* Priority is given to those who have the largest responsibilities to dependents.
- *The principle of general social value.* Priority is given to those believed to have the greatest social worth. Valuations of social worth may include prior contributions to society as well as potential contributions.

B. Egalitarian Principles

- *The principle of saving no one.* Priority is given to no one because none should be saved if not all can be saved.
- *The principle of medical neediness.* Priority is given to the medically neediest.
- *The principle of general neediness.* Priority is given to the most helpless or the generally neediest.
- *The principle of queuing.* Priority is given on a first-come, first-served basis.
- *The principle of random selection.* Priority is given to those selected by chance.

Only one of these egalitarian principles is absolute--the principle of saving no one. All of the others might be conjoined in any fashion. For example, in assigning priority to potential organ transplant recipients, a combination of queuing (first-come, first-served as represented by time on the waiting list) and possibility of medical success (as manifested by the closest histocompatibility) might be employed as methods of initial screening and final selection.

Choosing between individuals, deciding who will live and who will die, is both tragic and terrifying. The alternative is not to choose--thereby condemning all to death when not all can live. The following cases, illustrate the respective hazards of choosing and not choosing.

III. Paradigm Cases

A. *United States v. Holmes*

"Lifeboat ethics" cases are frequently used as paradigms for theoretical discussions of rationing dilemmas. The case of *United States v. Holmes* is an often-cited example of the decision-making process used in rationing lifeboat space to shipwreck survivors.

Holmes was a seaman aboard an American ship, the *William Brown*, which, in 1841, sank off of the coast of Newfoundland after striking an iceberg. Half of the passengers and all of the crew escaped aboard two lifeboats. One of the lifeboats, overloaded with survivors, began leaking after twenty-four hours. In order to prevent the vessel from sinking, members of the crew threw fourteen men overboard after solicitations for volunteers proved futile. The crew members' criteria for decision making prohibited the separation of spouses or the sacrifice of women survivors. Two women, sisters of one of the unfortunate fourteen, jumped overboard in company with their brother. Hours later, the survivors (except those thrown overboard) were rescued. Upon returning to Philadelphia, most of the crew disappeared. One crew member, Holmes, who had acted on orders from his mate, was tried for manslaughter. He was convicted of unlawful homicide by a jury, and sentenced to six months' hard labor.[4]

The sentence reflected the jurors' ambivalence about what degree of moral sanction to impose in such a dilemma. Although they convicted Holmes of manslaughter in the deaths of 14 people, the limited duration of the punishment signified a token sanction. In a later case analysis, legal scholar Edmond Cahn advocated not choosing as the proper course of action in such situations: "In a strait of this extremity, all

men are reduced--or raised, as one may choose to denominate it--to members of the genus, mere congeners and nothing else. Truly and literally, all were in the same boat, and thus none could be saved separately from the others. . . . For where all have become congeners, pure and simple, no one can save himself by killing another."[5] Cahn's position is one of absolute egalitarianism. Because he considers all to be equal, no one person can be sacrificed for the good of another.

Many would reject this valuation of pure equality over life. They would consider failing to choose when a choice must be made (which is, in itself a choice), or failing to use well-considered criteria as standards for decision making (as exemplified in the *Von Stetina* case below), a tragedy of equal dimensions as choosing who must live or die.

B. *Von Stetina v. Florida Medical Center*

Susan Von Stetina, a previously healthy 27-year-old woman, was injured in an automobile accident and taken to the emergency room of the Florida Medical Center, Fort Lauderdale, a designated trauma center. Her injuries included a complete transection of the pancreas and a fractured right femur. After the patient underwent a successful pancreatectomy (removal of the pancreas) and placement of leg traction, respiratory distress syndrome developed on the fourth post-trauma day, requiring intubation (insertion of a breathing tube), mechanical ventilation, and pharmacologically induced paralysis for control of ventilation. Over the next 48 hours her condition improved progressively but she remained ventilator dependent. There was objective improvement of the chest X-ray and arterial blood gas findings. During her second day in the intensive care unit [ICU], she was found to be severely bradycardic (slow heart rate) for an unknown period of time with an elevated arterial carbon dioxide partial pressure after 15 minutes of reinstituted artificial ventilation of 85 mm Hg (normal = 35-45 mm Hg). Although cardiopulmonary resuscitation was successful, she never regained consciousness and remains, several years later, in a nursing home with a tracheostomy (permanent breathing tube), gastrostomy (surgically placed abdominal feeding tube), and chronic anoxic brain injury (brain injury due to lack of oxygen), having made an otherwise complete recovery from her traumatic injuries. A lawsuit was filed on behalf of Ms. Von Stetina naming the hospital as the sole defendant. At the trial, evidence was presented indicating the patient had been accidentally disconnected from her ventilator for a prolonged period of time, with alarm systems apparently failing to detect the malevent until bradycardia was signaled on the cardiac monitor. During trial proceedings, the plaintiff presented a detailed analysis of all patients residing in the ICU and further showed that there were only three intensive care nurses (registered nurses) on duty and one licensed practical nurse "floating" from a hospital floor. The event occurred at approximately 3 a.m. At the beginning of the nursing shift, at 11 p.m., there were seven patients in the ICU, which expert testimony stated to be the limit that safely could be cared for by the existing resources. Despite this situation, the hospital continued to admit patients (totaling five additional) to the ICU between the hours of midnight and 6 a.m. The plaintiff presented evidence that the intensive care nurses were too busy with the new admissions arriving from the emergency room to deal adequately with the plaintiff. It was additionally argued that there were at least three other hospitals in the community that could have cared for the newly arriving admissions and that most probably those individuals could have been safely transported to the other facilities. Additional evidence was provided to indicate that one patient already residing within the ICU came close to meeting brain death criteria, and was, in fact, declared dead 36 hours later. Two others were to be electively discharged the following morning. Further evidence indicated that there was no available director of the ICU and that administrative mechanisms for dealing with a patient census out of proportion to the staffing capabilities of the unit were incomplete. Expert testimony was given that the patient required one-to-one nursing care. The jury ruled in favor of the plaintiff and awarded a verdict in the sum of $12,470,000. (The Supreme Court of Florida has subsequently returned the case for retrial because of the $4 million awarded for pain and suffering.)[6]

In this case, the absence of any attempt at patient selection (much less the application of formal patient-selection criteria) resulted in a situation that snowballed out of control. The consequences for Susan Von Stetina were disastrous. The consequences for the ICU staff members and hospital administrators who stood trial were expensive, embarrassing, and psychologically disturbing.

H. Tristram Engelhardt, Jr., and Michael Rie have identified three major problem situations in the allocation of resources in the ICU:

1. when admitting additional patients to the ICU will endanger current ICU patients by decreasing the standard of care delivered;
2. when potential admissions to the ICU appear to have greater possible benefit from ICU care than current ICU patients;
3. when the resources invested in the patient are disproportionate to the anticipated benefits.[7]

Although an ICU served as the setting for this particular case, such problems can and do arise in any healthcare setting.

IV. Procedural Problems

On the national level, an adequate examination of the policy issues surrounding allocation of healthcare resources has been hampered by a number of myths. These include the belief that in an affluent country like the United States the money is available to provide all of the necessary healthcare resources for those who need them. Even if public and political endorsement of funding reallocation from other major programs such as defense and education was possible, healthcare needs would still not be met. Many scarcities are not tied to fiscal restraints. For example, the limited availability of organs for transplant will continue irrespective of financial considerations. Also, technological advancements create their own inherent scarcities. As new drugs and devices are developed, tested, and marketed, their initial availability is limited.

Another myth involves the inefficiency of the healthcare delivery system. Proponents of this myth hold that; if bureaucratic waste and inefficiency were eliminated, there would be no need for rationing healthcare. Financial analysis does not support this argument. In the United States, bureaucratic waste accounts for about one-fifth of the cost of healthcare delivery. Its elimination would not allow for provision of the healthcare needed by the indigent or uninsured. Current organizational adaptions as healthcare institutions struggle for survival within the managed-care environment strain the traditional loyalties and interests of healthcare clinicians. Financial incentives to limit care (coupled with financial rewards for meeting capitation goals) place physicians and other clinicians in positions that they often find antithetical to the fiduciary patient-clinician relationship. Recently, the Joint Commission on Accreditation of Healthcare Organizations has added an organizational ethics component to its patient rights standards. Institutional policies that address organizational ethics should directly address issues such as conflicts of interest, adequate and accurate disclosure of financial data and incentives, and the fiscal relationship between healthcare providers and recipients.

The isolationist notion that our problems would be solved if we could generate a national "fix" for our healthcare system in the United States is naive. The healthcare needs of persons throughout the world have a direct economic, scientific, and medical impact on the healthcare delivery system in the United States. The resurgence of tuberculosis in the United States exemplifies these direct effects.

V. Historical Perspective

Rationing of healthcare services is not a new phenomenon. It is as old as medicine, necessitated by the shortage of resources such as nurses, physicians, drugs, organs, technology, and money. Relatively recent examples of scarce resources that have required rationing in this country include polio vaccine in the 1940s, penicillin in the 1940s and 1950s, and hemodialysis machines in the 1960s.

The development of penicillin is an interesting case study in allocation priorities. The medical historian Chester Keefer relates that in the summer of 1941 there was not enough penicillin in the United States to treat a single person. By the summer of 1942, there was an amount sufficient to treat only 10 patients. In early investigations, researchers were directed to choose test cases that "would yield the maximum information of value to the armed services."[8]

A notorious example of the use of utilitarian principles in patient selection involves the distribution of scarce penicillin supplies to American soldiers in North Africa during World War II. Not long after its discovery, limited amounts of penicillin were made available to American military leaders for the treatment of soldiers in North Africa. Rather than giving it in necessarily large doses to soldiers who were seriously wounded in combat, military leaders assigned priority to thousands of otherwise healthy soldiers who were infected with venereal disease. These men could be treated with smaller doses and restored more quickly to combat readiness.[9]

Rabbi Moses Tendler of Yeshiva University relates a similar distribution problem. In 1950, Rabbi Moshe Feinstein of New York City received an urgent transatlantic call from Rabbi Herzog, the chief Rabbi of Israel. An epidemic of bacterial meningitis had filled a ward of Hadassah Hospital, the largest hospital in the Middle East, with meningitis patients. The limited supply of available penicillin was not sufficient to meet the needs of all. How should this scarce resource be allocated? Rabbi Feinstein's advice was: "Give the first dose to the first patient you come to, the second dose to the second patient, and so on until your supply is gone."[10]

VI. Military Triage

One historical paradigm for patient selection is military triage. Triage (from the French verb *trier*, meaning to pick or sort) involves the most utilitarian (and perhaps the least agonizing) scheme of rationing at the level of the individual patient. The model for modern medical triage systems originated with the military application first accredited to Napoleon's chief surgeon, Baron Dominique Jean Larrey. A master of organization and efficiency, Larrey's priority was to begin surgery as soon after the injury occurred as possible. He devised a system of "ambulances" (a term referring to vehicles and personnel) to transport the wounded from the field. His primary selection criterion was the severity of the patient's injury, not the patient's rank or office (as had previously been the case).

It was not until World War II that battlefield triage efforts reflected more obvious utilitarian concerns by segregating wounded soldiers who needed lifesaving (or limb-saving) surgical intervention from those who merely needed first aid and could return to battle. Soldiers who required little treatment and were still capable of fighting were given priority.

Primary field triage was rendered obsolete during the Vietnam War because helicopters could evacuate all casualties. Patients generally were transported directly to surgical field hospitals, thus bypassing clearing stations. Modern military and civilian triage has become increasingly complex and involves more than "urgency prioritization." Current triage systems include not only types of prehospital transport but also the level of hospital care provided and the manner in which such care is assigned priority.[11]

VII. Principles and Methods

Rationing of healthcare has been defined as "the allocation of scarce healthcare resources among competing individuals."[12] It occurs when "not all care expected to be beneficial is provided to all patients."[13] Rationing of scarce resources such as personnel, equipment, organs, and space is an everyday occurrence on most units in most hospitals. The allocation of scarce resources goes beyond rationing, however, as is seen in the case of 13-year-old Michael Thompson, a trauma patient who was denied care for lack of health insurance (see Case 1 below). Quite often, patients who are denied resources are not in direct competition with another identified patient. They are denied services because of their inability to pay or because of criteria involving social worth. The overriding issue, therefore, is not one of rationing per se, but of patient selection. The two most important questions governing this area are: (1) What criteria should be used in making the selection? (2) Who should decide? A discussion of these two questions necessitates an examination of the underlying ethical principles.

Any consideration of individual or personal justice also involves questions of social justice. Theories of distributive justice examine the relationship between characteristics of persons as individuals and the distribution of benefits and burdens in society.[14] Some of the major tenets of distributive justice include:

- To each person an equal share.
- To each person according to need.
- To each person according to effort.
- To each person according to contribution.
- To each person according to merit.
- To each person according to free market exchanges.[15]

Earlier chapters of this book present cases in which principles such as autonomy and beneficence are in conflict with one another. This chapter begins with a discussion of the value conflicts inherent in tragic choices. It ends with the presentation of cases in which the tenets of distributive justice seem to collide. As with all ethical dilemmas, in cases of distributive justice there is no ultimately correct theoretical approach. The decision-making tools must fit the circumstances.

In the case involving rationing penicillin supplies to soldiers during World War II, the crux of the decision centered on future battlefield contributions of soldiers infected with venereal disease, not the medical needs of soldiers wounded in battle. While seemingly harsh and ungrateful, this decision reflected a triage mentality, an underlying utilitarian concern on the part of the military leaders: maximize the number of soldiers on the battlefield so as to win the war. Decision makers employed the principles of immediate usefulness and conservation by giving the drug to those who were most ready to return to combat and who needed the least amount of penicillin. Conversely, the advice given by Rabbi Feinstein regarding the treatment of meningitis patients at Hadassah Hospital reflected an egalitarian concern grounded in a particular religious perspective--let us avoid discriminating between persons, let us treat them all as equals. Thus, a method of chance or random selection was employed.

VIII. Criteria for Decision Making

Decision-making criteria might be subdivided into rules of exclusion and rules of final selection.[16] Rules of exclusion set minimum standards for patient selection. They provide a mechanism of initial screening that allows for selection of the largest possible pool of patients. They are generally less controversial than rules of final selection in that they are more inclusive and objective.

There are three categories of rules of exclusion: the constituency factor, the progress-of-science factor, and the prospect-of-success factor.[17] The *constituency factor* sets patient-centered boundaries such as geographic region, age group, and ability to pay. As might be expected, controversies regarding distributive justice often arise in this area. Patient selection based on ability to pay violates the standard of equal opportunity. Providing scarce organs to foreign nationals (such as illegal aliens) violates the justice-as-fairness standard for some persons. The question arises whether foreign nationals have the same moral claim on donated organs as U.S. citizens. Should a foreigner's ability to pay be a factor for consideration? The use of different selection criteria such as acuteness of patient's illness, need, probability of success, and ability to pay would each provide a different answer to this question.

The *progress-of-science factor* may exclude or admit patients in experimental trials based on particular characteristics such as disease processes, sex, or age. The *prospect-of-success factor* reflects a patient's medical acceptability. A major criticism of the use of medical acceptability as a sole criterion is that it often reflects hidden considerations involving social value. For example, concerns regarding a patient's ability to comply with a drug regimen may exclude persons with retardation or illiterate persons from consideration as potential transplant recipients.

Once a patient has entered the "pool," rules for final selection generally involve criteria having to do with social worth (number of dependents, compliance, willingness) or forms of chance (first-come-first served; lottery; or randomization). All of these decision-making criteria are, in certain circumstances, controversial or untenable.

"Choice by chance," says Joseph Fletcher, "is a contradiction in terms. To resort to sortilege (drawing lots) or casting dice or turning a card is, so to speak, a decision not to decide. It is a moral evasion of decision making and its anxieties, and as Kierkegaard said, 'To venture is to become anxious, but not to venture is to lose oneself. It is irresponsible, a rejection of the burden. Its refusal to be rational is a deliberate dehumanization, reducing us to the level of things and blind chance.' "[18]

Others, such as Rabbi Feinstein of New York or attorney Edmund Cahn advocate chance or not choosing as the most egalitarian, and consequently the most ethical, acts.

IX. The Physician as Gatekeeper

Competition for scarce healthcare resources has intensified as a result of the expanding population of aging patients in our society. The demand for healthcare services also is increased by the number of "salvageable" patients who survive previously life-threatening acute or chronic illness. In addition, there is the paradox of "advanced technology creating its own demand." This occurs when healthcare professionals who "are, after all, trained to prolong life, create a technological imperative that they use those techniques they have been trained to use."[19]

Approximately 75 percent of current U.S. healthcare expenditures are generated by physicians. Physician and bioethicist Edmund Pellegrino states:

This fact imposes a serious positive moral duty on the physician to use both the individual patient's and society's resources optimally. In the case of the individual patient, the physician has the obligation inherent in his promise to act for the patient's welfare, to use only those measures appropriate to the cure of the patient or alleviation of the patient's suffering. What the physician recommends must be effective (i.e., it must materially modify the natural history of the disease) and it must also be beneficial (i.e., it must be to the patient's benefit). . . . Physicians, therefore, have a legitimate and morally binding responsibility to function as gatekeepers. They must use their knowledge to practice competent, scientifically rational medicine. Their guidelines should be diagnostic elegance (i.e., using the right degree of economy of means in diagnosis) and therapeutic parsimony (i.e., providing just those treatments that are demonstrably beneficial and effective).[20]

The physician as gatekeeper to healthcare services is both an historical and a modern reality. Unfortunately, the manner in which healthcare resources are rationed is often inequitable. Authors of numerous studies (Crane,[21] Pearlman et al.,[22] Perkins et al.,[23] and Marshall et al.[24]) have reported on the biased and subjective nature of the patient selection process in intensive care units. Kilner reported that the relative importance of certain criteria for patient selection varied among medical directors of kidney dialysis and transplant facilities, depending on the scarcity of the resource. Age, ability to pay, and social value became important determinants of patient selection when resources were limited.[25]

In a now famous *Life* magazine story, journalist Shana Alexander was the first to reveal the use of questionable selection criteria in the allocation of hemodialysis. At Swedish Hospital in Seattle in the early 1960s, an anonymous lay committee was the first assembly in the country to allocate hemodialysis machines. The committee chose dialysis patients using such standards as church participation and Boy Scout leadership. Sex and racial preference were obvious, as were valuations of lifestyle and social worth. Most patients who received lifesaving dialysis were employed, married, white, male high-school graduates, aged 25 to 45.[26]

As discussed by the President's Commission for the Study of Ethical Problems in Medicine and Biomedical and Behavioral Research, healthcare is a primary social good rather than a "right."[27] It is directly related to opportunity, a value highly cherished in American society. Arbitrary deprivation of healthcare on the basis of ability to pay, social contribution, or expected social capacity diminishes opportunity. Although differences in lifestyle and the environment can affect health status, differences in the need for healthcare are primarily unpredictable and beyond an individual's control.

Authors of recent studies have found disturbing disparities in allocation based on differences in race, socioeconomic status, and gender. Williams and colleagues found undertreatment of African-American patients and overtreatment of Caucasian patients in the critical-care environment.[28] In examining healthcare provided to hospitalized Medicare patients, Kahn and her colleagues found that the quality of care provided to such patients is influenced by race, financial characteristics, and the type of hospital in which patients receive care.[29] Using data culled from the National Medicare Expenditure Survey, Seccombe and Amey found that:

1. The working poor are only one-third as likely to receive insurance from their employer as are the non-poor, and are over five times as likely to be without insurance from any source;
2. Employment characteristics are critical antecedents of employer-sponsored insurance and, as a set, explain variation in coverage

beyond that provided by human capital/socioeconomic factors; and
3. Most employment characteristics have a similar effect on the odds of coverage across income categories, except for unionization and minimum wages.[30]

Access to limited healthcare resources is not restricted to the treatment arena. Scarcities and inequities also exist within the domain of human subjects research. For example, in 1991, at the request of the National Institutes of Health, the Institute of Medicine of the National Academy of Sciences appointed a committee to investigate the perception that women were underrepresented as subjects of clinical research studies. The committee's report, *Women and Health Research*, cites the paucity of data that would evaluate these perceptions regarding the inclusion of women in clinical research.[31] The authors did, however, identify several specific areas in which women have been slighted as research subjects. These include heart disease, acquired immunodeficiency syndrome (AIDS), and the inclusion of women of childbearing potential in the early phases of drug trials. This perceived underrepresentation of women in clinical research led Congress, in June 1993, to pass the National Institutes of Health Revitalization Act, which requires that women and minorities be included in any federally funded research. Investigators designing studies that would exclude these research populations are required to provide sufficient justification for the exclusion.

X. Guidance

If we eliminate not choosing as an option, there is no absolute theoretical approach to choosing between persons. As stated previously, the method of choice in patient selection depends on the circumstances in which the decision is made. Use of the following tools for decision making may help clinicians who are faced with such choices:

1. Know as much about the case as possible. Try to obtain the facts firsthand.
2. Healthcare organizations should develop and adhere to formal (written) and prospective patient-selection policies (see Exhibit 12-1).
3. Institutional polices on organizational ethics should reflect thorough input from administrators,

---

Exhibit 12-1
Limiting Medical Care

Policy

We believe that we have a duty to treat every patient and to do no harm. No therapy will be initiated without the expectation that its medical advantages outweigh its burdens. Accordingly, when medical care or emergency treatments designed to prolong life are withdrawn or withheld, certain optional procedures that are not medically necessary may be omitted. These optional procedures include but are not limited to:

- critical unit care and cardiac monitoring
- intubation and assisted ventilation
- the administration of nutrition and hydration
- the administration of blood and blood products
- dialysis
- the administration of antibiotics
- laboratory studies
- radiologic and other diagnostic imaging procedures
- surgical procedures

This facility will provide the patient with spiritual and physical comfort. Certain obligatory procedures will be provided that may include but are not limited to:

- airway maintenance
- food and drink by mouth if tolerated
- medication and treatment for pain
- maintenance of body warmth
- bodily repositioning
- bodily cleanliness (including oral and eye care)
- verbal and tactile communication
- spiritual and psychological care

Source: Reprinted from J.F. Monagle and D.C. Thomasma, *Medical Ethics: A Guide for Health Professionals* (Rockville, Md.: Aspen Publishers, 1988), 440-41. Copyright 1988, J.F. Monagle and D.C. Thomasma. Used with permission.

---

clinicians, and ethics resources. They should explicitly address potential conflicts of interest and fiscal accountability.

XI. Cases for Further Study

Case 1: *Thompson v. Sun City Community Hospital* [32]

In 1984, Michael Thompson, a 13-year-old boy living in Sun City, Arizona, suffered a severe traumatic injury when a car fell off of its supporting jacks and pinned him against a wall. The local rescue squad provided emergency transport to a private hospital nearby. Michael arrived at the emergency room at Boswell Memorial Hospital at 8:22 p.m. His clinical presentation included severe lacerations of his left thigh accompanied by the absence of a pulse in his left leg. His toes on the left were dusky, cool, and clammy. Bone was visible at the lower end of the laceration near the knee.

Dr. Lipsky, the emergency room physician, began volume replacement with intravenous fluids, ordered blood for transfusion, and consulted an orthopedic surgeon. After his initial examination, the orthopedic surgeon consulted a vascular surgeon by phone. The medical consensus was that Michael needed emergency surgery. Once Michael's condition was stabilized, however, Dr. Lipsky informed Michael's mother that, "I have the shitty detail of telling you that Mike will be transferred to County (hospital)." Although she "begged" Dr. Lipsky not to send Mike to County Hospital, the transfer took place at 10:13 p.m.

Hospital administrators refused to admit Michael to Boswell Memorial because he lacked full insurance and had been determined to be "medically transferable." At County Hospital, Michael's condition deteriorated. Once he was restabilized, Michael underwent surgery at 1 a.m. The surgeons discovered a transected femoral artery, which they were able to successfully reanastomose. Because of the length of time that blood flow to his left lower extremity was impaired, however, Michael suffered considerable residual impairment of his left leg.

A Boswell Memorial Hospital administrator later testified in court that Michael was transferred for "financial reasons" and that the surgery could have been performed at Boswell Memorial.

Michael Thompson's case typifies the "dumping" syndrome that intensified during the 1980s as a result of efforts by hospitals and long-term care facilities to cut costs. Although the case borders on refusal of treatment by healthcare professionals, it really involves premature discharge. Although Michael Thompson was not in direct competition with another patient for a scarce resource, the care available to him was rationed based on a very specific criterion--his ability to pay.

[Source: G.J. Annas, "Your Money or Your Life: Dumping Uninsured Patients from Hospital Emergency Wards," *Public Health and the Law*, 76, no. 1 (1986): 74-77.

Case 2: "Two Cardiac Arrests, One Medical Team"

George Burnham and Donald Mattison were patients in adjoining rooms in the rehabilitation division of a state medical center. George was a 33-year-old, severely retarded man who had lived in state institutions since the age of three. His family had had no contact with him for over 20 years. George had been trained to feed himself and to keep himself reasonably clean, but at the age of 25 he had suffered a cardiac arrest that left him with some paralysis. After rehabilitation he only occasionally lacked bowel control. A second recent cardiac arrest left him semiparalyzed and totally incontinent. The chances of his regaining even his former level of continence, the staff felt, were hopeless.

Donald Mattison, a 48-year-old businessman, active in community and church affairs, married and the father of four, had suffered a minor stroke, which left him slightly paralyzed. In his six weeks on the rehabilitation ward he had regained almost total use of his arm and leg. His prognosis for full recovery seemed excellent.

The hospital has at least one cardiac-arrest team on duty 24-hours a day, and one crash cart in every patient area at all times. The possibility of simultaneous cardiac arrests seemed remote. If it were to happen, there would not be time to transfer an additional crash cart from another patient area, since the rehabilitation ward is served by an extremely slow elevator.

But in this case the improbable happened. George had a cardiac arrest at 3:00 one morning. Within four minutes the cardiac-arrest team had arrived in his room and was ready to begin work. At that very moment

Donald also had a cardiac arrest. Knowing of the simultaneous cardiac arrests, every team member hesitated. Two also knew both patients' histories; the others, including the team leader, did not. After a moment, the team leader said, "First come, first served. Let's go to work." With no further hesitation, the team began to resuscitate George.

Without the emergency aid, Donald died. George was resuscitated, but suffered yet another cardiac arrest at 8:20 the next morning. This time another team was unable to revive him, and he too died.

Did the team leader make the right decision in resuscitating George instead of Donald? Is "first-come, first-served" the proper principle to apply in such cases?

[Source: K.M. McIntyre and R.C. Benfari, "Two Cardiac Arrests, One Medical Team," *Hastings Center Report* (April 1982): 24-25.]

XII. Study Questions

1. What are the basic differences between consequentialist and egalitarian approaches to rationing?

2. Consider the dilemma faced by physicians at Hadassah Hospital in 1950--an outbreak of bacterial meningitis and a limited supply of penicillin with which to treat it. How should the penicillin have been allocated? By what criteria?

3. Persons who have been on waiting lists for heart or liver transplants are generally bumped up to the top of the list if their condition deteriorates and they have to be hospitalized (often in an intensive care unit). Given that such seriously ill patients who receive transplants have shorter survival rates than other, less severely ill patients who receive transplants, and that costs of transplanting severely ill patients are higher than for less sick patients, is moving sicker patients to the top of the waiting list justified in terms of fairness or wise in terms of use of resources such as scarce organs and money?

4. Consider Case 2, "Two Cardiac Arrests, One Medical Team." If you do not agree that "first-come, first-served" was the proper principle to apply in this case, what selection criteria would you propose?

Notes

1. W. Styron, *Sophie's Choice* (New York: Random House, 1979), 483.

2. J. Fletcher, *Humanhood Essays in Biomedical*

Ethics (New York: Prometheus Books, 1979), 51.

3. G.R. Winslow, *Triage and Justice* (Berkeley: University of California Press, 1982), 105-06.

4. *U.S. v. Holmes*, 1 Wall.Jr. 1, 26 Fed. Cas. 360 (E.D. Pa. 1842), 1-2.

5. E. Cahn, *The Moral Decision* (Bloomington, Ind.: Indiana University Press, 1955), 71.

6. H.T. Engelhardt, Jr. and M.A. Rie, "Intensive Care Units, Scarce Resources, and Conflicting Principles of Justice," *Journal of the American Medical Association* 255 (1986): 1159-64.

7. Ibid.

8. C. Keefer, *Penicillin: A Wartime Achievement in Advances in Military Medicine*, vol. 2, ed. E.C. Andrus et al. (Boston: Little, Brown, 1948), 717-22.

9. H.K. Beecher, "Scarce Resources and Medical Advancement," *Daedalus* 98 (Spring 1969): 279-80.

10. Personal communication from Rabbi Moses Tendler, Ph.D., Professor of Biology, Chair in Jewish Medical Ethics, Yeshiva University, New York, New York.

11. R.H. Cales and R.W. Helig, *Trauma Care Systems: A Guide to Planning, Implementation, Operation, and Evaluation* (Rockville, Md.: Aspen, 1986).

12. P.E. Dalb and D.H. Miller, "Utilization Strategies for Intensive Care Units," *Journal of the American Medical Association* 261 (1989): 2389-95.

13. H.I. Aaron and W.B. Schwartz, *The Painful Prescription: Rationing Hospital Care* (Washington, D.C.: Brookings Institution, 1984), 81.

14. T.L. Beauchamp and J.F. Childress, *Principles of Biomedical Ethics*, 3rd ed. (New York: Oxford University Press, 1989): 258.

15. Ibid., 261.

16. J.F. Childress, "Rationing of Medical Treatment," in *Encyclopedia of Bioethics*, vol. 4, W.T. Reich, ed., (New York: Free Press, 1978), 1414-19.

17. N. Rescher, "The Allocation of Exotic Medical Lifesaving Therapy," *Ethics* 79, no. 3 (1969): 173-86.

18. See note 2 above, pp. 50-51.

19. See note 9 above, p. 294.

20. E.D. Pellegrino, *Rationing Health Care in Medical Ethics: A Guide for Health Professional* (Rockville, Md.: Aspen, 1988): 263.

21. D. Crane, *The Sanctity of Social Life: Physicians' Treatment of Critically Ill Patients* (New York: Russell Sage Foundation, 1975).

22. R.A. Pearlman, T.S. Invi, and W.B. Canter, "Variability in Physician Bioethical Decision-Making," *Annals of Internal Medicine* 97 (1982): 420-25.

23. H.S. Perkins, A.R. Jonsen, and W.V. Epstein, "Providers as Predictors: Using Outcome Predictions in Intensive Care," *Critical Care Medicine* vol. 14, no. 2 (1986): 105-110.

24. M.F. Marshall et al., "The Influence of Political Power, Medical Provincialism and Economic Incentives on the Rationing of Surgical Intensive Care Unit Beds," *Critical Care Medicine* 20, no. 3 (1992): 387-94.

25. J.F. Kilner, "Selecting Patients When Resources Are Limited: A Study of U.S. Medical Directors of Kidney Dialysis and Transplantation Facilities," *American Journal of Public Health* 78, no. 2 (February 1988): 144-47.

26. D. Sanders and J. Dukeminier, "Medical Advance and Legal Lag: Hemodialysis and Kidney Transplantation," *UCLA Law Review* 15 (1968): 357-413.

27. President's Commission for the Study of Ethical Problems in Medicine and Biomedical and Behavioral Research, *Securing Access to Health Care* (Washington, D.C.: U.S. Government Printing Office, 1983).

28. J.F. Williams et al., "African-American and White Patients Admitted to the Intensive Care Unit: Is There a Difference in Therapy and Outcome?" *Critical Care Medicine* 23, no. 4 (1995): 626-36.

29. K.L. Kahn et al. "Health Care for Black and Poor Hospitalized Patients," *Journal of the American Medical Association* 27, no. 15 (1994): 1169-74.

30. K. Seccombe and C. Amey, "Playing by the Rules and Losing: Health Insurance and the Working Poor," *Journal of Health and Social Behavior*, 36 (1995): 168-81.

31. A.C. Mastroianni, R. Faden, and D. Federman ed., *Women and Health Research* (Washington, D.C.: National Academy Press, 1994), 64-67.

32. *Thompson v. Sun City Community Hospital*, 688 P.2d 605 141 Ariz. 597 (1984).

13

ECONOMICS, MANAGED CARE, AND PATIENT ADVOCACY

Edward M. Spencer, M.D.

Ethics distinguishes between desired and desirable goals.
--*AMA*, Economics and the Ethics of Medicine, *1936*

I. Introduction

This chapter explores the relationship between the economics of healthcare in the United States and ethical clinical practice within the healthcare system. A number of important questions direct this inquiry. What is today's healthcare system in the United States and how did it evolve? What are important economic considerations in the present system (particularly managed care) and how do they affect ethical medical care? What aspects of the system directly or indirectly affect decisions about patient care and are, therefore, of particular concern for clinical ethics?

In attempting to answer these questions, the chapter considers the following issues:

1. the relevant history and present composition of the healthcare system;
2. the major systemwide changes recently adopted or under active consideration;
3. the economic, social, and ethical considerations affecting the healthcare system of today and the near future; and
4. conflicts of obligation and interest imposed on healthcare professionals by changes within the system, and appropriate responses to these conflicts.

There is no doubt that economic factors are important in considerations of "justice" for all citizens, but is it reasonable to extend a consideration of economic issues to the care of individual patients and to clinical and ethical decision makers involved in this care? In spite of a previous focus on individual values in healthcare decision making, it is now obvious that the patient's income, savings, type and amount of insurance, membership in a particular managed-care program, as well as the clinician's need for appropriate income and need to recover costs of practice are important and sometimes critical factors in *all* clinical decision making. Add to these factors the healthcare institution's need to maintain its viability, the insurer's and managed-care organization's (MCO's) need to make adequate profit, and finally the government's need to maintain a viable political and social climate for its citizens (believed by most to include some attention to healthcare), and it can be appreciated that economic issues are among the most important considerations surrounding healthcare.

Rather than ignore economics in the ethics of clinical care, it behooves all clinicians, patients, and family members to consider it one of the most important factors affect ethical decisions for all patients, both as individuals and as group members. Economic issues are always there. These issues affect outcomes and the direction and results of decision making. Medical economics is an integral part of the context for appropriate decision making in clinical ethics.

Therefore, the aim of this chapter is to foster greater understanding of the economic factors affecting medical care and how these factors can be considered during concurrent case analyses and planning for care.

II. The U.S. Healthcare System Today

A. Historical Background

The United States has had a healthcare "system" for only a relatively short time. Prior to the Second World War, healthcare consisted mainly of individual encounters between a physician and patient. A majority of people completed their lives without an admission to a hospital, and some--particularly the rural poor--had no access to medical care at all. However, all of the fundamental aspects of today's health industry (physicians, hospitals, adequate training facilities, and research) were in place by the end of the war, with their future development dependent on the development of a system to manage and finance all aspects of healthcare.

Health insurance in the United States began in 1929, at Baylor University Hospital in Dallas, Texas, which initiated an insurance plan for schoolteachers in the area. Each teacher paid a small fee ($0.50 per month) and received a certain number of days of hospital care each year. Competing plans sponsored by other local hospitals soon began in the Dallas area. In 1932, a communitywide plan was developed in California, under which participating hospitals in a given geographic area agreed to provide services to any of the plan's subscribers. Hospitals in other areas soon developed similar communitywide plans, which subsequently became known as Blue Cross plans. In 1938, the American Hospital Association began to promote noncompetitive, community Blue Cross plans; by 1940, the overall nationwide enrollment in these plans was approximately 6 million subscribers.

These Blue Cross plans covered only hospitalization and offered a single community rate. Because the plans were begun as not-for-profit entities, they were exempt from taxes. In the early 1940s, physicians working with existing Blue Cross organizations

developed Blue Shield plans, which covered physicians' fees for certain services provided to hospital inpatients. Eventually most types of physicians' services, both inpatient and outpatient, came to be covered by Blue Cross/Blue Shield plans. With the participation of an ever-increasing number of commercial insurers, the health insurance industry soon became the "third-party payer" that exerted varying amounts of control over fees and prices and attempted to direct usage within the system.

In 1946, Congress passed the Hill-Burton Act, which helped local communities build and equip their own hospitals and, thereby, increased the number of hospital beds available and decreased the distance to hospital care for most of the U.S. population. The law expired in 1978, but by that time it had stimulated the building of 500,000 hospital beds, most of which were in small- to medium-sized communities.

Although there were attempts to institute national health insurance following World War II, it was not until 1965, when the Medicare and Medicaid bills were passed, that the federal government became intimately involved in the financing of healthcare.

Medicare, began as a proposal for limited health insurance for the elderly; during the legislative process, it developed into a more comprehensive package of benefits with coverage of major portions of the costs of hospitalization and physicians' fees. To ensure passage of the Medicare bill, it was necessary to include payment for hospitals on the basis of their per diem cost per patient and for physicians on the basis of their "usual, customary, and reasonable" fee. In addition, the task of administration of this program, including paying and auditing physicians and hospitals, was given to individual insurance companies. The choice of the particular insurance company to fulfil this administrative work was left to the hospitals and physicians.

Medicaid mandated healthcare insurance for those on welfare and for the medically indigent. The federal government and the states shared the costs of this program, with the states maintaining most of the authority to set the specific benefit package offered and to set payment amounts for hospital care and physicians' fees.

In the mid 1960s, the Johnson administration and Congress allocated funds to train more physicians, build more hospitals, and set up community health centers. Major additions to the funding for health-related research also occurred at this time.

By the mid to late 1980s, it was obvious that the initial estimates regarding the cost of Medicare and Medicaid were wildly optimistic and that, instead of stabilizing or decreasing the rate of increase of medical costs, these programs had actually led to a much greater rate of cost increases than had been anticipated.

Medicare and Medicaid have been responsible for many positive changes for the elderly and the poor. However, the adoption of a cost-based, fee-for-service reimbursement system for these programs stimulated increasing use of healthcare resources with concomitant ballooning of costs.

Several recent attempts at cost control have been made at the federal level with limited success. One notable example that received much attention was the institution of diagnosis related groups (DRGs), which mandated one specific payment amount for the total care of a Medicare patient with a particular diagnosis. Although it is believed that DRGs have had some slowing effect on rapidly escalating costs, they have not been demonstrated to be a reliable cost-control mechanism.

Accompanying the development of federal programs has been an increasing demand from unions and from non-union employees for healthcare benefits. Because expenses for employee healthcare benefits are not taxable for either the employer or the employee, this has been a financially appealing way for employers to increase compensation to employees.

All of these factors have led to a giant healthcare system with interrelated facets consumed 13.7 percent of the Gross Domestic Product (GDP) in 1994 or just under $950 billion. Although the rate of growth of healthcare expenditures has slowed somewhat during the past two years (6.4 percent growth in 1994),[1] it continues to increase at a rate greater than inflation. If it continues to grow in this manner, it could lead to financial catastrophe in the 21st century.

B. Present Situation

Observers have described the U.S. healthcare system as irrational, a patchwork, wasteful, and unjust. A closer look at some of the more obvious methods and results of this system will reveal the reasons for these attitudes and the resultant strong sentiment for instituting a method or methods for predictable control.

It is estimated that 40 million people (14 percent of the population) in the United States do not have health insurance of any kind and are not members of any group eligible for government-sponsored care. A small percentage of this group is economically secure and able to purchase healthcare directly, but most do not have access to ongoing medical care and receive care in a nonplanned, haphazard manner in emergency rooms, free clinics, and physicians' offices.

Approximately 14 percent of the U.S. GDP is healthcare expenditures. In 1994, Americans spent on average approximately $3,510 per person for healthcare while spending less than half that for education and approximately one-third of that amount for defense.[2]

Little wonder that there have been proposals for systemwide reform by a number of economists, healthcare professionals, and politicians, or that the Clinton administration in 1993-1994 attempted to reform the system by recommending to Congress the institution of a nationwide managed-care system with a number of important central governmental mandates aimed primarily at cost control. The planning for this major change was done by elite groups of "experts" behind closed doors with little or no input from the general public, so that opponents of this plan were able to capitalize on public suspicion and defeat it in Congress. That the system needs reform is a virtually uncontested conclusion. The best route to reform and its specifics, however, remain the basis of fundamental differences that are unlikely to be resolved soon.

Polls reveal that the public desires change in the healthcare system. Many individuals polled have articulated a fear of losing health insurance and being financially devastated by one or more illnesses. Most see universal access to healthcare as a positive societal goal and would like to see provision of a universal coverage plan, but are at the same time concerned about the costs involved in guaranteeing access to healthcare for all citizens.

Professional organizations such as the American Medical Association (AMA) have, until recently, paid little attention to economic considerations and their relationship to the ethical practice of medicine. Questions of whether a patient was able to pay for medical care, who was responsible for the payment, and whether it was ethical to refuse to treat a patient based on ability to pay were left to the individual practitioner or healthcare institution to decide. During the past few years, these issues have been addressed generally in professional codes, principles of practice, and ethical guidelines for the professions, but there has been little analysis of the effects of economic considerations.

Individuals outside the field of healthcare (economists, sociologists, political scientists, politicians, and representatives of the media) have led the way in questioning the relationship of the economics of practice to the ethics of practice. Physicians, nurses, other healthcare professionals, and their professional organizations have, in recent years, begun to consider these issues more fully. The AMA particularly has issued a number of recent position papers and opinions concerning healthcare economics generally, plus some suggestions for specific reform. In June 1992, the AMA House of Delegates, for the first time, called for all physicians to recognize their responsibility to care for indigent patients. In 1993, the AMA endorsed universal access to healthcare as a goal of the organization and has been a strong advocate for the government to provide a healthcare safety net for its citizens.[3]

C. Recent Changes

Before looking at major recent changes to the healthcare system, a brief overview of the causes of ever-increasing healthcare costs is in order. The Health Care Financing Administration (HCFA) uses the following method to simplify consideration of the causes of increased healthcare costs. HCFA divides the increases in healthcare costs into four different categories:

1. general inflation based on the overall increase in the Consumer Price Index;
2. population increase;
3. medical inflation based on the price increases in a defined "medical marketbasket"; and
4. intensity, which refers to new goods and services secondary to new technologies, new procedures, personnel, and other resources.[4]

Consideration of each of these categories separately adds to the understanding of the areas that must be adequately addressed if recent changes (such as the growth of managed care) are to be effective in meaningful control of the rise in costs, while at the same time maintaining or enhancing quality of care and increasing overall access to care.

Obviously, neither managed care nor any other systematic approach to healthcare delivery and financing can control the increase in healthcare costs attributable to general inflation. Institutions and individuals in the healthcare system must buy basic goods and services in the open market and must pay for these goods and services at a rate equivalent to that charged other individuals and institutions in the rest of the economy.

It is also true that no changes in healthcare delivery and financing will affect the increase in healthcare costs attributable to population increase. The growing population--particularly in the post-50 age group, which consumes healthcare resources at a greater rate than the rest of the population--will add significantly to the problems of controlling future healthcare costs.

The two causes of increasing healthcare costs that can be addressed are medical inflation and intensity of care. To date, much attention has been focused on medical inflation; intensity has been, if not ignored, at least given less attention than it may deserve. It has been politically popular to suggest that controlling drug prices and decreasing the costs of the bureaucracy surrounding healthcare financing (medical inflation) can lead to continued savings in healthcare costs. Managed care--which applies management techniques derived from business and industry to healthcare--has been positively portrayed in just such a manner, with particular attention to its effectiveness in decreasing bureaucratic inefficiencies inherent in the present system. However, neither politicians nor most managed-care representatives have called attention to the fact that the use of new and expensive technologies and techniques (intensity) must be controlled (in addition to medical inflation) in order to slow the escalating costs of healthcare. The rise in healthcare spending attributed to intensity, if allowed to continue without control, will soon be the major factor in the increase in healthcare costs.[5] If intensity is to be controlled, rationing in some form will by necessity be required. The word *rationing* as used here refers to limiting available interventions and/or treatments that may have real benefits for patients.

Major changes in the healthcare system that have been considered recently are:

1. managed care;
2. single payer;
3. individual, fee-based system accompanied by reform; and
4. state and local experiments.

1. Managed Care

What is managed care and how do managed-care organizations (MCOs) operate in managing the healthcare system? The concept of managed care is a contractual model of delivery and payment for medical care. MCOs integrate the different aspects of the system by developing contractual arrangements with each affected sector. MCOs contract with employers and governmental agencies for a certain level of healthcare benefits for employees or recipients of government benefits, thereby providing predictability for healthcare costs; they contract with providers (hospitals, clinicians, nursing homes, home health agencies, hospices, and so forth) for discounted fees for their subscribers or for a capitated rate (each subscriber's total healthcare needs are taken care of in return for one global fee within a specified time frame), thereby assuring providers a certain level of usage; also the MCO may act as primary insurer with employers and state agencies. In spite of attempts by some MCOs to enter the health insurance market for individuals, the majority of subscribers to MCOs are derived from contracts with employers, leaving the employee as the forgotten person in deciding upon benefit packages, participating providers, opportunity for choice, and other options for more freedom in directing his or her healthcare.

Even before the collapse of the Clinton plan in 1994, attention to managed care as the preferred method of cost control was increasing rapidly. A number of healthcare insurers, existing and newly formed managed-care companies, large and small employers, and certain state governments have encouraged institution of managed care as the best healthcare delivery and financing system possible at this time.

Therefore, since 1994, the number of MCOs and their healthcare "market penetration" has rapidly increased. Presently, more than 20 percent of the population of the US is enrolled in a health maintenance organization (HMO); these individuals receive all or most of their healthcare under the auspices of HMOs. HMOs are the most "managed" of the MCOs in that decisions concerning each enrollee's healthcare are made according to specific guidelines and made only by those approved by the HMO to make these decisions. More than two-thirds of physicians in this country are involved in managed care in some form.[6]

In spite of their similar mission of integrating the different aspects of the healthcare delivery system, no two MCOs are exactly alike. Some MCOs act as insurer and provider by owning and operating healthcare facilities and hiring, on a salary basis, all healthcare providers including physicians. These closed-panel HMOs, Kaiser-Permanente being the most prominent example, have, to date, done a good job of cutting wasteful costs while maintaining a satisfactory level of healthcare for most of their subscribers. Other MCOs contract with existing providers for services at a specified discounted fee. Still others hire certain providers (particularly primary-care physicians) as salaried employees and contract for other services from other providers (usually clinical specialists).

The clinician participating in a managed-care plan becomes a "preferred provider" for that plan and is listed with the plan as one of the providers from whom the plan subscribers can receive care. Providers may receive a yearly fee for each of the managed-care patients (capitation) in their practice, or a guarantee of a specified number of patients, or both. Otherwise, providers discount their fees to the plan's patients and may receive an incentive for using less of the plan's resources (such as fewer lab tests, X-rays, and referrals to specialists) or for adhering to certain guidelines that are believed to represent "quality care."

Most MCOs require some type of "gatekeeper" arrangement to prevent unnecessary use of healthcare resources. A primary-care physician is often designated as a gatekeeper, and he or she must approve all care covered by the particular managed-care plan. In other words, all diagnostic tests, including X-rays, and all referrals to medical specialists must be initiated by the gatekeeper or the plan will not pay for it. Some MCOs offer an economic incentive for the gatekeeper to approve spending less of the plan's resources.

Whether any managed-care plan, which includes a broad cross-section of patients, really saves money is still an open question. Some believe that the increase in bureaucracy in all MCOs and the dividends paid to stockholders of for-profit MCOs will cost more than the savings from efficient management techniques and lower fees.

2. Single Payer

A number of economists, politicians, and physicians have advocated changing the U.S. healthcare system to one in which the government is the only source of payment into the system. Canada has a healthcare system based on this concept. This type of system involves overt rationing and has been difficult to sell to the American public. Also, under this type of system, insurance companies--an important and powerful economic force in the United States--would no longer have any part in the healthcare payment business. With the public mindset against "socialized medicine" and the controls that accompany it, institution of a single-payer system is politically unthinkable now and will likely remain so unless the present movement toward managed care fails and cost increases become unbearable.

3. Individual Fee-Based System Accompanied by Bureaucratic Reforms

This particular option was the one most favored by Congress and organized medicine until the ascendancy of managed care. Focusing on bureaucratic reforms is unlikely to have significant long-term effect on cost increases; even with effective bureaucratic reform, the other factor that drives escalating costs--intensity--will continue to lead to spiraling costs.

4. State and Local Experiments

A number of states, cities, and other geographical and political entities are attempting major changes in one or more aspects of the healthcare system. For example, the state of Oregon has attempted to address the problem of access to healthcare by legislating universal access for its citizens whose individual incomes are below a certain level. This mandate for access was accompanied by the development of a list of medical problems and treatments, ranked in order of priority, for which the state would or would not pay under the new system. The state legislature passed this overt rationing scheme after several years of town and community meetings that were designed to educate all of Oregon's citizens about the necessity for such a system. The prioritization of the types of medical interventions for which the state will pay is the responsibility of a diverse citizens' panel that is required to be responsive to the citizens of Oregon. By early 1997, this program had not been fully implemented because of court challenges concerning possible discrimination under the plan. Other states and localities have attempted or are attempting similar interventions or interventions based on the concept of managed care.

Arguments concerning the direction and scope of additional changes in the healthcare delivery and financing system will certainly continue, but managed care is at present the prominent model for the delivery system and likely to remain so for the next several years. Whether it will prove to be responsive to the numerous problems inherent in healthcare delivery still remains to be seen. Any major shift from managed care toward either a system with greater central control (single payer) or a system driven more by market forces will require a social consensus concerning the proper direction, speed, and specific features of the desired reforms.

III. Economic, Social, and Ethical Considerations in Healthcare Reform

A. Fundamental Considerations Driving the Debate

Underlying any future debate concerning the effectiveness of managed care and the proper direction for changes are a number of fundamental attitudes and values. Because Congress and President Clinton seem to have decided to try incremental changes, and because numerous states are attempting statewide reforms, any number of the following individual and societal values and beliefs may affect these attempts at reform.

1. The Current System Is Perceived to Be Unfair

Many see healthcare as a fundamental right and consider that the government has an obligation to provide healthcare for its citizens in a manner that is fair. Although this concept is popular, it leads to a number of difficult questions such as the following:

- What is a "fair" method for allocating these fundamental resources?
- Can a system of basic healthcare for all that allows a higher level of care for those who can afford it (two-tiered system) be fair?
- Can one's accumulation of resources be considered a factor in deciding fairness?
- What other factors, if any, should be considered in the development of a fair system?
- Should governmental expenditures on healthcare take precedence over educational expenditures, expenditures for basic services, or expenditures for other services and responsibilities of the government?

2. The Free-Market System Should Be Allowed to Work

Many in our society believe that the free market is the best and fairest way to address economic problems. However, the existing healthcare system is influenced by many "non-free-market" factors--even outside the area of managed care--so that a return to a true free-market system is practically impossible.

Supporters of the free-market concept emphasize the importance of responsibility of individual patients for at least some of the costs of their care and actively support such reforms as "medical savings accounts," under which a portion of income could be set aside in a pre-tax account. This account could be invested at the direction of the owner and the proceeds of the account used to pay medical expenses; or, if the account is not used in this manner, it could be converted to other specified uses. Proponents of the free-market system believe that responsibility for a portion of one's healthcare costs would represent a deterrent to unwise usage of the system.

3. Controlling Development and Use of Technology Will Control Healthcare Costs

Increasing use of new techniques and technologies in recent years has been the most important factor in the escalation of healthcare costs, and this issue must be realistically addressed by any healthcare financing plan. If there is to be lasting control of the rapid increases in healthcare costs, this issue must be addressed fully and honestly.

4. Medical Research and Development Will Lead to Greater Efficiency and Lower Costs

Many believe that research will solve most healthcare problems and ultimately decrease costs. Research in this country has made great strides in the past several decades and is responsible for the fact that the U.S. healthcare system is considered to be one of the best, if not the best, in the world.

Research has solved many important healthcare problems and, in some areas, has led to decreasing costs. Research has also supported dramatic increases in new technologies and new drugs, which have led to major increases in healthcare costs. Whether the benefits afforded by these new technologies and drugs have been or will be worth the costs is a question that has received little attention.

Attention to research as an important factor in the increase of healthcare costs will be necessary in the development of any successful, lasting reform.

5. Medical Outcome Studies Will Demonstrate the "Best" Treatments and Thereby Increase Efficiency and Lower Costs

Managed care is focusing on results of medical outcome studies to determine the definition of "quality" medical treatment for specific disease processes. The goal is to develop "practical guidelines" from these studies, which will outline the most acceptable overall treatment protocol for each specific disease entity. Although practice guidelines, derived from appropriate outcome studies, may be of help, they can never be applied to all patients equally; individual physiological variations, value judgments about cost-benefit ratios of particular interventions, and possible mistakes in the outcomes studies themselves can point toward modification of the guidelines in particular cases. Also the costs of good outcome studies for even common illnesses may be prohibitive. Like DRGs in the 1980s, practice guidelines may be helpful but are unlikely to be "the answer."

6. Increased Spending for Preventive Medicine Will Decrease Overall Costs

Although spending on preventive medicine may increase the quality of life for many citizens, it will seldom lead to decreased overall costs in the health-care system.[7] Preventive-care interventions, particularly in adults, often lead to citizens with greater healthcare needs living longer and consuming more healthcare resources. Most individuals accept that this is beneficial for our society, but it does not lead to a systemwide decrease in costs.

7. Changes in End-of-Life Decision Making Will Decrease Overall Healthcare Costs

Emanuel and Emanuel published an important article, "The Economics of Dying," that challenged the premise that reforms in decisions about care at the end of life and palliative care will decrease costs. After studying the effects of the use of advance directives, hospice care, and fewer high-technology interventions, the Emanuels found that "cost savings due to changes in practice at the end of life are not likely to be substantial."[8]

8. The Costs of "Futile" Care Are Important Contributors to Overall Healthcare Costs

There is an ongoing debate concerning the proper definition of "futile" care and the necessity for the system to support such care (see "The Case of *Baby K*," Chapter 9). It may be that a consensus in society concerning this issue would decrease the costs of care for a few individuals at the end of their lives, but, based on the Emanuels' findings, it is unlikely to make a major difference in overall costs.

9. Education of Citizens Concerning Rights and Responsibilities Related to Healthcare Decision Making May Lead to Decreased Costs

Regardless of the direction and extent of future changes in the healthcare system and its financing, education of the public will be a necessary condition for the changes in the system to be effective and successful. An understanding of the system and its strengths and weaknesses is a prerequisite for the public to use the system well and efficiently.

B. Problem Areas

Certain diseases place a special economic burden on affected patients and society. Two conditions of this type are AIDS (acquired immunodeficiency syndrome) and Alzheimer's disease (AD). Other conditions that are costly, are difficult to control and treat, and manifest a risk to society may be afforded special consideration in the future; but AIDS and AD are at present the most well known, are the most feared, and have the greatest potential for quickly depleting healthcare resources.

1. AIDS

AIDS is a viral illness caused by the human immunodeficiency virus (HIV). This virus is transmitted via bodily fluid (mainly blood and semen), and it infects and ultimately destroys certain lymphocytes--white blood cells that are essential to maintaining immunity. This infection leads through a prolonged, gradually downhill course to death, which occurs on average 10 to 12 years after initial infection. AIDS is not a particularly easy infection to get, because it requires transmission of large amounts of the virus at one exposure or during multiple exposures. Its major mode of transmission is through sexual contact (both homosexual and heterosexual) with an infected person. Other modes of transmission are repeated intravenous drug use with shared needles, through transmission of the virus in utero to infants, and transmission from blood transfusions (this is rare today). Healthcare workers who have repeated exposures to inadvertent needle and scalpel skin punctures may be exposed to the virus. To date, no cure or preventive vaccine has been developed, although recent new and costly drugs are showing promise in significantly prolonging life and enhancing quality of life.

AIDS is a chronic disease (10 to 12 years from infection to death). There are a number of recognized specific and nonspecific treatment modalities that can slow the progression of the disease, treat the accompanying infections, and advance the general level of health of those with the disease. Unfortunately, many of these treatments are expensive, and even those of moderate cost must be continued over a long period of time. Methods of payment for this care are being considered in relation to systematic healthcare costs. There has been much attention paid to the possible development of a cure or preventive vaccine; however, this is unlikely to afford a solution in the next few years because the virus has characteristics that make development of a cure very difficult and of an effective vaccine problematic.

Ethical problems associated with this disease include considerations of confidentiality; responsibilities of those infected to inform sexual partners; possible risk in the workplace; and, most importantly, issues concerning the payment for the needed expensive care for a prolonged period.

The effect of the economic considerations associated with this illness on insurance coverage and payment for patient care was disputed in *Greenburg v. H & H Music Company*.

In 1988, J.W. McGann sued his employer (H & H Music Company) after the company, which was self-insured, had reduced lifetime benefits for AIDS treatments from $1,000,000 to $5,000. This reduction occurred shortly after McGann filed his first claim for benefits related to his treatment for AIDS. In his suit, McGann argued that H & H Music violated the Employee Retirement Income Security Act (ERISA), which prohibited employers from discriminating against an employee for exercising his or her right to an employee benefit. A lower court held that the company's decision was legitimately based on the need to contain costs, not on animosity toward McGann as an AIDS patient. The U.S. Court of Appeals for the Fifth District concurred and further ruled that self-insured employers are allowed

to rewrite their health insurance plans to save money. In refusing to hear the case, the U.S. Supreme Court let stand this ruling. Mr. McGann died in 1991.[9]

2. Alzheimer's Disease

Alzheimer's disease (AD) is another condition where current and expected future economic considerations generate ethical problems. AD is a degenerative disease of the brain and other nervous system tissue, which leads to a gradually increasing loss of normal cognitive function. The condition is generally associated with aging because its incidence and prevalence increase dramatically among people over the age of 70. In the United States, 10 percent of the population over the age of 65 has AD. This prevalence increases with age; approximately 50 percent of 85-year-olds have this disease. The direct cause of AD is unknown; there is no cure or means for prevention. Drugs developed to date only slightly ameliorate the symptoms of AD in selected patients, and they are costly. Significant disability accompanies this condition, and individuals with AD require, in most instances, a prolonged period of constant care.[10] The effects of this condition on the patient and the family can be devastating. A patient with advanced AD, who may live for a prolonged period, requires round-the-clock supervision and care. Few family members have the time or the will to undertake the care of an afflicted family member, and the responsibility for this care in the home must be shared.

Good nursing home care for these patients is becoming more available, but the costs continue to rise. In 1990, the Alzheimers Disease and Related Disorders Association estimated that the collective national costs of AD are between $80 billion and $90 billion yearly, with the costs increasing for each patient and the total number of patients expected to increase rapidly (the disease affects the fastest growing segment of U.S. society).[11]

Without a cure or hope for significant improvement, attention to social as well as medical management is crucial. A calm, safe, quiet, predictable environment can help patients with AD maintain comfort and dignity. How we can afford these amenities for all afflicted patients is the major question related to their care.

IV. Ethical Practice in the Managed-Care Arena

The U.S. healthcare system is in the process of significant change. Managed care and its different facets receive greater and greater attention from the political community, the media, and the citizenry in general. In considering the importance of managed care in the healthcare financing system, it should be noted that cost consciousness and prudence in the use of resources are related to fundamental ethical values. In discussing the importance of ethical values in healthcare reform Charles Dougherty stated:

It is important in and of itself to create a health care system that respects the dignity of all persons by guaranteeing a right to a basic level of health care, that shelters the inherently worthy activity of caring for others, and that serves the needs of those who are least well off. Creating a system that embodies these values will require that individualism be tempered by a greater focus on the common good, that serious cost containment measures be devised for the health care system, and that health care provision and decision making arrangements be created that are administratively simple and politically prudent. The debate on health care reform in the United States will be shaped by many political, professional, and economic factors. But if it is to result in a system worthy of the best American traditions, the debate must be shaped as well by serious attention to these ethical values.[12]

A. Professional Ethics and Managed Care

The traditional professional ethics of medicine has defined the duties of its practitioners in relation to activities that advance the best interest of the individual patient, within the context of a relationship based on mutual respect and trust. Professional ethical mandates of both medicine and nursing have, throughout the history of the professions, advocated a fiduciary duty to the patient. But what does this mean? Does this tradition require unlimited duty to advance the patient's interests, no matter the cost or the magnitude of the expected benefit? Is there any obligation toward society when such an obligation may be in conflict with a particular patient's interests? These questions are basic to each healthcare

professional's conceptualization of the profession and its ethical obligations.

William May suggests that, in approaching the ethical aspects of healthcare, the underlying relationship between the patient and physician (nurse or other healthcare professional) should be considered a covenant rather than a contract between equals. In discussing the distinction between contract and covenant, he states: "Contract and covenant, materially considered, seem like first cousins; they both include an exchange and an agreement between parties. But, in spirit, contract and covenant are quite different. Contracts are external; covenants are internal to the parties involved. Contracts are signed to be expediently discharged. Covenants have a gratuitous, growing edge to them that nourishes rather than limits relationships."[13]

The traditional view of the medical and nursing professions espoused by May has, during the past 20 years, undergone a change in emphasis. The American Nurses Association now asks that practitioners act as "client advocates," regardless of whether this is in line with the mandates of the physician or the parent institution.[14] The American Medical Association now expects physicians to provide "medical recommendations" and "discussion of options," with the patient having the final decision-making authority.[15] Both of these professions have, therefore, been moving toward a much greater involvement of patients in decisions affecting their care.

In more recent years, attention to a "caring" perspective as the primary ethical cornerstone for clinical care has returned. Francis W. Peabody, in 1925, gave, as a part of a group of lectures for medical students at the Harvard Medical School, a lecture entitled, "The Care of the Patient." The closing statement from this lecture demonstrates a commitment to caring at that time. Peabody said, "One of the essential qualities of the clinician is interest in humanity, for the secret of the care of the patient is in caring for the patient."[16]

This "caring" perspective has been embraced by many recent feminist thinkers and others. It has the advantage of combining the more useful aspects of a patient-centered outlook with a professional conscience and virtue outlook. In November 1992, Marie Kuffner, writing in *American Medical News*, emphasized that caring should be the primary attribute of the physician. She suggested that physicians begin "by focusing on the core values of our profession from which we receive our strength," and "emphasize our caring in our work," while remaining willing "to accept and fairly distribute the responsibility of care." She proposed an "agenda for caring" that includes caring for patients, caring for the profession, and caring for the community. She advocated that each physician begin to advance this agenda.[17]

Another aspect of the caring perspective as related to managed care has been advanced by Carlos Gomez:

> The seepage of this term [managed care] into common parlance should be a source of concern for several reasons. To begin with it distorts the vocabulary of medicine. "Patients," the people whom one aims to serve become "clients," or in even more distorted language, "enrollees." Where one could once speak of "caring for a patient," the new vernacular suggests that one "manage" their problems, i.e., that one enumerate, code, and rank their diseases. Clinics are described as parts of larger "cost centers," and their productivity is measured in terms of "outputs," i.e., billable diagnoses or procedures.
>
> To suggest that this is merely administrative language, that it is an accounting or managerial device and nothing more, misses the impact that this new paradigm has had, and is having, on clinical practice. The emphasis shifts, however imperceptibly, from a certain type of excellence in medical practice, to a certain type of efficiency in the management of medical problems. The danger we run here, and it is very real, is that we forget that people (especially people who are ill) are inherently messy, and getting messier (as they grow older) all the time. They resist, as if by sheer inertia, even the most ingenious of our efficiency schemes. Throughout this city, they arrive with their leaky, wheezing bodies, their multiple maladies, matched only by their multiple medicines, completely ignorant of their ICD-9 codes (or reimbursement rates). They arrive not wanting so much to be managed, I think, as to be cared for.[18]

What does the professional's duty to the patient, whether based on fiduciary responsibility, covenant, or caring, require in relation to the economic factors of medical care as defined within a managed-care system? In spite of the universal recognition of the obligation of the healthcare professional to the patient, there has never been a requirement for unlimited obligation regardless of the cost.

Consider how the time of a healthcare professional is allocated. The professional's most valuable asset is often his or her time, and no single patient is allowed unlimited access to this asset. If unlimited access to time were allowed, care could be limited to only one patient. This pattern of practice is unrealistic and not expected by patients or others in society. The covenant with patients involves an obligation to devote adequate time for attention to their immediate problem, their ongoing health concerns, and to patients as valued persons.

Professional medical decision making is part of a broader social and cultural context. To ignore or downplay any of the aspects of this context is to ignore important data necessary for good decision making. Economic considerations have become an ever-more important aspect of the cultural context of medical care and therefore need to be addressed in clinical decisions associated with case analysis or planning for care.

B. Specific Ethical Issues Related to Managed Care

Where and in what manner do different aspects of managed care affect individual, case-based ethical decisions and the planning for care of patients?

1. The Physician as Gatekeeper

The issue that is most often seen as a point of conflict for the physician is the dual responsibility of the "gatekeeper" in a managed-care system. The physician, as gatekeeper, has a responsibility to manage efficiently and conserve the MCO's resources, while at the same time maintaining his or her professional obligations to the patient.

Can a physician (or other healthcare professional) ever act ethically in this role? If patients are to be treated within a system in which all possible beneficial interventions are not available to all patients (and this has always been so), decisions must be made concerning what resources are available to which patients. If these decisions are made based on an analysis of expected benefit (or burden) for that particular patient, within the context of the availability (or lack thereof) of specific interventions or treatments within the plan, fairness and the obligation for fiduciary duty, as well as covenant and caring, can be fulfilled. In other words, a gatekeeping physician should be expected to consider the patient's best interest within the context of the healthcare economic system as well as within other more commonly considered contexts such as age, family situation, and belief systems. It is important that the patient understand the gatekeeping role, and that he or she be invited to discuss specific issues of concern related to the physician acting as a gatekeeper.

Gatekeepers who are provided economic incentives to reduce costs have an added ethical consideration. As professionals, they must continue to act for the patient within the system and never allow their own economic well-being to become a factor in decision making. This can be a difficult area and requires constant vigilance, but healthcare professionals should never perceive their role as being primarily focused on increasing their own income.

A related consideration is the question of who can better fit the role of gatekeeper. The patient's interests cannot be appropriately represented if a person only concerned with keeping down healthcare costs is in that role. Constant conflict between the patient's interests and the financial interests of the managed-care plan would be the expected result. As long as the gatekeeper physician's primary consideration is the patient's well-being, the physician may be able to enhance the patient's interests, when compared to others who could be designated as gatekeeper. If economic factors become the primary consideration, the physician is no longer acting in the patient's best interest and is practicing in an ethically untenable manner.

The gatekeeper's perceived dilemma corresponds to other areas of practice in which competing interests affect decisions. The allocation of a physician's time among a number of patients based on perceptions of relative need has already been mentioned. The need for limiting this valuable resource is completely acceptable and has been so throughout history. The physician, as gatekeeper, may therefore allocate other healthcare resources using the same ethical considerations as are used when allocating time with individual patients.

2. Incentives for Clinicians to Decrease the Use of an MCO's Resources

Managed care has introduced a number of new terms and redefined other terms in describing the MCO's mechanism for paying clinicians and its economic incentives for clinicians. Clinicians may be rewarded financially for being more efficient and using smaller amounts of the MCO's resources when compared to other participating physicians. Clinicians may be paid via salary (HMO), according to a capitated rate, or via discounting of normal fees. There may be withholding of a predetermined percentage of each clinician's income throughout a time period, which is paid to the more efficient clinicians at the end of this period.

None of these methods for determining clinicians' compensation from the MCO is inherently unethical, but each requires attention and, if indicated, a defined mechanism for addressing the following issues. To define efficiency only in terms of cost saving rather than quality of care is shortsighted and potentially problematic. During contract negotiations, each clinician should pay close attention to this issue and make sure that efficiency is defined in a manner that will lead toward the best in patient care and not toward possible harmful shortcuts. A salaried clinician is less likely to have ethical problems related to compensation, unless the salary is tied to other issues that could adversely affect patient care. A clinician paid according to a capitated rate has a strong economic incentive to cut corners, because the clinician can keep all moneys not spent on patient care. Clinicians practicing under a capitated plan must remain constantly vigilant to prevent possibilities of economic gain or loss from becoming an issue in clinical decisions. Discounting of fees can be a problem if it leads to attempts to decrease the access of such patients or to favoring patients who are paying the undiscounted fee. Withholding a percentage of all fees and then disbursing this money based on excellence of clinical care is to be commended, while distributing this money only on the basis of perceived cost savings should be resisted.

Whatever the cost-saving mechanisms that affect particular clinicians, disclosure of these mechanisms to all affected patients is a valuable first step and should encourage the necessary vigilance to ensure that decisions about patient care are not being made to enhance the clinician's income. A willingness to discuss these payment mechanisms openly with affected patients and family members should also lead to a more trusting relationship. Disclosure will not force a clinician to ignore his or her own financial situation when considering decisions about patient care, but it will be a constant reminder of problematic areas.

3. External Mandates

How should a participating clinician respond to mandates from the MCO that are required for the physician to remain a provider, but that may lead to questionable patient care?

Some MCOs require that the participating clinicians not disclose to patients all information that could affect their care. Some MCOs have refused to allow discussion of availability of expensive drugs that could be of benefit, availability of beneficial treatments, availability of talented clinicians not participating in the MCO, or the financial incentives mentioned above. Obviously, clinicians should address these issues before signing a participatory agreement with any MCO. If issues such as these occur after the contract has been signed, the clinician must decide which should take precedence--the MCO's interests or the interests of one or more individual patients. These questions are similar to those concerning the gatekeeper's dilemma. Clinicians have a responsibility to further the interests of the MCO, hospital, nursing home, hospice, or other institution where they attend patients as long as these interests do not conflict with those of the patients. When there is a conflict between the institution's interests and the interests of the patient, it is expected that the professional will consider the duty to the patient as primary. Thus, it may become necessary to "fight the system." The only acceptable primary purpose for any MCO or other healthcare organization must be good clinical care. If, in the opinion of the clinician, mandates from the MCO adversely affect care generally or care for a specific patient, the clinician has an obligation to call attention to this mandate and attempt to have it changed.

A court case illustrating this problem is *Wickline v. State of California:*

A middle-aged woman had surgical removal and graft replacement of an occluded descending aorta in the lower abdomen. This surgery was necessary because the occlusion was blocking blood flow to her lower extremities. A clot formed in the graft shortly after the surgery and was removed during a second operation. Five days, later another operation was necessary to sever some of the nerves to the blood vessels of the right leg so that these vessels could dilate further and enhance blood flow to this leg. These complications were not considered unusual and, following the operations, the patient's physicians believed that she was doing well. Payment for the patient's medical care was through Medi-Cal, California's Medicaid plan. Under this plan, a hospital stay of 11 days was authorized. The patient's physicians believed that her complicated medical course required eight additional days of hospital care, and they asked for an extension. A nurse working for Medi-Cal reviewed the case and believed that a shorter extension was indicated. The nurse discussed this matter with the Medi-Cal physician-consultant, who had final decision-making authority; he approved only a four-day extension, and the patient was discharged at the end of this time (nine days following her last operation). The physicians involved in the patient's care all acquiesced to the Medi-Cal time limitation.

Six days, later the patient returned to her physician's office complaining of increasing pain in her right leg. Three days following this visit, she became much worse and was hospitalized on an emergency basis. Examination showed probable recurrence of the blood clot in the right leg, and her leg was subsequently amputated.

The patient sued the State of California but did not wish to sue her physicians. The state argued that the physicians did not protest the decision to discharge the patient and were therefore liable for the injury rather than the state. The physicians responded with statements to the effect that they had tried to protest in other cases but had been rebuffed and that they did not have time to buck the system when they had little hope of making a difference.

The court concluded that the state had "carelessly and negligently" abandoned the patient by requiring discharge from the hospital prior to the time recommended by her physicians. On appeal, the court held that third-party payers can be held legally accountable when decisions that cause harm to the patient result from defects in implementation of cost containment methods, but also "that the physician who complies without protest with limitations imposed by a third-party payor cannot avoid ultimate responsibility for the patient's care."[19]

4. Confidentiality

How the MCO handles confidential information related to specific patients is an important ethical issue. Most MCOs accumulate and collate data on their plan's subscriber population in order to identify "risk" and to enhance outcome studies. These data are often transmitted to employers, because the employer is entitled to this information by law (Employee Retirement Income Security Act). It is important for clinicians, the MCO, and the employer to develop a method to protect information about individual patients, so that it can never be used to influence decisions in the workplace. All patients should be informed about which information will be disclosed to their employer and about all mechanisms that have been developed to protect confidential information.

Confidentiality of information concerning clinician-providers in the MCO may also be a problem. Accumulation of confidential data concerning providers may lead to "profiling" of the clinician-provider based on economic factors--particularly the provider's ability to save the MCO's resources. These profiles may be used in the selection (hiring) and deselection (firing) of professional providers within the plan. Criteria that incorporate this information in the provider profile may put pressure on the provider to emphasize economic considerations rather than clinical appropriateness in healthcare decision making.

5. Duty to Change the System?

Do clinicians have any obligation to change the healthcare system? If the system is not conducive to good medical care for the clinician's patients, then the clinician has an obligation to try to change the system as a part of his or her obligation to the pa-

tients. But does the clinician have a special obligation as a citizen to change the system to one that he or she believes will be more beneficial for society? An answer to this question is less clear.

It can be argued that clinicians' superior knowledge of the important clinical factors that should be considered in all healthcare decisions makes them uniquely qualified to attempt to improve the system for their patients, for society, and for themselves. Activism in this arena is fraught with difficulty, because it requires commitment of time and other resources with no guarantees of success. However, many physicians, nurses, and others believe that it is a part of the duty of the professional to try to improve the environment in which decisions about medical care are made. At a minimum, physicians should have knowledge of the system and its effects on patient care and should educate patients about these issues.

V. Guidelines for Clinicians

The issues related to ethical practice within the healthcare system are difficult issues. They involve values of clinicians, individual patients, and society in general. There are honest differences in these values and presently there is no social consensus. Ethical concepts held by individual healthcare professionals; codes of professional societies; policies of healthcare institutions; and the laws, court decisions, and commission guidelines are often helpful and should be considered in actual decision making.

The following guidelines are a brief compilation of some of the available information:

1. Clinicians should understand the present healthcare system and its effects on individual decisions about patient care and attempt to transmit this information to their patients.
2. Clinicians should maintain their professional integrity and maintain allegiance to their professional duties. This does not mean that every professional must agree with all of the present tenets of the profession, but that clinicians should be aware of their primary professional duties and attempt to fulfil them. They should continue to be an advocate for the care that reasonably advances the best interest of their patients.
3. Clinicians should be willing to challenge the system when it is in a patient's best interest to do so.

4   Clinicians should understand that the healthcare system competes with other important needs of society (such as education and defense), and that it is the function of society as a whole to decide how and where its resources will be spent. To help in this decision making, each clinician may join in the necessary discussions and clarify any misunderstandings or myths.

VI. Final Thoughts

Beneficial change in the healthcare system will require attention to all of the problems mentioned above--not just by political and social groups, but by the populace in general. Changes already instituted and under active consideration may lead to a more efficient system. Managed care may help keep down costs, and universal access--with the government being the insurer of last resort--may be politically possible soon. However, other important issues must be considered. Before lasting, fundamental changes can occur, it is necessary to address control of research, a public education program that addresses fundamental assumptions and responsibilities of patients and a reemphasis on professionalism in education of clinicians. It is obvious that economic factors do matter in ethical medical care. How they matter now and how they will matter in the future are basic questions that must be addressed. The expectation that the citizens of the United States will ever reach complete consensus on these issues is unrealistic. However, it should be possible to introduce methods that will support an ongoing conversation about these matters. This conversation should enable all to have a voice in the decision making, and should lead the way to the development of a working system that will enhance ethical patient care.

VII. Case for Further Study: "Who Is Responsible for This Patient?"

An 85-year-old female was brought to the emergency room for a "kidney problem" by a niece who lives nearby. According to the niece, the patient also has diagnoses of Parkinson's disease and progressive dementia and takes some type of medication daily when "she doesn't forget." The niece also reported that the patient's family had unsuccessfully attempted to place her in a nursing home. The patients 86-year-old spouse is the only caregiver at home, and he is in deteriorating health. The patient's two children, both of whom live some distance away, have families and responsibilities of their own, and are not able to care for the patient.

The patient's "kidney problem" was found to be a simple urinary tract infection without complication, so an appropriate oral antibiotic was prescribed and the niece was told to take the patient home and see to it that the patient received the medication. The niece refused because she felt that the patient could not be cared for properly at home. Hospital personnel contacted the husband and told him that the patient would be returning home and would need to be cared for there. The husband said that no one would be at home if the patient returned and told the emergency room staff to place her in a nursing home. The patient refused placement; she was considered capable of giving or withholding informed consent, but was physically unable to meet her own needs. The physicians in the emergency room wanted to admit this patient to the hospital until the situation could be clarified by the social work department. The hospital has recently been sanctioned by Medicare for allowing too many "unnecessary" admissions. What should be done? Can consideration of the financial situation of the hospital be a legitimate part of the decision making? Who is responsible for this patient?

[Source: E. Conrad, Chairman of the Ethics committee at Johnston Memorial Hospital, Abingdon, Virginia.]

VIII. Study Questions

1. Do you agree "that economic issues are among the most important considerations surrounding healthcare"? Why or why not?
2. Is some type of rationing of healthcare in the U.S. inevitable? Explain.
3. Do you believe "managed care" in its present form can support ethical healthcare?
4. What should be done to address the healthcare costs of Alzheimers Disease and AIDS? What do we as a society owe severely demented individuals?
5. Should physicians and nurses be actively involved in the administration and financing of the healthcare system?

Notes

1. K.R. Levit, H.C. Lazenby, and L. Sivarajan, "Health Care Spending in 1994: Slowest in Decades," *Health Affairs* 15, no. 2 (Summer 1996): 131-41.

3. Ibid., 131-33.

3. Council on Ethical and Judicial Affairs, *Code of Medical Ethics Current Opinions with Annotations* (Chicago: American Medical Association, 1996), 147-48.

4. T.A. Massaro, "Impact of New Technologies on Health Care Costs and on the Nations Health," *Clinical Chemistry* 36 (1990): 1612.

5. Ibid., 1612-14.

6. "InterStudy's Competitive Edge Industry Report," in "Publications and Reports," *Health Affairs* 15, no. 3 (Fall 1996): 273.

7. W. Gaylin, "The Clinton Plan Ignores Our Real Health-Care Problems," *Medical Economics* 71, no. 4 (21 February 1994): 30-44.

8. E. Emanuel and L. Emanuel, "The Economics of Dying," *New England Journal of Medicine* 330, no. 8 (1994): 540-44.

9. *Greenburg v. H&H Music Co.* 503 U.S. 958 (1992) as reported in L. Fleck and S. Lind, "In the Courts," *Hastings Center Report* 23, no. 1 (1993): 3.

10. Alzheimers Disease and Related Disorders Association, *Alzheimers Disease Statistics* (Chicago: Alzheimers Disease and Related Disorders Association, 1990).

11. Ibid.

12. C.J. Dougherty, "Ethical Values at Stake in Health Care Reform," *Journal of the American Medical Association* 17 (1992): 262.

13. W. May, "Code, Covenant, Contract or Philanthropy," *Hastings Center Report* 5, no. 34 (1975): 34.

14. American Nurses Association, *Code for Nurses*, (Kansas City, Mo.: American Nurses Association, 1985).

15. See note 3 above. ("Principles of Medical Ethics and Fundamental Elements of the Patient-Physician Relationship," *xiv, xxxiv-xxxv*).

16. F.H. Peabody, "The Care of the Patient," *Journal of the American Medical Association* 88 (1927): 881.

17. M.G. Kuffner, "Agenda for Caring," *American Medical News*, 16 November 1992.

18. C.F. Gomez, "Your Words and Mine: Managing Other People's Misery," *Albemarle Medical News* 1, no. 4, (Winter 1992): 1.

19. *Wickline v. State of California*, 183 Cal.App.3d 1064, 228 Cal.Rptr. 661 (1986).

References

Califano, J.A. Jr. *America's Health Care Revolution.* New York: Random House, 1986.

Council on Ethical and Judicial Affairs, American Medical Association. *Code of Medical Ethics: Current Opinions and Annotations.* Chicago: American Medical Association, 1996.

Ginzberg, E., *American Medicine: The Power Shift.* Totowa, N.J.: Rowman and Allanheld, 1985.

Health Care Financing Administration, *National Health Expenditures, 1986-2000.* Washington, D.C.: Division of National Cost Estimates, Office of the Actuary, Health Care Financing Administration, 1988.

Project Hope, *Health Affairs.* Chevy Chase, Md.: Project Hope, Fall, 1992.

SECTION III

RESOURCES FOR ETHICS COMMITTEES

14

ETHICS SERVICES IN HEALTHCARE ORGANIZATIONS

John C. Fletcher, Ph.D. and Edward M. Spencer, M.D.

I. Introduction

Healthcare organizations (HCOs) today must have effective programs to address ethical problems in patient care and organizational life. To meet this goal three resources are required:

1. ethically informed clinicians;
2. a well-supported ethics program that addresses patient care and organizational ethics; and
3. good morale in the organization.

The main subject of this chapter is the development of the second resource, an ethics program with services for clinical and organizational ethics. However, these three resources are interdependent and mutually reinforcing.

A. Ethically Informed Clinicians

As discussed in Chapters 1 and 2, clinicians are the primary moral problem solvers in patient care. A "clinician" is anyone who interacts with patients and their families within the goals of a plan of care (for example, physicians, nurses, social workers, chaplains, or other healthcare professionals). An ethics program's top priority is to educate clinicians for moral problem solving. Patient care ethics (Chapters 3 through 12) and issues of economic and organizational integrity (Chapter 13) are two overlapping are-

nas for education for clinicians. Administrators, physician-"gatekeepers," case managers, and others also become moral problem solvers in cases where economic issues provoke ethical problems in patient care.

B. Healthcare Ethics Services

This chapter explains how to develop and evaluate a well-supported ethics program in a HCO. The top priority of an ethics program is to serve clinicians and patients. For several reasons, it is recommended that HCOs grow from a "committee" framework to a "program" with services for clinical staff, patients, and the community.

1. The Place of Ethics Programs

With some difficulty, ethics programs are gradually becoming a part of the culture of healthcare. There are crucial differences between an ethics committee and an ethics program. Services are hard to associate with a committee but not with a program. Committees are more expendable than programs. Committees can be abolished by decision of boards or administrators.

What is the place of an ethics program in healthcare? Ethics programs are analogous to social work. The level of social work services might be reduced for cost savings, but a HCO with no social work activities would be deficient. Ethics programs are evolving to a similar status in HCOs. The Joint Commission on Accreditation of Healthcare Organizations (JCAHO) accredits 90 percent of U.S. hospitals and at least 30 percent of the nursing homes. HCOs that ignore JCAHO's requirements for ethics services (discussed more fully below) do so at their own peril, because Medicaid and Medicare payments are dependent on accreditation. However, HCOs are wise to strengthen their ethics programs before JCAHO requires it, because ethics programs meet complex needs that cannot be addressed by individual clinicians.

2. Larger Vision

Another reason to aim toward an ethics program is that it requires a larger vision than a committee. Understanding the history and scope of ethics activities and how these connect with an extensive literature, nationally significant cases, and the work of national commissions requires a larger vision.

It is "everybody's business" in a HCO to support an ethics program. However, the HCO's administration and board have a special duty to evaluate the quality of the process to address ethical issues in patient care as well as the infrequent "ethics emergency." A poorly addressed ethics emergency can, figuratively speaking, bring an institution to its knees.[1] The board's task is twofold: (1) to ensure that adequate resources --trained leadership and financial support--exist to support an ethics program and (2) to hold accountable to reasonable standards those who "do ethics"--moral problem solving--in the name of the HCO.

3. Resistance

A programmatic direction can reduce resistance, especially by physicians. Physicians tend to understand "ethics" to raise only issues about character or the integrity of professional relationships. Believing that an ethics committee will intrude into these matters, physicians often oppose the committee. The development of "ethics services" or "clinical ethics services" provides a clearer message of the purpose of the program.

C. Organizational Morale

The organization's morale involves a shared sense of common purpose and usefulness. Morale influences the climate within which clinicians and administra-

tors perceive all types of ethical problems. This resource is more fully discussed below in the final section on "organizational ethics."

D. Precis of Chapter

The chapter begins with a history of various types of ethics committees. It then describes the major problems that weaken ethics committees in patient care and a strategy to remedy these problems. It recommends adopting standards for committee operations and standards for education and training of committee members and others to provide services, including case consultation (see Appendix 2). The four main services of an ethics program (ethics education, policy development, ethics case consultation, and targeted research) and some legal concerns are discussed as well as the topic of "organizational ethics." Regional bioethics networks, discussed in the concluding part, are a base from which to create partnerships with HCOs for education and training to accomplish these goals. Creating educational partnerships through regional networks to help orient, educate, and train those who serve ethics programs must become priorities of the clinical ethics community (see Chapter 1) and of the bioethics movement in the United States and Canada.[2]

II. Know the History: The Evolution of Healthcare Ethics Committees

Leaders in HCOs and of ethics programs need to know the national and local history of ethics committees. Jonathan Moreno fully describes the interesting "prehistory" of healthcare ethics committees.[3] Earlier committees were instituted to make decisions about eugenic sterilization, access to abortion, and selection of patients for dialysis. This story need not be told here. Insofar as healthcare ethics committees are an expression of a movement to reform an older medical ethics that espoused physicians' paternalism and secrecy in the care of patients, their history is deeply linked to reform of the ethics of research with human subjects. One cannot understand the history of reforms in the ethics of patient care apart from reforms in research with human subjects or reforms in the education of healthcare professionals.

More and more frequently, ethics programs are assigned the responsibility of providing education and support to members of various types of ethics committees in today's larger HCOs. Knowing the history of ethics committees is part of the education and training of members of all of these committees.

A. Research with Human Subjects

Reform of the ethics of research with human subjects marks the beginning of contemporary ethics committees. Human subjects research raises large ethical issues of voluntary informed consent and conflicts between moral claims on physicians and scientific claims on researchers.

Federal policy and law mandated the institutional review board (IRB), the first type of ethics committee; this reform was a response to serious ethical problems in research with human subjects, first exposed in the 1960s when civil rights and other movements had the nation's attention.[4] Controversial research projects such as the following were exposed to moral debate beyond the research community, giving birth to "bioethics":[5]

- Tuskegee (Public Health Service, Centers for Disease Control), 1932-1972
- Thalidomide and Food and Drug Administration, 1962
- Jewish Hospital Cancer Study, 1963
- Baboon-to-human Heart Transplant, 1964
- Willowbrook Hepatitis Study, 1965
- Beecher article, 1966
- "Tea Room Trade," 1967
- Fetal research, 1973

These studies were widely considered to have exceeded acceptable risks or violated the norms of informed consent. In this period, government slowly became an advocate of "prior group review" by IRBs as government officials and the public painfully learned that reforms were sorely needed to protect human subjects. Several public scandals in research ethics, cited below, led to change.

The federal government not only learned slowly from these crises but had a large blind spot about the ethics of research conducted by its own agencies. This is evident in the long-lived study, begun in 1932, of untreated syphilis in African-American males in Macon County, Alabama (Tuskegee Study). The study was conducted by the Public Health Service and the

Centers for Disease Control.[6] Government researchers disguised the diagnosis of syphilis as "bad blood" and described research activities, such as lumbar punctures, as "special treatment." The researchers withheld available treatments from the subjects even after investigators learned in 1943 that penicillin could be used to treat syphilis. It was not until 1972 that the study was finally stopped, after a journalist published a story about it.[7] The terrible moral legacy of this study lives on. Many African Americans are distrustful of research activities today, especially any concerned with acquired immunodeficiency syndrome (AIDS); they cite "Tuskegee" as the main reason for their distrust and fear.[8]

Reform began with two major steps. In 1966, the Public Health Service mandated a local process of prior group review of any research project that involved human subjects.[9] Ethics review had to occur before scientific peer review at the National Institutes of Health (NIH) could begin. This was a controversial policy decision. Prior to 1966, researchers had almost total power to design and conduct clinical research, subject to norms of professional integrity and informed consent.[10] It became clear that the research community, acting alone, was not able to protect human subjects. It was necessary for researchers to share the power to involve persons in research with others who had no self-interest in the specific project under consideration.

Congress took the second step in 1974, creating a national commission to recommend federal regulations to protect human subjects.[11] This law also required that all institutions and entities supported by federal funds practice prior review through a local IRB. The IRB had to have at least one outside member who was not a scientist and at least one female member. Because the NIH and other government agencies were not subject to the 1966 policy, the new law also applied to them. (The blind spot evident in the history of the Tuskegee study had delayed and hindered reform of research activities within the NIH itself.[12])

This transition to shared decision making--between scientists, their interdisciplinary peers, and the public--took several years with research scandals exploding along the way. Today, there are more than 2,000 IRBs in the United States in public and private sectors. In 1994-1995, revelations by the secretary of the U.S. Department of Energy prompted a review of the ethics of radiation research in the post-World War II period by the President's Advisory Committee on Human Radiation Experiments.[13] This national review confirmed that ionizing radiation research was conducted without the informed consent of some subjects, including some pregnant patients. The advisory committee also made a number of recommendations to improve the quality of today's IRBs.[14]

B. Education of Healthcare Professionals and Other Ethics Committees

In the 1970s, concern turned to improving education of healthcare professionals in the humanities and ethics in order to balance the heavy emphasis on the biological and medical sciences. At that time, few schools had more than occasional lectures on ethical issues. Many schools of medicine and nursing have since changed their curriculums and created new faculty positions in medical humanities and ethics. Today, all U.S. medical schools have some teaching in medical ethics, and many have a separate required course or teach the topic in tandem with another required course.[15]

In addition to IRBs, other types of committees began to focus on different ethical issues in research. In the 1980s, the ethics of research with animals came under scrutiny, due in part to the influence of Singer's argument about "specieism." Singer argued that specieism justifies animal research from a premise that humans are superior in every way to animals, and he linked this view to racism and sexism.[16] Although his argument is foreign to researchers, it contributed to widespread public concern to prevent unnecessary pain and harm to animals in research. Federal law now requires each HCO doing such research to have an ethics committee for prior review of proposed projects with most species of animals.[17]

In the late 1980s, reformers identified the need to develop another form of ethics committee to conduct local investigations of allegations of misconduct and fraud in medical science. Although there is ongoing debate about the definition of scientific misconduct,[18] the tradition of self-regulation today requires impartiality in the investigation of allegations. Also, the federal government now requires a course in research ethics for trainees in the biological and medical sciences who are supported by federal training funds.[19]

As a consequence of this history, many teaching hospitals and academic medical centers have four types of ethics committees:

1. an IRB for prior group review of research that involves human subjects;
2. a committee for prior group review of proposed animal research;
3. a committee to assist with formal inquiries into allegations of research fraud and education of trainees; and
4. an interdisciplinary committee for ethical issues in patient care.

One of the main tasks of ethics programs is to support and nurture the work of these committees. Large hospitals are not the only HCOs that have committees of the fourth type. Small hospitals, nursing homes, home health agencies, and hospices also have them.

C. Evolution of Healthcare Ethics Committees

In the late 1970s, healthcare ethics committees began to focus on ethical issues in patient care. Why did these groups emerge? In an important discussion of consensus in clinical ethics,[20] Moreno views healthcare ethics committees as creatures of a period of reform and changing consensus in medical ethics. The cornerstone of traditional medical ethics was an "impregnable" doctor-patient relationship, presumably based upon trust (see Chapter 15). The ascendancy of the legal and ethical doctrine of informed consent (see Chapter 6) required physicians to respect the freedom and equality of the patient. Moral consensus regarding respect for patient autonomy, initially framed in the context of research ethics, extended to and transformed the old medical ethics. However, proponents of the new medical ethics also wanted to preserve the beneficence-based duties and professional integrity of physicians. It would have been degrading to the profession to view physicians as mere tools of patient autonomy. Moreno understands ethics committees as an attempt to promote and "troubleshoot" a new consensus with two key elements: an emphasis on patient self-determination and a continuing defense of physicians' beneficence.

The interdisciplinary and community composition of committees and their patient-centered mission confirm Moreno's insights. In terms of social history in a liberal democracy, ethics committees are functionally required to mediate a difficult compromise in medical ethics.

The early committees were mainly forums for debate and resources for clinicians with difficult cases. Legal cases such as Karen Ann Quinlan (1976) (see Chapter 9) and cases involving handicapped infants such as Infant Doe of Bloomington, Indiana (1982) and Infant Doe of New York (1983) (see Chapter 10) sparked widespread debate and drew attention to ethics committees as avenues for conflict resolution. Other authors thoroughly describe these early ethics debates.[21] The President's Commission for the Study of Ethical Problems in Medicine and Biomedical and Behavioral Research recommended in 1983 that courts be used only as a last resort to resolve decisions for incompetent patients who required medical treatment.[22] Mindful of these new ethics committees, the commission recommended that HCOs were responsible "to ensure that there are appropriate procedures to enhance patients' competence, to provide for the designation of surrogates, to guarantee that patients are adequately informed, to overcome the influence of dominant institutional biases, to provide review of decision making, and to refer cases to the courts appropriately."[23]

The commission saw committees as protectors of the interests of incapacitated patients in the context of decisions to forgo life-sustaining treatment (see Chapter 9). The Commission stated: "the medical staff, along with the trustees and administrators of healthcare institutions, should explore and evaluate various formal and informal administrative arrangements for review and consultation, such as 'ethics committees,' particularly for decisions that have life-or-death consequences."[24]

A few states have mandated healthcare ethics committees. Maryland's law, first passed in 1985 and amended in 1987, requires each licensed hospital and long-term care facility to have a "patient care advisory committee" for guidance on request in cases involving choices to forgo life-sustaining treatment.[25] New Jersey began requiring ethics committees in 1990.[26] Hawaii does not require ethics committees but recognizes their place in decision making in patient care.[27] Hawaii also gives legal protection to physicians who consult an ethics committee and take their advice. Neither Maryland nor New Jersey provides such a shield for physicians, although Maryland's law

provides legal immunity for ethics committee members who make recommendations "in good faith."

An ethics program, or its functional equivalent, is now required of HCOs for JCAHO accreditation. In 1991, JCAHO required a "mechanism" for "the consideration of ethical issues arising in the care of patients and to provide education to caregivers and patients on ethical issues in health care."[28] This rule was later reworded to require a "functioning process to address ethical issues" in both patient rights and organizational ethics.[29] (see Appendix 1 for 1997 standards) JCAHO's involvement has dramatically increased the spread of ethics committees in hospitals. In 1989, approximately 75 percent of U.S. hospitals with more than 200 beds and 25 percent of those with fewer than 200 beds had an ethics committee.[30] By 1992, 51 percent of all hospitals responding to a survey by the American Hospital Association had a committee.[31] Today, between 80 and 90 percent of all U.S. hospitals, the number accredited by JCAHO, presumably have an ethics committee. Possibly as many as 25 to 30 percent of nursing homes now accredited by JCAHO have an ethics committee, which represents an increase over the number reported in an earlier national survey.[32]

The needs of ethics committees in nursing homes and hospitals are similar in some important respects, although the physical characteristics of nursing homes and their residents create a "moral ecology" that is somewhat different from hospitals. From this premise, Hoffman and colleagues have created an outstanding written resource for nursing home ethics committees.[33] Home healthcare ethics committees and teams is yet a third major type of ethics program. Fry-Revere and colleagues have produced the single best resource for the arena of home healthcare ethics.[34]

III. The Condition of Healthcare Ethics Committees Today

Today, healthcare ethics committees are in one of two conditions:

1. in a "failure-to-thrive" condition; or
2. evolving from a "committee" to a "program" with services for patient care issues.

To some degree, most of the nation's healthcare ethics committees are failing to thrive. Each committee has a great deal of room for improvement.

A. Failure to Thrive

A national survey of healthcare ethics committees in 1988 found that, in their early stage, ethics committees defined their tasks as educating themselves and clinical staff about ethical issues in patient care, developing policy guidelines, and providing consultation services on request.[35] At the time of this survey, the most widely used manual for ethics committees also recommended this threefold mission.[36] We urge a departure from this now narrow definition.

Despite widespread consensus about the tasks of ethics committees, another survey reported that many committees were marginal and suffering from "failure to thrive."[37] This condition, which is still common today, is characterized by the following traits:

- Members are ill educated and untrained for tasks.
- Members feel isolated, vulnerable, and marginal.
- The committee is unsupported by leadership and without a budget.
- The committee's services are unknown to the clinicians who most need them.
- The committee is not consulted for significant ethical problems or is not consulted about preventing these problems.
- Family members and patients are infrequent users.

There are several key causes of this condition. The most weighty causes, which are not a fault of the committee are (1) the lack of educational and training opportunities for members and (2) disagreement in the clinical ethics community about the appropriateness of standards for quality and performance of the committee's services.[38]

Ethics committees began as a voluntary effort in a competitive medical marketplace without the educational and training infrastructure that would secure their place and development in healthcare. As a result, a weak committee usually does not have the collective will to press the HCO's leaders for stronger support and funding. (The issue of education and training is discussed more fully below.) Also, the bioethics movement and the academic community have not put as high a priority on ethics services as on teaching and research.

Ethics committees' generic weakness is no secret and is communicated clearly to clinicians. Clinicians' resistance to using committees can be well grounded in some cases. Clinicians may genuinely lack information about why the committee exists and how it can serve them. In the early "committee" stage, the group can present an unappealing and even threatening face to clinicians. If members do no serious study or training for their tasks, clinicians are right to be concerned that committee deliberations will be thin or out of touch with the clinical ethics and health law literature.

In addition, sensitive clinicians may be concerned about privacy and the rights of patients. Some committees make decisions about difficult cases "behind closed doors" at the request of clinicians who approach the committee without notifying the patient or surrogate decision makers.[39] The committee may not follow or even be aware of standards of due process.[40] The degree of respect for confidentiality and privacy is difficult to judge, but ethics consultants can easily obtain patients' charts without patients' knowledge. Some committees provide consultation on cases through individuals who have had no advance training for the role other than their experiences in healthcare.

Further, clinicians who use data to request services cannot fail to note the paucity of controlled studies showing any benefits of ethics consultation.[41] The few published empirical studies have major methodologic flaws.[42] Case reports[43] and evaluations of satisfaction[44] focus on physicians who requested ethics case consultation. Plans for controlled, multi-institutional studies of the efficacy of ethics consultations are in the early stages.[45] The lack of good studies has lowered expectations about the work of committees and may have increased physicians' skepticism about contacting ethics committees in ethically troubling cases.

In addition, physicians may be legally wary of contacting committees. They mistakenly, but understandably, fear that their choices will be legally bound by a committee's recommendation. In HCOs where the committee is weak and marginal, observant clinicians may also see a potential for "ethics disasters" waiting to happen. Poorly led committees or arbitrary decision making are invitations to lawsuits. Lawsuits are a predictable result of violating simple rules of due process or overreaching an educational and advisory role.[46] Six lawsuits in which ethics committees or consultants were named or negatively implicated are reviewed later in this chapter.

Role conflicts between the ethics committee, legal officers, and risk managers can add to a committee's passivity and confusion. The committee's role can be displaced by legal and risk-management concerns. Macklin describes a situation in which legal fears undermined an ethics committee's efforts to shape a hospital policy for pregnant women whose beliefs as Jehovah's Witnesses led them to refuse blood transfusions.[47] A committee can abdicate its mission in ethics to risk-management concerns.[48]

As a result of these problems, there is more criticism of ethics committees[49] and of ethics consultation in the context of committees[50] than praise in the literature. Healthcare ethics committees do not enjoy a good reputation. What are the remedies for "failure to thrive"?

B. Strategies for Change

1. Local Strategies: A Programmatic Goal

Various local (institutional) and regional strategies may prove to be effective.[51] The local strategy is to transform the committee's role in the HCO. The goal is to develop the committee into an ethics program that offers services, has its own internal resource persons, and has a budget for operations. The local strategy requires the following steps:

- With support of the HCO leadership, create a work plan that sets the goal that the committee will evolve to a new programmatic stage.
- Identify two or more persons in the HCO who desire to make clinical ethics part of their career goals and invest in their training and education.
- Adopt and implement standards for quality in the operations of the committee and its services (see Appendix 2).
- Adopt and implement standards for education and training of committee members (see Appendix 2).
- Adopt and implement higher standards for those

who provide ethics consultation (see Appendix 2).
- Develop a capacity for program evaluation and targeted research.
- Join in partnership with others to create a regional or statewide network[52] to support the effort to address the problems of ethics committees.

2. Regional Strategies: Programs for Education and Training in Clinical Ethics

The local strategy will be ineffective without a larger regional or statewide strategy. The larger strategy needs two activities: (1) short-term education and training and (2) long-term education and training.

a. Short-Term Education and Training[53]

The first activity is a conference for education and training of local resource persons, chairpersons, and key committee members. The model is one of brief leadership training with a time commitment of no more than five or six days.

During the conference, these resource persons develop a plan to move to or strengthen their local ethics program. The event gives local HCOs an opportunity to select candidates as resource persons and send them into training. These resource persons' assignment is unambiguous: they are expected to develop a plan, return to the institution, and implement the plan. It is important, of course, that the leadership of the HCO share the same intent for the program as do the resource persons. The educational aims of the short-term event include the following:

- review of the history of healthcare ethics committees and their present situation;
- review of the potential of ethics programs in HCOs with a candid analysis of one's own situation;
- study of the major ethical obligations and problems facing clinicians, patients, and HCOs today, including managed care and economic issues (Chapters 3 through 13);
- careful assessment, with the assistance of guest speakers, of the best examples of the four ser-

vices of ethics programs (education, policy development, consultation, and targeted research);

- interaction with clinicians who have benefited from the services of an ethics program and who are articulate about ethical issues;
- discussions of specific issues in healthcare law (decision making about treatment at the end of life, informed consent, patient capacity, advance directives, and so forth);
- daily seminars on the practical aspects of starting or strengthening an ethics program;
- participation in several "mock" ethics consultations for practice and reflection;
- consideration of ways one's HCO and ethics program could respond to the "organizational ethics" requirement of JCAHO;
- sharing with other participants and instructors the elements of a one-year work plan before returning to the HCO.

b. Long-Term Education and Training

The second activity in a regional strategy consists of a long-term education and training program in clinical ethics. Ideally this program should be conducted on a graduate level with qualified faculty. This strategy requires a partnership that consists of the following groups:

- a university-based clinical ethics center with an outreach program and a graduate program offering the M.A. in clinical ethics;
- adjunct regional faculty qualified to teach courses;
- a university division of continuing education;
- regional or statewide bioethics networks; and
- HCOs willing to share costs with participants whom they sponsor.

Within this partnership, three types of programs can be offered: (1) a program that thoroughly introduces ethics committee members to the content of clinical ethics and the services of an ethics program, (2) a longer program of studies and clinical training that prepares the HCO's resource persons in much more depth than the short conference, (3) a master's level program in clinical ethics for professionals who not only want to serve an HCO's ethics program but also wish to teach within the region and beyond.

These interdependent local and regional activities will provide the support system needed by health-

care ethics committees. The partnerships for education and training need to be created regionally and cooperatively by the professional community in healthcare ethics. The ideal outcome would be accreditation of regional and statewide education and training programs in clinical ethics by the relevant professional societies. Accreditation of education and training programs will help the field of healthcare ethics pass milestones recognized by the larger community and society.

Certification or licensing of individuals to do clinical ethics is an unreasonable goal, considering the diverse professional backgrounds of those involved in ethics programs. Certification is unnecessary because ethics services are not reimbursed in any healthcare system, although the costs of ethics services are allocated in the daily patient charges. Ethics services are contributed by the HCO, as are pastoral care and social work. The most important reason to oppose certification is that it would undermine the premise that clinicians are the primary moral problem solvers in the clinical setting.

IV. The Services of an Ethics Program

With support from the HCO and educational and training opportunities from the clinical ethics community of the region, it is possible to make a transition from the committee stage to a functional ethics program. A full ethics program for the HCO consists of seven components. Four of these are "services" for issues related to patient care, which can also be developed and extended to organizational ethics. These four services are indicated with an asterisk (*).

1. an interdisciplinary ethics committee,[54] reporting to the HCO's governing body with a mission statement specifying that it shall provide or oversee the provision of the services outlined below (For recommended guidelines on the committee's mission, composition, and functions, see Appendix 2.);
*2. education in clinical ethics for the clinicians who serve patients in the HCO and for the community that is served by the HCO
*3. assistance to the HCO and the community with policy development--on request or at the initiative of the ethics committee;
*4. ethics case consultation, on request, to assist with ethical problems that arise in patient care;

*5. resources for program evaluation and targeted research aimed to prevent ethical problems in the HCO or community that affect patient care;
6. at least two resource persons, selected from clinicians or other professionals in the HCO to receive advanced education in clinical ethics and to be compensated for time serving the ethics program; and
7. a process for addressing issues in organizational ethics and offering services in this area that parallel and complement the services described above.

There are no data on how many ethics committees have made a transition to programs that provide all of these services, including organizational ethics. Some HCOs have made the transition.[55] The four services of clinical ethics are discussed below, with special attention to case consultation and targeted research. These services can best be organized by a division of labor among members of the ethics program and its resource persons. Even in a small HCO, it is unfair and unrealistic to expect everyone to engage in all services.

A. Ethics Education

It is a commonplace concept that an ethics program ought to provide education for the professional staff and community on issues in ethics and healthcare law. Whether education is a "service" depends on how well it meets the needs of those who participate. By planning good educational events and courses, committee members also continue to educate themselves. Smaller HCOs can increase educational effectiveness by planning jointly and cooperatively with other HCOs in the region on the most important and costly courses and events. In larger HCOs, such courses can become a routine part of the orientation and continuing education of clinicians. Clinicians need the opportunity to study and discuss basic clinical ethics and healthcare law in their local or regional settings. The framework of a basic course in clinical ethics for healthcare professionals can be adapted from problem-based typology on which this textbook is based (see Chapter 1).

Each HCO's ethics committee can also provide an open and inviting forum to which individuals or groups can bring ethical issues for study, debate, and discussion. Maintaining a fair-minded forum requires skills in moderating debate that can easily be divisive and deteriorate into *ad hominem* comments. Good planning and leadership skills are required. Ethics education must also address major ethical and legal controversies in a timely way. The most critical controversies today include the following:

- unresolved ethical issues of justice in lack of access to adequate primary and preventive healthcare for one-sixth of the U.S. population;
- moral effects of managed-care practices on the clinician-patient relationship;
- the moral and legal debate about physician-assisted suicide;
- results of the Study to Understand Prognosis and Preferences for Outcomes and Risks Treatment (SUPPORT) study (see Chapters 1 and 9) and their implications for decision in critical care and making advance directives;
- disputes about medical futility and community/regional policy needs;
- issues of genetic testing in individuals and protection from "genetic discrimination";
- confidentiality and privacy issues, particularly in view of the on-line medical record;
- issues raised by pregnant patients, especially in regard to refusal of treatments or procedures beneficial for the fetus;
- clinicians' roles in addressing problems of physical abuse in families;
- use of chemical or physical restraints in long-term care of the elderly;
- rights of cultural and religious minorities who reject Western traditions of medicine; and
- alternative forms of healthcare and their place in a plan of care.

An effective ethics program has a long-term and an annual plan for education in clinical ethics for clinicians, patients, surrogates, and the larger community. Regular courses in clinical ethics and healthcare law combined with special events cosponsored by the HCO and the ethics program work best. Regular offerings afford the best opportunities to evaluate adult learning. The "easy way out" of education is to rely only on special events and outside speakers.

The following objectives should be incorporated into the plan for an ethics education program:

- Conduct needs assessments among relevant groups.
- Involve members of groups to be served in program planning.
- Attempt to reach entire HCO community.
- Extend education to community served by HCO.
- Distribute cases or materials prior to course or event.
- Begin and end sessions on time.
- Use recognized and well-informed teachers.
- Recruit and briefly train small-group discussion leaders.
- Plan for evaluation prior to teaching course or event.
- Evaluate and communicate findings to participants and leaders.

Chapters 3 through 14 of this text can be adapted to a weekly course for fall, spring, or summer. Another format for small settings is a monthly "ethics lunch" with discussion of a previously distributed case. Such a session can be conducted entirely as a group discussion with a summary at the end.

Significant new legal or ethical cases or laws create other opportunities for education. When such a case occurs, inservice education is an excellent format for all staff to raise questions and express their doubts and concerns. The services of policy development and ethics consultation provide other obvious educational opportunities.

B. Policy Development

Assisting clinicians and the HCO with policy development is a service that also uses skills in education and consultation. A service presumably benefits the persons or groups served. The greatest experiential tests of policies is whether they are understood, are followed, and guide actions in difficult cases. An important distinction ought to be made between policy and guidelines. A *policy* prescribes what should or must be done, assigns responsibilities for decisions and actions, and details procedures to be followed. *Guidelines*, by contrast, only advise or suggest approaches and allow for interpretive latitude to recognize the complexities of clinical situations.

Some policies for the HCO serve as a bridge between federal/state regulations and standards of practice within the institution. Clinicians, surrogates, and patients need specific guidance on such matters. The ethics program serves as a resource for policy study and for drafting proposed guidelines and policies concerning ethical issues. Authorities in the HCO receive the results of these studies and the recommendations of the ethics committee. Among the issues for which JCAHO requires policy statements and guidelines are:

- the HCO's process for addressing ethical issues in patient care and in organizational life;
- informed consent to treatment;
- use of family and/or surrogate decision makers;
- decisions to participate in research or clinical trials;
- refusal of medically indicated treatment;
- advance directives;
- pain management;
- decisions to withhold resuscitative services;
- decisions to forgo life-sustaining treatment;
- decisions about care and treatment at the end of life;
- confidentiality of information;
- privacy and security of patients' property;
- resolution of complaints;
- procurement and donation of organs and other tissue; and
- patients' access to medical records.

Additional issues that require specific policies or guidelines are: Jehovah's Witnesses' refusal of blood transfusion; informed-consent practices in the context of human immunodeficiency virus (HIV) testing; maternal-fetal conflicts; the status of preexisting do-not-resuscitate (DNR) orders in the context of an operative procedure, including dialysis; and counseling parents who want to donate organs of live-born anencephalic infants.

Leaders in the HCO should refer study of these and other issues to the ethics committee as the first step in developing policies that have a bearing on ethical issues and problems. The committee's work is to draft, debate, and recommend language for such policies and guidelines to the administration and governing body. The HCO's description of the ethics committee's role should recognize the committee's responsibility to recommend specific needs for policy initiatives to the HCO's authorities, rather than only entering the policy arena by request. An ethics committee has no authority to make policy, but it has the standing to recommend new directions for policy and should provide data to support recommendations.

The process of developing policy can be educational for the participants, and members of the ethics committee can serve as consultants and educators for the policy planning group. The steps outlined below can be considered by members of ethics programs serving in this role.

1. *Form a policy design team.* Organize a policy development team with representatives from the ethics committee and representatives of groups who have requested the policy, will need it, and will be most affected by it. Define the need or problem and identify others who should be consulted.
2. *Understand the problem.* Collect necessary information to clarify the issues, focus on relevant values and principles, and study paradigm cases.
3. *Identify policy options.* Be able to offer justifications for each option and practical significance for consideration of policy and guidelines.
4. *Provide feedback to key persons.* Convene representatives from the group(s) most affected by the proposed policy or guidelines. Seek consensus on what would be a policy improvement.
5. *Select among policy alternatives.* Prepare final presentation to key stakeholders, summarizing the need, how the proposed policy was conceptualized, quantitative and qualitative information, criteria for selecting among the options, the proposed policy statement, financial impact (if relevant), and a communications plan.
6. *Implement the policy.* Create an evaluation method, including indicators of the effectiveness of the policy and how data will be collected. Identify who is responsible for the evaluation and establish timelines for regular review.

C. Ethics Case Consultation

A long tradition of medicine encourages requesting consultation[56] for a problem in patient care. Physicians traditionally sought ethical guidance from their peers or trusted clergy advisers.[57] The founders of some medical humanities and bioethics programs,

although not physicians, were expected to consult on difficult cases.[58] The service of ethics case consultation (ECC) is a recent development in patient care. The first conference on ECC met in 1985.[59] Tulsky and Fox have critically reviewed a large literature on ethics consultation.[60]

The scope of ECC services is widening beyond patient care to include issues in cases provoked by managed healthcare systems. Decision makers also include administrators, case managers, gatekeepers, and so forth. Cases in which practice guidelines and cost-effectiveness strategies impinge on physician-patient relationships will increasingly be subjects for ECC.

1. Models for Ethics Case Consultation

There are three major models for providing ECC (see Exhibit 14-1). ECC by an ethics committee, with large variation, is the most prevalent model. Some committees provide ECC by the chairperson assembling an ad hoc team of members and others, depending on the clinical issues and the type of ethical problem(s). Some committees identify a subgroup or teams of members who are on-call for ECC. Other committees meet as a whole to consider cases. A second model is an ethics consultation service (ECS) with wide variation in membership and patterns of accountability. A third model relies on individual consultants who may or may not report to an ethics committee or to a source of authority within the HCO. These differences reflect lack of consensus among HCOs and in the field of clinical ethics about the goals of ECC, access to consultation, documentation, and credentialing of consultants. A joint task force of two professional societies is studying the question of credentialing for ECC and will make recommendations in 1997.[61]

A conference on ECC, supported by a grant from the Agency for Health Care Policy and Research, convened in 1995 to develop consensus for a long-term project to evaluate ECC.[62] After extensive debate and revisions, the 28 participants reached consensus on a statement of purpose and goals of ECC, as shown in Exhibit 14-2. A report of the process used to reach the consensus appears elsewhere.[63]

This consensus statement is a point of departure for regional and statewide bioethics networks and HCOs to discuss standards, education, and training.

Exhibit 14-1
Models for Ethics Case Consultation

Model 1: Ethics Committee
  A.   Chair assembles ad hoc team of members and others, depending on the features of the case.
  B.   Identified subgroup or teams of members are on-call.
  C.   Whole committee meets to consider all cases.

Model 2: Ethics Consultation Service
  A.   ECS is a mixture of committee members and others; it reports to the ethics committee.
  B.   ECS includes members not on the ethics committee; it reports to ethics committee.
  C.   An independent ECS reports to medical staff or to no one.

Model 3: Individual Consultant
  A.   Under contract to HCO
  B.   Part of a firm under contract to HCO
  C.   Under contract to the HCO's ethics committee

The interdependence and linkage of different elements of an ethics program is evident in the statement (such as ECC, education, policy development, and being a good bridge to authority when necessary).

2. Indications for an Ethics Case Consultation

When is an ethics consultation indicated? Some typical indications are when the requester finds that she or he is:

- an interested party to a dispute caused by an ethical problem;
- genuinely conflicted about the moral options;
- lacking information or informed opinion about an ethical issue; or
- mistrusted by patients or surrogates, who perhaps have threatened to sue.

The first three reasons could also be reasons for a patient or surrogate to request ECC.

Other situations could also call for ECC. For example:

- A rare or novel problem arises (for example, the *Baby K* case, Chapter 9).
- The patient is incapacitated, no surrogates or family can be found, and an important decision about treatment must be made.

- A clinician proposes action that colleagues believe is ethically unjustified.
- A patient or surrogate demands a treatment or action that clinicians believe is ethically unjustified.
- An iatrogenic error has harmed a patient, who remains uninformed along with other family members.

Clinicians, sharing important decisions with the patient or surrogate, are the primary moral problem solvers in such situations. But to whom can they confidently turn for assistance? Decision makers need assurance that consultants are adequately prepared for such situations and will not dominate decisions of those with standing to make a judgment. Consultants should be familiar with their proper roles by education, training, and experience. However, the reality is that readiness for ECC and quality of performance varies widely.

3. Scope and Quality in Ethics Case Consultation

Issues of scope of ECC and quality of performance can be addressed together. What is the proper scope of ECC? What are examples of role confusion? What counts as a good ethics consultation? What are the legal risks of ECC? ECC's scope is usually limited to requests for help with ethical problems in a "specific

---

Exhibit 14-2
Consensus Statement on Definition and Goals of Ethics Case Consultation

Ethics consultation is a service provided by an individual consultant, team, or committee to address the ethical issues involved in a specific clinical case. Its central purpose is to improve the process and outcomes of patient care by helping to identify, analyze, and resolve ethical problems.

To guide the evaluation of ethics consultations services, we propose the following goals:

1. To maximize benefit and minimize harm to patients, families, healthcare professionals and institutions by fostering a fair and inclusive decision making process that honors patient/proxy preferences and individual and cultural value differences among all parties to the consultation.
2. To facilitate resolution of conflicts in a respectful atmosphere with attention to the interests, rights, and responsibilities of those involved.
3. To inform institutional efforts at quality improvement, appropriate resource utilization, and policy development by identifying the causes of ethical problems and to promote practices consistent with the highest ethical norms and standards.
4. To provide education in healthcare ethics to assist individuals in handling current and future ethical problems.

Source: J.C. Fletcher and M. Siegler, "What Are the Goals of Ethics Consultation? A Consensus Statement," *The Journal of Clinical Ethics* 7, no. 2 (Summer 1996): 125. Copyright © 1996, The Journal of Clinical Ethics, Inc. Used with permission.

---

clinical case" (that is involving the care of an identified patient). The scope of ECC is somewhat elastic. It can extend to policy development, especially on very controversial issues. Many of the same skills and knowledge required for ECC in patient care are needed in consultation with groups that must develop policy when their members are divided in their views. Speaking now only of the clinical setting, violations of boundaries occur if an ECC service or consultant formally responds to requests for the following:

- professional assessment of the benefits/burdens of specific medical tests, treatments, or procedures (refer to the proper source of expertise);
- professional assessment of a patient's decision-making capacity (refer to liaison-consultation psychiatry, clinical psychology, neurology, as appropriate);
- requests for legal advice (refer to risk management or the proper attorney);
- issues of a clinician's competence (refer to chief of medical or nursing staff);
- issues of sexual or emotional harassment (refer to designated official or supervisor, unless the supervisor is the accused, then go higher);
- issues of child, spouse, or elder abuse (refer to the designated protection service); or

- an ethical problem in a location outside of the ECC service's designated responsibility (refer to most suitable ECC service or person).

No boundaries are violated by brief, informal discussion of such requests, while respecting rules of confidentiality ("please do not mention names"). One must have a sound factual basis for effective referral. There must also be room for "ethics conversations" with persons on an informal basis, while respecting confidentiality.

Issues of quality in ECC can be addressed at two levels: (1) guidelines for HCO ethics programs and (2) standards for consultants in specific cases. These two levels are interactive, but for purposes of analysis they may be separated. We recommend for consideration the Virginia Bioethics Network's (VBN) guidelines for HCO ethics consultation programs (see Appendix 2). Education and training programs for ECC can also consider the usefulness of these guidelines, which respect the diversity in models of ECC. Three premises underlie the VBN guidelines:

1. Diversity among HCOs in the United States and Canada requires a variety of approaches to ECC.
2. Multidisciplinary participation is an important value and safeguard.

3. Standards for education and training for ECC must be higher than standards to prepare an ethics committee member for his or her role.

A high standard of education and training for those who are to do ECC is necessary due to the challenging nature of the activity and its high visibility. A major error by a poorly informed ethics consultant may adversely affect a particular patient, one or more staff members, or the entire institution.

4. Legal Concerns

What are the risks of liability to those who serve in ECC? Several recommendations are set forth below.

*   It is prudent to assure in writing those who do ECC that the HCO's liability insurance carrier covers them and pays legal fees for defending them should they be sued for their role in a case.
*   There must be a sound process to approve and appoint those who provide ECC. Skills and knowledge of effective professionals in other fields do not directly translate into those needed for ECC. For this reason, the HCO's board needs assurance that those who do ECC have adequate education and training. The HCO can be a partner in facilitating such opportunities.
*   Members of ethics committees should be careful but not fearful of adverse legal consequences. There are risks involved for anyone in patient care, but compared to the risks of physicians and nurses, the risks to ethics consultants are not significant.[64]

Authorities in health law in the United States[65] and Canada[66] have described the grounds on which ethics consultants could be sued for negligence or violating the rights of patients. They emphasize the difficulty that exists in establishing a standard of care for ECC, which will persist due to issues of diversity. Lawsuits in clinical ethics are rare, but suits can and do arise.

There are at least four reasons why ethics committees or consultants to date have been named in suits and judicially criticized:

1. A committee or its consultants strongly take sides in cases; the cases may have varying degrees of complexity (for example, *Bouvia, Baby K*).
2. A committee or its consultants give approval to a process in which a physician takes unilateral action to withdraw life-sustaining treatment over the objections of surrogates, (for example, *Gilgunn, Rideout*).
3. A committee chairperson intervenes in the plan of care of a terminally ill patient without consultation with surrogates (for example, *Bland*).
4. A committee, backed by hospital policy, is part of a process in which DNR orders are written over the objections of the patient's surrogate (for example, *Bryan*).

To date, ethics committees or consultants have been named in at least five lawsuits and criticized by a federal judge in a sixth. Below, each case is described with comments. Except for the *Bouvia* and *Baby K* cases, all were disputes about medical futility. Ethics services and futility disputes are discussed below (also see Chapter 9).

a. *Bouvia v. Superior Court*

Beginning in 1983 at the age of 25, Elizabeth Bouvia, a quadriplegic suffering from cerebral palsy and painfully severe arthritis, was involved in legal proceedings that upheld physicians' forcefully feeding her by artificial means that she refused. The dispute was daily news for months. She became a patient at Los Angeles County High Desert Hospital in 1985. The ethics committee of that hospital, apparently without dissent, supported her physician's decision to force-feed her by a nasogastric tube. Her physicians believed that her failure to eat more was a suicidal attempt to starve herself to death. She claimed that she was eating as much as she could. Bouvia had been examined by a psychiatrist and found to be a capable decision maker. In 1986, a California court of appeals found in her favor and overturned an earlier court decision siding with her physician and the hospital. The appeals court ordered the feeding tube removed, and stated:

Elizabeth Bouvia's decision to forego medical treatment or life-support through a mechanical means belongs to her. It is not a medical decision for her physicians to make. Neither is it a legal question whose soundness is to be resolved by lawyers or judges. It is not a conditional right subject to approval by ethics committees or courts of law. It is a moral and philosophical decision that, being a competent adult, is hers alone.[67]

After the tube was removed, Bouvia and her attorney sued the hospital and the physicians for monetary damages. She learned that her physicians had stated that the ethics committee was as responsible as they were, and she filed an amended complaint against each member of the committee as a defendant.[68] Bouvia never served the committee members and voluntarily dropped the suit to avoid publicity[69] (see Chapter 7 for a discussion of the case).

The main lesson of the *Bouvia* lawsuit for ethics committees is about strongly taking sides in a moral problem. The degree of complexity of the issues in this case is debatable. For many, the case is easy. A competent patient has a clear, negative right to refuse any form of unwanted treatment, regardless of its life-saving effect. The case is harder for those who make distinctions between feeding and hydration and other forms of life-sustaining treatment. However, regardless of debate about degrees of complexity, ethics committees and consultants should guard against taking sides and being coopted by physicians. Their role is to provide education and offer consultation about all moral options in a case.

b. *In Re Baby K*

In 1992, an ethics committee at Fairfax Hospital in Virginia had a role in the *Baby K* case (see Chapter 9). A federal court judge criticized the committee's participation. The critique will alert plaintiff's attorneys and other interested parties to the criticisms that can be made of ethics committees.

At the physicians' request, a team of the ethics committee met with Baby K's mother, who demanded life-sustaining measures for a newborn with anencephaly. The staff of the neonatal intensive care unit viewed these measures as futile and as violations of their professional integrity. A three-person team (family practitioner, psychiatrist, and minister) was unsuccessful in resolving the dispute. Their ECC chart note stated that care was "futile" and advised that the hospital "attempt to resolve this through our legal system" if, after a waiting period, no change occurred in Baby K's mother's position. Judge Hilton wrote in his opinion that "treating physicians requested the assistance of the Hospital's 'Ethics Committee' in overriding

the mother's wishes."[70] He may have put quotation marks around the committee's name to deride their taking sides and their failure to give due attention to the moral arguments for the mother's position. Judge Hilton's ruling that the Emergency Medical Treatment and Active Labor Act (EMTALA) required the hospital to provide emergency ventilatory treatment for Baby K's periodic apnea (Baby K was by then residing in a nearby nursing home) was upheld by the Fourth Circuit Court of Appeals.[71] The U.S. Supreme Court declined to hear an appeal by the hospital, Baby K's father, and the guardian *ad litem*. Again, the lesson for ECC is to avoid taking sides in a morally complex case.

c. *Bryan v. Stone et al.; Bryan v. Rector and Visitors of the University of Virginia*

Bryan, the executrix of the estate of a 53-year-old patient who died at the University of Virginia (UVa) Hospital on 25 February 1993, brought two lawsuits.

The patient had undergone surgery at a regional county hospital on 14 December 1992 for a perforated pyloric ulcer with peritonitis secondary to ingestion of mineral oil. Her postoperative course was very poor: acute respiratory distress syndrome, sepsis, bilateral pneumothoraxes, a code followed by stroke, and inability to wean from a ventilator. She was transferred to UVa for evaluation and further treatment on 5 February. Her condition worsened, and computed tomography (CT) scan revealed a massive left cerebrovascular stroke. In addition, her multiple infections were not responsive to antibiotics, and she had massive subcutaneous emphysema and kidney failure. Her family, speaking through her husband, demanded that "everything be done" including cardiopulmonary resuscitation (CPR). The medical team concluded that CPR for this patient, who by then had seven chest tubes, would be ethically and medically inappropriate.

The house staff asked for ethics consultation shortly after the patient was transferred to UVa, but the patient's husband and family would not consent to ECC. It is UVa's policy that no formal consultation can be offered without consent of patients or surrogates. However, the Ethics Consultation Service (ECS) continued to communicate informally with the medical team about the issues in the case.

The dispute about CPR persisted. The house staff strongly resisted the prospect of CPR for this patient. The attending physician attempted to mediate. When the patient's husband refused to meet with the ECS or come to the hospital to discuss the question, the attending physician requested formal assistance from the ethics committee. The hospital's policy is that the chair of the committee can, in such a situation, convene an ad hoc advisory group to assist clinicians. Further, acting under a 1992 amendment to the UVa Medical Center's DNR policy, the ad hoc group recommended a plan that began with consultation with other noninvolved physicians about the family's request for CPR and the potential for transferring her care to one of them. If other physicians evaluating the request for CPR deemed it to be futile, the plan included writing a DNR order and an order to withhold CPR for reasons of medical futility.

Two other physicians were consulted. Each came to the same conclusion that the attending physician had reached about the futility of CPR. The patient was too critically ill to attempt a transfer out of the hospital. Subsequently, the attending physician wrote a DNR order, informed the patient's husband, and documented his objections. The medical team continued to communicate with the patient's husband by telephone. The patient died eight days after the DNR order was written.

Later, a dispute arose between the hospital's billing department and the family. Risk Management at UVa believes that the aggravation over billing was the primary causation for an ensuing suit. The patient's total bill was approximately $105,000, and her insurance paid for all but about $2,000. The family, already bitter over the outcome of the case, received repeated bills with a final notice that the unpaid bill would be turned over to a collection agency. They turned the letter over to their attorneys, who sought and received the medical record. Within the report was a report from the Ethics Committee chairperson about the consultation and recommendation supporting writing a DNR order.

In a context of this unresolved grievance and the wake of court decisions in the *Baby K* case, the family's attorneys filed two suits. A suit in county court alleged that the attending physician and the members of the ad hoc group had violated the patient's religious beliefs and specifically some conditions of the Virginia Health Care Decisions Act (see Chapter

9).[72] A second suit, filed in federal court, alleged that the patient had died as a result of withholding emergency treatment in the form of CPR. In the wake of the *Baby K* decisions, the plaintiffs charged that the hospital had violated EMTALA, aided by the ethics committee's ad hoc advisory group.

The suit in county court was dismissed "with prejudice," meaning that it could not be refiled. The Fourth Circuit Court of Appeals upheld a district court's dismissal of the federal suit. The federal court held that EMTALA was not violated, since the patient died after a 12-day period in the hospital.[73] This important ruling clarified the Fourth Circuit's interpretation of EMTALA following the *Baby K* case. It ruled that the patient had received "stabilizing treatment" during the entire hospital stay, and the court made no comment about the DNR order. The hospital policy permitting DNR orders in such controversies was adopted after a 1992 amendment to the Virginia Health Care Decisions Act stipulated that physicians are not required to prescribe or render treatment that the physician determines to be "medically or ethically inappropriate."[74] The law requires that a good-faith effort be made to transfer the patient to the care of another physician; because of this patient's hopeless condition, should could not be transferred outside the hospital.

d. *Gilgunn v. Massachusetts General Hospital*

Capron discussed the ethical and legal significance of this important case.[75] In brief, a 71-year-old woman in very poor health broke her hip in a fall. Before she could undergo orthopedic surgery she suffered seizures followed by brain damage and coma. Her daughter, the surrogate of choice, informed physicians that her mother would have "wanted everything done." After several weeks, the medical team desired to stop treatment that they considered futile. The hospital's optimum care committee was one of the earliest types of patient care ethics committees in the nation; it was a small group that confined its scope mainly to intensive care. The committee's chair was a psychiatrist with a long-standing practice of advocating DNR orders when incapacitated and hopelessly ill patients had lengthy stays in the intensive care unit (ICU) and families demanded that "everything be done."[76] The chair persuaded the attending physician to write a DNR order, which the attending physician later revoked when the daughter protested. The chair then supported a subsequent attending physician's decision to write a DNR order. The chair and committee did not meet with the surrogate. After a DNR was written, the attending physician gradually extubated the patient over the surrogate's objections. The patient died, and her daughter sued for violations of her, rather than the patient's rights. A trial court jury sided with the hospital.[77] The decision is now on appeal to a higher court.

Capron is correct in his criticism of the intervention of the physician-chairperson of the optimal care committee. The committee did not act as an ethics committee but, in Capron's words, "in the style of a medical consultant." None of the mediational and educational benefits of ECC were evident in the process used in this case.

e. *Estate of James Davis Bland v. Cigna Healthplan of Texas, et al.*

This suit was brought by the family of a patient with AIDS for intentional infliction of emotional harm due to decisions made by the chair of the ethics committee that were associated with the manner of the patient's death.[78] The case also figured prominently in a 1995 article about managed care and medicine in Texas.[79]

Bland was a registered nurse who understood that he had a terminal illness and would die soon. In July 1993, he was admitted to Houston's Park Plaza Hospital's ICU and placed on a respirator. He was given a paralytic drug to make him comfortable, and the respirator took over his breathing function. Afraid of suffocating if he was taken off the respirator, he asked his physician to allow him to die peacefully while being ventilated. His physician agreed, and the patient soon lapsed into a coma.

The physician explained his plan to the family, who understood and agreed to a DNR order on the condition that the patient remain on the respirator. Bland's physician then withdrew from the case and turned over care to a Cigna primary-care physician. After a few days, the medical director of Cigna contacted the chair of the ethics committee, a pulmonologist. The Cigna official raised questions about the patient's stay in the ICU and whether he could be moved. The chair of the ethics committee went to the unit, presumably in the role of a physician--but not the patient's physician--without consulting the patient's original physician or the patient's family. He did discuss the care plan with the Cigna primary-care physician. As a result of the intervention by the pulmonologist/ethics committee chair, the patient was removed from the respirator by a respiratory therapist and died shortly thereafter.[80] The circumstances of Bland's death and the involvement of the pulmonologist/ethics committee chair were not discussed with the family. They learned the facts from documents prepared for another lawsuit brought by Bland's original physician against Cigna. The suit by Bland's family was settled out of court for an undisclosed amount.

Questions arise about the Cigna official's motives and the actions of the ethics committee chair in this case. These questions cannot be answered without more knowledge of the facts. Was the motive for contact cost savings or the appropriate level of care for a moribund patient? If the former, the chair should not have permitted the contact by the official. It is inappropriate for an insurance company official to contact an ethics committee except to identify an ethical problem in the care of a patient.

Even if the pulmonologist believed that he was confining his role to that of physician, he appears to have violated the interests of the patient's family. The Cigna primary-care physician may have abdicated his role by permitting the pulmonologist to go to the patient's room and initiate a process leading to removal of the ventilator with no discussion with the family. If this act occurred, it is morally problematic, because it is a well-established social practice that physicians should share such crucial decisions with surrogates. The act was legally questionable in the light of decision-making criteria required by the Texas Natural Death Act.[81] In today's society, physicians do not have the moral authority unilaterally to withdraw life supports, even from a hopelessly ill patient. To be morally valid, this action requires discussion and agreement from surrogates or legally authorized representatives of the patient, because this action contributes to the timing and circumstances of the patient's death.

The legal authority of physicians to withdraw life supports unilaterally is unsettled and controversial, as shown in *Gilgunn*. Physicians' authority to write DNR orders unilaterally is still controversial, as shown by *Bryan*, but is more settled than withdrawing life supports, as shown by the next case, *Rideout*. However, if it is true in *Bland* that an ethics committee chairperson was the main figure in the decision to remove the patient from the ventilator, without consultation with surrogates, this action should be viewed as a serious violation of the role of ethics committees and a failure of the HCO to take precautions to prevent such conflicts. It is a guideline of the Virginia Bioethics Network, for example, that an ethics consultant should make other arrangements and avoid taking a consultation in a unit where he or she regularly practices (see Appendix 2).

An alternative course of action in *Bland* was that the care plan drawn up by Bland's first physician could have been reviewed in the context of an ethics consultation requested by the Cigna primary-care physician with the consent and participation of the original physician and family (if they were willing to participate in such a meeting). Also, the original physician and the Cigna primary-care physician could have prevented the original problem by supervising a more rapid process of withdrawing life-support measures with control of distress by analgesics.[82]

f. *Rideout v. Hershey Medical Center*

Brianne Rideout, a two-year-old patient with a brain stem glioblastoma (a malignant tumor), had neurosurgery at Johns Hopkins University Hospital. She was admitted to the emergency department of the Hershey Medical Center in Pennsylvania on 6 April 1992. While at Hershey, she lapsed into a stupor and required assistance to breathe. By 13 April, she had a tracheostomy and was placed on a ventilator. Physicians regarded her condition as incurable, but her parents favored aggressive treatment.

Then began a period of negotiation regarding home care or hospital care. Home care was ruled out due to inadequate wiring for a ventilator. By 20 May, the patient's parents learned that her insurance coverage would soon be depleted and Medicaid was needed to cover costs. The next day, the ethics committee met at the request of the patient's physician (without the parents present) to discuss the case, and the committee supported a decision to write a DNR order. On 22 May, when they were informed of this decision, the Rideouts stated that they were opposed because it meant giving up on the child's life. A search began for an appropriate alternate site without success. On 12 July, the child's pupils became fixed and

dilated for the first time. On 13 July, her physician decided, based on discussions with the ethics committee and in the light of the patient's deteriorating condition, to remove the ventilator.

On 14 July, her physician informed the Rideouts that he would withdraw the ventilator that day. The chair of the ethics committee met with the parents to confirm the decision. Following this meeting, the parents complained to the patient advocate, who persuaded the physician and ethics committee chair to delay to allow legal consultation. Nonetheless, the removal was scheduled for 11:00 a.m. on 15 July. The parents sought a judicial order to stop this action and secured the services of an attorney. The hospital had asked local police to be present to prevent disorder. While the parents were in the office of the patient advocate speaking with their attorney by phone, the physician removed the ventilator. The hospital's chaplain communicated the action to the Rideouts. Hearing this, they rushed to her room. They were described in their complaint as being hysterical and crying that their daughter was being murdered. They requested that the ventilator be reconnected, but the physician declined to do so. Mr. Rideout reportedly had an acute asthma attack. The patient died two days later, in the presence of her parents.

The Rideout's 11-count complaint raised common-law, statutory, and constitutional claims, each of which the hospital contested.[83] On 29 December 1995, a three judge panel overruled the medical center's challenge to claims that by stopping the ventilator over the parents' wishes, the hospital committed an assault and battery on the child, negligently and intentionally inflicted emotional distress on the parents, and impinged parental rights rooted in the free exercise of religion.[84] The panel refused to rule out punitive damages. The hospital won arguments that it did not violate constitutional privacy and liberty interests and that EMTALA was not violated. The panel's decision meant that the parents were free to continue their lawsuit in a jury trial.

The *Rideout* case has the classic features of a futility dispute. The Hershey ethics committee may have erred in the process of the case in two respects. First, was it good practice to meet originally with the physician without notifying and inviting the parents? An opportunity to engage and involve them was missed. Second, later in the case, was it good practice for the chair to meet with the parents for the purpose of notifying them that the decision to withdraw would be carried out? Closing out morally acceptable options is not the role of an ethics committee. There were two other options available, even at that point: (1) transfer the patient to an alternate site or, failing that, (2) to seek a court's concurrence with the decision to withdraw.

At the deepest level, the Hershey ethics committee appears to have strongly taken sides with a physician and hospital authorities against the patient's parents. The alternative stance is to offer only consultation, education, and mediation about the morally acceptable options. Also, the committee appears to have been a party to a unilateral decision to remove a ventilator over the parents' objections. In such a situation, the ethics committee's role should be confined to searching for other morally acceptable alternatives to such a morally dubious action. If that search fails, then the physician and hospital should seek the help of a court in resolving the dispute. Physicians and ethics committees are not the final arbiters of futility disputes until our society works out fairer approaches to allocation of expensive healthcare resources. The institutions of law must be involved to ensure the highest standards of impartiality.

Bland and *Rideout* pose serious legal challenges to ethics committees or their chairpersons who strongly take sides and who advocate unilateral decision making in situations involving treatment at the end of life. These cases also bear upon the question of the competence and perspective of those who do ECC. A court has not yet asked the question: "For what exactly is an ethics consultant (or a team acting for a committee) responsible and accountable?" Based on the evolution of these cases, such a question can be expected.

5. The Consultant's Competence and Perspective

The consultant's role in each case calls for competence in two areas: moral diagnosis and education. Depending on the circumstances, the role also calls for skills in mediation and being a trustworthy bridge to authority. Every full ethics consultation has a five-part history:

1. the threshold of the case and the consultant's entry;

2. the consultant's assessment;
3. moral diagnosis and education;
4. goal setting, decision making, and implementation; and
5. evaluation.

a. Perspective

The consultant's perspective ought to value a good process in ECC over the "right" solution to the moral problems in the case. The ethics consultant is not the agent of a higher societal power who is authorized to take over disputes and make decisions. Ethics consultants at most represent healthcare ethics, an interdisciplinary field with services to offer, one of which is ECC. Ethics consultants serve decision makers with standing in the case. Their obligation as moral diagnosticians and educators is to probe the complexity of the ethical problems in the case.

Real differences do exist between views of ECC that emphasize outcomes and views that emphasize process.[85] Proactive consultants advocate for their point of view and recommend what ought to be done in a case. Process-oriented consultants favor being educators over being moral advocates. They restrain desires to determine the outcomes of cases and are willing to leave such decisions to those with legitimate moral and legal power to make them. Proactive ECC is likely to be paternalistic and assumes too much power and responsibility for outcomes. If it is good to avoid the old medical paternalism, why is neopaternalism in ECC desirable except for a rare "ethics emergency?" And, as in *Bland* and *Rideout*, consultants' taking sides cases can result in lawsuits.

b. Criteria for Entering a Case

If a consultation is indicated, the consultant enters the case using criteria in the HCO's protocol for ECC. Entry criteria for ECC are recommended in the VBN guidelines in Appendix 2. The two most important entry criteria are briefly covered below.

1. *Notify the attending physician.* If the attending physician has not requested the consultation, he or she should be promptly notified, preferably by the person who requests consultation. If the person who requests consultation wants anonymity

(usually because of fear of the attending physician), he or she should solve this problem prior to entry. An option is to persuade someone else to request the consultation openly or persuade the caller of protection by the institution's policy on this matter. Some attending physicians may refuse ECC for their own reasons. However, an open access policy for ECC requires a process for the chairperson of the ethics committee to have authority to respond to refusals of consultation, review the attending physician's reasons, and resolve the problem of how the consultation will proceed.

2. *Obtain the consent of patient or surrogate.* In most circumstances, respect for the patient's privacy requires consent for the ethics consultation, prior to the ethics consultant's seeing the patient's chart. The patient's or surrogate's consent is required because ethics consultants are not part of the healthcare team and they will have access to private and confidential information. Ideally, the attending physician introduces the consultant(s) to the patient or surrogate.

After entry, the ethics consultant first reviews the assessment and moral diagnosis made by clinicians or makes a fresh assessment of the issues. The consultant can then guide the process through efforts to resolve the problem(s) and an evaluation. The steps needed for an adequate ECC are outlined in Exhibit 14-3. These steps are adapted from the case method discussed in Chapter 2. The contents of Exhibit 14-3 are comprehensive and cover the relevant issues in the types of cases in which ECC is involved. The consultant needs the knowledge, skills, and experience to use the elements in the outline that are relevant to the case at hand. The consultant must have the competence to use this process in cooperation with decision makers in the case. Again, opportunities for education, training, and supervision must be created regionally by the clinical ethics community.

D. Targeted Research: From Crisis-Orientation to Prevention

Strengthened ethics programs create larger opportunities to serve. An advanced service to a HCO and its community is research aimed to prevent chronic ethical problems. So-called targeted research aims at the causes of recurrent problems rather than

crisis reactions to their symptoms and consequences. Targeted research is a good example of the influence of quality improvement on healthcare ethics. Wolf expertly reviewed arguments for quality improvement in ethics.[86] Adapting lessons from the "quality revolution in medicine"[87] will help ethics programs mature and promote more professional relationships with those to be served. Teichholz discussed the relevance of the work of Deming and others in industry to the quality improvement movement in medicine.[88] By focusing on structure, process, and outcome, quality assurance has been transformed from a formerly "policing" function to one in which the "emphasis is now on finding common denominators and asking what the overall process is and whether it can be improved, not on what is wrong in any individual case."[89] This emphasis could help the condition of ethics services evolve from crisis-orientation to prevention. Clinical ethics was shaped in the crucible of acute-care medicine of the 1970s and 1980s. It is not surprising that its role has largely been crisis-oriented. Clinical ethics must perform well in crises or "ethics emergencies," but it will fail if it remains in this posture.

Ethics services need a two-level strategy informed by reliable knowledge about causation. Strategy at an immediate level aims to identify, analyze, and assist in resolving ethical problem(s) that obstruct planning for the care of patients. Strategy at a higher level aims at interim and long-term prevention of remediable causes of ethical problems. Some human conditions underlie and contribute to ethical problems and cannot be "prevented" (for example, contingency, ambiguity, freedom to choose values, finitude, and death itself). However, some causes of ethical problems can be ameliorated. The SUPPORT (see Chapters 1 and 9) truly opens doors for further research into the causes of ethical issues in critical care. Some of these causes may be:

- failure to assess promptly the goals of treatment in patients with poor prognosis;
- toleration of lengthy stays on ventilators without discussion of alternatives;
- lack of training and practice in advance-care planning;
- lacking a prior plan to identify and treat surrogate decision makers;
- structural and power arrangements (for example, leaving decisions about when to initiate discus-

Exhibit 14-3
Elements of an Ethics Consultation

I. Consultant's assessment
  A. What is the patient's medical condition?
    1. Identification of medical problems
    2. Diagnosis/diagnostic hypotheses
    3. Predictions and uncertainties regarding prognosis
      a. What are the prospects for full or partial recovery?
      b. Is the patient terminally ill?
    4. Provisional formulation of goals of treatment and care
    5. Recommendations for treatment and reasonable alternatives
  B. What are the relevant contextual factors?
    1. Demographic facts: age, gender, education
    2. Life situation and life style of patient
    3. Family relationships
    4. Setting of care: home or institution
    5. Socio-economic factors (such as insurance coverage)
    6. Language spoken
    7. Cultural factors
    8. Religion
  C. Is the patient capable of decision making?
    1. Legally incompetent (for example, child, court determination of incompetence)
    2. Clearly incapacitated (for example, unconscious)
    3. Diminished capacity (for example, depression or other mental disorder interfering with understanding or judgment)
    4. Fluctuating capacity
    5. Prospects for enhancing capacity
  D. What are the patient's preferences?
    1. Understanding of condition
    2. Views on quality of life
    3. Values relevant to decision making about treatment
    4. Current wishes for treatment
    5. Advance directives
    6. Reasons for seeking treatment regarded as medically inappropriate or for refusing treatment regarded as medically indicated
  E. What are the needs of the patient as a person?
    1. Psychic suffering and possible interventions for relief
    2. Interpersonal dynamics
    3. Resources and strategies for helping patient cope
    4. Adequacy of home environment for care of patient
    5. Preparation for dying
  F. What are the preferences of family/surrogate decision makers?
    1. Competence as surrogate decision maker
    2. Judgment and evidence of relevant patient preferences
    3. Opinions on quality of life of patient
    4. Opinions on best interest of patient
    5. Reasons for seeking treatment regarded as medically inappropriate or refusing treatment regarded as medically indicated
  G. Are there interests other than, and potentially competing with, those of the patient?
    1. Interests of family (for example, concerns about burdens of caring for patient, disagreements with preferences of patient)
    2. Interests of fetus
    3. Scarce resources and competing needs for their use
    4. Interests of healthcare providers (for example, professional integrity)
    5. Interests of healthcare organization

Exhibit 14-3, continued

    H.   Are there issues of power or conflict in the interactions of the key actors in the case that should be addressed?
        1.   Between clinicians and patient/family
        2.   Between patient and family
        3.   Between family members/surrogates
        4.   Between members of the healthcare team (for example attending physicians and house staff, physicians and nurses)
    I.   Have all the parties involved in the case had an opportunity to be heard?
    J.   Are there institutional factors contributing to moral problems posed by the case?
        1.   Work routines
        2.   Fears of malpractice/defensive medicine
        3.   Biases favoring disproportionately aggressive treatment or neglect of treatable conditions
        4.   Cost constraints/economic incentives

II. Consultant's moral diagnosis and educational aims
    A.   Examine how the moral problem in this case is being framed by the participants. Does this framework need to be reconsidered and replaced by an alternative understanding?
    B.   Identify and rank the range of relevant moral considerations.
    C.   Identify any relevant institutional policies pertaining to the case.
    D.   Consider ethical standards and guidelines, drawing on consensus statements of commissions and interdisciplinary or specialty groups. Educate using these resources.
    E.   Consider similar cases and discussions in the literature that might shed light on the analysis and resolution of moral problems in the case. Educate using these cases and literature.
    F.   Identify the morally acceptable options for resolving the moral problem(s) posed by the case? Educate about these options.

III. Goal setting, decision making, and implementation
    A.   Consider or reconsider and negotiate the goals of treatment and care for the patient.
    B.   Consider ideas (hypotheses) for possible interventions to meet the needs of the patient and resolve moral problems.
    C.   Deliberate regarding merits of alternative options for resolving the moral problem.
    D.   Endeavor to resolve conflicts.
    E.   Negotiate acceptable plan of action.
    F.   If negotiations and ethics consultation fail to achieve satisfactory resolution, consider judicial review.
    G.   Implement plan of action.

IV. Evaluation
    A.   Current Evaluation
        1.   Is the plan of action working? If not, why not?
        2.   Do the observed results of implementing the plan indicate the need for a modification of the plan?
        3.   Have conditions changed in a way that suggests the need to rethink the plan?
        4.   Are interactions between clinicians and the patient or surrogate helping to meet the needs of the patient, to respect the patient as a person, and to serve the goals of the plan of care?
        5.   Are there relevant interests, institutional factors, or normative considerations that have not been adequately addressed in planning for the care of the patient?
    B.   Retrospective Evaluation
        1.   What opportunities for resolving the moral problem were missed?
        2.   How did the care received by the patient match up to standards of good practice?
        3.   What factors contributed to a less than optimal resolution of the problems posed by the case?
        4.   Was the process of problem solving satisfactory in this case?
        5.   What might have been done to improve the care of the patient?
        6.   Are there desirable changes in institutional policy, feasible changes in the clinical environment, or educational interventions that might help to prevent or better resolve the moral problems posed by similar cases?

sion about changing the goals of treatment completely to attending physicians); and

- lack of financial incentives to promote timely discussion and decision making.

Futility disputes are clear examples of the failure of conventional approaches in clinical ethics that prove the need for a two-level strategy. The lawsuits reviewed above are important in this regard. Even if the lawsuits had been avoided by better communication and mediation, the disputes would not have been prevented. Clinicians and HCOs are attempting to resolve and prevent bedside disputes about futile treatment by means of ethics committees, hospital policies, and the courts. Although well intended, these are interim approaches and unstable as true prevention. Ethics consultation or institutional policies that address such disputes have only minor preventive effects. When ineptly provided, albeit with good intentions, such efforts can do harm. One mark of a futility dispute is that the surrogates do not trust ethics consultants or anyone associated with the HCO. For this reason, a better first-level alternative may be to enlist the help of respected leaders in the community as mediators of such disputes and to ask the disputants to abide by their recommendations as a last resort prior to seeking judicial review.

In the long run, futility disputes can only be resolved by reform of allocation of treatments and procedures in healthcare. The root causes of disputes about futile treatment lie in the economic needs of a "supply-state" healthcare policy to support a huge investment in acute-care and critical-care medicine.[90] Failure to reform the policy results in the following:

- the phenomenon of "strangers treating strangers" with desperate life-prolonging measures in acute-care and ICU settings;
- a lack of lifelong preventive care and primary-care medicine for Americans; and
- mistrust of healthcare professionals and medicine among members of underserved and disadvantaged groups, who are more likely not to believe what physicians say about futile treatment and to demand that "everything be done" in a catastrophic illness or at the end of life.

Remedying these causes requires long-term reform of the healthcare system and higher-quality life-long medical care for all Americans. We will continue to experience futility disputes as long as the U.S. health policy remains heavily weighted on the side of supply and disadvantaged groups are underserved. Reform of allocation and global budgeting combined with ethically acceptable practices of rationing at the bedside are sources of prevention of futility disputes.

V. Organizational Ethics: Whose Responsibility?

In addition to a strong ethics program with services, organizational morale is important for moral problem solving. Good organizational morale depends on several factors, which can be represented as concentric circles. The largest circle is the way persons are treated in their interactions with those in authority, especially over performance evaluation and job security. The second is the example set by the HCO's leaders in relationships with one another and with those who serve patients. Does trust and openness prevail in relations between the board of directors, the administration, and the medical and nursing staffs? Clinicians find it hard to be open and share decisions with patients where antagonism, secrecy, or a high level of suspicion exists. Another significant factor is the integrity of the business practices of the organization and its interactions with other organizations in the region. A final factor is the organization's responses to larger forces--economic, social, and political--at work in the society. Is the HCO guided by a broad vision of its role and responsibilities? Is there a shared statement of vision and values that is periodically reexamined and renewed?

Healthcare ethics committees to date have mainly addressed issues in patient care. This stance must be balanced by attention to ethical issues raised by organizational and economic forces. As Reiser wrote in an important article: "Institutions have ethical lives and characters just as their individual members do."[91] JCAHO has published new rules about "organizational ethics,"--issues that concern the integrity of the HCO (see Appendix 1).

JCAHO requires members to establish and maintain "structures to support patient rights . . . based on politics, procedures, and their philosophical basis, which makes up the framework that addresses both patient care and organizational ethical issues . . ."[92] JCAHO rules specifically require a process to examine ethical issues in marketing, admissions, discharge, billing, relationships with third-party payers and managed-care plans, as well as a "code of organizational ethics" to address each of these areas. JCAHO rules can best be met by a HCO's ethics program with two arms: patients' rights and organizational ethics.

Development of effective services in patient care ethics is a useful precedent for services in organizational ethics. Ethical analysis of healthcare systems draws upon some of the ethical concepts used in this text but requires a different set of skills in describing the context of ethical problems that arise for healthcare and managed-care organizations as such. The tasks of organizational ethics are:

- to provide a forum for discussion and education in issues of organizational ethics for clinical and administrative staff, concerned patients or their surrogates, and members of the larger community (these issues include marketing, admissions, transfer, discharge, and billing practices; relationships with healthcare professionals, third-party payers, managed-care companies, and educational institutions; as well as other issues that may arise);
- to do policy studies on request and make recommendations for institutional guidelines to address various ethical issues in the life of the organization and its relationships with others; and
- to provide a process for consultation concerning ethical problems that arise in the life of the organization.

Examples how such ethical issues can arise are:

- An employee, patient, or member of the community questions the veracity of statements the HCO has made in marketing and advertising activities.
- A particular managed-care contract contains restrictions on patient services or treatments that appear to HCO physicians to compromise what in the best medical interests of patients.
- A patient and a primary-care physician complain together that the patient's discharge was premature and based on financial considerations.
- A HCO physician who is removed from the roster of by a health insurer's managed-care plan for criticizing the company's policies and not for poor performance complains of unfair treatment.

- A patient with significant chronic disease has been assigned a new primary-care physician and complains about the lack of continuity of care.

Organizational ethics services could follow some of the practices used by an ECS in patient care:

- Any involved employee, patient, surrogate, or potential patient may ask for consultation regarding an ethical issue in the life of the organization.
- After identifying the ethical issue(s) that need consideration, an organizational ethics subcommittee provides a process for consultation, education, and mediation (if needed) concerning the morally acceptable options and ways to resolve the problem(s). The consultation is advisory only.
- The organizational ethics subcommittee reports all of its consultations to the ethics committee, respecting rules of confidentiality and privacy where these apply.

HCOs with well-developed ethics programs for patient care already have the experience in moral problem solving to examine concerns of organizational ethics. Different skills and knowledge of the HCO's business and institutional life are needed, but the process of moral problem solving in these areas is not essentially different from that in patient care settings. In the future, more problems will arise that call for skills and knowledge of both arenas.

Notes

1. Three examples of poorly addressed, costly "ethics emergencies" with large public relations and legal problems for each hospital were: (1) the Fitzgerald case at the Alexandria, Virginia hospital, (2) the Angie Carder case at the George Washington University Hospital, and (3) the Baby K case at Fairfax Hospital. The Fitzgerald case is described in B. Hosford, *Bioethics Committees* (Rockville, Md.: Aspen, 1986), 5-8. The Carder case is reported in G.J. Annas, "She's Going to Die: The Case of Angela C," *Hastings Center Report* 18, no. 1 (1988):23-25. The Baby K case is discussed by G.J. Annas, "Asking the Courts to Set the Standard of Emergency Care," *New England Journal of Medicine* 330 (1994): 1542-45; and J.C. Fletcher, "The Baby K Case: Ethical and Legal Considerations of Disputes about Fu-

tility," *BioLaw* 2, no. 11 (1994): S219-38.

2. Bioethics as a social movement is discussed in J.C. Fletcher, "The Bioethics Movement and Hospital Ethics Committees," *Maryland Law Review* 50, no. 3 (1991): 859-94; also see J.D. Moreno, *Deciding Together* (New York: Oxford University Press, 1995): 143-59.

3. See note 2 above, Moreno, pp. 93-97.

4. D. Rothman, *Strangers at the Bedside* (New York: Free Press, 1991).

5. For a discussion of thalidomide, see *Thalidomide* 89th Cong., 2d sess., 1966, S. Rept. 1153, 8-2. For a discussion of the Jewish Hospital for Chronic Diseases Cancer Study, see E. Langer, "Human Experimentations: New York Affirms Patients' Rights," *Science* 151 (1966): 663-65. For a discussion of the baboon-to-human heart transplant, see J.D. Hardy, "Heart Transplantation in Man," *Journal of the American Medical Association* 188 (1964): 1132-35. For discussions of the Willowbrook study, see S. Krugman et al., "Infectious Hepatitis Detection of Virus During the Incubation Period and in Clinically Inapparent Infection," *New England Journal of Medicine* 261 (1959): 729-34; S. Goldby, "Experiments at the Willowbrook State School," *Lancet* 1 (1971): 749. For the Beecher article, see H.K. Beecher, "Ethics and Clinical Research," *New England Journal of Medicine* 74 (1966): 1354-60. For discussion of "Tea Room Trade" deceptive social research, see L. Humphreys, *Tea Room Trade: Impersonal Sex in Public Places* (Chicago: Aldine, 1970); D.P. Warwick, "Tearoom Trade: Means and Ends in Social Research," *Hastings Center Report* 1, no. 1 (1973): 24-38. On fetal research, see "Live Abortus Research Raises Hackles of Some, Hopes of Others," *Medical World News,* 5 October 1973, 32-36; V. Cohn, "NIH Vows Not to Fund Fetus Work," *Washington Post*, 13 April 1973, A1.

6. J.H. Jones, *Bad Blood*, 2nd ed. (New York: Free Press, 1991).

7. Ibid., 204. Jones relates the way Jean Heller, an Associated Press writer, got the story and published it on 25 July 1972 in the *Washington Star*.

8. V. Gamble, "A Legacy of Distrust: African Americans and Medical Research," *American Journal of Preventive Medicine* 9, no. 6 (1993): 35-38 (suppl).

9. Surgeon-General, U.S. Public Health Service, Department of Health, Education, and Welfare, "Investigations Involving Subjects, Including Clinical Research: Requirements for Review to Insure the Rights and Welfare of Individuals," PPO no. 129, Revised Policy, 1 July 1966. In 1974, Congress passed the National Research Act (pub. L. No. 93-348) requiring that all research involving human subjects receive prior group review by an institutional review board.

10. These two norms--professional integrity and informed consent--are the core of the traditional practices embodied in the Nuremberg Code, along with the requirement for previous animal experiments. See P.M. McNeill, *The Ethics and Politics of Human Experimentation* (New York: Cambridge University Press, 1993), 42.

11. National Research Act, (Pub. L. No. 93-348), 88 Stat. 348 (1974).

12. J.C. Fletcher and F.G. Miller, "The Promise and Perils of Public Bioethics," in *The Ethics of Research Involving Human Subjects: Facing the 21st Century*, H.Y. Vanderpool, ed. (Frederick, Md.: University Publishing Group, 1996), 155-84.

13. C.M. Spicer, "Fallout from Government-Sponsored Radiation Research." *Kennedy Institute of Ethics Journal* 4 (1994):147-54; Advisory Committee on Human Radiation Experiments, *Final Report* (Washington, D.C.: U.S. Government Printing Office, 1995).

14. See note 13 above, Advisory Committee, pp. 818-22.

15. Of 125 U.S. medical schools responding to a 1994-1995 survey, 61 had a separate required course in medical ethics, 94 offered medical ethics as part of an existing required course, and all said that there was at least an elective on the topic. Association of American Medical Colleges, *Institutional Profile System Ranking Report* (unpublished report, 1994-1995).

16. P. Singer, *Animal Liberation* (New York: Avon, 1977).

17. R.A. Whitney, "Animal Care and Use Committees: History and Current National Policies in the United States," *Laboratory Animal Science* 37 (January 1987): 18-21.

18. U.S. Department of Health and Human Services, Commission on Research Integrity, *Integrity and Misconduct in Research* (Washington, D.C.: U.S. Government Printing Office, 1995, publication number 1996-746-425).

19. R.E. Bulger, E. Heitman and S.J. Reiser, ed., *The Ethical Dimensions of the Biological Sciences* (New York: Cambridge University Press, 1993); R. L. Penslar, ed., *Research Ethics: Cases and Materials* (Bloomington, Ind.: University of Indiana Press, 1995).

20. See note 2 above, Moreno, p. 36.

21. The first published article about ethics committees was by a physician, K. Teel, "The Physician's Dilemma. A Doctor's View: What the Law Should Be,"

Baylor Law Review 27 (1975):6-9. Later and extensive discussions are in R.E. Cranford and E.A. Doudera, "The Emergence of Institutional Ethics Committees," in *Institutional Ethics Committees and Health Care Decision Making*, R.E. Cranford and E.A. Doudera, ed. (Ann Arbor, Mich.: Health Administration Press, 1984), 5-21; also see B. Hosford, *Bioethics Committees*, (Rockville, Md.: Aspen, 1986).

22. President's Commission for the Study of Ethical Problems in Medicine and Biomedical and Behavioral Research, *Decisions to Forego Life-Sustaining Treatment* (Washington, D.C.: U.S. Government Printing Office, 1983): 153-60.

23. Ibid., 4.

24. Ibid., 5.

25. *Annotated Code of Maryland*, section 19-373 (Supp. 1994).

26. *New Jersey Administrative Code*, 8: 43-4.15 (1992); *New Jersey Statutes Annotated*, sec. 2A: 84A-22.10 (West 1994) (establishing priviledge).

27. *Hawaii Revised Statutes Annotated*, sec. 663-1.7 (1995) (extending peer review priviledge to ethics committee).

28. Joint Commission on Accreditation of Healthcare Organizations, *Accreditation Manual for Hospitals* (Oakbrook Terrace, Ill., JCAHO: 1992).

29. Joint Commission on Accreditation of Healthcare Organizations, *Standards, Rights, Responsibilities, and Ethics* (Oakbrook Terrace, Ill., JCAHO, 1995).

30. American Hospital Association, *1992 Statistical Guide* (Chicago: AHA, 1992). Data were collected in 1989. Of 2,071 hospitals with more than 200 beds, approximately 518 did not have a committee; of 4,649 with fewer than 200 beds, 3,487 did not have a committee. Smaller hospitals were more likely to lack a committee.

31. J.C. Fletcher and D.E. Hoffman, "Hospital Ethics Committees: Time to Experiment with Standards," *Annals of Internal Medicine* 120 (1994): 335-38.

32. G. Glasser, N.R. Zweibel, and C.K. Cassel, "The Ethics Committee in the Nursing Home: Results of a National Survey," *Journal of the American Geriatrics Society* 36 no. 2 (1988): 150-56.

33. D.E. Hoffman, P. Boyle, and S.A. Levenson, *Handbook for Nursing Home Ethics Committees* (Washington, D.C.: American Association of Homes and Services for the Aging, 1995).

34. S. Fry-Revere, J. Sorrell, and M. Silva, ed., *Ethics and Answers in Home Health Care*, (Leesburg, Va.: Regis Group, 1995).

35. R.F. Wilson et al., "Hospital Ethics Committees: Are They Evaluating Their Performance?" *HEC Forum* 2 (1993): 449-55.

36. J.W. Ross et al., ed., *Handbook for Hospital Ethics Committees*, (Chicago: American Hospital Association, 1986).

37. D.E. Hoffman, "Evaluating Ethics Committees: A View from the Outside," *Milbank Quarterly* 71 (1994): 4-40.

38. See note 31 above.

39. B. Lo, "Behind Closed Doors: Promises and Pitfalls of Ethics Committees," *New England Journal of Medicine* 317 (1987): 46-50.

40. S. Fry-Revere, "Some Suggestions for Holding Bioethics Committees and Consultants Accountable," *Cambridge Quarterly of Healthcare Ethics* 2 (1993): 449-55; S.M. Wolf, "Ethics Committees and Due Process: Nesting Rights in a Community of Caring," *Maryland Law Review* 50 (1991): 798-858.

41. J.A. Tulsky and B. Lo, "Ethics Consultation: Time to Focus on Patients," *American Journal of Medicine* 92 (1992): 343-45.

42. J.A. Tulsky and E. Fox, "Evaluating Ethics Consultation: Framing the Questions," *The Journal of Clinical Ethics* 7, no. 2 (Summer 1996): 109-15.

43. C.M. Culver, *Ethics at the Bedside* (Hanover, N.H.: University Press of New England, 1990).

44. H.S. Perkins and B.S. Saathoff, "Impact of Medical Ethics Consultations on Physicians: An Exploratory Study," *American Journal of Medicine* 85 (1988):761-65; J. LaPuma et al., "An Ethics Consultation Service in a Teaching Hospital: Utilization and Evaluation," *Journal of the American Medical Association* 260 (1988): 808-11.

45. E. Fox and J.A. Tulsky, "Evaluation Research and the Future of Ethics Consultation," *The Journal of Clinical Ethics* 7, no. 2 (Summer 1996): 146-49.

46. In the *Baby K* case, which did not involve a lawsuit against an ethics committee, federal judge Clarence Hilton ruled that the mother's "treating physicians requested the assistance of the Hospital's 'Ethics Committee' in overriding the mothers' wishes" (see Chapter 9). Judge Hilton placed the quotation marks around 'Ethics Committee' in order to deride the committee's actions. *In Re Baby K*, 832 F.Supp. 1022 (E.D. Va. 1993).

47. R. Macklin, *Enemies of Patients* (New York: Oxford University Press, 1993), 212-29.

48. G.J. Annas, "Ethics Committees: From Ethical Comfort to Ethical Cover," *Hastings Center Report* 21, no. 3 (May-June 1991):18-21.

49. For criticisms of ethics committees, see J.D.

Moreno, "Ethics by Committee: The Moral Authority of Consensus," *Journal of Medicine and Philosophy*, 14 (1988): 411-32; J.D. Moreno, "What Means This Consensus? Ethics Committees and Philosophic Tradition," *The Journal of Clinical Ethics* 1, no. 1 (Spring 1990): 38-43; M. Siegler, "The Progression of Medicine: From Physician Paternalism to Patient Autonomy to Bureaucratic Parsimony," *Archives of Internal Medicine* 145 (1985): 713-15; J.C. Fletcher, "Ethics Committees and Due Process," *Law, Medicine & Health Care* 20 (1992): 291-93.

50. For criticisms of ethics consultation, see G. Scofield, "The Problem of the Impaired Clinical Ethicist," *Quality Review Bulletin* 18, no. 1 (1992): 26-32; G. Scofield, "Ethics Consultation: The Least Dangerous Profession," *Cambridge Quarterly of Healthcare Ethics* 2 (1993): 417-48; J.C. Fletcher, "Commentary: Constructiveness Where It Counts," *Cambridge Quarterly of Healthcare Ethics* 2 (1993): 426-34; J. La Puma and D.L. Schiedermayer, "Ethics Consultation: Skills, Roles, and Training," *Annals of Internal Medicine* 114 (1991): 155-60; J. La Puma, E.R. Priest, "Medical Staff Privileges for Ethics Consultants: An Institutional Model," *Quality Review Bulletin* 18 no. 1 (1992): 17-20; J.C. Fletcher, "Needed: A Broader View of Ethics Consultation," *Quality Review Bulletin* 18 no. 1 (1992): 12-14.

51. This statement is based on six years of experience in "Developing Hospital Ethics Programs" (DHEP), an outreach training and education program of the Center for Biomedical Ethics, University of Virginia. An external evaluation of the first group of 10 hospitals (1990) to participate in DHEP, funded by the Greenwall Foundation (New York) in 1992, showed clearly that DHEP had succeeded in eight of the 10 hospitals. M.N. Smith et al., "Evaluation of Effectiveness of Developing Hospital Ethics Programs--A Project to Help Community Hospitals to Strengthen Institutional Ethics Programs," University of Virginia, Center for Biomedical Ethics, 1993. DHEP has served more than 150 hospitals and nursing homes to help them develop stronger ethics programs.

We write "may prove to be effective" because the statewide and regional plan in Virginia and bordering states for Programs of Education and Training in Clinical Ethics (PETCE) are to be implemented in September 1997 and have yet to pass the tests of quality control and adequate funding.

52. Statewide and regional bioethics networks are organized in some parts of the nation. These groups have several functions: (1) public education, (2) clearinghouse for regional issues, and (3) mutual support and encouragement of ethics committees. Well-developed networks provide educational and training opportunities for ethics committee members. Some have graduate education in clinical ethics. Networks with efforts of this kind are in Florida, Maryland (Baltimore), Michigan, Minnesota, Ohio, New Mexico, New York City, North Carolina (Charlotte), Pennsylvania (Pittsburgh), Virginia, West Virginia, and Wisconsin.

53. In Virginia, the short-term educational event is "Developing Hospital Ethics Programs," (see note 51 above), a six-day program offered twice a year. The long-term program is "Programs of Education and Training in Clinical Ethics" (see note 51 above), which will be offered in two regions of Virginia to ethics committee members (6 credit hours), to candidates for a certificate in clinical ethics (12 to 15 credit hours plus a one-week summer residency at the University of Virginia), and to individual enrolled in a master's degree program (24 to 27 credit hours plus two one-week summer residencies at the University of Virginia.)

54. Significant literature on ethics committees includes: E. Doudera and R. Cranford, *Institutional Ethics Committees and Health Care Decision Making* (Ann Arbor, Mich.: Health Administration Press, 1985); R.P. Craig, C.L. Middleton, and L.J. O'Connell, *Ethics Committees: A Practical Approach* (St. Louis, Mo.: Catholic Health Association, 1986); G.A. Kanoti and J.K. Vinicky, "The Role and Structure of Hospital Ethics Committees," in *Health Care Ethics*, ed. G.R. Anderson and V.A. Glesnes-Anderson (Rockville, Md.: Aspen, 1987): 293-307; J.W. Ross et al., ed., *Handbook for Hospital Ethics Committees* (Chicago: American Hospital Association, 1986). See notes 33 and 34 above for literature on ethics committees in nursing homes and home health agencies.

55. Information is available from HCOs that have made this transition. These include large, medium sized, and small hospitals, as well as a few long-term care facilities (Duke University Medical Center, Durham, N.C.; Johnston Memorial Hospital, Abingdon, Va.; Mary Washington Hospital, Fredericksburg, Va.; University of Virginia Medical Center, Charlottesville, Va.; Camelot Health and Rehabilitation Center, Harrisonburg, Va.).

56. The Hippocratic writings direct physicians in doubt about a patient or "in the dark through inexperience" to urge "the calling in of others, in order to learn by consultation the truth about the case, and . . . that there may be fellow workers to afford abundant help." See "Selections from the Hippocratic Corpus," in *Eth-*

ics in Medicine, S.J. Reiser, A.J. Dyck, and W.J. Curran, ed. (Cambridge, Mass.: Massachusetts Institute of Technology Press, 1977); 5-9. Thomas Percival's *Medical Ethics*, first published in 1803, urged British physicians to seek help by consultation with others about problems in long and difficult cases; see T. Percival, *Medical Ethics*, 3rd ed. (Oxford, England: John Henry Parker, 1849). Percival prescribes approaches to the resolution of conflict between physicians who disagree, when these conflicts threaten the best interest of the patient. The first (1847) and latest (1990) code of ethics of the American Medical Association also direct physicians to seek consultation. See American Medical Association, "First Code of Medical Ethics," in *Ethics in Medicine*, ed. S.J. Reiser, A.J. Dyck, and W.J. Curran (Cambridge, Mass.: Massachusetts Institute of Technology Press, 1977), 26-34; American Medical Association, *Current Opinions of the Judicial Council* (Chicago: AMA, 1990). These codes refer to medical problems for which consultation is needed, but they do not exclude seeking help with ethical problems.

57. I.N. Trainin and F. Rosner, "Jewish Codes and Guidelines," in *Encyclopedia of Bioethics*, ed. W.T. Reich (New York: Free Press, 1978), 1428-30; C.E. Curran, "Roman Catholicism," in *Encyclopedia of Bioethics*, 1522-34.

58. A.R. Jonsen, "Can an Ethicist be a Consultant?" in *Frontiers in Medical Ethics*, ed. V. Abernethy (Cambridge, Mass.: Ballinger, 1980); M. Boverman and J.C. Fletcher, "The Evolution of the Role of an Applied Bioethicist in a Research Hospital," in *Research Ethics*, ed. K. Berg and K.E. Traney (New York: Alan R. Liss, 1983), 131-58.

59. This conference, cosponsored by the National Institutes of Health (NIH) and the University of California at San Francisco, was convened at the NIH in 1985. Conference papers and other contributions were published in J.C. Fletcher, N. Quist, and A.R. Jonsen, ed., *Ethics Consultation in Health Care* (Ann Arbor, Mich.: Health Administration Press, 1989). In 1986, the Society for Bioethics Consultation was founded to study ethics consultation in healthcare and support the continuing education of ethics consultants (Society for Bioethics Consultation, Stuart Youngner, M.D., President, c/o Department of Medicine, University Hospitals, 2074 Abington, Cleveland, Ohio 44106).

60. Tulsky and Fox reviewed the small and weak empirical core of this literature, see note 42 above. Older literature reviews are by T. Pruzinsky, "Definition and Evaluation of Biomedical Ethics Consultations: An Annotated Bibliography," *BioLaw* 2, no. 29 (1989):

S221-29; D. Anzia, F. Miedema, and J. LaPuma, "Ethics Consultation: An Annotated Bibliography," *Newsletter of the Society for Bioethics Consultation* (Spring 1991): 3-5. Two important discussions are: J. LaPuma and D. Schiedermayer, *Ethics Consultation: A Practical Guide* (Boston: Jones and Bartlett, 1994); and F.E. Baylis, ed., *The Health Care Ethics Consultant* (Totowa, N.J.: Humana Press, 1994). See a review of these books in J.C. Fletcher: "The Consultant's Credentials," *Hastings Center Report* 25 (July-August 1995): 39-40.

61. The Society for Bioethics Consultation (SBC) and the Society for Health and Human Values (SHHV) cosponsor this task force, funded by a grant from the Greenwall Foundation and contributions from many ethics centers and networks. The task force is codirected by Robert Arnold, M.D., and Stuart Youngner, M.D., Mark Aulisio, Ph.D., is project coordinator. The task force will report its conclusions in 1997.

62. Papers from this conference appeared in *The Journal of Clinical Ethics* 7, no. 2 (Summer 1996).

63. J.C. Fletcher and M. Siegler, "What Are the Goals of Ethics Consultation? A Consensus Statement," *The Journal of Clinical Ethics* 7, no. 2 (Summer 1996): 122-26.

64. L.J. Nelson, "Legal Liability in Bioethics Consultation," in *Healthcare Ethics Services*, ed. M.F. Marshall, J.C. Fletcher, and E.M. Spencer (Dordrecht, The Netherlands: Kluwer, in press).

65. J.A. Robertson, "Clinical Medical Ethics and the Law: The Rights and Duties of Ethics Consultants," in *Ethics Consultation in Health Care*, ed. J.C. Fletcher, N. Quist, and A.R. Jonsen (Ann Arbor, Mich.: Health Administration Press, 1989), 157-72, especially 166.

66. L. Lowenstein and J. DesBrisay, "Liability of Health Care Ethics Consultants," in *The Health Care Ethics Consultant* ed. F. Baylis (Totowa, N.J.: Humana Press, 1994): 133-61.

67. *Bouvia v. Superior Court*, 179 Cal. App. 3d 1127, 225 Cal. Rptr. 297, (1986). The entire *Bouvia* case is well-reported, except for the involvement and suit against the committee, in G.E. Pence, *Classic Cases in Medical Ethics*, 2nd ed. (New York: McGraw-Hill, 1995), 41-47.

68. "Bouvia Sues Hospital Ethics Committee," *Hospital Ethics* 3, no. 1 (1987): 13-14; L.J. Nelson, "Legal Liability of Institutional Ethics Committees to Patients," *Clinical Ethics Report* 6, no. 4 (1992): 1-8.

69. C. Blades and M. Curreri, "Law, Ethics, and Health Care: An Analysis of the Potential Legal Liability of Institutional Ethics Committees," *BioLaw* 2, no. 33 (1989): S317-26. Nelson, see note 68 above, also

cites a personal communication with the late Richard Scott, Bouvia's attorney at the time.

70. *In re Baby K*, 832 F.Supp. 1022 (E.D. Va. 1993). This case and the ethics committee's role is discussed at length in J.C. Fletcher, "Bioethics in a Legal Forum: Confessions of an 'Expert Witness,' " *Journal of Philosophy and Medicine* 22, no. 4, (in press).

71. *In re Baby K*, 16 F.3d 590 (4th Cir. 1994).

72. Virginia Health Care Decisions Act of 1992, *Virginia Code Annotated*, sec. 54.1-2981-2991 (Michie 1994).

73. *Bryan v. Rectors and Visitors of the University of Virginia*, 95 F.3d 349 (4th Cir.1996).

74. See note 72 above.

75. A.M. Capron, "Abandoning a Waning Life," *Hastings Center Report* 25 no. 4 (1995): 24-26.

76. T.A. Brennan, "Incompetent Patients with Limited Care in the Absence of Family Consent," *Annals of Internal Medicine* 109 (1988): 819-25.

77. *Gilgunn v. Massachusetts General Hospital*, No. 92-4820, Suffolk Co., Mass., Super. Ct. (April 1995); G. Kolata, "Court Ruling Limits Rights of Patients," *New York Times*, 22 April 1995, A1.

78. *Estate of James Davis Bland v. Cigna Healthplan of Texas; Kenneth Lawrence Toppell, M.D.; Milton Thomas, M.D.; and Park Plaza Hospital*, District Court of Harris County, Tex., 11th Dist. No. 93-52630 (1995).

79. M. Swartz, "Not What the Doctor Ordered," *Texas Monthly* (March 1995): 86-89, 115-132.

80. In describing his action and the process by which the patient was removed from the respirator, according to the pulmonologist's deposition, he went to the room and changed the settings on the patient's ventilator, observed him breathing on his own, and then returned the ventilator to the previous settings. The pulmonologist testified that a respiratory therapist was called who "put him on a T-tube . . . on twenty-eight percent oxygen." *(Estate of) James Bland v. Cigna Healthplan of Texas*, 2 No. 790732: 118-19.

81. Natural Death Act, *Vernon's Texas Codes Annotated* 672.001 (1992).

82. T. Gillian and T.A. Raffin, "Withdrawing Life Support: Extubation and Prolonged Terminal Weans Are Inappropriate," *Critical Care Medicine* 24, no. 2 (1996): 352-53.

83. *Marlene and Tyrone Rideout v. Hershey Medical Center*, No. 96-5260, Court of Common Pleas, Dauphin County, Pa. (December 1995).

84. *Rideout v. Hershey Medical Center*, No. 96-5260, Court of Common Pleas, Dauphin County, Pa. (December 1995). The court decision is discussed in W.P. Murphy, "Hospital Faces Liability for Cutting Life Support," *Pennsylvania Law Weekly* 19, no. 3 (1996):1, 22.

85. For a range of views, see J. LaPuma and D. Schiedermayer, *Ethics Consultation: A Practical Guide* (Boston: Jones and Bartlett, 1994); F.E. Baylis, ed., *The Health Care Ethics Consultant* (Totowa, N.J.: Humana Press, 1994); J.C. Fletcher, "The Consultant's Credentials," *Hastings Center Report* 25 (July-August 1995): 39-40; J.C. Fletcher and H. Brody, "Clinical Ethics: Elements and Methodologies," in *Encyclopedia of Bioethics*, 2nd ed., W.T. Reich, ed. (New York: Simon & Schuster MacMillan, 1995), 399-404.

86. S.M. Wolf, "Quality Assessment of Ethics in Health Care: The Accountability Revolution," *American Journal of Law & Medicine* 20 (1994): 107-28.

87. A. Relman, "Assessment and Accountability: The Third Revolution in Medical Care," *New England Journal of Medicine* 319 (1988): 1220-23.

88. L.N. Teichholz, "Quality, Deming's Principles, and Physicians," *Mount Sinai Journal of Medicine* 35 (1993): 350-58.

89. Ibid, p. 351.

90. L.R. Jacobs, "Politics of America's Supply State," *Health Affairs* 14, no. 2 (1995): 143-57.

91. S.J. Reiser, "The Ethical Life of Health Care Organizations," *Hastings Center Report* 24, no. 6 (1994): 24-45.

92. Joint Commission on Accreditation of Healthcare Organizations (JCAHO), *Standards on Patient Rights and Organization Ethics*, reproduced in this volume as Appendix 1.

15

PROFESSIONAL ETHICS

Edward M. Spencer, M.D.

. . . If I fulfil this oath and do not violate it, may it be granted to me to enjoy life and art, being honored with fame among all men for all time to come; if I transgress it and swear falsely, may the opposite of this be true.
--The Hippocratic Oath

I will do all in my power to maintain and elevate the standard of my profession.
--The Florence Nightingale Pledge

I. Introduction

Since the late 1960s, the ethics of patient care in the United States has developed along two pathways that have at times been parallel and at other times divergent. One of these pathways, contemporary bioethics, began in the mid-to-late 1960s with ethical questions concerning human research. From the beginning, contemporary bioethics developed outside of organized medicine; it involved academic philosophers, theologians, and attorneys, along with a few interested physicians and other clinicians. After addressing ethical problems associated with research on humans, the field of bioethics continued to develop with the organization of bioethics centers and groups, received a significant boost from several very public court cases (*Quinlan*, *Conroy*, and *Cruzan*), and was publicly legitimized by the formation of the President's Commission for the Study of Ethical Problems in Medicine and Biomedical and Behavioral Research. The reports of the President's Commission became the foundation of the major accepted societal guidelines for decision making concerning ethical is-

sues related to medical care, particularly those decisions affecting medical care at the end of life.

Presently, bioethicists are concerned with theoretical and practical considerations of general issues and specific problems in ethics. Largely based on concepts of "rights" or "principles," the field of bioethics directly and indirectly influences clinical ethics (which entails the practical application of bioethics theory to specific situations involving the care of patients.) Contemporary bioethics is an impetus for the formation of institutional ethics committees, for the institution of programs of ethics education and ethics consultation in healthcare settings, and for many other aspects of the ethics of patient care in healthcare institutions. Other chapters in this text draw upon bioethics for their theoretical base.

The second pathway, which is more traditional and clinician-based, is commonly called "professional ethics." In the past, this conceptualization of medical ethics has guided physicians, nurses, and other clinicians when they encountered a situation described as an "ethical problem." Rather than focusing on rights or principles, this stream of medical ethics focuses largely on maintaining the professional integrity of the individual clinician and his or her profession, and it has been externally documented in the form of professional codes.

Professional codes, with a basis in tradition, are seen as the guiding beacons for the behavior of practitioners. The codes involve advice and direction, both specific and general, concerning the proper manner of responding to a defined problem or circumstance. In addition, the codes define certain fundamental character traits of the professional practitioner.

How decisions concerning clinical care are perceived, discussed, and acted upon is directly determined by which of these differing perspectives is held to be authoritative. Contemporary bioethics emphasizes patient autonomy and resultant individual rights as primary determining factors. When using contemporary bioethics as the basis for decision making, clinical decisions require conversations and the sharing of authority. However, the final authority to make these decisions rests with the patient, and this can lead to a clinician-patient relationship based on contractual considerations rather than on trust.

The professional ethics perspective concentrates on the clinician as moral agent. It asks, "What kind of a person should I be to fulfill my professional obligations?" rather than, "What should I do and how should it be done?" Contemporary bioethics perceives an ethical problem as a case or situation with a discernable, consistent answer. Professional ethics perceives these problems as deviations from accepted professional norms or as a lack of proper attention by a conscientious professional, which has led or may lead to difficulty for the patient or a professional colleague.

As attention to contemporary bioethics has gradually increased during the past 30 years, the potential for confusion has also increased. There is an unavoidable tension between the bioethics viewpoint and the professional ethics viewpoint, particularly when one attempts to decide what is right in an actual situation. Should an institutional ethics committee be concerned only with issues involving patients' rights, or should it also be concerned with issues of professional integrity? Should a physician, who is struggling with an ethical issue, look to pronouncements from contemporary bioethics or to his or her obligations as a professional for help in understanding and addressing the problem? These and similar questions illustrate this tension and confusion.

Professional organizations, such as the American Medical Association (AMA), have actually contributed to the confusion by not clearly distinguishing between bioethics and professional ethics in their work. The Council for Ethical and Judicial Affairs (CEJA), AMA's group that interprets its *Code of Medical Ethics* and issues *Current Opinions* on subjects of ethical importance, has attempted to consolidate the two positions by incorporating the viewpoint of contemporary bioethics into its code. CEJA recently added a new section to the code called "Fundamental Elements of the Patient-Physician Relationship," and it defined these fundamental elements in terms of the patients' rights rather than the more traditional physician's obligations.[1] In a number of its opinions on ethical issues, CEJA has addressed bioethics issues, has used the language of bioethics, and has appealed directly to contemporary bioethics for the foundational authority for the particular opinion. In doing so, the council has gone beyond its mandated role of interpreting the *Code of Medical Ethics* and defining an ethical physician via opinions about the physician's obligations in specific circumstances.

CEJA's own confusion in distinguishing between bioethics and professional ethics is demonstrated by its recent turnabout in its opinions relating to using the organs of anencephalic infants for transplantation. This issue is an appropriate one for CEJA to consider, because as long as anencephalic infants are defined by society as "human" and "alive," the physician's traditional obligation for protection pertains. This position was the crux of the opinion issued in 1988.[2] However, the 1988 opinion was radically revised in March 1992. The following statement from the 1992 opinion demonstrates the complete reversal of the earlier position: "It is ethically permissible to consider the anencephalic as a potential organ donor, although alive still under present definitions of death."[3]

Instead of questioning society's definition concerning the humanity of the anencephalic infant, CEJA reversed a primary obligation of physicians (to protect the patient) with that single opinion. Predictably, there was significant disagreement with this action in the AMA House of Delegates and elsewhere; CEJA issued another opinion in 1996, reversing the 1992 opinion and reverting back to the 1988 position that requires determination of death prior to using the organs of anencephalic infants for transplantation.[4] This reversal demonstrates a lack of understanding within the AMA itself of the important differences between contemporary bioethics and professional medical ethics, in that a bioethics issue (defining the humanity of an anencephalic infant) was equated with interpreting the *Code of Principles of Medical Ethics* to define clearly the obligations of an ethical physician to anencephalic infants.

Whether there can ever be a realistic accommodation between these differing perspectives concerning the ethics of clinical care is still an open question. The attempts toward accommodation to date have fallen far short of being effective in decreasing the tension naturally present between these two viewpoints. Contemporary bioethics--with its influence on courts and legislatures, its strong backing from most of academia, and its fundamental position emphasizing patients' rights--seems to be ascendent at present. However, our society still shows a strong desire for a relationship between a clinician and patient based on trust rather than on negotiation grounded in "rights." The ideal of the old-fashioned doctor still seems to strike a chord in most people, and people seldom question the desirability of healthcare professions that adhere to a fundamental internal ethos.

This chapter explores the history and fundamentals of the professional ethics viewpoint specifically for physicians and nurses. It points out the value of this viewpoint for individual patients and society and calls attention to some problematic areas. Finally, it briefly explores some possible areas of accommodation and coexistence between traditional professional ethics and contemporary bioethics.

II. Historical Background

A. Professional Medical Ethics

The Code of Hammurabi was the first known code of conduct for medical practitioners. Conceived by the Babylonians about 2000 B.C., it set forth in considerable detail the conduct demanded of a physician. Because it was very specific for that time and culture, it has not continued as a practical set of professional guidelines and is only of interest for historical reasons.

Portions of the body of work attributed to the Hippocratic School such as the Hippocratic Oath, on the other hand, have continued to the present time as a basic statement of principles upon which the prac-

tice of medicine should rest. This statement of principles was likely conceived in the fifth century B.C. Unlike the Code of Hammurabi, the Hippocratic Oath set out in brief form a general statement of ideals which protected patients by appealing to the finer instincts of the physician without imposing sanctions.

I swear by Apollo the Physician and Ascleplus and Hygela and Panakela and all the gods and goddesses, making them my witnesses, that I will fulfill according to my ability and judgment this oath and this covenant:

To hold him who has taught me this art as equal to my parents and to live my life in partnership with him, and if he is in need of money to give him a share of mine, and to regard his offspring as equal to my brothers in male lineage and to teach them this art, if they desire to learn it, without fee and covenant; to give a share of precepts and oral instructions and all the other learning to my sons and to the sons of him who has instructed me and to pupils who have signed the covenant and have taken an oath according to the medical law, but to no one else.

I will apply dietetic measures for the benefit of the sick according to my ability and judgment; I will keep them from harm and injustice.

I will neither give a deadly drug to anybody if asked for it, nor will I make a suggestion to this effect. Similarly I will not give to a woman an abortive remedy. In purity and holiness I will guard my life and my art.

I will not use the knife, not even on sufferers from stone, but will withdraw in favor of such men as are engaged in this work.

Whatever houses I may visit, I will come for the benefit of the sick, remaining free of all intentional injustice, of all mischief, and in particular of sexual relations with both female and male persons, be they free or slaves.

What I may see or hear in the course of the treatment or even outside of the treatment in regard to the life of men, which on no account one must spread abroad, I will keep to myself holding such things shameful [unspeakable] to be spoken about.

If I fulfill this oath and do not violate it, may it be granted to me to enjoy life and art, being honored with fame among all men for all time to come. If I transgress it and swear falsely, may the opposite of all this be true.[5]

Other civilizations since Ancient Greece have developed written principles concerning the practice of medicine, but the Oath of Hippocrates (modified in the 11th century A.D. to eliminate reference to pagan gods) has remained as an expression of ideal conduct for the physician. The distinguishing aspects of the Hippocratic Oath are its strong emphasis on beneficence toward the patient, on the physician's acquisition and maintenance of competence, and on certain self-serving practices to limit admission into the profession.[6]

Following Hippocrates and other early Greek philosophers, the development of the professional ethics of medicine is linked to traditional values associated with the Christian, Jewish, and Islamic religions. These ties fostered the development of compassion and other humane ideals in addition to the competence and beneficence emphasized by the Greek codes.

Al-Ruhawi, an Islamic physician, wrote what is probably the earliest systematic treatise on medical ethics in the Arabic world in the eighth century A.D. In this treatise, al-Ruhawi tempered the ideals of the Greeks and the Islamic prophets with concrete judgments arising from bedside practices. His efforts to give realistic guidelines for action, derived from basic religious and philosophical tenets within the context of the everyday problems faced by the physician, are quite modern in their outlook.[7]

Isaac Israeli, a Jewish physician and contemporary of al-Ruhawi, also wrote extensively. His works include *The Book of Admonitions to the Physicians*. These admonitions, although written within the Jewish tradition, are notably secular and include issues such as thorough knowledge, attention to patients' needs, and prompt response. The admonitions relied on ancient authorities including those from the Hippocratic tradition, and emphasized the healing power of nature. Jewish religious ideals were sustained in the provocative and sobering, *Daily Prayer of a Physician*, attributed to Moses Maimonides, a physician and philosopher of the late 12th century. This prayer begins with references to the creation of the human body by God and its purpose as the envelope of the soul. The prayer's major theme is a request for help and support for the physician as he works to benefit mankind. It asks for inspiration leading to love of

the art of medicine and God's creatures. It asks for confidence from patients so as to ensure compliance with the physician's counsel. It also asks that the physician's soul be receptive to education, be gentle and calm, and be forgiving of the arrogance of others.[8]

In their search for professional ethics, Christian physicians attempted to reconcile the ideals of the Hippocratic tradition with their religious values. The physician was looked upon as an agent of God, with God as the ultimate healer. More practically, the physician was urged to be modest, chaste, and humble, as well as charming and affable (the latter two were hardly religious ideals). As fundamental sources of ideals, medieval physicians ignored neither the Greek philosophical legacy nor the Christian Church and its teachings, but many did attempt to apply these ideals to contemporary practice in a practical way.[9]

In this fashion, professional medical values became enmeshed with religious values. As an alternative to the priesthood, medicine was also a profession to which one could be "called," and the physician was seen as a conduit for God's power to heal the sick.

The next significant contribution to the development of modern professional medical ethics was made by the English physician, Thomas Percival, when he published his *Code of Medical Ethics* in 1803. This was a "scheme of professional conduct relative to hospitals and other charities." Percival followed the Hippocratic tradition and included such admonitions as physicians must "keep heads clear and hands steady" by observing constant temperance. Percival's code emphasized professional etiquette.[10]

The first items of discussion at the initial meeting of the American Medical Association (AMA) in 1847 were the establishment of a code of ethics and the creation of minimum requirements for medical education. Certain state medical societies had formal written codes of conduct prior to the development of the AMA code, but these tended to be provincial. The AMA's *Principles of Medical Ethics* was based on Percival's code to a larger extent than any of the previously established state codes. To some extent, the AMA code was used to exclude those who were trained in other schools or philosophies of medical practice. In general, the language and concepts of the original AMA code remained unchanged until recently. It included matters of professional etiquette as well as principles related to the care of patients.

In 1957, the AMA revised the format of the *Principles* to include 10 short sections, preceded by a preamble that "succinctly express[es] the fundamental concepts embodied in the present [1955] Principles." When presenting this change to the AMA House of Delegates, the AMA Judicial Council stated: "every basic principle has been preserved; on the other hand, as much as possible of the prolixity and ambiguity which in the past obstructed ready explanation, practical codification and particular selection of basic concepts has been eliminated."[11] In 1977, the Judicial Council recommended that the *Principles* be revised "to clarify and update the language, to eliminate reference to gender, and to seek a proper and reasonable balance between professional standards and contemporary legal standards in our changing society."[12]

The Judicial Council of the AMA has subsequently been renamed the Council on Ethical and Judicial Affairs (CEJA). This is the body responsible for interpreting and recommending changes in the *Code of Medical Ethics*, for investigating general ethical conditions and all matters pertaining to the relations of physicians to one another or to the public, and for making recommendations to the House of Delegates (the ruling body of the AMA) or the constituent associations (those organizations that comprise the membership of the AMA including state medical societies).

The present *Code of Medical Ethics* consists of four related parts: (1) "Principles of Medical Ethics," which is the fundamental statement of the core principles of the code; (2) "Fundamental Elements of the Patient-Physician Relationship," which was first published in 1990 as a report of CEJA and was updated in 1994; (3) "Current Opinions," which reflect the application of the principles to more than 135 specific ethical issues in medicine (it is here that CEJA has gone well beyond its mandate and addressed bioethics issues); and (4) "Reports" on issues of importance and interest prior to or concurrent with the issuance of an opinion.[13]

The AMA's "Principles of Medical Ethics" are as follows:

PREAMBLE:

The medical profession has long subscribed to a body of ethical statements developed primarily for the benefit of the patient. As a member of this profession, a physician must recognize responsibility not only to patients, but also to society, to other health professionals, and to self. The following Principles adopted by the American Medical Association are not laws, but standards of conduct which define the essentials of honorable behavior for the physician.

I. A physician shall be dedicated to providing competent medical service with compassion and respect for human dignity.

II. A physician shall deal honestly with patients and colleagues, and strive to expose those physicians deficient in character or competence, or who engage in fraud or deception.

III. A physician shall respect the law and also recognize a responsibility to seek changes in those requirements which are contrary to the best interests of the patient.

IV. A physician shall respect the rights of patients, or colleagues, and of other health professionals, and shall safeguard patient confidences within the constraints of the law.

V. A physician shall continue to study, apply and advance scientific knowledge, make relevant information available to patients, colleagues, and the public, obtain consultation, and use the talents of other health professionals when indicated.

VI. A physician shall, in the provision of appropriate patient care, except in emergencies, be free to choose whom to serve, with whom to associate, and the environment in which to provide medical services.

VII. A physician shall recognize a responsibility to participate in activities contributing to an improved community.[14]

B. Professional Nursing Ethics

Contemporary bioethics has involved nurses from the beginning. The nursing profession and its major organizations have supported the clinical activities of bioethics much more than has the medical profession. The development of bioethics came at a time of significant change in attitudes toward the basic concepts of nursing professional ethics as defined by the initial codes of the American Nurses Association. It may be that the changes in attitude toward nursing ethics meshed with perspectives in contemporary bioethics and that the timing was right for a symbiosis of the nursing profession and those involved with contemporary bioethics. Nurses may also have seen that the rights-based concepts that were being advanced by contemporary bioethics would, if generally accepted, lead to a greater sharing of clinical power by physicians and an advancement in the power allotted to nurses.

The origin of professional nursing ethics is usually attributed to Florence Nightingale and her concepts of responsible obedience to the physician as developed during the Crimean War (1854-1857). Nightingale is known as the founder of modern nursing because of her organizational work during the Crimean War; her subsequent activities, including founding the Nightingale Nursing School in 1860; and her concepts of preventive medicine developed in a 1893 paper. In this famous work, she exhorted that it was important to treat the sick person rather than the disease, that prevention is much better than cure, that hospitalization does not necessarily lead to health, and that nursing must hold to its ideals as represented in the Nightingale Pledge.[15] The Nightingale Pledge is as follows:

> I solemnly pledge myself before God and in the presence of this assembly; To pass my life in purity and to practice my profession faithfully; I will abstain from whatever is deleterious and mischievous and will not take or knowingly administer any harmful drug. I will do all in my power to maintain and elevate the standard of my profession and will hold in confidence all personal matters committed to my keeping and family affairs coming to my knowledge in the practice of my calling. With loyalty I will endeavor to aid the physician in his work, and devote myself to the welfare of those committed to my care.[16]

Nightingale's emphasis on the duty of the nurse to obey the physician has become an anachronism. However, scrutiny of her writings reveals that she did not call for blind obedience; instead she advocated responsible obedience with the needs of the patient being a primary consideration.

From the mid-1970s until recently, the major guiding concept in the professional ethics of nursing

has been "client advocacy." This line of thought developed at that particular time for a number of reasons: decreasing esteem for physicians; the beginnings of feminism, consumerism, and patients' rights movements; and an overall climate of increasing self-determination for patients and for healthcare professionals--including nurses but excluding physicians. Client advocacy emphasizes the autonomy and rights of the patient, as does contemporary bioethics; it is based on a freely expressed contract between the professional and the patient, which is in contrast to the earlier emphasis on care and beneficence with the physician as the final decision-making authority.[17]

Recently, some writers have focused renewed attention on caring as an important aspect of the nurse-patient encounter. Sally Gadow, a prominent proponent of this position in nursing, has written that care is the supreme covenant between the nurse and patient and that care is the moral basis for the nurse-patient relationship.[18] Adeline Falk Rafael has attempted to combine the concepts of caring and power into a single concept that she calls "empowered caring." She sees this idea as moving beyond "power over" others to include power that enables others. She believes that empowered caring should be grounded in knowledge and driven by caring. Neither Gadow or Rafael envisions a return to the traditional subservient position of the nurse to the physician.[19]

The American Nurses Association originally adopted its code of ethics in 1950. This code was extensively revised in 1976 and its preamble modified slightly in 1985. Both the 1976 and 1985 revisions reflect the changing role of the nurse in society, reflect the changes in the nurse's relationship with the physician, and codify the concept of client advocacy in nursing.[20] The following extract is taken from the 1985 *Code for Nurses*:

1. The nurse provides services with respect for human dignity and the uniqueness of the client unrestricted by considerations of social or economic status, personal attributes, or the nature of health problems.
2. The nurse safeguards the client's right to privacy by judiciously protecting information of a confidential nature.
3. The nurse acts to safeguard the client and the public when health care and safety are affected by

the incompetent, unethical, or illegal practice of any person.

4. The nurse assumes responsibility and accountability for individual nursing judgments and actions.

5. The nurse maintains competence in nursing.

6. The nurse exercises informed judgment and uses individual competence and qualifications as criteria in seeking consultation, accepting responsibilities, and delegating nursing activities to others.

7. The nurse participates in activities that contribute to the ongoing development of the profession's body of knowledge.

8. The nurse participates in the profession's efforts to implement and improve standards of nursing.

9. The nurse participates in the profession's efforts to establish and maintain conditions of employment conducive to high quality nursing care.

10. The nurse participates in the profession's effort to protect the public from misinformation and misrepresentation and to maintain the integrity of nursing.

11. The nurse collaborates with members of the health professions and other citizens in promoting community and national efforts to meet the health needs of the public.[21]

III. Defining the Professional and the Professional Practice

What is a "profession"? The definitions vary widely, but most include the following elements:

1. advanced training;
2. well-defined and circumscribed role;
3. continuing education;
4. control over admission to the profession;
5. responsibility to specified individuals (patients) and to the particular group defined by the "profession";
6. devotion to humanistic ideals; and
7. a well-defined group of necessary virtues and moral rules that define the ethical parameters of the profession.

Some definitions mention a specific or nonspecific duty to society, the secondary nature of compensation for the work of the professional, and other elements.

Robert Orr, a physician and teacher of ethics to medical students, has written: "In the classic sense being a professional implies a publicly declared vow of dedication or devotion to a way of life. It implies a special knowledge not available to the average person; it is an unequal relationship. But with that special knowledge comes a special responsibility. It is thus a fiduciary relationship in that the possessor of knowledge has a responsibility of altruism, and the recipient of the special knowledge may thus trust the professional. In other words a professional is a trustworthy trustee."[22]

A. Physicians as Professionals

Allen Dyer, a psychiatrist and author, has stated that the medical profession is defined either by the knowledge and technical expertise of the physician or by the ethics of the professional group, specifically the fiduciary commitments of the doctor-patient relationship. This distinction between knowledge and ethics is anti-Hippocratic and would once have been unthinkable. From a traditional Hippocratic perspective, knowledge is a very personal quality that cannot be separated from the values of the knower or user of that knowledge. However, scientific medicine has been so successful as a purveyor of technological knowledge that it has become much easier to uncouple expertise and ethical responsibility. Indeed it is easier to imagine medicine as merely the application of technology and to view medical service as a commodity and the medical profession as a business.[23]

It is the increasing acceptance of the separation of clinical competence from compassion and caring for the patient that has, to some extent, fostered the development of contemporary bioethics as a field separate from the medical profession. And it is this attitude that is feared, even looked upon with horror, by many in the profession. For most physicians, the medical profession is still defined by its internal ethics, specifically the ethic of human service. They believe that attention to appropriate professional ethical issues by professional organizations and attention to proper individual ethical decisions guided by their own professional and personal conscience are all that is needed to ensure the ethical practice of medicine. Many physicians see no need for "outsiders" such as academic ethicists to be involved in the decision-making process in the clinical setting.

B. Professional Ethics and Medical Practice

Views regarding the practice of medicine can be classified as one of three types: (1) the scientific or technological model; (2) the participatory or community model; and (3) the classical or Hippocratic model.[24] A brief description of each of these models follows, along with discussion of the future of physicians as professionals under each of these models.

The last 30 years have witnessed the development and the beginning of the decline of the scientific model of medical practice. This model is based on a mechanistic view of medical practice and treats the doctor as a biotechnician. In this mode, medicine is susceptible to economic and legal control, and "informed consent" as a contract is the major limiting factor. This model has not been satisfying for most practitioners, and it has left patients with a less-than-encouraging view of the profession and its work. Its major advantage, if it can be called that, has been to increase dramatically the use of complicated technology and the amount paid for it. Many people see this model as an aberration and wish a return to a more humanistic approach to medical practice. This particular model contributed to the early development of contemporary bioethics, because the traditional professional ethics was ignored or downplayed under this model.

A second model, the community or participatory mode of practice, is based on the concept of equal individual worth and community-based ideals; it requires cooperation between the physician, other clinicians, and the patient and family. It is best represented by the concept of "shared decision making" as defined by the President's Commission for the Study of Ethical Problems in Medicine and Biomedical and Behavioral Research.[25] It gives equal importance to the physician and patient and emphasizes cooperation. It exists unhappily with the more analytic mechanisms of regulation of the law and is more comfortable in consensus-seeking endeavors.

The classical model of medical practice is based on Hippocratic ideals and begins with the ultimate worth of the doctor's activities (a calling). It depends, to some extent, on mysticism or at least on beliefs that cannot be proved. The medical profession is seen as a closed discipline whose practitioners regard their work--the relief of human suffering--as their highest duty. The physician and patient are unequal, as are

the physician and others involved in the care of the patient. This model is not comfortably responsive to outside regulation whether moral, legal, or bureaucratic. It is embodied in the quotations derived from the writings of Hippocrates: "Life is short and Art is long; the occasion fleeting; experience fallacious and judgement difficult; the physician must not only be prepared to do what is right himself, but also to make the patient, the attendants and the externals cooperate"[26]; and "the physician is the servant of his Art."[27]

The Hippocratic, classical ideal is broad enough to encompass ideas from research science; patient-centered but physician-directed medicine; a guild approach to practice and knowledge; and, in large measure, all of the modern approaches to healthcare. It is not broad enough to include a patient or society-dominated approach or even a partnership.

Although the Hippocratic ideal of medical practice has been highly criticized recently, it continues as the basic ideal of medical practice for many, both in and out of the profession. This ideal is the foundation for professional ethics in medicine; until very recently, it has been the only authority upon which the professional codes have been built.

Historically, this ideal represents the first time that the power to heal was vested in a practitioner who was not also a shaman with the power to harm. According to the late anthropologist Margaret Mead, the Hippocratic Oath marked one of the turning points in the history of man. Mead says:

> For the first time in our tradition there was a complete separation between killing and curing. Throughout the primitive world the doctor and the sorcerer tended to be the same person. He, with power to kill had power to cure, including especially the undoing of his own killing activities. He who had power to cure would necessarily also be able to kill. With the Greeks the distinction was made clear. One profession was dedicated completely to life under all circumstances, regardless of rank, age, or intellect--the life of a slave, the life of the Emperor, the life of a child.[28]

The value of traditional medicine as a conservative cultural institution in a time of rapid fundamental changes in other major institutions is also mentioned as an important positive aspect of the traditional Hippocratic ideal.

The major criticisms of the Hippocratic ideal of medical practice are:

1. Hippocratic medicine does not fully address rights of patients and emphasizes relationships of physicians to one another.
2. The Hippocratic ideal opposes abortion and euthanasia, and modern technology such as prenatal diagnosis, organ transplants, and heart/lung machines are difficult to fit into this schema.
3. This ideal is basically paternalistic.

These criticisms tend to be based only on the Hippocratic Oath and other writings attributed to Hippocrates and do not consider the more common position of the modern practicing physician--that is, the Hippocratic Oath and subsequent codes should serve as professional beacons that guide the professional course. If legitimate moral ideals are confused with imperatives, they may not be recognized as goals toward which one might strive, but rather held as mandates to which one must adhere.

In specific defense of the Hippocratic ideal as compared to the other models, the following arguments have been advanced:

1. High technology is inadequate to address the needs of many patients (the scientific model is inadequate).
2. Autonomy and rights of the patient should not always be paramount in medical decision making (professional obligations and responsibility should be considered).
3. The oath and subsequent codes are reminders and are not meant to be a specific set of rules.
4. Paternalism and self-determination are not mutually exclusive (for example, a wise parent encourages autonomy in the child).
5. With the classical model, if there is a conflict between the best interests of the patient and those of the physician, the best interests of the patient are to have preference.

What are the attributes of the physician required by each of these models? The scientific model requires only a knowledgeable and honest scientist. The community model requires a cooperative, socially aware, and analytic clinician who attends to many aspects of living in his or her practice and is committed to the patient's rights in clinical decision making. The required attributes for the classical model seem at first to be more complex. Religious and/or mystical perspectives have in the past been associated with this mode of practice, but they have become less important in recent years. The physician may or may not be religious and still adhere to this mode of practice. Integrity and character are the major determinants of the ideal physician in the classical model.

C. Professional Integrity

Theologian Stanley Hauerwas has said, "Integrity, not obligation, is the hallmark of the moral life."[29] Integrity is an integration of beliefs about values and purposes by which lives are conducted. It is the psychosomatic integration of mind and body including emotions. Integrity is required of the physician practicing under all of the aforementioned models of medical practice. It is most closely associated with the classical model and is the basis for the professional ethics under this model.

The integrity of medicine as a profession and of its practitioners as professionals with professional ideals depends not only on applicable rules and principles, but also on the professional physician and his or her character. The application of professional ethics in medical care depends on this personal integrity of the individual practitioner.

D. The Concept of Medical Practice

What of the concept of "medical practice" and its effects on professional integrity and ethics? The concept has come to mean an organized activity that has within it certain standards of excellence independent of the uses to which that practice may be put by society. In other words when one is engaged in a practice there are internally set norms of excellence to which one must adhere. The integrity of the profession and of the individual professional is maintained through this concept.[30] A professional practice is a method for maintaining the tenets of the profession and the virtues of the individual professional by reminding the practitioners and the public that a practice does in fact exist.

Certain controversial issues have arisen in relation to the integrity of a medical practice and the ethical aspects of certain decisions and activities within this context. Two of the more important of these issues, the concept of futility and its relationship to clinical decision making and the professional's right to refuse to include certain types of patients in his/her practice, are important examples of practice-related controversies.

E. Futility

What is futile medical care and how should this concept be considered in relation to the integrity of a professional and his or her practice?

The AMA defines futility in strictly physiological terms--that is, the treatment will not have the desired physiologic effect.[31] (For example, penicillin for a viral sore throat is futile treatment; if cardiopulmonary resuscitation can not be expected to restore cardiopulmonary function, then it is also futile treatment).

A second, more common, conceptualization of futility is that an intervention is futile if it fails to produce any benefit for the patient. (Here, consideration of quality of life as defined by the patient and/or the patient's surrogate come into play.)

A third definition of futility advanced by Howard Brody, a physician-ethicist at Michigan State University School of Medicine, is that a treatment is futile if it fails to achieve any reasonable purpose of treatment, which can occur in three circumstances:

1. the probability of benefit is unacceptably low;
2. the magnitude of benefit is unacceptably small; and
3. the harm is much too great relative to any benefit.[32]

The definition that one uses is important because, in our society, an intervention that is considered "futile" is often not ethically or legally required and is, therefore, optional.

The integrity of medicine as a profession requires that members of the profession have the authority to determine what counts as truth in the area of professional expertise. The physician has the obligation and authority to decide, within the confines of good professional practice, whether a treatment possibility should be considered. If this authority is to have meaning, it must extend to decisions concerning the futility of specific interventions--particularly when con-

sidered under the strict physiologic definition of futility. Based on the same arguments, the physician as a professional has the authority to make decisions concerning futility, when defined as a lack of benefit or lack of therapeutic reasonableness, as long as the physician makes the decision after consideration of the patient's life plan. Brody argues that this is a professional decision that affects the patient's quality of life (as do essentially all professional decisions) but, when made in the context of knowledge of the patient and his or her values, is a proper decision for the physician and would be improper for anybody else outside a professional practice.[33]

In spite of these arguments, this matter is far from settled and the debate continues. Physician and ethicist Edward Pellegrino, discussing the concept of futility, has written:

It has been and continues to be useful, however, because it exposes the need for carefully weighing the limits of both physician and patient autonomy, the explicit meaning of participation, and the relative reliability and moral weight of objective medical and subjective value determinations. Underlying these issues are deeper philosophical questions about the nature of medical knowledge, the relationship between fact and value and the moral status of the physician's conscience in a pluralistic and democratic society like ours, which so highly prizes individual autonomy.[34]

F. Professional Refusal

Another area of controversy affecting the professional integrity of the physician and his or her practice is that of refusing to accept a particular patient into the practice. (This notion is stated in AMA "Principles of Medical Ethics" as, "A physician shall, in the provision of appropriate medical care, except in emergencies, be free to choose whom to serve, with whom to associate, and the environment in which to provide medical services."[35]

Some physicians have been criticized for refusing to see patients with certain diseases, such as acquired immunodeficiency syndrome (AIDS), or for refusing to see patients based on their financial status. Are these criticisms warranted? How can behavior, which on the face of it seems "unjust," be defended as a fundamental tenet necessary to maintain the integrity of the profession and its members?

Although society licenses professions and allows them to operate within certain parameters, society has been loath to try to change fundamental internal professional tenets. The tendency has been to allow professions to develop their own standards for practice and maintain these standards through self-regulation or methods prescribed by the profession.

The medical profession, through the AMA and other professional organizations, defends its stand concerning allowing physicians to choose who shall be admitted to their practice based on the necessity to maintain the practice as an individually controlled entity, and on physicians' civil rights as individuals. Within this context, the reasons for refusing to accept certain specific patients or patients belonging to a particular group must be ethically defensible. Consider the following example: A pediatrician refuses to write a prescription for the parent of one of her 10-year-old patients on the basis that she is not as knowledgeable concerning adult patients and is therefore not as competent to treat this parent are other, easily accessible, physicians in the immediate area. She could be prescribing less than optimum treatment when optimum treatment is available. This refusal is based on professional concepts of competence that are necessary to maintain the integrity of the profession and, as such, is ethical.

A less clear situation occurs when a person with a particular medical-payment mechanism is refused entry into the professional practice solely on the basis of the method of payment. It has not been uncommon for some physicians to refuse to admit Medicaid and/or Medicare patients to their practices. Their reasons for this refusal include:

1. significant increase in paperwork and regulatory burdens with these patients;
2. increased external regulation of interactions with these patients;
3. a personal political philosophy that contends that Medicaid or Medicare is a form of governmental control of medical practice and that it is therefore antagonistic toward good patient care; and

4. a significant decrease in income from this group of patients that requires shifting costs to other patients, which many consider unfair.

When the physician continues his/her obligation to attend all people as patients in an emergency, and when adequate care is available elsewhere, this sort of refusal has been considered minimally acceptable. In defending such a refusal, physicians have correctly pointed out that they, under most conditions, are not allowed to treat Medicaid and Medicare patients for free or for a minimal reduced fee. Bureaucratic requirements must be met for these patients, or legal sanctions against the physician can be instituted.

Does a professional practice's refusal to accept certain patients contradict the professional ethical standard that patients should be treated without regard to income or ability to pay? If the refusal is based on reasons other than decreased payment for services, if there are other available avenues for the patient to receive adequate care, and if the physician would treat individual patients in this payment class under the same conditions as his or her other patients and without regard to income or payment, then many believe that this refusal is ethical and should be supported. Refusal based only on economic factors would not likely be considered ethical by any professional body.

What about refusal to treat certain patients based on their particular disease? A number of professional practices do not accept patients with AIDS. The stated reasons include:

1. lack of expertise to treat;
2. other patients' fear of patients with AIDS;
3. fear of possible transmission of the disease to staff and self;
4. fear of decreased income; and
5. fear of negative social reactions.

There is little question that the first of these reasons, lack of expertise, is ethically sound unless the physician is guilty of not maintaining or achieving standard competence. All of the other reasons are questionable, because the patient's well-being and needs are a secondary consideration to the well being and needs of others or of the practice.

The AMA Council on Ethical and Judicial Affairs states: "A physician may not ethically refuse to treat a patient whose condition is within the physician's realm of competence solely because the patient is (HIV) seropositive. The tradition of the AMA since 1847 is that: when an epidemic prevails, a physician must continue his labors without regard to his own health."[36]

IV. Legal Considerations

The impersonal view of physicians that can be seen with the technological model seems firmly established in most aspects of the law. In recent decisions, the courts have permitted advertising among physicians and have modified the historical professional ethics mandate to maintain absolute confidentiality. In *Tarasoff v. Regents of the University of California*, the court ruled that physicians are required to ignore patient confidentiality if significant harm to a specific person could likely be prevented.[37] There are now mandatory reporting requirements for a number of clinical situations and mandatory review of medical records by numerous others in governmental and insurance reimbursement plans. Whether any or all of these legal requirements for breeches of confidentiality are beneficial is still an open question.

Other individual court decisions (such as *Quinlan, Cruzan,* and *A.C.*) that primarily concern decision making at the end-of-life seem to favor the community model of practice. These decisions have made specific reference to the advantages of hospital ethics committees and the consideration of serious end-of-life decisions by all interested parties.

Few recent court decisions favor the classical model except to use certain codes as the behavioral standard to which a practitioner must adhere.

V. Advice for Professional Students

What advice can be given to students of clinical professions, particularly medical students, concerning their duties to patients, to their profession, to society, and to themselves? Should they be concerned only with the contemporary bioethics viewpoint and its focus on patients' rights, or should they adhere to a more traditional concept of obligation to the patient above all as the primary determinant of ethical sound-

ness? These questions are not easily answered, and the answers depend upon many factors including current law, other ethical parameters sanctioned by society, professional ethical mandates, and the conscience and character of the individual student.

Student clinicians should study and learn what these societal and professional mandates require, and the historical and other reasons for these requirements (the focus of this text). Students should observe and listen to and discuss with others, within and outside of the profession, these issues and how they do and should affect medical care. Students should consider what their chosen profession has meant historically, what they believe it means now, and how they would like to see it meet future ethical challenges. Finally, students should attempt to know themselves, be self-critical, and use their innate character as a basis for thinking about and developing their conscience and personal ethical outlook toward the profession generally and toward their relationship to the profession and the patients it serves.

There are no magic lists of virtues, principles, case studies, or codes that will guarantee success. The search for the ethics of clinical care is a continuing process that can never be totally completed, so looking for one "answer" should be discouraged. Education based on this textbook and similar texts and courses can be used as a beginning, but professional and personal ethical education should continue throughout one's professional career.

Albert Jonsen has written: "At a time when the genuine nobility of medicine is compromised and threatened from within and without, at a time when many of medicine's younger practitioners either have forgotten or have never learned the ethos of noblesse oblige, the challenge is the choice of an ethos--or rather the renewed commitment to an ethos."[38]

VI. Final Considerations

Beginning in the 1960s, society demanded a change from the traditional mode of medical practice, in which physicians were making newly possible life-and-death decisions for patients without inquiring about their values and desires. The pendulum swung from physician-dominated clinical decisions to patient-dominated decisions. Patient autonomy and the patient's right to make decisions became the most important aspect of the relationship, and the move from the physician as a trusted ally to the physician as a provider began.

Following this lead, contemporary bioethics paid almost exclusive attention to the application of principles (particularly patient autonomy and the rights encompassed by this autonomy) as the foundation for proper ethical decision making and neglected the medical professional--both as an individual and as a member of a profession.

Our society appears to have embraced many of the methods and concepts of contemporary bioethics. Whether it still sees value in the traditional methods of addressing professional ethical problems is an open question. In spite of the strong growth of decision-making analysis and processes associated with contemporary bioethics, there is still a reluctance to dismiss the tradition of professional ethics. Many believe this dismissal would lead to further decrease in the trusting relationship desired by many patients and their physicians. The recent perceived loss of some of the traditional virtues associated with the "old-fashioned family doctor" has caused consternation. Some also fear that, as the influence of traditional professional ethics diminishes, professional devotion to competence and compassion may also decrease.

This issue of the authority of professional ethics is not just academic; the future direction of the medical profession and the attitudes of society toward physicians and, indirectly, toward other clinicians hang in the balance. Should medicine receive its mandates on the ethics of medical care based on specific principles and procedures imposed by society, or should physicians and other clinical professionals concentrate on developing a stronger and more responsive professional ethics of their own?

A fusion of these pathways is unlikely because their perspectives are so different. However, it may be possible to develop a positive coexistence that relegates the larger societal issues associated with medical care (such as the definition of death, the regulation of information and processes from the Human Genome Project, and issues related to financing medical care) to the bioethics community for consideration (with appropriate input from the profession but no authority for the final decision), and allows traditional professional ethics to continue to define an ethical clinician in terms of his or her professional obligations.

Edmund Pellegrino recently addressed the issue of the importance of maintaining a traditional professional ethics for medicine. In commenting on the present-day relevance of the Hippocratic Oath, he stated: "This is no mere academic skirmish. Its practical consequences affect all of society and all of us as physicians and citizens. No human being can escape the reality of being sick and being cared for. All must seriously contemplate what a divided profession without a common set of moral commitments would mean. Most important, we are obligated to ask how patients might fare in the hands of a profession with its moral fabric in tatters."[39]

Notes

1. Council on Ethical and Judicial Affairs of the American Medical Association, "Fundamental Elements of the Patient-Physician Relationship," in *Code of Medical Ethics* (Chicago: AMA, 1996), *xli-xliii*.

2. Council on Ethical and Judicial Affairs of the American Medical Association, "Anencephalic Infants as Organ Donors," *Reports* (Chicago: AMA, December 1988).

3. Council on Ethical and Judicial Affairs of the American Medical Association, "Anencephalic Infants as Organ Donors," in *Current Opinions* (Chicago: AMA, March 1992).

4. Council for Ethical and Judicial Affairs of the American Medical Association, "Anencephalic Neonates as Organ Donors," in *Current Opinions* (Chicago: AMA, June 1996).

5. J. Areen et al., *Law, Science and Medicine* (Mineola, NY: Foundation Press, 1984), 273.

6. Hippocrates, *The Theory and Practice of Medicine* (New York: Philosophical Library, 1964).

7. M. Levey, "Medical Ethics of Medieval Islam with Special Reference to Al-Ruhawi's Practical Ethics of the Physician," *Transactions of the American Philosophical Society* 57, part 3 (1967): 18-94.

8. C.R. Burns, *Legacies in Ethics and Medicine* (New York: Neale Watson Academic Publications, 1977), 145-70.

9. Ibid., 181-203.

10. C. Leake, *Percivals Medical Ethics* (Baltimore, Md.: Williams & Wilkins, 1927).

11. Council on Ethical and Judicial Affairs of the American Medical Association, *Code of Medical Ethics, Current Opinions and Annotations* (Chicago: AMA, 1996), *xi*.

12. Ibid.

13. American Medical Association, *Constitution and Bylaws of the American Medical Association* (Chicago: AMA, 1993), 36-40.

14. See note 11 above, p. *xiv*.

15. N.J. Bishop and S. Goldie, *A Bio-Bibliography of Florence Nightingale* (London: International Council of Nurses, 1962).

16. C.A. Quinn and M.D. Smith, *The Professional Commitment: Issues in Ethics and Nursing* (Philadelphia, Penn.: W.B. Saunders, 1987), 179.

17. G.L. Husted, and J.H. Husted, *Ethical Decision making in Nursing* (St. Louis, Mo.: Mosby-Yearbook, 1991), 27-38.

18. S. Gadow, "Covenant Without Cure: Letting Go and Holding On in Chronic Illness," in *The Ethics of Care and the Ethics of Cure: Synthesis in Chronicity*, ed. J. Watson and M. Ray (New York: National League of Nursing, 1988).

19. A.R.F. Rafael, "Power and Caring: A Dialectic in Nursing," *Advances in Nursing Science* 19, no. 1 (1996): 3-17.

20. American Nurses Association, *Code for Nurses* (Kansas City, Mo.: ANA, 1985).

21. American Nurses Association, *Perspectives on the Code for Nurses* (Kansas City, Mo.: ANA, 1985), 45-46.

22. R.D. Orr, "Personal and Professional Integrity in Clinical Medicine," *Update* 8, no. 4 (1992): 1-3.

23. A. Dyer, *Ethics and Psychiatry: Toward Professional Definition* (Washington, D.C.: American Psychiatric, 1988), 4-5.

24. J.M. Jacob, *Doctors and Rules* (New York: Routledge, 1988).

25. President's Commission on the Study of Ethical Problems in Medicine and Biomedical and Behavioral Research, *Making Health Care Decisions* vol. 1 (Washington, D.C.: U.S. Government Printing Office, 1982).

26. *Hippocratic Writings*, G.E.R. Lloyd, ed., J. Chadwick and W.N. Mann, tran. (New York: Penguin Books, 1978), 206.

27. Ibid.

28. M. Levine, *Psychiatry and Ethics* (New York: George Brazilier, Inc., 1972) 324-25.

29. S. Hauerwas, *Community and Character* (Notre Dame, Ind.: University of Notre Dame Press, 1981), 48.

30. H. Brody, *The Healer's Power* (New Haven, Conn.: Yale University Press, 1992), 174.

31. Council on Ethical and Judicial Affairs of the American Medical Association, "Guidelines for Appropriate Use of Do-Not-Resuscitate Orders," *Journal of the American Medical Association* 265 (1991): 1800-01.

32. See note 30 above, p. 176.

33. Ibid., 178-82.

34. E. Pellegrino, "Ethics," *Journal of the American Medical Association* 270, no. 2 (1993): 203.

35. See note 12 above, p. *xiv*.

36. Ibid., 157.

37. *Tarasoff v. Regents of the University of California*, 131 Cal.Rptr. 14, 551 P.2d 334 (1976).

38. A. Jonsen, *The New Medicine and the Old Ethics* (Cambridge, Mass.: Harvard University Press, 1990), 78.

39. E.D. Pellegrino, "Ethics," *Journal of the American Medical Association* 275, no. 23 (June 1996): 1807-09.

APPENDICES

APPENDIX 1

Joint Commission Standards on Patient Rights and Organization Ethics

The following is an edited version of the Joint Commission on Accreditation of Healthcare Organizations (JCAHO) Standards on Patient Rights and Organization Ethics from the 1997 Accreditation Manual for Hospitals. Examples of "Evidence of Performance" for each standard and "Specific Scoring Rules" have been deleted from this text.

OVERVIEW

The *goal* of the patient rights and organization ethics function[1] is to help improve patient outcomes by respecting each patient's rights and conducting business relationships with patients and the public in an ethical manner.

Patients have a fundamental right to considerate care that safeguards their personal dignity and respects their cultural, psychosocial, and spiritual values. These values often influence patients' perception of care and illness. Understanding and respecting these values guide the provider in meeting the patients' care needs and preferences.

A hospital's behavior towards its patients and its business practices has a significant impact on the patient's experience of and response to care. Thus, access, treatment, respect, and conduct affect patient rights. The standards in this chapter address the following processes and activities:

- Promoting consideration of patient values and preferences, including the decision to discontinue treatment;
- Recognizing the hospital's responsibilities under law;
- Informing patients of their responsibilities in the care process; and

- Managing the hospital's relationships with patients and the public in an ethical manner.

FLOWCHART

Practical Application

The following example illustrates all components of the flowchart for *Patient Rights and Organization Ethics*, including the rights that the hospital protects on behalf of the patient, and the hospital's ethical practices. First, the patient's rights to access, treatment, and respect:

A 4-year-old girl is severely injured by an automobile. En route to the hospital, she is managed by the emergency physician staff via radio-telephone. Hospital staff are aware that she will be taken directly to a trauma room, so her access to care and treatment will not be hindered by check-in procedures; her parents will take care of these later.

As soon as the emergency medical technicians arrive at the hospital, they report the child's condition and care since the accident, her current physiological status, and the results of efforts to determine her name and her parents' names and address. The child's hospital treatment team takes over, and is responsible for continuously assessing the patient's critical vital functions and treating all life-threatening conditions.

When the child's parents arrive, they are informed of their daughter's condition; according to the trauma room protocol, a member of the child's treatment team speaks with them as soon as possible after the patient's arrival and every 30 minutes thereafter. The protocol is designed to meet the patient's treatment needs and to respect the right of the family[2] to be involved in the care process.

The hospital also has in place procedures that address the organization's ethical practices.

Since the family belongs to a health maintenance organization (HMO), the hospital follows the HMO's procedures for notifying the child's primary care physician. The child's stay in the hospital, from her arrival at emergency service to her discharge from the pediatric unit, is evaluated as part of the hospital's utilization management program, and her length of stay in each unit is compared with data from an external utilization management service.

The child's condition does not respond to the prescribed medication, but the physician staff believes she can be helped by one of the hospital's medication clinical trials. Before placing the child in the trial, however, they fully inform her parents and obtain their consent. If the child had no hope of recovery, staff members would have asked her parents if they wished to donate her organs or tissues.

As the child approaches discharge, it appears she will need a specially made prosthetic device. Although the device is not available in the hospital, it is available from a wholly owned subsidiary of the hospital. The staff informs the parents of this relationship while the referral is being planned and asks if there is any other prosthetic group practice they wish to use. They also check to see if the HMO requires them to use a particular practice.

STANDARDS

The following is a list of all standards for this function. They are presented here for your convenience without footnotes or other explanatory text.

RI.1	The hospital addresses ethical issues in providing patient care.
RI.1.1	The patient's right to treatment or service is respected and supported.
RI.1.2	Patients are involved in all aspects of their care.
RI.1.2.1	Informed consent is obtained.
RI.1.2.1.1	All patients asked to participate in a research project are given a description of the expected benefits.
RI.1.2.1.2	All patients asked to participate in a research project are given a description of the potential discomforts and risks.
RI.1.2.1.3	All patients asked to participate in a research project are given a description of alternative services that might also prove advantageous to them.
RI.1.2.1.4	All patients asked to participate in a research project are given a full explanation of the procedures to be followed, especially those that are experimental in nature.
RI.1.2.1.5	All patients asked to participate in a research project are told that they may refuse to participate, and that their refusal will not compromise their access to services.
RI.1.2.2	The family participates in care decisions.
RI.1.2.3	Patients are involved in resolving dilemmas about care decisions.
RI.1.2.4	The hospital addresses advance directives.

RI.1.2.5	The hospital addresses withholding resuscitative services.
RI.1.2.6	The hospital addresses forgoing or withdrawing life-sustaining treatment.
RI.1.2.7	The hospital addresses care at the end of life.
RI.1.3	The hospital demonstrates respect for the following patient needs:
RI.1.3.1	confidentiality;
RI.1.3.2	privacy;
RI.1.3.3	security;
RI.1.3.4	resolution of complaints;
RI.1.3.5	pastoral counseling;
RI.1.3.6	communication.
RI.1.3.6.1	When the hospital restricts a patient's visitors, mail, telephone calls, or other forms of communication, the restrictions are evaluated for their therapeutic effectiveness.
RI.1.3.6.1.1	Any restrictions on communication are fully explained to the patient and family, and are determined with their participation.
RI.1.4	Each patient receives a written statement of his or her rights.
RI.1.5	The hospital supports the patient's right to access protective services.
RI.2	The hospital has a policy and procedures, developed with the medical staffs' participation, for the procuring and donation of organs and other tissues.
RI.3	The hospital protects patients and respects their rights during research, investigation, and clinical trials involving human subjects.
RI.3.1	All consent forms address the information specified in RI.1.2.1.1 through RI.1.2.1.5; indicate the name of the person who provided the information and the date the form was signed; and address the participant's right to privacy, confidentiality, and safety.
RI.4	The hospital operates according to a code of ethical behavior.
RI.4.1	The code addresses marketing, admission, transfer and discharge, and billing practices.
RI.4.2	The code addresses the relationship of the hospital and its staff members to other health care providers, educational institutions, and payers.
RI.4.3	In hospitals with longer lengths of stay, the code addresses a patient's rights to perform or refuse to perform tasks in or for the hospital.

Please note: Examples of implementation offer various strategies, activities, or processes that can be used to comply with the standards. They are not requirements.

These examples are simply ideas for your organization to consider. Scorable requirements are included only in the standards and intent statements.

STANDARD

RI.1   The hospital addresses ethical issues in providing patient care.

Intent of RI.1

A mere listing of patient rights cannot guarantee that those rights are respected. Rather, a hospital demonstrates its support of patient rights through the processes by which staff members interact with and care for patients. These day-to-day interactions reflect a fundamental concern with and respect for patients' rights. All staff members are aware of the ethical issues surrounding patient care, the hospital's policies governing these issues, and the structures available to support ethical decision making.

The hospital establishes and maintains structures to support patient rights, and does so in a collaborative manner that involves the hospital's leaders and others. The structures are based on policies, procedures, and their philosophical basis, which makes up the framework that addresses both patient care and organizational ethical issues, including the following:

a. The patient's right to reasonable access to care;
b. The patient's right to care that is considerate and respectful of his or her personal values and beliefs;
c. The patient's right to be informed about and participate in decisions regarding his or her care;
d. The patient's right to participate in ethical questions that arise in the course of his or her care, including issues of conflict resolution, withholding resuscitative services, forgoing or withdrawal of life-sustaining treatment, and participation in investigational studies or clinical trials;
e. The patient's right to security and personal privacy and confidentiality of information;
f. The issue of designating a decision maker in case the patient is incapable of understanding a proposed treatment or procedure or is unable to communicate his or her wishes regarding care;
g. The hospital's method of informing the patient of these issues identified in this intent;
h. The hospital's method of educating staff about patient rights and their role in supporting those rights; and
i. The patient's right to access protective services.[3]

Example of Implementation for RI.1

Patient rights processes may include a variety of strategies, such as using an established ethics committee, a for-

malized ethics forum, ethics consultations, or any combination of these or other methods. There are a number of ways hospitals may address implementing an ethics process to deal with ethical issues. For example:

● A hospital has policies and procedures in place describing how a full-time bioethics consulting staff addresses the issues listed in the intent.
● A hospital has 24-hour access to an external consulting service to help resolve ethical issues.
● A small, rural medical center has access to the ethics service of a large medical center.
● Staff members are educated on recognizing ethical issues.
● Staff members are either skilled in the hospital's policies addressing ethical decision making or have access to appropriate support mechanisms, such as an ethics committee.
● Patients and their families are informed of how to gain access to the ethics committee and the process for ethical issues resolution.
● The corporate entity of a multihospital system establishes policies and procedures that explain the ethics process for dealing with an ethical issue required for each subentity based on the patient populations served. Each subentity establishes specific policies and procedures and reports its activity to the corporate entity.
● A hospital serving a Native American population has policies and procedures based on law and customs. The policies and procedures reflect the specific population's needs to address ethical care issues.

STANDARD

RI.1.1   The patient's right to treatment or service is respected and supported.

Intent of RI.1.1

A hospital provides care in response to a patient's request and need, so long as that care is within the hospital's capacity, its stated mission and philosophy, and relevant laws and regulations. When a hospital cannot provide the care a patient requests, staff fully inform the patient of his or her needs and the alternatives for care. If it is necessary and medically advisable, the hospital transfers the patient to another organization. The transfer has to be acceptable to the receiving organization.

Example of Implementation for RI.1.1

The hospital's policies and procedures for admission to and transfer from the facility are based on the patient's need for services, including the hospital's ability to provide those services. The hospital's mission statement reflects its policies and procedures of patient care. The hospital uses a formal process for the prompt and safe transfer of the patient to another organization when the hospital cannot meet the patient's request or care needs. It is obvious that economics are not the sole motivator for transferring a patient. Instead, it is clear that the decision is based on the hospital's ability to provide the type and quality of care the patient needs, including availability of resources needed to treat a specific condition or disease. In addition, the hospital's policies and procedures address withholding or withdrawal of treatment in case the patient or legally designated representative decides to do so.

The hospital's responsibility to provide access to care is governed by The Americans with Disabilities Act (ADA) and other applicable law and regulation.

STANDARD

RI.1.2   Patients are involved in all aspects of their care.

Intent of RI.1.2

Hospitals promote patient and family involvement in all aspects of their care through implementation of policies and procedures that are compatible with the hospital's mission and resources, have diverse input, and guarantee communication across the organization. Patients are involved in at least the following aspects of their care:

- Giving informed consent;
- Making care decisions;
- Resolving dilemmas about care decisions;
- Formulating advance directives;
- Withholding resuscitative services;
- Forgoing or withdrawing life-sustaining treatment; and
- Care at the end of life.

To this end, structures are developed, approved, and maintained through collaboration among the hospital's leaders and others.

Patients' psychosocial, spiritual, and cultural values affect how they respond to their care. The hospital allows patients and their families to express their spiritual beliefs and cultural practices, as long as these do not harm others or interfere with treatment.

Examples of Implementation for RI.1.2

Services for patients are provided in such a way as to respect and foster their sense of:

- dignity;
- autonomy;
- positive self-regard;

- civil rights; and
- involvement in their own care.

The patient's involvement includes:

- perceptions of his or her own strengths, weaknesses, and resources;
- relevant demands of his or her environments; and
- the requirements and expectations for participation by service providers and the patient.

STANDARD

RI.1.2.1   Informed consent is obtained.

Intent of RI.1.2.1

Staff members clearly explain any proposed treatments or procedures to the patient and, when appropriate, the family. The explanation includes:

- potential benefits and drawbacks;
- potential problems related to recuperation;
- the likelihood of success;
- the possible results of nontreatment; and
- any significant alternatives.

Staff members also inform the patient of:

- the name of the physician or other practitioner who has primary responsibility for the patient's care;
- the identity and professional status of individuals responsible for authorizing and performing procedures or treatments;
- any professional relationship to another health care provider or institution that might suggest a conflict of interest;
- their relationship to educational institutions involved in the patient's care;
- any business relationships between individuals treating the patient, or between the organization and any other health care, service, or educational institutions involved in the patient's care.

Example of Implementation for RI.1.2.1

The medical staff, in collaboration with others, develops a formal process to guide and support the following:

- Documenting the disclosure process (for example, discussions with the patient relative to the specific benefits and drawbacks of the treatment or procedure, including impact on daily living activities and alternate therapies, when available);
- Availability of translation services when appropriate;

- Availability of appropriate audiovisual aids;
- A method to assess and document evidence of patient understanding; and
- Documents of patient consent for procedures.

STANDARDS

RI.1.2.1.1   All patients asked to participate in a research project are given a description of the expected benefits.

RI.1.2.1.2   All patients asked to participate in a research project are given a description of the potential discomforts and risks.

RI.1.2.1.3   All patients asked to participate in a research project are given a description of alternative services that might also prove advantageous to them.

RI.1.2.1.4   All patients asked to participate in a research project are given a full explanation of the procedures to be followed, especially those that are experimental in nature.

RI.1.2.1.5   All patients asked to participate in a research project are told that they may refuse to participate, and that their refusal will not compromise their access to services.

Intent of RI.1.2.1.1 Through RI.1.2.1.5

When patients are asked to participate in an investigational study or clinical trial, they need information upon which to base their decision. The hospital protects patients and respects their rights during research, investigation, and clinical trials involving human subjects by:

- giving them information to make a fully informed decision;
- describing expected benefits;
- describing potential discomforts and risks;
- describing alternatives that might also help them;
- explaining procedures to be followed;
- explaining that they may refuse to participate, and that their refusal will not compromise their access to the hospital's services.

The hospital has policies and procedures for providing patients with this information.

STANDARD

RI.1.2.2   The family participates in care decisions.

Intent of RI.1.2.2

Care sometimes requires that people other than (or in addition to) the patient be involved in decisions about the patient's care. This is especially true when the patient does not have the mental or physical capacity to make care decisions, or when the patient is a child. When the patient cannot make decisions regarding his or her care, a surrogate decision maker[4] is identified. In the case of an unemancipated minor, the family or guardian is legally responsible for approving the care prescribed. The patient has the right to exclude any or all family members from participating in his or her care decisions.

Example of Implementation for RI.1.2.2

The hospital has outlined situations, with help from legal counsel, in which the family or surrogate decision maker needs to be included in the decision-making process. Legal counsel provides direction in such cases. Policies and procedures guide clinicians in the proper format for medical record entries.

STANDARD

RI.1.2.3   Patients are involved in resolving dilemmas about care decisions.

Intent of RI.1.2.3

Making decisions about care sometimes presents questions, conflicts, or other dilemmas for the hospital and the patient, family, or other decision makers. These dilemmas may arise around issues of admission, treatment, or discharge. They can be especially difficult to resolve when the issues involve, for example, withholding resuscitative services or forgoing or withdrawing life-sustaining treatment. The hospital has a way of resolving such dilemmas and identifies those who need to be involved in the resolution.

Examples of Implementation for RI.1.2.3

1. The hospital has a multidisciplinary committee or designated individual who reviews and assesses reports of dilemmas in patient care (for example, between family members) and applies hospital policies and procedures to help in conflict resolution.
2. Hospital policy directs clinicians to refer family members to appropriate clergy or other organization spiritual advisor for consultation when the issue of withholding resuscitative services arises.

STANDARD

RI.1.2.4   The hospital addresses advance directives.[5]

Intent of RI.1.2.4

The hospital determines whether a patient has or wishes to make advance directives. The hospital also ensures that health care professionals and designated representatives honor the directives within the limits of the law and the organization's mission, philosophy, and capabilities. For example, if a patient elects to donate organs at the end of life, the organization must have a process to honor that directive. In the absence of the actual advance directive, the substance of the directive is documented in the patient's medical record. The lack of advance directives does not hamper access to care. The hospital, however, provides assistance to patients who do not have an advance directive but wish to formulate one.

Example of Implementation for RI.1.2.4

The hospital's policies and procedures require that a patient be told his or her right to make advance directives. The discussion is facilitated by authorized staff members who have specific training in this area or by the attending physician. The course of discussion, including any educational materials used, and its outcome is documented in the medical record. The patient or surrogate decision maker may review and modify the advance directives any time throughout the episode of care.

STANDARDS

RI.1.2.5   The hospital addresses withholding resuscitative services.

RI.1.2.6   The hospital addresses forgoing or withdrawing life-sustaining treatment.

Intent of RI.1.2.5 and RI.1.2.6

Decisions about withholding resuscitative services or forgoing or withdrawing life-sustaining treatment are among the most difficult choices facing patients, families, health care professionals, and hospitals. No single process can anticipate all of the situations in which such decisions must be made. All the more reason why it is important for the hospital to develop collaboratively a framework for making these difficult decisions.

The framework:

- helps the hospital identify its position on initiating resuscitative services and using and removing life-sustaining treatment;
- ensures that the hospital conforms to the legal requirements of its jurisdiction;
- addresses situations in which these decisions are modified during the course of care;
- offers guidance to health professionals on the ethical and legal issues involved in these decisions and de-

creases their uncertainty about the practices permitted by the hospital.

The decision-making process is applied consistently, and the lines of accountability are clear. To ensure this, it is vital that a guiding process be formally adopted by the hospital's medical staff and approved by the governing body.

Example of Implementation for RI.1.2.5 and RI.1.2.6

The medical staff and others develop policies and procedures on advance directives. These are approved by the governing body. The clinician refers to the policies and procedures for guidance when a decision must be made to withdraw life-sustaining treatment or withhold resuscitative services.

STANDARD

RI.1.2.7   The hospital addresses care at the end of life.

Intent of RI.1.2.7

Dying patients have unique needs for respectful, responsive care. All hospital staff are sensitized to the needs of patients at the end of life. Concern for the patient's comfort and dignity should guide all aspects of care during the final stages of life.

The hospital's framework for addressing issues related to care at the end of life provide for:

- providing appropriate treatment for any primary and secondary symptoms, according to the wishes of the patient or the surrogate decision maker;
- managing pain aggressively and effectively;
- sensitively addressing issues such as autopsy and organ donation;
- respecting the patient's values, religion, and philosophy;
- involving the patient and, where appropriate, the family in every aspect of care; and
- responding to the psychological, social, emotional, spiritual, and cultural concerns of the patient and the family.

Effective pain management is appropriate for all patients, not just for dying patients.

Examples of Implementation for RI.1.2.7

1. The patient, family, or surrogate decision makers are involved in every aspect of the patient's care at the end of his or her life. The hospital uses a formal process to support this involvement. Policies and proce-

dures guide clinicians in the appropriate format for medical record entries.

2. The hospital may use as its basis acute pain management guidelines that reflect the state of knowledge on pain management and are published by the Agency for Health Care Policy and Research.

STANDARDS

RI.1.3	The hospital demonstrates respect for the following patient needs:
RI.1.3.1	confidentiality;
RI.1.3.2	privacy;
RI.1.3.3	security;
RI.1.3.4	resolution of complaints;
RI.1.3.5	pastoral counseling;
RI.1.3.6	communication.
RI.1.3.6.1	When the hospital restricts a patient's visitors, mail, telephone calls, or other forms of communication, the restrictions are evaluated for their therapeutic effectiveness.
RI.1.3.6.1.1	Any restrictions on communication are fully explained to the patient and family, and are determined with their participation.

Intent of RI.1.3 Through RI.1.3.6.1.1

Communication and information are important areas of rights and respect for patients. The hospital has a way of providing for:

- effective communication[6] for each patient served, including the hearing and speech impaired;
- the patient's right to privacy and security;
- the patient's right to confidentiality of information; and
- the patient's right to voice complaints about his or her care, and to have those complaints reviewed and, when possible, resolved.

Generally, patients have the right to expect unrestricted access to communication. Sometimes, however, it may be necessary to restrict visitors, mail, telephone calls, or other forms of communication as a component of a patient's care (for example, to prevent injury or deterioration in the patient, damage to the environment, or infringement on the rights of others). The patient is included in any such decision.

Communication restrictions are explained in a language the patient understands. For an unemancipated minor or patient under guardianship, applicable law determines who is legally entrusted to act in the patient's best interest. Clinical justification of such restrictions is documented in the medical record.

For many patients, pastoral counseling and other spiritual services are an integral part of health care and daily life. The hospital is able to provide pastoral counseling services for patients who request them.

Example of Implementation for RI.1.3.1

Policies and procedures, based on applicable law and regulation, address confidentiality of patient information. The patient is informed of the hospital's policy on confidentiality at the time of admission.

Examples of Implementation for RI.1.3.2

- Partitioning in patient rooms give privacy and respect without visual obstruction to the nursing staff.
- Cubicle curtains in the emergency area give visual privacy.
- Spacing of stretchers and examination areas in the emergency area gives auditory privacy.
- Patients are interviewed out of the hearing range of other patients in the waiting room at outpatient sites.
- Procedures for bathing, positioning, and the use of the bed pan and bedside commodes are developed to ensure patient privacy and comfort in all situations.
- Locked storage areas are available for patients to secure some personal items; however, patients are encouraged on admission not to store valuables on hospital premises.

Example of Implementation for RI.1.3.4

The hospital has a formal process for reviewing patient complaints and helping to resolve conflicts. This process includes a plan to inform patients and their families of their right to make complaints and how to go about having them resolved. This process also involves a patient advocate or representative who reviews the complaint and consults with the appropriate hospital staff (for example, nursing, medical staff, housekeeping). Those issues that cannot be resolved in this manner are referred to the hospital administration for intervention.

Example of Implementation for RI.1.3.5

Hospitals respect and provide for each patient's right to pastoral counseling. It is recognized that services for patients' spiritual needs may be provided by clergy or certified chaplains as well as individuals who are not ordained or certified. Therefore, services are provided or available in a variety of ways.

For example, a small community hospital may maintain a list of clergy who have consented to be available to the hospital's patients in addition to visiting their own parishioners. A larger hospital, such as an academic health center or a Veterans Administration medical center, may have a department of clinical pastoral counseling. The larger hospitals may employ qualified clinical chaplains who have graduated from an accredited Master of Divinity degree program. These departments may or may not provide services that are considered part of the patient care process. When pastoral counseling services are included in the patient care service provision, the right to provide documentation of pastoral or spiritual services in the patient's medical record is determined by the hospital.

The position description for the director of a clinical pastoral counseling department may specify that the individual is currently a competent Certified Clinical Chaplain and meets any current legal requirements for licensure, registration, or certification stated in the position description. Clinical chaplains assess and treat patients using individual and group interventions to restore or rehabilitate spiritual well-being. Clinical chaplains counsel individuals who are experiencing spiritual distress, as well as their families, caregivers, and other service providers, about their spiritual dysfunction or the management of spiritual care.

STANDARD

RI.1.4　　Each patient receives a written statement of his or her rights.

Intent of RI.1.4

Admission to the hospital can be a frightening and confusing experience for patients, making it difficult for them to understand and exercise their rights. A written copy of the hospital's statement of patients' rights is given to patients when they are admitted and is available to them throughout their stay. This statement is appropriate to the patient's age, understanding, and language.

The hospital may also post a copy of its patients' rights document in public areas accessible to patients and their visitors. When written communication is not effective (for example, the patient cannot read or the patient's language is rare in the patient population served), the patient is informed again of his or her rights after admission, in a manner that he or she can understand.

STANDARD

RI.1.5　　The hospital supports the patient's right to access protective services.

Intent of RI.1.5

When the hospital serves a patient population that often needs protective services (that is, guardianship and advocacy services, conservatorship, and child or adult protective services), it has ways of helping patients' families and the courts determine a patient's need for special services, such as guardianship. An independent assessment

ensures that the patient's best interests are of primary concern. When the services are especially pertinent to the population served by the hospital, the patient is given, in writing:

- a list of names, addresses, and telephone numbers of pertinent state client advocacy groups such as the state survey and certification agency, the state licensure office, the state ombudsman program, the protection and advocacy network, and the Medicaid fraud control unit; and
- information regarding the patient's right to file a complaint with the state survey and certification agency if he or she has a concern about patient abuse, neglect, or about misappropriation of a patient's property in the facility.

The hospital has policies and procedures that address all the issues described above.

STANDARD

RI.2　　The hospital has a policy and procedures, developed with the medical staffs' participation, for the procuring and donation of organs and other tissues.

Intent of RI.2

Any hospital procuring human organs or tissues is a member of the appropriate procurement organization and follows its rules and regulations. For nonfederal hospitals, this organization is the Organ Procurement and Transplantation Network established under section 372 of the Public Health Service Act. For Department of Defense hospitals, Veterans Affairs medical centers, and other federally administered health care facilities, the appropriate organizations are designated by the respective agency.

Policies and procedures for organ and tissue procurement and donation include the following elements:

- Identification of the organ or tissue procurement agency with which the hospital is affiliated;
- Criteria for identifying potential organ and tissue donors;
- Procedures for notifying the family of each donor of the option to donate, and for recording their decision;
- Discretion and sensitivity to the circumstances, beliefs, and desires of the families of potential donors;
- Procedures for directly notifying appropriate organ procurement organizations and tissue banks when an organ (specifically, a heart, kidney, liver, lung, or pancreas) or other tissue is potentially available--that is, before the patient dies (in Department of Defense hos-

pitals, Veterans Affairs medical centers, and other federally administered health care agencies, notification is carried out according to procedures approved by the respective agency);

- Written documentation showing that the patient or family accepts or declines the opportunity for the patient to become an organ or tissue donor; and
- Records of potential organ donors whose names have been sent to organ or tissue procurement organizations.

These policies and procedures are developed with medical staff participation.

STANDARDS

RI.3   The hospital protects patients and respects their rights during research, investigation, and clinical trials involving human subjects.

RI.3.1   All consent forms address the information specified in RI.1.2.1.1 through RI.1.2.1.5; indicate the name of the person who provided the information and the date the form was signed; and address the participant's right to privacy, confidentiality, and safety.

Intent of RI.3 and RI.3.1

A hospital that conducts research, investigations, or clinical trials involving human subjects knows that its first responsibility is to the health and well-being of the individual patient. To protect and respect patients' rights, the hospital always:

- reviews all research protocols in relation to the hospital's mission statement, values, and other guidelines;
- weighs the relative risks and benefits to the subjects;
- obtains the subject's consent.

Because the patient's decision to participate in clinical trials or research needs to be based on his or her competency and sound information, the following items are documented in the patient's record:

- The name of the person who provided the information; and
- The date the form was signed.

When research procedures are complete, the principal investigator does everything possible to eliminate any confusion, misinformation, stress, physical discomfort, or other harmful consequences the participant may have experienced as a result of the procedures.

STANDARDS

RI.4   The hospital operates according to a code of ethical behavior.[7]

RI.4.1   The code addresses marketing, admission, transfer and discharge, and billing practices.

RI.4.2   The code addresses the relationship of the hospital and its staff members to other health care providers, educational institutions, and payers.

Intent of RI.4 Through RI.4.2

A hospital has an ethical responsibility to the patients and community it serves. Guiding documents, such as the hospital's mission statement and strategic plan, provide a consistent, ethical framework for its patient care and business practices.

But a framework alone is not sufficient. To support ethical operations and fair treatment of patients, a hospital has and operates according to a code of ethical behavior. The code addresses ethical practices regarding:

- marketing;
- admission;
- transfer;
- discharge; and
- billing, and resolution of conflicts associated with patient billing.

The code ensures that the hospital conducts its business and patient care practices in an honest, decent, and proper manner.

Example of Implementation for RI.4 Through RI.4.2

A hospital's governing body reviews a proposed relationship before entering a contractual agreement with a provider of services. The proposed contract is approved or rejected based on best-bid practices and the potential for conflict of interest. Marketing materials only reflect the services available and the level of licensure and accreditation. All initial patient billing is itemized and includes dates of service. The hospital has a formal process to review patient or other payer questions about charges expeditiously and resolve a conflict or discuss a question without real or perceived harassment.

Admission and transfer policies are not based on patient or hospital economics. Only patients whose specific condition or disease cannot be safely treated at the hospital are diverted, refused admission, or transferred to another hospital.

STANDARD

RI.4.3   In hospitals with longer lengths of stay, the code addresses a patient's rights to perform or refuse to perform tasks in or for the hospital.

Intent of RI.4.3

Patients are encouraged to take responsibility for their own living quarters. In addition, patients may be offered the opportunity to perform work for the organization (for example, patient work therapy programs in grounds keeping or the library) that does not endanger the patient, other patients, or staff. If the hospital asks longer-stay patients to perform such tasks (work), the patient has the right to refuse. If the patient agrees to perform tasks for the organization

- the work is appropriate to the patient's needs and therapeutic goals;
- the organization documents the patient's desire for work in the plan of care;
- the plan specifies the nature of the services performed and whether the services are nonpaid or paid;
- compensation for paid services is determined based on the work performed, whether the work would be otherwise done by a paid employee, and the applicable wage and hourly standards in the community for the work; and
- the patient agrees to the work arrangement described in the plan of care.

The intent of this standard does not extend to the patient's care of his or her body, maintenance of his or her room or space, or the patient's preparation of his or her own meals.

ADDITIONAL EXAMPLES OF IMPLEMENTATION

Following are additional examples of implementation for this function. The examples address four general categories:

- Hospital type;
- Discipline;
- Regulatory or legal requirements; and
- Compliance issues.

The hospital type, discipline, and regulatory or legal requirements categories are also broken down into subcat-

egories. This chapter may not have examples for each category or subcategory at this time. However, examples may be provided in the future.

As you read through these examples, please keep in mind that in addition to the examples that are directly applicable to your hospital setting, other examples in this section may provide you with additional insight. Therefore, we encourage you to read through all the examples in this section.

Examples by Hospital Type

These examples address one or more of the following subcategories: small or rural, government, public, private or community, academic medical center, and specialty hospitals, such as rehabilitation, psychiatric, pediatric, and chronic disease.

Small or Rural Hospital--Example for RI.4 Through RI.4.2.
A small hospital develops a plan to identify and implement a code for ethical behavior. An ad hoc committee--composed of two members each from governance, senior executive leadership, the medical staff, nursing, social services, and the business office--is appointed and given the responsibility for developing a code.

The first step in the committee's work plan is to ask the local university's resource center to do a literature search for existing codes of ethics for the health care professions, organization development literature, and business literature. The committee reviews the articles found and identifies codes that include activities appropriate to the hospital's services and business practices.

The committee develops an outline for its own code by identifying key phrases that can be reasonably related to business ethical practices that are common in each of the codes. Several meetings are devoted to developing the structure of the hospital's code of ethical behavior. The structure or draft outline is reviewed by staff members in the various groups represented by members of the ad hoc committee over a one-month time period.

The results of this review are then considered by the ad hoc committee, whose members wordsmith a full draft of the code. This draft is passed before all involved groups --governance, senior management, medical staff, nursing, social services, and business--and department heads.

Department heads are asked to discuss the draft code with their staff and to provide feedback to the ad hoc committee within a month. The discussions result in further revisions. Once complete, the code is adopted and approved by the hospital's governing body and published in the hospital newsletter. An article about the code is also published in the local newspaper. Because of widespread community support, the hospital's leaders decide to share their experience with developing such a code by submitting articles for publication in professional journals.

Academic Medical Center--Example for RI.2. Specially trained members of the hospital's bioethics staff act as counselors for the families of potential organ or tissue donors and interface with the appropriate agencies.

Specialty Hospital--Psychiatric Hospital--Example for RI.1. In a hospital providing biopsychosocial care and treatment services, the statement of patient rights promotes their vision, which respects and fosters the patient's sense of:

- dignity;
- autonomy;
- positive self-regard;
- civil rights; and
- involvement in his or her care.

The patient's involvement includes:

- perceptions of his or her strengths, weaknesses, and resources;
- relevant demands of his or her environment; and
- the requirements and expectations for participation by service providers and the patient.

This also includes educating patients regarding their:

- psychiatric;
- physical; and
- functional diagnoses and prognoses.

The communication of information regarding assessment and treatment options facilitates comprehension and understanding and elicits the patient's active participation in forming his or her rehabilitation plan.

Examples by Discipline

These examples address one or more of the categories found in the:

- Applicability of the Standards to Specific Individuals and Departments' matrix found in the "How to Use This Manual" chapter.

Physicians--Example for RI.1.2.1. Any patient scheduled for needle lung biopsy is informed of the risks and alternatives and has agreed to the procedure. Their consent is documented in the medical record according to hospital policy.

Examples Covering Regulatory or Legal Requirements

These examples address one or more regulatory or legal requirements at the federal, state, county, city, municipal, or local level.

Federal. Americans with Disabilities Act--Examples for RI.1.3.6.

1. The hospital has a formal process that ensures effective communication with patients through demonstrated patient understanding. The hospital has a library of educational material that includes anatomical models and other visual aids.

   - The hospital has access to translators or translation services when necessary.
   - The hospital's switchboard has Telecommunications Device for the Deaf (TDD) access. Telephones in patient rooms, as appropriate, are supplied with voice amplification devices.
   - Patients have or have access to written copies of their rights provided at the time of admission or whenever requested.
   - Patient information is available in braille or on audiocassette.

2. An off-site ambulatory diagnostic radiology department that serves a large Hispanic population provides interpreters. All signs that are posted are printed in both English and Spanish to accommodate the Hispanic population.

National Institutes of Health--Examples for RI.3. A proposal requesting the hospital's participation in an experimental surgical implantation procedure is presented to the institutional review board (IRB). The board approves participation based on the:

- project's compatibility with the hospital's mission;
- its staff expertise;
- available resources; and
- positive benefits to its patients.

In addition, the IRB has developed a patient consent form and policies that govern the conduct of participation.

The materials presented to the patient are written in the patient's primary language and have understandable explanations.

When a patient has been selected for participation in an investigational study, research project, or clinical trial, he or she is informed of the focus of the activity as it relates to his or her care. Directed by an informed consent process developed by the IRB, the patient is allowed to refuse participation and ensured that the decision will in no way effect the quality of his or her care.

Office for Protection from Research Risk/National Institutes of Health--Example for RI.1.2.1. The hospital determined that it would use a set of criteria developed by the Office of Protection from Research Risk/National Institutes of Health (OPRR/NIH) (see the "Suggested Readings and

Other Resources" section of this chapter for full citation) to define activities that constitute research.

- The intent of the activity is to produce information that will contribute to generalizable knowledge, rather than to produce information for internal use in the management of individual patients or in the assessment and improvement of processes within the organization.
- When research is undertaken, an institutional review board is established and used throughout the conduct of the study.
- The results of the activity are or will be published.

Local, Municipal, City, County, State. State--Example for RI.1.2.5. In New York state, DNR [do-not-resuscitate] policies are not required for ambulatory care sites.

Examples Addressing Compliance Issues

These examples address compliance issues that reflect the top frequently cited standards. This chapter may have more than one example addressing compliance issues if more than one frequently cited standard appears in the chapter.

Examples for RI.1.2.1--Consent as a Process. A hospital-sponsored birthing center process includes prenatal consent for care and delivery and emergency procedure consent for cesarean-section should the need arise. A form exists that documents the patient's consent for her entire care process including prenatal care, labor and delivery care, and any surgical consent discussions that occur between the caregiver and the patient and her family. However, the patient does not sign a separate surgical consent form.

As long as a patient is fully informed and indicates that he or she understands what is being discussed, the primary caregiver (for example, the physician) can document the discussion and the patient's expressed understanding and consent. (See definition for "advance directives" in the notes that addresses both documents and documentation of the patient's preferences.)

Examples for RI.4--Ethical Behavior. A network component hospital is given direction to base its code of ethical behavior on its mission and show in the hospital's annual budget and strategic planning process documents how the code is used as a framework for ethical business practices.

Examples for RI.1.2.4--Advance Directives as Both Documentation and Process. The intent of RI.1.2.4 includes the following sentence: In the absence of the actual advance directive, the substance of the directive is documented in the patient's medical record. In the absence of a copy of an existing advance directive, what does the hospital have to document in the patient's medical record and how would the hospital and the patient's care providers use such docu-

mentation? Does the documentation of the patient's wishes without the actual advance directive place the hospital at increased risk?

The principles embodied in this standard and its intent statement are:

- The right of the patient to express his or her wishes regarding treatment at any point in the care process;
- The responsibility of the hospital to document the wishes of the patient and ensure that the patient's physician is aware of those wishes;
- The documentation in the patient's medical record can be through the insertion of existing or newly completed formal directives, the recording of the patient's description of the content of the directives, or the recording of the patient's wishes irrespective of the existence of a formal directive;
- While state law, legal precedent, and hospital policy may influence how the patient's wishes are carried out, the right of the patient to make his or her wishes known and have the wishes documented is protected by the hospital.

These principles and the types of documentation are illustrated as follows:

1. The patient is admitted and does have a copy of his or her existing advance directive that is placed in the medical record.
2. The patient is admitted but does not have a copy of his or her existing advance directive. The person who is responsible for determining the existence of an advance directive as designated in hospital policy (for example, the admitting nurse or physician), should respond as follows:

- First, make arrangements to immediately obtain a copy of the existing advance directive.
- Second, the patient may be offered assistance in completing a new written advance directive(s).
- Third, the hospital designee may inform the patient that he or she may verbalize treatment preferences. That is, the patient may explain the "substance" of his or her original advance directive including treatment preferences, preferred surrogates, and statements regarding his or her wishes concerning a minimum quality of life. If a patient chooses to verbalize treatment choices, the conversation is documented in the patient's medical record and the patient's physician is informed.

The patient may at any point make clarifications, modifications, or revocations of the directive(s). Such conversations should be documented in the patient's medical record, and the patient's physician should be informed.

The Joint Commission is not suggesting that the hospital obtaining of a verbal description of a written existing advance directive is necessarily the same, under any applicable law, as that of actual possession by the hospital of the actual document.

3. A patient is admitted with no advance directive. The patient is offered the opportunity to execute an advance directive. If the patient chooses to make a written advance directive, a copy should be made part of his or her medical record, and the original document should be given to the patient or to the patient's surrogate if the patient has lost decisional capacity at the time of discharge.
4. If the patient does not wish to make a verbal or written advance directive, this decision is noted in the patient's medical record.

In all of the above cases, if the patient is capable of making decisions, the advance directive, whether verbal or written, is not in effect. However, if the patient lacks or loses the ability to make decisions, the physician should refer to the advance directive document or documentation and, within the limits of the law and the organization's mission, philosophy and capabilities, honor the patient's wishes by writing appropriate orders. Such orders might address palliative care, forgoing or withdrawing life-sustaining treatment, or DNR orders.

In summary, whether or not the patient has a written advance directive, health care professionals should record conversations with patients about treatment preferences and choice of surrogate in the patient's permanent medical record. Within the limits of the law and the hospital's mission, philosophy, and capabilities, these directives and choices are then honored as a verbal advance directive in the event that the patient loses the ability to make treatment decisions.

In all events, the patient has the right to change his or her mind regarding any written or verbal advance directive. The hospital or other health care organization must have a mechanism in place to honor any changes that the patient wishes to make in his or her advance directive.

SUGGESTED READINGS AND OTHER RESOURCES

Appelbaum PS: Advance directives for psychiatric treatment. *Hospital and Community Psychiatry* 42(10):983-4, 1991.

Discusses the impact advance directives are beginning to have on psychiatric care. Defines the two types

of advance directives--instruction and proxy--and describes the advantages and disadvantages of both. Explains how new statutes in various states encourage the use of health care proxies. Presents issues raised by the use of advance directives in psychiatric treatment.

Downing BT: A multilingual model for training health care interpreters. Paper presented at the National Conference on Health and Mental Health of Soviet Refugees, Chicago, Dec 10-12, 1991. (Reprints from author: Bruce T. Downing, PhD, Associate Professor and Chair, Department of Linguistics, University of Minnesota.)

Addresses the need for trained and skilled interpreters to handle the growing refugee population in the United States. Uses a multilingual model that has been implemented at the University of Minnesota as an example to demonstrate how quality training for interpreters can be provided, and to present the benefits of competent interpreters to both the patient and the health care provider.

The Bilingual Medical Interview I, The Bilingual Medical Interview II. Videotapes available through Boston Area Health Education Center, 818 Harrison Avenue, Boston, MA 02118, (617) 534-5258.

Illustrate effective utilization of medical interpreters. Present common barriers to conducting the medical interview.

Emanuel EJ, Emanuel LL: Proxy decision making for incompetent patients: An ethical and empirical analysis. *JAMA* 267:2067-71, Apr 15, 1992.

Discusses the current endorsement and justification of proxy decision making. Presents theoretical and empirical objections to proxy decision making, and offers solutions to the problems these objections address.

Friedman E: *Choices and Conflict: Explorations in Health Care Ethics*. Chicago: American Hospital Publishing, Inc, 1992.

Examines timely ethical issues for health care professionals, such as patient rights issues, rising costs, increasing cultural diversity, "high tech" death, and ethics and public policy. Contains 28 articles written by leading health care attorneys, ethicists, sociologists, physicians, and nurses.

Friedman RJ: Scientific and ethical consideration in human clinical experimentation. *South Med J*, 85:917-22, Sep 1992.

Reviews the ethical codes and guidelines of human clinical experimentation, and examines their underlying ethical principles. Provides examples of neglected ethical principles in the pursuit of scientific knowledge. Presents standards for ethical research design.

Jecker NS, Pearlman RA: Medical futility: Who decides? *Arch Intern Med* 152:1140-1144, Jun 1992.

Discusses the futility of medical treatment under certain conditions, and who is responsible for judging this futility. Addresses the issue of who should be authorized to decide whether a patient receives nutrition and hydration.

Meeker T: Decision Tree: A process for determining when to withdraw or continue life-sustaining medical treatment. *Health Prog* 74:48-51, Mar 1993.

An ethicist presents a modified version of the "decision tree" in Guidelines for State Court Decision Making in Life-Sustaining Medical Treatment Cases (1992). Provides two medical cases to illustrate how the decision tree can assist in making life-sustaining medical treatment decisions.

OPRR: *Protecting Human Research Subjects Institutional Review Board Guidebook*. National Institutes of Health Office of Extramural Research, Office for Protection from Research Risks, 1993.

Provides information for Institutional Review Boards (IRBs) regarding the regulations that govern research with human subjects. Containing regulations, relevant institutional documents, and forms, this guidebook is particularly useful for new IRB members.

Paridy N: Complying with the Patient Self-Determination Act: Legal, ethical, and practical challenges for hospitals. *Hospital and Health Services Administration* 38:287-296, Summer 1993.

Discusses PSDA history, why it came into being, its provisions, how to comply with it, and what can happen if a health care provider fails to comply.

Q&A: Hospitals and Advance Directives. American Hospital Association, 1993.

Designed to answer questions that may arise as hospitals develop or revise their advance directives policies or procedures. Developed by the AHA Technical Panel on Biomedical Ethics to assist hospitals in addressing issues of PSDA implementation.

Ross JW, et al: *Handbook for Hospital Ethics Committees*. Chicago: American Hospital Publishing, Inc, 1993.

Examines the nature and purpose of ethics com-

mittees. Provides suggestions for defining the roles and responsibilities of committee members.

Shields JM, Johnson A: Collision between law and ethics: Consent for treatment with adolescents. *Bull Am Acad Psychiatry Law* 20 (3):309-23, 1992.

Uses case examples to address some of the legal, ethical, and treatment issues of adolescent treatment when parental consent is problem-filled. Outlines the components of informed consent, and discusses the issue of the competence of minors to provide informed consent.

Solomon MZ, et al: Decisions near the end of life: Professional views on life-sustaining treatments. *Am J Public Health* 83:14-23, Jan 1993.

Presents the results of a five-hospital survey designed to determine whether or not clinicians agree with national recommendations regarding the care of patients near the end of life, and how they themselves view the issues. Reveals a gap between the views of the practicing clinicians and the prevailing guidelines. Analyzes these differences and suggests strategies for bridging the gap and improving the care of patients near the end of life.

Values in Conflict, Resolving Ethical Issues in Health Care, Second Edition. Chicago: American Hospital Association, 1994.

Designed to guide organizations in the development of policies, educational programs, and guidance mechanisms to support the resolution of value conflicts in the health care field.

Weber LJ: The business of ethics: Hospitals need to focus on managerial ethics as much as clinical ethics. *Health Prog* 71:87-8, 102, Jan-Feb 1990.

Presents four key values in business decisions and practices. Examines the two main approaches in contemporary business ethics and discusses the attention to conflict of interest.

Wolkon GH, Lyon M: Ethical issues in computerized mental health data systems. *Hospital and Community Psychiatry* 37:(1):11-6, 1986.

Addresses the ethical issues surrounding computerized mental health records. Claims that paper systems and automated systems share similar dangers, and similar steps must be taken to protect them. States that the same ethics and laws related to privacy, confidentiality, and privilege apply to both paper and electronic files.

NOTES

The source for the JCAHO *Standards on Patient Rights and Organization Ethics* is: © 1997 *Accreditation Manual for Hospitals.* Oakbrook Terrace, IL: Joint Commission on Accreditation of Healthcare Organizations, 1997, pages RI-1 to RI-32. Reprinted with permission.

1. *Function*--A goal-directed, interrelated series of processes, such as patient assessment or patient care.

2. *Family*--The person(s) who plays a significant role in the patient's life. This may include an individual(s) not legally related to the patient, but who has been identified as playing a significant role. This person(s) is often referred to as a surrogate decision maker if authorized to make care decisions for a patient should the patient lose decision-making capacity.

3. *Protective services* determine the need for protective intervention, correct hazardous living conditions or situations in which vulnerable adults are unable to care for themselves, and investigate evidence of neglect, abuse, or exploitation. Such services for children help families recognize the cause of any problems and strengthen parental ability to provide acceptable care. Protective services can include guardianship and advocacy services, conservatorship, state survey and certification agency, state licensure office, the state ombudsman program, the protection and advocacy network, and the Medicaid fraud control unit.

4. *Surrogate decision maker*--Someone appointed to act on behalf of another. Surrogates make decisions only when an individual is without capacity or have given permission to involve others.

5. *Advance directives*--Written or verbal statements made by the patient indicating treatment wishes in the event the patient becomes incapacitated. Advance directives may include living wills, durable powers of attorney, or similar documents or documentation conveying the patient's preferences.

6. *Effective communication*--Any form of communication (for example, writing or speech) that leads to demonstrable understanding.

7. The hospital may have one code of ethical behavior or multiple codes addressing the issues identified in RI.4.1 through RI.4.2.

APPENDIX 2

Recommendations for Guidelines on Procedures and Process and Education and Training to Strengthen Bioethics Services in Virginia

Virginia Bioethics Network:
John C. Fletcher, Ph.D.,
Edward M. Spencer, M.D.,
Sigrid Fry-Revere, J.D., Ph.D., and
Cavin Leeman, M.D.

PREAMBLE AND MISSION STATEMENT

The Virginia Bioethics Network (VBN) is an organization of institutional and individual members whose mission is to promote education in bioethics and to strengthen bioethics services in the healthcare institutions and organizations of the Commonwealth. To this end, the Board of Directors of the VBN desires to begin an eight month's process of consultation with its members and others about recommendations of guidelines for:

1. procedures and process for ethics committees and their activities; and
2. education and training for ethics committee members and ethics consultants.

An earlier draft of this document was discussed at the Annual Meeting of VBN on October 27-28, 1994, and the changes recommended at that meeting are incorporated in this document. At that meeting the Guidelines portion (as indicated by bold type) was approved by the VBN Board. The present document, or a revised version, will be "on the table" for discussion by each member institution and others during the next eight months. At the 1995 Annual Meeting, a final version should be ready for adoption by the VBN. The VBN desires the greatest degree of local and regional participation in shaping these recommendations.

The VBN makes these recommendations to the boards and professional staffs of healthcare institutions and organizations in Virginia.[1] The authority to use or improve on the recommendations clearly lies within the boards of these organizations. Local and regional forms of self-regulation in providing bioethics services is preferable to regulations imposed by government or courts. However, since ethics committees are involved with patients' rights, healthcare organizations that neglect the issue of standards for bioethics services take a large risk.

The values underlying these guidelines concern:

1. insuring a fair and open process for ethics committees' deliberations; and
2. equipping ethics committee members and consultants with education and training for tasks that relate to improving quality in decisionmaking about ethical issues that arise in patient care.

Besides consultation about these recommendations with institutions and professionals in Virginia, the VBN will consult with the Joint Commission on Accreditation of Healthcare Organizations (JCAHO), the Society for Bioethics Consultation, and other interested and involved groups.

The Procedure and Process Guidelines focus on the rights of patients and responsibilities of clinicians and healthcare organizations in reference to the activities of their ethics programs. The guidelines are framed to satisfy minimal requirements and allow for flexibility in implementation in large and small organizations.[2]

The Education and Training Guidelines also are framed to satisfy minimal requirements and allow for flexibility and choice in implementation. The guidelines are goal-oriented statements and the methods to accomplish the goals are purposely not specified.

Specific examples are included to help organizations in deciding how to implement the guidelines. These examples need to be considered from the perspective of each organization and used in fulfilling the guidelines for that organization within a specific time frame. The examples may be used as an ideal toward which an organization can strive or as a menu from which certain parts can be selected to fulfill the guidelines. In the Education Guidelines section there are also some suggestions as to how an institution can ascertain whether the basic guidelines are being followed and evaluate its present position and progress in maintaining these guidelines.

GUIDELINES FOR PROCEDURE AND PROCESS

INTRODUCTION

A main purpose of these guidelines is to help assure fairness in the provision of bioethics services, which include education, policy development, and a process for ethics consultation. In reference to the latter service, there are many acceptable procedures for conducting ethics consultations and the VBN has no intention of limiting procedural options beyond recommending those elements of process essential for assuring fairness of whatever procedures are in place for ethics consultation. Therefore the guidelines will apply equally whether the focal point of an organization's bioethics consultation service is an ethics committee, a single consultant, or a consultation team. The method(s) used to fulfil the guidelines will vary from institution to institution and, in any particular institution, may not totally correspond to the examples which follow each guideline.

Keep in mind that the guidelines are general recommendations to be applied to all institutions, and that the method which each individual institution chooses to fulfil each guideline will, by necessity, vary with institutional type, size, and level of development of its ethics program.

Following each guideline is either a short discussion of the guideline or specific examples of recommendations which may be used to fulfil the goals stated in the guideline.

The following guidelines and examples represent two levels of information addressing implementation of procedure and process for institutional ethics programs. The guidelines represent the more general level which is applicable to all healthcare institutions and organizations. The examples following each guideline represent the specific policy and procedural aspects of bioethics services which a number of bioethics programs have found reasonable and useful. These examples are however only that, examples, and are not meant to represent policies which must be adopted. If desired by particular healthcare institutions, the examples may be considered an ideal toward which an ethics program may strive.

GUIDELINE I: AN INSTITUTIONAL ETHICS PROGRAM SHOULD HAVE ITS FUNCTIONS CLEARLY DEFINED BY A MISSION STATEMENT AND/OR WRITTEN POLICIES

Important bioethics service functions sponsored by institutional ethics programs include:

1. educating healthcare staff on bioethics issues;
2. assisting in policy development on bioethics issues;
3. organizing and carrying out community education on bioethics topics either individually or as a member of a bioethics network; and
4. assisting patients, patient's families, and healthcare staff in making and/or dealing with difficult ethical decisions relevant to patient care. The type and degree of commitment of an institutional ethics program to each of these functions should be addressed in the mission statement and/or specific policies.

Specific example of mission statement. "Patients, their families and healthcare staff are frequently confronted with difficult ethical issues. In order to meet their needs for discussion and clarification of ethical issues, [name of institu-

tion] has established an institutional ethics program which sponsors certain bioethics services. These services include acting as a forum for discussion of ethical issues, education concerning ethical issues and problems, and the facilitation of ethical decisionmaking in specific cases. To further its goals the institutional ethics program will consult with patients, patient's families, and staff; make institutional policy recommendations; and offer education on bioethics issues. The bioethics program will work to maximize options for those making difficult ethical decisions but will not seek to impose the moral preferences of its members on patients, patient's families or staff."

GUIDELINE II: AN INSTITUTIONAL ETHICS PROGRAM'S STRUCTURE AND OPERATING RULES, AS DEFINED BY THE MISSION STATEMENT AND SPECIFIC POLICIES, SHOULD ASSURE FAIRNESS AND ACCOUNTABILITY TO THOSE WHO USE THE BIOETHICS SERVICES

Specific examples.

1. The ethics committee should be a multispecialty committee with representatives from all of the important clinical areas of the institution. In addition one or more representatives from the community at large, who can reflect the community's values, should be afforded full membership on the committee. Attention to gender, ethnic, and religious diversity in selecting members of the ethics committee is desirable.
2. The ethics committee should be an integral part of the structure of the institution and have a defined responsibility within this structure. The ethics committee's authority should be derived from the institutional entity (medical staff, administration or board of directors) to which it reports.
3. The ethics committee should have a specific schedule for regular meetings and have a defined written procedure for placing items on the agenda of the regular meetings. All committee members and staff members, who may wish to have an item placed on the agenda of the regular ethics committee meeting, should be aware of this procedure. Accurate minutes of all ethics committee meetings should be maintained.
4. The ethics committee should have a specific method for calling a special meeting of the committee for timely consideration of particular ethical issues. This method should be widely known and easily available to the healthcare and administrative staff. Consideration may be given to patients and families who wish to have specific issues discussed by the ethics committee.
5. The ethics committee should have specific policies concerning qualifications for membership, appoint-

ment procedure, time frame for appointments, methods and reasons for removal of a committee member prior to completion of his/her term (any method for removal of a committee member must minimally meet the same procedural standards as outlined in the policies of the committee or group which is directly responsible for the activities of the committee), and acquisition and disbursement of operating funds.

6. The ethics committee should have a specific and well-defined procedure for consideration and development of institutional policies bearing upon the ethics of clinical care in the institution.

GUIDELINE III: AN INSTITUTIONAL ETHICS PROGRAM WHICH UNDERTAKES ETHICS CONSULTATION AS A PART OF ITS BIOETHICS SERVICES MUST ASSURE THAT ANY ETHICS CONSULTATION PROCEEDS IN A MANNER WHICH CONFORMS TO MINIMAL STANDARDS OF FAIRNESS AND ACCOUNTABILITY

Such minimal standards include defined methods for

1. access to consultation,
2. timely notice of consultation,
3. consultation process,
4. documentation of consultation, and
5. review (evaluation) of consultations.

Specific examples.

1. The ethics committee (or other appropriate body) should develop a protocol which addresses the entire process of ethics consultation and this protocol should be followed during all ethics consultations.
2. One member of an ethics consultation team or the single consultant should have completed all of the educational and training requirements to be specified as a "qualified consultant" (see Educational and Training Guidelines)
3. If ethics consultation is provided by more than one consultant, the consultation group or team should not consist entirely of persons with the same professional background. Possible exceptions and the acceptable reasons for the exceptions could be addressed in the ethics consultation protocol or in the rules and regulations of the ethics committee.
4. The ethics committee (or similar group) should be responsible for all ethics consultations and should review all consultations in a timely manner.
5. Ethics consultation should be focused on the clarification of options, education about the ethical issues represented by the options, and mediation where necessary. Specific moral advice as to a particular outcome should be avoided by the consultants, so that the ap-

propriate decisionmakers can make the decision(s) that are most fitting for them. No ethics consultation should involve voting.

6. Any healthcare provider directly involved in a patient's care should be able to request a consultation without fear of intimidation or punishment. Likewise any patient, patient's surrogate or family member may request a consultation. The ethics committee or the administration should take steps to inform patients, families, and healthcare staff of the availability of ethics consultation.
7. The patient or the patient's surrogate and the patient's attending physician should be notified of a consultation request. (But also see example 12, below.) Only the patient or his/her surrogate has the authority to veto a consultation.
8. Strict attention to confidentiality should be maintained during the entire consultation process. This includes getting permission from the patient or surrogate prior to reading the patient's chart as well as fully explaining the consultation process to the patient or surrogate. (But also see example 12, below.)
9. A good-faith effort should be made to notify and invite to the consultation meeting the patient's treating physician(s), and all healthcare staff and family members involved in the patient's care, as well as any person with legal authority to make healthcare decisions for the patient.
10. When the consultation process involves a meeting of the participants in the case, the meeting should proceed with certain guidelines in place including: the appropriate decision makers are present, the consultant explains the purpose and parameters of the meeting, the goal of maintaining confidentiality is emphasized, each person present will be allowed to state his/her thoughts concerning the case, and limits concerning length of meeting, issues to be discussed, and goals of the meeting will be set at the beginning of the meeting.
11. All consultations shall be documented by a brief note in the patient's chart giving an overview of the issues and recommendations (if any) which the consultation process addressed. A complete record of each consultation including the ethics committee review and any available follow-up information should be kept by the bioethics service.
12. There should be an informal process for addressing and discussing ethics issues of importance to the clinical staff without instituting the formal process specified above. This informal process may be activated by one or more clinical staff members because of concerns about a specific clinical case and need not involve notification or participation of all parties mentioned above. However the case itself should only be

discussed generally. Maintaining confidentiality concerning a case during this process is of utmost importance. Whether or not the names, specific aspects of the case, and information in the chart should be available to the ethics consultant(s) as a part of the informal process depends upon the nature of the inquiry, upon the culture of the institution and upon who is doing the consultation. This informal process should be considered an educational service.

13. If, in a particular case, complaints concerning the ethics consultation process or the ethics consultant(s) develop, there should be a mechanism in place for consideration of these complaints and for alternative consideration of the case, if needed.

GUIDELINE IV: A BIOETHICS PROGRAM SHOULD EVALUATE AND REVIEW ITS SERVICES
Specific examples of methods for review.

1. A bioethics service should appoint a member to periodically review the records of the service and report to the service as to possible methods for improvement.
2. A reviewer with no connection to the bioethics service or the institution should be employed to review the bioethics service at specified intervals. (Other VBN members can complete this review.)
3. A bioethics service may wish to undertake one or more surveys of staff members and/or patients and families to ascertain satisfaction levels with the activities of the service and suggestions for improvement.

RECOMMENDED GUIDELINES FOR EDUCATION AND TRAINING OF ETHICS COMMITTEE MEMBERS

Membership in an institutional ethics committee requires a commitment to acquire and maintain a level of education needed to fulfill the obligations of a particular ethics committee as outlined in its mission and as understood by the patients, clinical staff, and administrative staff of the institution. Ethics committee functions include:

1. discussion and recommendations concerning institutional policy issues which bear on ethical clinical care,
2. acting as a forum for discussion of specific ethical problems or dilemmas,
3. sponsorship of an ongoing educational program for the institutional staff, patients, and community, and
4. sponsorship of an appropriate method for those patients, family members, and staff members with an ethical problem to receive help in addressing their problem.

Research and networking activities are also functions of certain ethics committees.

GUIDELINE I: EVERY ETHICS COMMITTEE MEMBER SHOULD, WITHIN AN APPROPRIATE TIME FRAME (E.G., ONE YEAR), HAVE COMPLETED THE EDUCATION NECESSARY FOR HIM/HER TO FUNCTION AS A KNOWLEDGEABLE AND EFFECTIVE MEMBER OF THE COMMITTEE BASED ON THE COMMITTEE'S STATED MISSION AND GOALS

A. Education for ethics committee members should be aimed at providing a basic understanding of goals and activities of the particular ethics committee and its relationship to the parent institution and surrounding community.
B. Education for ethics committee members should lead to an understanding of acceptable processes for consideration of clinical ethics issues and problems as well as a basic knowledge of the parameters (legal and cultural) within which ethically appropriate decisions can be reached.

Specific examples. The following are examples of educational subjects which may be used to fulfill Guideline I.

1. History of institutional ethics committees generally and of the ethics program in the particular institution.
2. Mission and scope of ethics committees generally and of the particular institution's ethics committee.
3. Methods of analyzing ethics problems.
4. Procedure and Process Guidelines affecting the operation of the ethics committee.
5. Specific ethical obligations in clinical care including disclosure, assessment of capacity, informed consent process, confidentiality, truthfulness.
6. Clinical ethical issues including refusal of treatment, forgoing life-sustaining treatment, controversial reproductive choices, access and cost issues, death and dying issues, and others, including how diverse cultural and religious traditions affect decision making.
7. Legal issues bearing upon the ethical considerations of clinical care.

Evaluation of fulfillment of Guideline I. There are several techniques which may be used to evaluate whether Guideline I is being met. Which technique or method is appropriate for a specific ethics committee should be left for that committee--in concert with the board of the institution or organization--to decide. The most important factor in evaluating the education of ethics committee members is their demonstrated effectiveness in addressing the tasks of the committee. Possible methods for evaluation include:

1. Internal evaluation of adequacy of educational level of committee members in relation to assigned tasks.
2. Adherence to a specified educational curriculum.
3. Internal or external testing of knowledge.
4. . Outside evaluation of educational curriculum and/or effectiveness of committee members.

Ethics consultants. A higher standard of education and training for those who are to be designated ethics consultants is necessary because of the challenging nature of the task as well as the high visibility and importance of this activity. A major error by a poorly informed ethics consultant may adversely affect a particular patient, one or more staff members, or the entire institution.

GUIDELINE II: ALL ETHICS CONSULTANTS, PRIOR TO ACCEPTING PRIMARY RESPONSIBILITY FOR ETHICS CONSULTATION, SHOULD MEET REQUIREMENTS ADOPTED BY THE PARENT

These requirements should include those educational and training elements which assure that the ethics consultant fully understands the ethics consultation process in the particular institution, is comfortable in the clinical setting, and has the requisite knowledge of clinical ethics and health-care law.

Specific examples. The following are examples of educational and training activities which may be used to fulfil Guideline II.

1. Fulfill Guideline I with added attention to ethics consultation.
2. Course or courses focused on the clinical setting and its language.
3. One or more basic or advanced clinical ethics courses.
4. Lectures, or courses focused on principles and practice of ethics consultation including consideration of history, different models, evaluation techniques, and relationship to other professional endeavors.
5. Involvement in real or mock consultations as a trainee or participant/observer, with supervision from consultants with experience.
6. Training sessions devoted to skills in communication and group leadership, individual and group dynamics, mediation, and self-awareness.

Evaluation of fulfillment of Guideline II. Evaluation of ethics consultation and the educational and training activities associated with it is at an early stage of develop-

ment and is therefore difficult. Nevertheless each institution should attempt to evaluate this activity in some manner which seems appropriate in reference to the goals of consultation in the institution. One or more of the following examples of evaluation methods may be used to evaluate specific ethics consultants or ethics consultation generally.

1. Internal or external testing of the knowledge and/or level of expertise of the ethics consultant.
2. Internal review of each ethics consultation and the consultant's knowledge and ability in relation to the consultation. This can be done by the ethics committee or another designated body.
3. Observation of ethics consultant by external evaluators with recognized experience in ethics consultation.
4. Surveys of levels of satisfaction with ethics consultants or of their effectiveness in relation to specific desired processes.
5. Acceptance of demonstrated competence in another institution.

GUIDELINE III: ALL PERSONS WHO ARE DESIGNATED AS FACULTY FOR THE EDUCATION AND TRAINING NECESSARY TO FULFILL GUIDELINES I AND II SHOULD HAVE KNOWLEDGE AND/OR TRAINING IN THE AREA WHICH HE/SHE WILL TEACH AND HAVE DEMONSTRATED HIS/HER ABILITY TO TEACH IN THIS AREA

Recommendations for teaching faculty:

A. For an initial orientation of new ethics committee members: It is recommended that someone conducting this teaching have:
    1. At least one year's experience as an ethics committee member or chairperson;
    2. Attended and evaluated two prior orientations;
    3. Assisted with one prior orientation; and
    4. Completed at least the education to fulfill Guideline I.
B. For teaching required to fulfill Guideline I for education of ethics committee members, it is recommended that each faculty member for this activity have:
    1. At least two years' experience as an ethics committee member or chairperson;
    2. Completed the recommended education and training for ethics committee members in Guideline II; and
    3. Assisted in the teaching of the education to fulfill Guideline I for ethics committee members at least once.
    4. The legal component of this educational activity

should be taught or supervised by an attorney admitted to the bar in Virginia or on the faculty of an accredited law school in Virginia.

C. For the teaching needed to fulfill Guideline II for education for ethics committee members and consultants, it is recommended that each faculty member for this activity have:

1. At least two years' experience as an ethics committee member or chairperson;

2. Completed the education required for Guideline II for ethics committee members and consultants;

3. Provided ethics consultation effectively in a healthcare institution or organization; and

4. Assisted in the teaching designed to fulfill Guidelines I and II at least once;

5. The legal component of this educational activity should be taught or supervised by an attorney admitted to the bar in Virginia or on the faculty of an accredited law school in Virginia.

D. For the teaching of pathophysiology and medical terminology associated with fulfilling Guideline II, it is recommended that each faculty member for this activity have:

1. Either the M.D. or R.N. degree; and

2. Either assisted in the teaching of this material at least once, or demonstrated skill in teaching persons who are not clinicians.

NOTES

1. The resources of VBN will be made available to member institutions, both to consult on the application of these recommendations to the unique situation of an individual institution, and to assist, where possible, in the development of appropriate training for ethics committee members and ethics consultants.

This version of the guidelines was adopted at the Annual Meeting of VBN on 31 October 1995.

2. The VBN makes these recommendations recognizing that they will be flexibly used. For example, it initially may be desirable to "grandfather" some committee members, ethics consultants, and/or faculty members, in recognition of the work which they have been doing prior to the adoption of standards for bioethics services. Also, institutions have sufficient discretion to permit exceptions to standards for persons who present education and training equivalent, although not identical, to the standards.

APPENDIX 3

*Two Course Outlines and
Additional Readings*

I. A Semester Course Outline for Medical and Nursing Students

A. "Introduction to Clinical Ethics"
(13 2-Hour Sessions)

This course outline is adapted from a course taught each semester at the University of Virginia. In the fall semester, the students are from diverse disciplines and backgrounds that always include physicians, nurses, ethics committee members, and laypersons from the local community. In the spring semester, the course is required for first-year medical students.

Clinical ethics concerns the identification, analysis, and resolution of ethical problems that arise in planning for the care of patients. This course deals with ethical problems that occur frequently in the clinical setting as well as with issues of access, costs, and allocation. The course is designed to maximize the use of the textbook, *Introduction to Clinical Ethics*, and the cases and the information on legal trends that accompany the chapters. The course emphasizes the ethical responsibilities of clinicians in planning for the care of their patients.

The best format for the course is to spend a majority of contact hours in small discussion groups--co-led by persons who have taken the course at least once and who have talent for Socratic teaching. Some plenary sessions are needed to begin the course and to involve clinicians, patients, and family members who are willing to share their experiences in an actual case.

The philosophy of the course is explained in the Preface and Chapters 1 and 2 of the textbook. One source of this philosophy is expressed in the report of a Dartmouth College conference on planning a curriculum for medical school courses in ethics: C.M. Culver et al., "Basic Curricular Goals in Medical Ethics," *New England Journal of Medicine* 312 (1985): 253-56.

At the course's end, students should demonstrate the following abilities:

1. to identify clearly clinicians' ethical obligations in each case and the ethical problems involving patients (Chapters 3 through 13) that clinicians face most frequently in training and practice;
2. to understand the history of these obligations and problems and see them as opportunities to provide optimal care for patients and families whose lives have been disrupted by illness, pain, and suffering; and
3. to be able to use a case method (Chapter 2) that is designed:
   a. to prevent ethical problems through planning for the optimal care of patients;
   b. to be a process of practical deliberation about ethical problems, when they do arise, that brings major ethical considerations and principles to bear upon the decisions to be made;
4. to be familiar with the services of a clinical ethics program and how to access these resources; and
5. to discuss their ethical concerns as clinician-trainees in relation to their supervisors and patients.

The objectives listed above are especially designed to meet the needs of clinicians. When the course is offered to meet the needs of clinicians and members of ethics committees in healthcare organizations (HCOs), a substitute for the fifth objective is:

5. to enable members of ethics committees, especially those involved in education and consultation for ethical problems involving patients, to understand their role and the knowledge and skills required for their tasks.

B. Assigned Readings

The textbook should be available well before the first session, as students should prepare by reading the Preface and Chapter 1 before session 1.

C. Assigned Viewing

The videotape of "Dax's Case" is recommended for use prior to the session on refusal of treatment (session 5). Viewing time is 58 minutes. This video is widely available, and it can be ordered by calling the Kennedy Institute of Ethics Library (1-800-MED-ETHX).

D. Plenary Sessions

The textbook is designed to help course planners avoid the need for lectures. An initial plenary session can present the goals of the course, the plan for grading and assignments, an overview of the philosophy of the course, and the four-part case method discussed in Chapter 2. It is also possible to hold a brief plenary session to launch each class, if there is an adequate supply of clinicians/patients/family members who have been involved in the particular ethical problem being discussed and are willing to share their experience with the class. Ample time is needed in small groups, which should be co-led by persons who have taken the course at least once and have talent for teaching.

Participants need time in small groups to examine and express their views. Problems such as patient refusal of treatment, death and dying, or forgoing life-sustaining treatment may be the most likely sources of plenary sessions. A plenary session must be thoroughly planned, and if guests are invited to present, a prior planning meeting of all concerned is advisable.

E. Grading

One method of grading is to have small-group leaders read all written assignments and grade all the students in their groups. Either a letter grade or a pass/fail grade can be derived from three sources:

1. 30 percent for preparation, participation, and attendance in small group discussion. Students should notify their group leaders when they know that they will be absent.
2. 40 percent for two written assignments during the course. The first is a case analysis using the method explained in the text. The second is a paper on death and dying or a related topic. Students will receive the case two weeks before it is due. The written assignments should be no more than 2,500 words per paper (10 pages, double spaced).
3. 30 percent for final paper or examination, by student choice. A final paper is not to exceed 20 word-processed, double-spaced pages, properly researched and referenced. The subject should be selected with the advice of the group leader. A final examination--to use the four-part method in analyzing one of two new cases--is a two-hour, take-home, open-book exam.

To use this approach, group leaders need a grading key for evaluating the scope and content of case-study assignments. The course director should write such a key for the first assignment and for the two cases on the final examination. The key should represent the course director's best effort at an adequate analysis of a case, using the method in Chapter 2.

F. A Semester Course Schedule

Session 1 **Plenary--Introduction to the Course: 1 hour.**
Small groups 2 hours. (Reading: Preface, Chapters 1 and 2)

Session 2 **Confidentiality and Privacy**
(Reading: Chapter 3)

Session 3 **Communication, Truthtelling, and Disclosure**
(Reading: Chapter 4)

Session 4 **Capacity and Informed Consent**
(Reading: Chapters 5 and 6)

Session 5 **Refusal of Treatment**
(Reading: Chapter 7; assign paper 1)

Session 6 **Death and Dying**
(Reading: Chapter 8; assign paper 2)

Session 7 **Forgoing Life-Sustaining Treatment**
(Reading: Chapter 9; paper 1 due)

Session 8 **Newborns, Infants, and Children**
(Reading: Chapter 10)

Session 9 **Reproductive Issues**
(Reading: Chapter 11; paper 2 due)

Session 10 **Patient Selection**
(Reading Chapter 12)

Session 11 **Economics, Case Management, and Patient Advocacy**
(Reading: Chapter 13)

Session 12 **Professional Ethics**
(Reading: Chapter 15)

Session 13 **Summary and Review**
(Final examination handed out)

G. Suggested Additional Readings

Some instructors may want to assign additional readings. The readings below were selected to meet two criteria: historical value and value to clinicians. The readings are listed chronologically by topic.

1. Respecting Privacy and Confidentiality (Chapter 3)

M. Siegler, "Confidentiality in Medicine--A Decrepit Concept," *New England Journal of Medicine* 307 (1982): 1518-21.

J.C. Beck, ed., *Confidentiality Versus the Duty to Protect: Foreseeable Harm in the Practice of Psychiatry* (Washington, D.C.: American Psychiatric Press, 1990).

B. Freedman, "Violating Confidentiality to Warn of a Risk of HIV Infection: Ethical Work in Progress," *Theoretical Medicine* 12 (1991): 309-23.

C. Grady, J. Jacob, and C. Romano, "Confidentiality: A Survey in a Research Hospital," *The Journal of Clinical Ethics* 2, no. 1 (Spring 1991): 25-30.

American College of Medical Genetics, "Statement on Storage and Use of Genetic Materials," *American Journal of Human Genetics* 57, no. 6 (1995): 1499-500.

Midwest Bioethics Center, Task Force on Health Care Rights for Minors," Health Care Treatment Decision-Making Guidelines for Minors," *Bioethics Forum* 11, no. 4 (1995): A1-A16.

2. Communication, Truthtelling, and Disclosure (Chapter 4)

J. Vogel and R. Delgado, "To Tell the Truth: Physicians'

Duty to Disclose Medical Mistakes," *UCLA Law Review* 28 (1980): 52-94.

J. Katz, *The Silent World of Doctor and Patient* (New York: Free Press, 1984).

E.J. Cassell, *Talking with Patients* (Boston: Massachusetts Institute of Technology Press, 1985).

H.L. Hirsh, "The Physician-Patient Relationship: The Art and Science of Communication," *Medical Law* 5 (1986): 477-88.

D.H. Novack et al., "Physicians' Attitudes toward Using Deception to Resolve Difficult Ethical Problems," *Journal of the American Medical Association* 261, no. 20 (1989): 2980-85.

K.H. Brown, "Information Disclosure: I. Attitudes toward Truth-Telling," in W.T. Reich, ed., *Encyclopedia of Bioethics*, 2nd ed. (New York: Simon & Schuster MacMillan, 1995), 1221-25.

A. Jameton, "Information Disclosure: II. Ethical Issues," in W.T.Reich, ed., *Encyclopedia of Bioethics*, 2nd ed. (New York: Simon & Schuster MacMillan, 1995), 1225-32.

3. Determining Patients' Capacity to Share in Decision Making (Chapter 5)

J.F. Drane, "Competency to Give an Informed Consent," *Journal of the American Medical Association* 252 (1984): 925-27.

P.S. Appelbaum and T. Grisso, "Assessing Patients' Capacities to Consent to Treatment," *New England Journal of Medicine* 319 (1988):1635-38.

B. Lo, F. Rouse, and L. Dorbrand, "Family Decision Making on Trial: Who Decides for Incompetent Patients?" *New England Journal of Medicine* 322 (1990): 1228-32.

D. Brock and S. Wartman, "When Competent Patients Make Irrational Choices," *New England Journal of Medicine* 322 (1990): 1595-99.

V. Ho, "Marginal Capacity: The Dilemmas Faced in Assessment and Declaration," *Canadian Medical Association Journal* 152, no. 2 (1995): 259-63.

L.J. Schneiderman, H. Teetzel, and A.G. Kalmanson, "Who Decides Who Decides? When Disagreement Occurs Between the Physician and the Patient's Appointed Proxy about the Patient's Decision-Making Capacity," *Archives of Internal Medicine* 155, no. 8 (1995): 793-96.

4. The Process of Informed Consent (Chapter 6)

A.J. Rosoff, *Informed Consent: A Guide for Health Care Professionals* (Rockville, Md.: Aspen, 1981).

F.A. Rozovsky, *Consent to Treatment: A Practical Guide* (Boston: Little, Brown, 1984).

R. Faden and T.L. Beauchamp, (New York: Oxford University Press, 1986).

W.J. Morton, "The Doctrine of Informed Consent," *Medicine and Law* 6 (1987): 117-25.

H. Brody, "Transparency: Informed Consent in Primary Care," *Hastings Center Report* 19 (1989): 5-9.

R.M. Arnold and C.W. Lidz, "Informed Consent: IV. Clinical Aspects of Consent in Health Care," in W.T. Reich, ed. *Encyclopedia of Bioethics*, 2nd ed. (New York: Simon & Schuster MacMillan, 1995), 1250-56.

5. Treatment Refusals by Patients and Clinicians (Chapter 7)

R. Macklin, "Consent, Coercion, and the Conflict of Rights,"*Perspectives in Biology and Medicine* 20 (1977): 360-71.

A.M. Capron, "The Right to Refuse Medical Care," in W.T. Reich, ed., *Encyclopedia of Bioethics*, 1st ed. (New York: MacMillan and Free Press, 1978), 1498-507.

P.S. Appelbaum and L.H. Roth, "Patients Who Refuse Treatment in Medical Hospitals," *Journal of the American Medical Association* 250 (1983): 1296-301.

J.E. Connelly and C. Campbell, "Patients Who Refuse Treatment in Medical Offices," *Archives of Internal Medicine* 147 (1987):1829-33.

R. Masters and S.F. Marks, "The Use of Restraints," *Rehabilitation Nursing* 15, no. 1 (1990): 22-25.

G.J. Annas, "Patients' Rights," in W.T. Reich, ed., *Encyclopedia of Bioethics*, 2nd ed. (New York: Simon & Schuster MacMillan, 1995),1925-27.

L.E. Kopolow, "Mental Patients' Rights," in W.T. Reich, ed., *Encyclopedia of Bioethics*, 2nd ed. (New York: Simon & Schuster MacMillan, 1995), 1927-33.

L.B. Weinstein, "The Right to Refuse Treatment," *American Journal of Nursing* 95, no. 8 (1995): 52-53.

6. Death and Dying (Chapter 8)

S.H. Wanzer et al., "The Physician's Responsibility toward Hopelessly Ill Patients," *New England Journal of Medicine* 310, no. 15 (1984): 955-59.

Anonymous, "It's Over Debbie," *Journal of the American Medical Association* 259 (1988): 272.

W. Gaylin et al., "Doctors Must Not Kill," *Journal of the American Medical Association* 259 (1988): 2139-40.

S.H. Wanzer et al., "The Physician's Responsibility toward Hopelessly Ill Patients: A Second Look," *New England Journal of Medicine* 320, no. 13 (1989): 844-49.

T.E. Quill, "Death and Dignity: A Case of Individualized Decision Making," *New England Journal of Medicine* 324 (1991): 691-94.

D. Callahan, *The Troubled Dream of Life* (New York: Simon & Schuster, 1993).

F.G. Miller and H. Brody, "Professional Integrity and Physician-Assisted Death," *Hastings Center Report* 25 (1995): 8-17.

T.E. Quill, *A Midwife through the Dying Process* (Baltimore, Md.: Johns Hopkins University Press, 1996).

7. Forgoing Life-Sustaining Treatment (Chapter 9)

R.A. McCormick, "To Save or Let Die: The Dilemma of Modern Medicine," *Journal of the American Medical Association* 229 (1974): 172-75.

President's Commission for the Study of Ethical Problems in Medicine and Biomedical and Behavioral Research, *Deciding to Forgo Life-Sustaining Treatment* (Washington, D.C.: U.S. Government Printing Office, 1983).

J. Lynn and J.F. Childress, "Must Patients Always Be Given Food and Water?" *Hastings Center Report* 13 (October 1983): 17-21.

R.F. Weir and L. Gostin, "Decisions to Abate Life-Sustaining Treatment for Nonautonomous Patients," *Journal of the American Medical Association* 264 (1990): 1846-53.

A. Meisel, "The Legal Consensus about Forgoing Life-Sustaining Treatment: Its Status and Prospects," *Kennedy Institute of Ethics Journal* 2, no. 4 (1992): 309-45.

R.M. Veatch, "Forgoing Life-Sustaining Treatment: Limits to the Consensus," *Kennedy Institute of Ethics Journal* 3, no. 1 (1993): 1-19.

D.P. Sulmasy and J. Sugarman, "Are Withholding and Withdrawing Therapy Always Morally Equivalent," *Journal of Medical Ethics* 20, no. 4 (1994): 218-22.

R.D. Truog, "Progress in the Futility Debate," *The Journal of Clinical Ethics* 6, no. 2 (Summer 1995): 128-32.

8. Decisions about Treatment in Newborns, Infants, and Children (Chapter 10)

R.S. Duff and A.G.M. Campbell, "Moral and Ethical Dilemmas in the Special Care Nursery," *New England Journal of Medicine* 289 (1973): 890-94.

R. Weir, *Selective Treatment of Handicapped Newborns: Moral Dilemmas in Neonatal Medicine* (New York: Oxford University Press, 1984).

Hastings Center Research Project on the Care of Imperiled Newborns, "Imperiled Newborns," *Hastings Center Report* 17, no. 6 (1987): 5-32.

L.J. Nelson, "Perinatology/Neonatology and the Law: Looking Beyond Baby Doe," *Yearbook of Pediatrics* (1988): 5-10.

L.M. Kopelman, T.G. Irons, and A.E. Kopelman, "Neonatologists Judge the 'Baby Doe' Regulations," *New England Journal of Medicine* 318, no. 11 (1988): 677-83.

L.J. Nelson and R.M. Nelson, "Ethics and the Provision of Futile, Harmful, or Burdensome Treatment to Children," *Critical Care Medicine* 20 (1992): 427-33.

R.F. Weir, "Infants. III. Ethical Issues," in W.T. Reich, ed., *Encyclopedia of Bioethics*, 2nd ed. (New York: Simon & Schuster MacMillan, 1995), 1206-13.

A.M. Dellinger and P.C. Kuszler, "Infants. IV. Public Policy and Legal Issues," in W.T. Reich, ed., *Encyclopedia of Bioethics*, 2nd ed. (New York: Simon & Schuster MacMillan, 1995), 1214-21.

9. Reproductive Choices (Chapter 11)

D. Callahan, "The Abortion Debate: Is Progress Possible?" in S. Callahan and D. Callahan, *Abortion: Understanding Differences* (New York: Plenum, 1984), 309-24.

V.E. Holder, J. Gallagher, and M.T. Parsons, "Court-Ordered Obstetrical Interventions," *New England Journal of Medicine* 316 (1987): 1192-95.

L.J. Nelson and N. Milliken, "Compelled Medical Treatment of Pregnant Women," *Journal of the American Medical Association* 259 (1988): 1060-66.

B.K. Rothman, *Recreating Motherhood* (New York: W.W. Norton, 1989).

P.R. Reilly, *The Surgical Solution: A History of Involuntary Sterilization in the United States* (Baltimore, Md.: Johns Hopkins University Press, 1991).

D. Wikler and N.J. Wikler, "Turkey Baster Babies: The Demedicalization of Artificial Insemination," *Milbank Quarterly* 69, no. 1 (1991): 5-25.

J.A. Robertson, *Children of Choice: Freedom and the New Reproductive Technologies* (Princeton, N.J.: Princeton University Press, 1994).

J.D. Arras and J. Blustein, "Reproductive Responsibility and Long-Acting Contraceptives," *Hastings Center Report* no. 1 (1995): S27-S29.

10. Patient Selection: Tragic Choices (Chapter 12)

H.E. Aaron and W.B. Schwartz, *The Painful Prescription: Rationing Hospital Care* (Washington, D.C.: Brookings Institution, 1984).

G. Annas, "Your Money or Your Life: Dumping Uninsured Patients from Hospital Emergency Wards," *Public Health and the Law* 76, no. 1 (1986): 74-77.

H.T. Engelhardt, Jr. and M.A. Rie, "Intensive Care Units, Scarce Resources, and Conflicting Principles of Justice," *Journal of the American Medical Association*

255 (1986): 1159-64.

M.F. Marshall et al., "Influence of Political Power, Medical Provincialism, and Economic Incentives on the Rationing of Surgical Intensive Care Unit Beds," *Critical Care Medicine* 20 (1992): 387-94.

M. Strosberg et al., ed., *Rationing America's Medical Care: The Oregon Plan and Beyond* (Washington D.C.: Brookings Institution,1992).

L.M. Fleck, "Just Caring: Health Reform and Health Care Rationing," *Journal of Medicine and Philosophy* 19, no. 5 (1994): 435-43.

11. Economics, Case Management, and Patient Advocacy (Chapter 13)

P. Starr, *The Social Transformation of American Medicine* (New York: Basic Books, 1982).

B.L. Hillman, M.V. Pauly, and J.J. Kerstein, "How Do Financial Incentives Affect Physicians' Clinical Decisions and the Financial Performance of Heath Maintenance Organizations?" *New England Journal of Medicine* 321 (1989): 891-95.

J.J. Finnerty and J.V. Pinkerton, "Ethical Considerations of Managed Care," *Obstetrical and Gynecological Survey* 48 (1993): 699-706.

E.H. Morreim, *Balancing Act: The New Ethics of Medicine's New Economics* (Washington, D.C.: Georgetown University Press, 1995).

E.J. Emanuel and N.N. Dubler, "Preserving the Physician-Patient Relationship in the Era of Managed Care," *Journal of the American Medical Association* 273, no. 4 (1995): 323-29.

C.M. Clancy and H. Brody, "Managed Care: Jekyll or Hyde?" *Journal of the American Medical Association* 273, no. 4 (1995): 338-39.

12. Ethics Services in Healthcare Organizations (Chapter 14)

J.C. Fletcher, N. Quist, and A.R. Jonsen, ed., *Ethics Consultation in Health Care* (Ann Arbor, Mich.: Health Administration Press, 1989).

J.D. Moreno, "What Means This Consensus? Ethics Committees and Philosophic Tradition," *The Journal of Clinical Ethics* 1, no. 1 (Spring 1990): 38-43.

B. Hoffmaster, B. Freedman, and G. Fraser, *Clinical Ethics: Theory and Practice* (Clifton, N.J.: Humana Press, 1989).

G.J. Agich and S.J. Youngner, "For Experts Only? Access to Hospital Ethics Committees," *Hastings Center Report* 21, no. 5 (1991): 17-25.

J. LaPuma and D. Schiedermayer, *Ethics Consultation: A Practical Guide* (Boston: Jones and Bartlett, 1994).

F.E. Baylis, ed., *The Health Care Ethics Consultant* (Totowa, N.J.: Humana Press, 1994).

S.J. Reiser, "The Ethical Life of Health Care Organizations," *Hastings Center Report* 24, no. 6 (1994): 24-45.

13. Professional Ethics (Chapter 15)

M. Siegler and H. Osmond, "Aesculapian Authority," *Hastings Center Studies* 1 (1973): 41-52.

E. Pellegrino, "Toward a Reconstruction of Medical Morality: The Primacy of the Act of Profession and the Fact of Illness," *Journal of Medicine and Philosophy* 4 (1979): 32-56.

A. Relman, "The Future of Medical Practice," *Health Affairs* 2 (1983): 5-19.

A.R. Jonsen, *The New Medicine and the Old Ethics* (Cambridge, Mass.: Harvard University Press, 1990).

H. Brody, *The Healer's Power* (New Haven, Conn.: Yale University Press, 1992), chapters 11, 12, 13, and 16.

J.P. Kassirer, "Managed Care and the Morality of the Marketplace," *New England Journal of Medicine* 333, no. 1 (1995): 50-52.

II.   A Course for Ethics Committees

The textbook can be used as an orientation for new ethics committee members or as a self-education course. At least two formats are useful:

1. a one-day retreat of at least six working hours, followed by a series of weekly or monthly sessions; or
2. a series of educational sessions in regular monthly (or differently scheduled) meetings of the committee.

In either setting, use of the textbook is most effective when sessions are co-led by experienced clinicians (physicians or registered nurses). The retreat format is outlined below. If the latter method is used, one can simply begin with Chapters 1, 2, 14, and 15, and adapt some of the elements suggested in the retreat format to use in committee meetings.

Before a one-day retreat, assign Chapters 1, 2, 14, and 15 for background reading. The retreat can be divided into three working sessions, combining plenary sessions with breakout groups. The breakout groups should ideally be composed of volunteers for subcommittees, organized to carry out the functions of the committee described in Chapter 14: education (including forum activities), policy development, and case consultation. Only very advanced committees may be ready to attempt a fourth function, targeted research.

Session I. 9:00 a.m. - 9:45 a.m.
"The Evolving Role and Responsibilities of Ethics Committees"

Prepare and use attached handout for Session 1, also drawing on prior reading of Chapters 14 and 15.

The leader can cover the material in the handout, referring to the mission of the ethics committee as "the major resource group to support clinical ethics in the institution," and to the main tasks of the committee as: education in clinical ethics, policy studies and policy review, and case consultation (primarily prospective cases).

9:45 a.m. - 10:15 a.m. Discussion of the Committee's Mission Resources: Chapters 14 and 15 plus handout

Session 2. 10:30 a.m. - 11:15 a.m. "Introduction to Case Study" Resources: Chapters 1 and 2

Prepare handouts of Exhibit 2-1 (Chapter 2), the outline of the four-part approach to case analysis.

The leader can explain this approach to case study, by emphasizing the plan of care before explaining the four-part method. Leaders can present a case that occurred in their institution for discussion or use another case from the textbook (e.g., "Code Him until He's Brain Dead!" (Chapter 9).

11:15 a.m. - 12:15 p.m. Divide into work groups with the preassigned case, with a task to work through the four-part method. Return at 12:15 p.m. to report on outcomes of discussion, asking two final questions for plenary discussion:

1. What is the best outcome of this case for all concerned?
2. What are the obstacles to our being able to provide ethics consultation for decision makers in such a case?

Session III. 1:15 p.m. - 2:15 p.m.
"Developing a Work Plan for the Ethics Committee" (Chapter 14)

Divide up into three working groups: education, policy development, and ethics case consultation. A reporter for each working group should take legible notes.

Each group has the task of proposing a work plan for the year for itself. If the ethics committee is large (more than 12 to 15 members), the members may design a plan to meet more often in subgroups than as a whole committee. One option is to meet twice a month in subgroups and quarterly as a whole group.

The education group will plan to continue self-education for the committee and develop a program on clinical ethics for the entire healthcare organization. Material from Sections I and II of the textbook is relevant to both questions.

The policy group must conduct an inventory on all existing institutional policies with ethics content, and submit a plan that sets priorities for new policy areas that need study. The plan should contain an element of evaluation of existing policy statements (e.g., those that are adequate and still up-to-date, those that need updating, and those that are inadequate and need complete revision). This group will want to ask the institution's administration for their suggestions. Material from Section I of the textbook may be relevant to policy review or development.

The ethics consultation group will need to do the following:

1. recommend an interim method to deliver emergency consultation before a full plan is in effect;
2. sketch the elements of a proposal for education and training of those members most interested in consultation;
3. communicate with other ethics committees to secure their protocols for case consultation; and
4. identify and invite members of the clinical staff to meetings to present past cases (without identifiers) for which consultation may have helped.

2:30 p.m. - 3:00 p.m. The three working groups report back to the whole group. The entire group develops an overall work plan for the institution. (Save each reporter's notes to compile a record.)

3:00 p.m. - 3:15 p.m. (Adjourn)
Subsequent meetings of the committee can use Chapters 3 through 13 of the textbook as background reading for more specific education to be conducted. It is generally effective to open each educational session with a case that embodies the problem that is the subject of the chapter.

B. Handout for Session I (see next page)

The Evolution of Patient Care Ethics: Ethics Committees in Healthcare Organizations

I. Introduction: Know Your History

A. Bioethics, (*bios* is Greek for "life"--life sciences):
   A 1960s social movement and new interdisciplinary field. Why? (1) complex ethical problems in research, healthcare, and public health (e.g., dialysis, transplants, genetics, prolongation of life, behavioral research, etc.) and (2) increasing respect for autonomy and protection of research subjects and patients.[1]

B. The "beginnings of bioethics"
   1. Joseph Fletcher, (Morals and Medicine), 1954
   2. Seattle Dialysis Committee; 1963
   3. Research ethics controversies

C. Older history: medical ethics, nursing ethics, Roman Catholic and Jewish traditions in medical ethics

D. Two major societal values in bioethics:
   1. Sharing power and decision making
   2. Using more foresight in applying technology

E. To many physicians, "ethics" means only issues of character, professional relationships, etc.

II. Four Stages of Concern--With Four Social and Institutional Changes

A. Stage 1: Ethics in research with human subjects
   1. Nazi research (*The Nuremberg Code*, 1947); absolute rule of informed consent; prior animal research; conscience of the researcher; no prior group review.
   2. Famous cases of abuses of power in research[2]
      a. Tuskegee Study (Public Health Service, Centers for Disease Control), 1932-1972
      b. "Cold War" radiation studies, 1950-1960
      c. Thalidomide and Food and Drug Administration, 1962
      d. Jewish Hospital cancer study, 1963
      e. Baboon-to-human heart transplant, 1964
      f. Willowbrook hepatitis study, 1965
      g. Beecher article, 1966
      h. "Tea Room Trade," 1967
      i. Fetal research, 1973
   3. The first "ethics committees" in research: Surgeon-General's order on prior group review (July 1966)
   4. Institutional review board (IRB) required by National Research Act (1974) to review projects involving human subjects for (1) risk/benefit issues, (2) plan to obtain voluntary informed consent/assent, (3) issues in selection of subjects, and (4) confidentiality and privacy issues.

B. Stage 2: Education of healthcare professionals in ethics/humanities/religious concerns (1968 to the present)
   1. Pioneers: J. Katz; E. Pellegrino; T. Hunter

   2. Society for Health and Human Values (1968)
   3. Hastings Center (1969); Kennedy Institute of Ethics (1971); Parkridge Center (1987)
   4. Ethics and medical humanities programs in medical and nursing schools, residency training
   5. Medical school courses in ethics (1995): Curriculum change--new positions

C. Stage 3: Patient care--clinical ethics (1976 *Quinlan* case to present)
   1. Ethical obligations in the care of each patient
      a. Privacy and confidentiality
      b. Communication, truthtelling, disclosure
      c. Determining the patient's capacity to make decisions
      d. Informed consent
   2. Ethical problems that may arise in patient care
      a. Refusal of medically indicated treatment
      b. Decision to forgo life-sustaining treatment in incapacitated adults
      c. Terminal illness (limits of comfort care; assisted suicide/euthanasia)
      d. Reproductive choices, abortion, etc.
      e. Decisions about treatment involving imperiled newborns, infants, and children
      f. Access to and containing costs of healthcare
      g. Rationing at the bedside
      h. Managed care and advocacy of patients
   3. Hospital and nursing home ethics committees
      By 1989, 75 percent of U.S. hospitals with more than 200 beds and 25 percent of hospitals with fewer than 200 beds had an ethics committee.[3] In a 1992 survey, the American Hospital Association found that of 5,916 respondent hospitals, 3,015 (51 percent) had a committee.[4] By 1996, 90 percent of hospitals had ethics committees, reflecting JCAHO's accreditation rate. Perhaps 15 to 25 percent of U.S. nursing homes have committees.
   4. Chronological history: Ethics committees are recommended by:
      a. State supreme court decisions: *Quinlan* decision,1976[5]
      b. The President's Commission, 1983[6]
      c. The American Medical Association[7]
      d. The American Hospital Association[8]
      e. Ethics committees recommended for implementation of Patient Self-Determination Act, 1991[9]
   5. Ethics committees are required by:
      a. State law in Maryland, Hawaii, New York (pending), and Pennsylvania (pending)[10] for all licensed hospitals and long-term care facilities.
      b. The Joint Commission on Accreditation of

Healthcare Organizations requires members to have a "functioning process to address ethical issues."[11] A functioning and well-supported ethics committee satisfies this requirement; an ethics program exceeds it.

6. Failure to thrive--Hospitals and nursing home ethics committees often lack the resources needed for their mission to provide bioethics services. An evaluation[12] of ethics committees in the Mid-Atlantic region showed "a failure to thrive." Such committees may have the following characteristics:

   a. The committee is unsupported and unfunded by institutional leadership.
   b. The committees is unknown to those who need it most.
   c. The committee is unconsulted in true "ethics emergencies."
   d. The committee members are poorly informed and untrained for tasks.
   e. The committee is without a mission statement or work plan.

7. Some committees still suffer seriously from lack of support, education, and focus, or if they have received some help, the members function in a "crisis mode." HCOs need a well-supported institutional program served by one or two resource persons. Patient care ethics services include these features:

   a. A multidisciplinary ethics committee with some community members (How shall members be oriented and educated for their tasks?);
   b. An educational program for clinicians, trainees, and students, and for members of the community that covers the most frequent ethical and legal problems in the clinical encounter (How shall they become equipped for this task?);
   c. A process for developing policy and guidelines that address ethical issues in the clinical setting and in the HCO's organizational life (How shall members become equipped for this task?);
   d. A process for ethics consultation at the bedside with a second tier of conflict resolution in the ethics committee (How shall consultants be selected, trained, and appointed?[13]);
   e. A way to evaluate program outcomes and to conduct research on ethical problems in the clinical setting;
   f. At least one (preferably two) resource persons.

8. Present status: Committees can be found between

"failure to thrive" or "living from crisis to crisis" (or some of both); need to "respond to JACHO's Organization Ethics Initiative"; in a significant identity crisis.

D. Stage 4: Strengthening local patient care ethics services and organization ethics by regional networks and educational partnerships

1. Regional bioethics networks: needed for the educational and training infrastructure that single institutions cannot provide for themselves. Networks are growing in the United States.

2. The Virginia Bioethics Network (functions)
   a. public education on bioethical issues
   b. propose standards for clinical ethics services to boards of HCOs
   c. services to HCOs, including educational programs
   d. orientation and basic education of new institutional ethics committee members
   e. continuing education of institutional ethics committee members
   f. advanced education for ethics consultation
   g. support and continuing education for persons interested in clinical ethics

3. Contacts for regional bioethics networks
   a. Virginia Bioethics Network: Walter Zirkle, M.D. (703) 433-4100 or Edward M. Spencer, M.D. (804) 982-3970.
   b. Minnesota Network of Hospital Ethics Committees: R.E. Cranford, M.D. (612) 347-2430.
   c. New Jersey Citizens for Biomedical Ethics: Mary Strong (201) 277-3858.
   d. Bioethics Resource Group of Charlotte, North Carolina: Katherine Thompson (704) 332-4421.
   e. Richmond (Virginia) Consortium for Biomedical Ethics: Matthew Jenkins (804) 788-8736.
   f. Bioethics Network of Hampton Roads (Virginia) Melissa Warfield, M.D. (804) 628-7462.
   g. West Virginia Network of Hospital Ethics Committees: Alvin Moss, M.D. (304) 293-7618.
   h. Washington (D.C.) Metropolitan Bioethics Network: Joan H. Lewis, (202) 682-1581.
   i. Institutional Ethics Committee Resource Network of Maryland: Diane E. Hoffman, J.D. (301) 328-7191.

4. Society for Bioethics Consultation: Stuart Youngner, M.D., President. c/o Department of Medicine, University Hospital, 2074 Abingdon, Cleveland, Ohio 44106, (216) 844-3429.

Notes

1. D. Rothman, *Strangers at the Bedside* (New York: Free Press, 1992).

2. On the Tuskegee Study, see J.H. Jones, *Bad Blood*, 2nd ed. (New York: Free Press, 1993); on radiation studies, see *Final Report: Advisory Committee Report on Human Radiation Experiments* (Washington, D.C.: U.S. Government Printing Office, 1995); on thalidomide, see Senate Report No. 1153, 89th Congress, 2d Session 8-25, 1966; on the Jewish Hospital cancer study, see E. Langer, "Human Experimentations: New York Affirms Patients' Rights," *Science* 151 (1966): 663-65; on baboon to human heart transplant, see J.D. Hardy, "Heart Transplantation in Man," *Journal of the American Medical Association* 188 (1964): 1132-35; on the Willowbrook hepatitis study, see S. Krugman et al., "Infectious Hepatitis Detection of Virus during the Incubation Period and in Clinically Inapparent Infection," *New England Journal of Medicine* 261 (1959): 729-34; S. Goldby, "Experiments at the Willowbrook State School," *Lancet* 1 (1971): 749; for Beecher's article H.K. Beecher, "Ethics and Clinical Research," *New England Journal of Medicine* 274 (1966): 1354-60; on the Tea Room Trade (deceptive social research), see L. Humphreys, *Tea Room Trade: Impersonal Sex in Public Places* (Chicago: Aldine, 1970); D.P. Warwick, "Tearoom Trade: Means and Ends in Social Research," *Hastings Center Report* 1, no. 1 (1973): 24-38; on fetal research, see "Live Abortus Research Raises Hackles of Some, Hopes of Others," *Medical World News* (5 October 1973), 32-36; V. Cohn, "NIH Vows Not to Fund Fetus Work," *Washington Post*, 13 April 1973, A1.

3. *1992 Statistical Guide* (Chicago: American Hospital Association, 1992). The data were collected in 1989. These numbers mean that of 2,071 hospitals with more than 200 beds, approximately 518 did not have a committee; of 4,649 with fewer than 200 beds, 3,487 did not have

a committee. Outreach efforts need to focus on smaller hospitals.

4. J.C. Fletcher and D.E. Hoffman, "Ethics Committees: Time to Experiment with Standards," *Annals of Internal Medicine* 120 (1994): 335-38.

5. *In re Quinlan*, 70 N.J. 10, 355 A.2d 647, cert. denied, 429 U.S. 922 (1976).

6. President's Commission for the Study of Ethical Problems in Medicine and Biomedical and Behavioral Research, *Decisions to Forgo Life-Sustaining Treatment* (Washington, D.C.: U.S. Government Printing Office, 1983), 160.

7. American Medical Association, "Guidelines for Ethics Committees in Health Care Institutions," Judicial Council Report E., adopted December 1984 Interim Meeting. Reprinted in J.W. Ross, *Handbook for Hospital Ethics Committees* (Chicago: AHA, 1986), 112.

8. American Hospital Association, "Guidelines: Hospital Committees on Biomedical Ethics," Approved by American Hospital Association General Council, 27 January 1984. Reprinted in Ross, see note 7 above, p. 110.

9. M.L. White and J.C. Fletcher, "The Patient Self-Determination Act: On Balance, More Help than Hindrance," *Journal of the American Medical Association* 266, no. 3 (1991): 410-12.

10. See note 4 above, p. 335.

11. Joint Commission on Accreditation of Healthcare Organizations, "Patient Rights and Organization Ethics," in *1995 Standards, Rights, Responsibilities, and Ethics* (Oakbrook Terrace, Ill.: JCAHO, 1994).

12. D.E. Hoffman, "Regulating Ethics Committees in Health Care Institutions--Is it Time?" *Maryland Law Review* 50 (1991): 746-67.

13. The Society for Bioethics Consultation and the Society for Health and Human Values have a joint task force to study the need and feasibility of certification of persons who provide ethics consultation.

APPENDIX 4

Resources in Clinical and Biomedical Ethics

The purpose of this appendix is to introduce readers some important published books, manuals, and resources in clinical ethics, and to different perspectives in bioethics. The contents are introductory and not a full survey.

Full-length books in clinical ethics are far fewer than those in bioethics. The number of published articles and book chapters on specific topics in clinical ethics, such as informed consent or death and dying, is huge. The National Library of Medicine's on-line services of MEDLINE and BIOETHICSLINE provide bibliographic resources in articles and book chapters from 1973 to the present. Specific literature searches can be ordered without charge by calling 1-800-MED-ETHX, the Kennedy Institute of Ethics Library at Georgetown University.

This appendix has three sections: resources in clinical ethics, perspectives in bioethics, and resources recommended for libraries that serve ethics programs in healthcare organizations.

Section I on clinical ethics has two parts. Part A is a chronological selection of important textbooks, manuals, and other works. Part B lists "casebooks" for clinical ethics to help students and ethics consultants search for similar cases when doing case analysis. Some resources listed in Part A also have good collections of cases for discussion. They are identified with an asterisk (*).

Section II is a selection of works in bioethics that have significance for clinical ethics. These works represent different perspectives and approaches. Some important books by physician-ethicists are also included.

Section III is for individuals and committees that are in charge of planning and acquisitions for libraries. It lists journals, books, and encyclopedias useful to members of a healthcare ethics program.

I. Resources in Clinical Ethics

A. Textbooks, Manuals, and Collections of Papers

J.W. Ross, C. Bayley, V. Michel, and D. Pugh, ed., *Handbook for Hospital Ethics Committees* (Chicago: American Hospital Association, 1986).

An early resource for hospital ethics committees, which was revised and updated in 1993.

T.F. Ackerman, G.C. Graber, C.H. Reynolds, and D.C. Thomasma, ed., *Clinical Medical Ethics: Exploration and Assessment* (Lanham, Md.: University Press of America, 1987).

This volume of essays originated from a meeting in 1982 at the University of Tennessee. The work is still fresh and interesting today, especially from the perspective of philosophy and teaching medical ethics. Some of the early views of the first generation of teachers and consultants in clinical ethics (in addition to the editors) are in this volume (for example, Jonsen and Brody). Critical essays by Nielsen and Caplan are "musts" for those who do graduate study in clinical ethics or want to start hospital ethics programs.

R.L. Zaner, *Ethics and the Clinical Encounter* (Englewood Cliffs, N.J.: Prentice Hall, 1988). Paperback.

This book is by a philosopher who became, to his surprise, the resident bioethicist at Vanderbilt University Hospital. It combines history, philosophy, and ethics in a very interesting study of the ethical problems faced by physicians and those who attempt to help them understand these problems.

*B. Brody, *Life and Death Decision Making* (New York: Oxford University Press, 1988).

An important work by a clinically based philosopher who espouses a pluralistic approach to moral reasoning. The book is notable for its many cases to demonstrate the method for moral deliberation that Brody recommends.

B. Hofmaster, B. Freedman, and G. Fraser, ed., *Clinical Ethics: Theory and Practice* (Clifton, N.J.: Humana Press, 1989).

A set of conference papers that presents Canadian and American perspectives.

J.C. Fletcher, N. Quist, and A.R. Jonsen, *Ethics Consultation in Health Care* (Ann Arbor, Mich.: Health Administration Press, 1989).

A collection of papers from the first national conference on ethics consultation in healthcare, convened in 1985 by the National Institutes of Health and the University of California at San Francisco.

*R.A. Kane and A. Caplan, *Everyday Ethics: Resolving Dilemmas in Nursing Home Life* (New York: Springer, 1990).

This book is an excellent resource for ethical issues in nursing home life. The cases illustrate the major differences between ethical issues that arise in acute and long-term care.

*C.M. Culver, ed., *Ethics at the Bedside* (Hanover, N.H.: University Press of New England, 1991).

A collection of essays about difficult cases by ethics consultants, who detail the complexities and frequent failures of their activities.

*A.R. Jonsen, M. Siegler, and W.J. Winslade, *Clinical Ethics: A Practical Approach to Ethical Decisions in Clinical Medicine*, 3rd ed. (New York: McGraw-Hill, 1992). Paperback.

The earliest textbook in clinical ethics, now in its third edition. It was designed to be used by clinicians as a handbook and reference work. The text was written by three pioneers in the field who represent the fields of ethics, medicine, and psychiatry/law. This work helped to define the activity of clinical ethics as the "identification, analysis, and resolution of moral problems that arise in the care of a particular patient." Their "four-quadrant" approach to case analysis is an alternative to the four-step approach described in Chapter 2.

J. Buckman, *How to Break Bad News: A Guide for Health Professionals* (Baltimore, Md.: Johns Hopkins University Press, 1992).

Although this book is not directly on ethical issues, it contains many helpful sections for ethics consultants, who often work in conditions of emotional stress and grief.

*N.N. Dubler and D. Nimmons, *Ethics on Call* (New York: Harmony Books, 1992).

Written by a resident attorney-ethicist in a New York hospital, this book reads like an adventure story. The difference is that it is true. Many detailed cases discussed here.

*R. Macklin, *Enemies of Patients* (New York: Oxford University Press, 1993).

Macklin has served as bioethicist at Einstein College of Medicine for many years. In this book, she carefully distinguishes law from ethics, and through the use of many fascinating cases, she shows how the fear of liability and the need for cost-containment have influenced hospital administrators, risk managers, ethics committees, and physicians to take positions contrary to patient-centered decision making.

J.F. Drane, *Clinical Bioethics* (Kansas City, Mo.: Sheed & Ward, 1993). Paperback.

This book is by a veteran bioethicist who helped to start many ethics committees in rural areas of Pennsylvania. The chapters make an excellent textbook to orient a new ethics committee.

F.E. Baylis, *The Health Care Ethics Consultant* (Totowa, N.J.: Humana Press, 1994).

The results of a consensus development process among clinical ethicists in Canada. The effort is to describe the education, skills, and character traits needed for "doing ethics" in clinical settings.

*J. LaPuma and D. Schiedermeyer, *Ethics Consultation: A Practical Guide* (Boston: Jones and Bartlett, 1994).

Two of the most experienced physician-ethics consultants describe their requirements for skills, training, and clinical appointment. The book has an outstanding collection of cases and a good bibliography.

*J.C. Ahronheim, J. Moreno, and C. Zuckerman, *Ethics in Clinical Practice* (Boston: Little, Brown, 1994).

A very useful reference that clearly explains key concepts in clinical ethics and contains a collection of 32 cases. This book is similar to this textbook in its attempt to bridge between the "standard" academic view in bioethics and the clinical setting.

D.E. Hoffman, P. Boyle, and S.A. Levenson, *Handbook for Nursing Home Ethics Committees* (Washington, D.C.: American Association of Homes and Services for the Aging, 1995).

The best written resource for ethics committees in long-term care. It meets the needs of small or large facilities, and the legal-regulatory aspects are soundly researched and written.

S. Fry-Revere, J. Sorrell, and M. Silva, ed., *Ethics and Answers in Home Health Care* (Leesburg, Va.: Regis Group, 1995).

The only published resource for ethics committees in home health agencies and visiting nurses associations.

J.D. Moreno, *Deciding Together* (New York: Oxford University Press, 1995).

The director of the program in bioethics and humanities at State University of New York in Brooklyn discusses the strengths and weaknesses of consensus decision making in ethics committees and consultation. A first-rate examination of an important issue in the field. He includes many creative reflections on work in the social and behavioral sciences.

*B. Lo, *Resolving Ethical Dilemmas: A Guide for Clinicians* (Baltimore, Md.: Williams & Wilkins, 1995). Paperback.

Written by the director of the program in medical ethics at the University of California at San Francisco, this is possibly the best book in the field to address physicians' skepticism about the usefulness of ethics as a field in patient care. Ethics consultants and committees may find his brief and well-documented chapters useful as handouts in cases and meetings. Highly recommended.

*K.V. Iverson, A.B. Sanders, and D. Mathieu, *Ethics in Emergency Medicine* 2nd ed. (Tucson, Ariz.: Galen Press, 1995).

An important book for teaching and use with emergency department personnel and critical care, with many interesting and useful cases.

B. Anthologies of Cases and Casebooks

R.M. Veatch, *Case Studies in Medical Ethics* (Cambridge, Mass.: Harvard University Press, 1977).

A volume with 112 cases in medical and research ethics.

R.M. Veatch and S. Fry, *Case Studies in Nursing Ethics* (Philadelphia: J.B. Lippincott, 1987). Paperback.

Background articles and chapters for a course in clinical ethics for nursing students, well arranged by the authors.

C. Levine, ed., *Cases in Bioethics* (New York: St. Martin's Press, 1989). Paperback.

A selection of cases, with discussions on various sides of the issues, from the Hastings Center Report, by a former editor of the journal.

T.M. Perlin, *Clinical Medical Ethics: Cases in Practice* (Boston: Little, Brown, 1992).

B.J. Crigger, ed., *Cases in Bioethics* (New York: St. Martin's Press, 1992). Paperback.

A collection of cases from the Hastings Center Report, with discussion on various sides of the issues, by an editor of the journal.

G.E. Pence, *Classic Cases in Medical Ethics*, 2nd ed. (New York: McGraw-Hill, 1994.)

Pence reconstructed the cases that have helped to shape contemporary medical ethics, with philosophical, legal, and historical backgrounds. The cases include: Karen Quinlan, Elizabeth Bouvia, mercy killing in Holland, Louise Brown (the first child born who was conceived by in vitro fertilization), the Baby M case, the trial of Dr. Edelin, the Baby Jane Doe case, research with human subjects, and cases about individual rights versus the public good.

R.M. Veatch and H.E. Flack, *Case Studies in Allied Health Ethics* (Upper Saddle River, N.J.: Prentice-Hall, 1997).

Discussion of more than 100 cases involving ethical issues facing allied health professionals (for example, nutritionists, respiratory therapists, occupational therapists, and so on).

II. Perspectives in Bioethics

A. Historical Perspective

D.J. Rothman, *Strangers at the Bedside: A History of How Law and Bioethics Transformed Medical Decisionmaking* (New York: Basic Books, 1991). Paperback.

This is the first extensive history of bioethics and covers the period 1960 to 1970 with precision. An indispensable resource for "the beginnings of bioethics."

B. Legal Perspective

G.J. Annas, *Standard of Care: The Law of American Bioethics* (New York: Oxford University Press, 1993).

In a collection of his best essays and articles on specific controversies, Annas advocates a view that "American law, not philosophy or medicine, is primarily responsible for the agenda, development and current state of American bioethics."

C. Family Perspective

*H.L. Nelson and J.L. Nelson, *The Patient in the Family* (New York: Routledge, 1995).

A very important book on why bioethics cannot neglect families and the place of families in decision making. This book fills an important void in bioethics that is clearly relevant to clinical ethics.

D. Teaching Perspectives

R. Purtilo, *Ethical Dimensions in the Health Professions*, 2nd ed. (Philadelphia: W.B. Saunders, 1993).

An excellent book for teaching students with many helpful exercises and outlines.

J.D. Arras and B. Steinbock, *Ethical Issues in Modern Medicine*, 4th ed. (Mountain View, Calif.: Mayfield, 1995).

Perhaps the best annotated anthology of readings in bioethics for graduate and undergraduate courses. This book covers everything.

R.M. Veatch, ed., *Medical Ethics*, 2nd ed. (Boston: Jones and Bartlett, 1997).

Excellent and full essays on many topics of relevance to clinical ethics.

E. Theological Perspectives

I. Jacobovitz, *Jewish Medical Ethics* (New York: Bloch Publishing, 1958).

P. Ramsey, *The Patient as Person* (New Haven, Conn.: Yale University Press, 1970).

P. Ramsey, *Ethics at the Edges of Life* (New Haven, Conn.: Yale University Press, 1978).

W.F. May, *The Physician's Covenant* (Philadelphia: Westminister, 1983).

R.A. McCormick, *Health and Medicine in the Catholic Tradition* (New York: Crossroad, 1984).

S. Hauerwas, *Suffering Presence: Theological Reflections on Medicine, the Mentally Handicapped, and the Church* (Notre Dame, Ind.: Notre Dame University Press, 1986). Paperback.

S.E. Lammers and A. Verhey, *On Moral Medicine: Theological Perspectives in Medical Ethics* (Grand Rapids, Mich.: Eerdmans, 1987).

B.M. Ashley and K.D. O'Rourke, *Health Care Ethics: A Theological Analysis*, 3rd ed., (St. Louis, Mo.: Catholic Health Association of the United States, 1989).

G.P. McKenny and Jonathan R. Sande, ed., *Theological Analyses of the Clinical Encounter* (Dortrecht, The Netherlands: Kluwer Academic Publishers, 1994).

F. Consequentialist Perspectives

J.F. Fletcher, *Morals and Medicine* (Princeton, N.J.: Princeton University Press, 1954).

J.F. Fletcher, *Humanhood: Essays in Biomedical Ethics* (Buffalo, N.Y.: Prometheus Books, 1979). Paperback.

P. Singer, *Practical Ethics*, 2nd ed., (New York: Cambridge University Press, 1996). Paperback.

G. Principlism

*R.M. Veatch, *A Theory of Medical Ethics* (New York: Basic Books, 1981).
Veatch aims to replace conventional professional medical ethics with a theory of a new universal base for medical ethics: a triple contract with a hierarchy of

principles. An important contribution to the development of principlism.

T.L. Beauchamp and J.F. Childress, *Principles of Biomedical Ethics*, 4th ed., (New York: Oxford University Press, 1994). Paperback.
This perspective bridges many religious and philosophical traditions with a theory that employs four ethical principles arising from a "common morality." It has been the dominant theory at work in bioethics.

E.R. Dubose, R. Hamel, and L.J. O'Connell, ed., *A Matter of Principles* (Valley Forge, Penn.: Trinity Press International, 1994).
A volume full of criticism and support for principlism.

H.T. Engelhardt, Jr., *The Foundations of Bioethics*, 2nd ed. (New York: Oxford University Press, 1995).
A new edition by a theorist who relies on three principles for an ethical approach to issues with "moral strangers" and a conservative theological approach with "moral companions."

H. Casuistry

A.R. Jonsen and S. Toulmin, *The Abuse of Casuistry* (Berkeley, Calif.: University of California Press, 1988). Paperback.
A history of casuistry, the art of giving advice to the morally perplexed by the study and use of cases. The authors credit contemporary medical ethics, especially done in public by national commissions and other bodies, for the renewal of case-oriented ethics. Jonsen also discusses casuistry in the preface to *Clinical Ethics* (see above), as well as in an important article, "Case Analysis in Clinical Ethics," *The Journal of Clinical Ethics* 1, no. 1 (Spring 1990): 63-65.

I. Feminist Perspectives

C. Gilligan, *In a Different Voice* (Cambridge, Mass.: Harvard University Press, 1982). Paperback.

H.B. Holmes and L.M. Purdy, ed., *Feminist Perspectives in Medical Ethics* (Bloomington, Ind.: Indiana University Press, 1992).

N. Noddings, *Caring* (Berkeley, Calif.: University of California Press, 1984).

S. Sherwin, *No Longer Patient: Feminist Ethics and Health Care* (Philadelphia: Temple University Press, 1992).

S. Wolf, ed., *Feminism and Bioethics* (New York: Oxford University Press, 1996).

J. Virtue Ethics

J.L. Drane, *Becoming a Good Doctor: The Place of Virtue and Character in Medical Ethics* (Kansas City, Mo.: Sheed & Ward, 1988).

E.D. Pellegrino and D.C. Thomasma, *For the Patient's Good* (New York: Oxford University Press, 1988).

A.R. Jonsen, *The New Medicine and the Old Ethics* (Cambridge, Mass.: Harvard University Press, 1990).

K. Works by Physicians

J. Katz, *The Silent World of Doctor and Patient* (New York: Free Press, 1984).

L. Kass, *Towards a More Natural Science: Biology and Human Affairs* (New York: Free Press, 1985).

E.J. Cassell, *The Nature of Suffering and the Goals of Medicine* (New York: Oxford University Press, 1991).

T.A. Brennan, *Just Doctoring: Medical Ethics in the Liberal State* (Berkeley, Calif.: University of California Press, 1991).

E.J. Emanuel, *The Ends of Human Life: Medical Ethics in a Liberal Polity* (Cambridge, Mass.: Harvard University Press, 1991).

H. Brody, *The Healer's Power* (New Haven, Conn.: Yale University Press, 1992).

III. Resources Recommended for Library Purchases

A. Journals

Hastings Center Report. Published bimonthly by the Hastings Center, 255 Elm Road, Briarcliff Manor, N.Y. 10510. $46 for individuals, $37 for full-time students, and $60 for institutions and libraries. Telephone (914) 762-8500.

Back issues of the *Hastings Center Report*, dating from 1987 forward, will also be valuable.

The Journal of Clinical Ethics. 12 S. Market Street, Ste. 300, Frederick, Md. 21701. $119 for institutions and libraries. Telephone (800) 654-8188.

Law, Medicine, and Ethics. Received free of charge to all members of the American Society of Law and Medicine, 765 Commonwealth Avenue, Suite 1634, Boston, Mass. 02215. Annual subscription fee is $50.

BioLaw. A legal and ethical reporter on medicine, health care, and bioengineering. Published by University Publications of America, 4520 East-West Highway, Bethesda, Md. 20814. Members of the Society for Bioethics Consultation receive a special rate of $100 off the list price. (301) 657-3200.

Cambridge Quarterly of Healthcare Ethics, published four times a year. Institutional rate $94. Order from Cambridge University Press, 40 W. 20th St., New York, NY 10011-4211.

HEC Forum, a publication for healthcare ethics committees.

B. Other Journals

Journal of Medicine and Philosophy
Bioethics
Journal of Medical Ethics
Kennedy Institute Journal of Ethics

C. Commission Reports, Encyclopedias, Health Law

Publications of the President's Commission for the Study of Ethical Problems in Medicine and Biomedical and Behavioral Research.

Many of the reports published by the commission (which was established by Congress in 1978) are considered landmarks in biomedical ethics. Below is a list of the commission's publications. Stock numbers of the most important reports for clinical ethics are included for documents available from the U.S. Government Printing Office, Washington, D.C. 20402. Telephone (202) 783-3238.

Deciding to Forego Life-Sustaining Treatment. 1983. O-402-884.

Defining Death. 1981. 040-000-00451-3.

Making Health Care Decisions, vol. 1. 1982 - 1983. 040-000-00459-9.

Screening and Counseling for Genetic Conditions. 1983. 040-000-00461-1.

Securing Access to Health Care, vol. 1. 1983. 040-000-00474-2.

Splicing Life. 1983. 040-00-00464-5.

Summing Up. 1983. 040-000-00475-1.

W.T. Reich, ed., *Encyclopedia of Bioethics*, 2nd ed. (New York: Simon & Schuster Macmillan, 1995), 5 vols. Telephone (800) 257-5755.

    An outstanding work with more than 400 entries on virtually every subject in bioethics. A required purchase for undergraduate and graduate students.

L. Walters and T.J. Kahn, ed., *Bibliography of Bioethics*, (Washington, D.C.: National Reference Center for Bioethics Literature, Kennedy Institute of Ethics, Georgetown University, Washington, D.C. 20057).

    Issued annually since 1975. Corresponds to the BIOETHICSLINE database in the MEDLINE system.

A. Meisel, *The Right to Die* (Colorado Springs, Colo.: Wiley Law Publications, 1993).

    This book costs $125, but it is unrivaled for coverage of the health law issues raised by forgoing life-sustaining treatment. Subsequent appendices and commentaries are also regularly published.

International Directory of Bioethics Organizations (Washington, D.C.: Kennedy Institute of Ethics, Georgetown University, Washington, D.C. 20057, 1994).

    A guide to 150 bioethics organizations in the United States and to many in Canada and other nations.

American Medical Association, Council on Ethical and Judicial Affairs, *Code of Medical Ethics. Current Opinions with Annotations*, 1996 - 1997 ed. (Chicago: American Medical Association, 1996).

INDEX